Culinary Nutrition:
The Science and Practice
of Healthy Cooking

Culinary Nutrition: The Science and Practice of Healthy Cooking

Jacqueline B. Marcus, MS, RD, LD, CNS, FADA
President/Owner
Jacqueline B. Marcus and Associates
Food and Nutrition Consulting
Highland Park, Illinois USA

AMSTERDAM • BOSTON • HEIDELBERG • LONDON
NEW YORK • OXFORD • PARIS • SAN DIEGO
SAN FRANCISCO • SINGAPORE • SYDNEY • TOKYO

Academic Press is an imprint of Elsevier

Academic Press is an imprint of Elsevier
225 Wyman Street, Waltham, MA 02451, USA
The Boulevard, Langford Lane, Kidlington, Oxford, OX5 1GB, UK

Notices
Knowledge and best practice in this field are constantly changing. As new research and experience broaden our understanding, changes in research methods, professional practices, or medical treatment may become necessary.

Practitioners and researchers must always rely on their own experience and knowledge in evaluating and using any information, methods, compounds, or experiments described herein. In using such information or methods they should be mindful of their own safety and the safety of others, including parties for whom they have a professional responsibility.

To the fullest extent of the law, neither the Publisher nor the authors, contributors, or editors, assume any liability for any injury and/or damage to persons or property as a matter of products liability, negligence or otherwise, or from any use or operation of any methods, products, instructions, or ideas contained in the material herein.

Library of Congress Cataloging-in-Publication Data
Marcus, Jacqueline B.
 Culinary nutrition : the science and practice of healthy cooking / Jacqueline B. Marcus.
    p. cm.
 Includes index.
 ISBN 978-0-12-391882-6
 1. Nutrition. 2. Diet. 3. Minerals in human nutrition. 4. Proteins in human nutrition. 5. Vitamins in human nutrition. I.Title.
 QP141.M2565 2012
 612.3--dc23

                                                                                    2012027603

British Library Cataloguing-in-Publication Data
A catalogue record for this book is available from the British Library.

For information on all Academic Press publications
visit our website at http://store.elsevier.com

Printed and bound by CPI Group (UK) Ltd, Croydon, CR0 4YY
Transferred to digital print 2012

Working together to grow
libraries in developing countries

www.elsevier.com | www.bookaid.org | www.sabre.org

ELSEVIER   BOOK AID International   Sabre Foundation

Contents

v

ABOUT THE AUTHOR

Jacqueline B. Marcus, MS, RD, LD, CNS, FADA, TheFitFoodPro, is President/Owner of Jacqueline B. Marcus and Associates Food and Nutrition Consulting in Highland Park, IL, USA. Jacqueline is an internationally-recognized food and nutrition consultant, instructor, speaker and writer. She chaired two culinary nutrition programs at hospitality and culinary arts schools; taught food and nutrition at local and national colleges and universities; presented at national and international meetings and authored and professional and consumer books, chapters and articles.

Thanks to Grace Natoli-Sheldon for the beautiful food photography; Annie E. Lin, MS, RD for editorial assistance and nutrition expertise; Chef Kyleigh Beach for recipe testing and food styling; Chef Jaclyn Kolber for nutrient analysis, Mason Marcus for illustrations, Steven L. Baron for legal counsel; the food and nutrition professionals highlighted in Chapter 12 for their collegiality, and the Elsevier publication team for their steadfast support.

A special thanks to Harvey, Meredith, Morgan and Mason Marcus—examples of culinary nutrition in practice.

Jacqueline B. Marcus, MS, RD, LD, CNS, FADA

February, 2013

The Nutrition, Food Science and Culinary Connection
Integrating Nutrition, Food Science and the Culinary Arts

INTRODUCTION

People have integrated nutrition, food science and cooking since the beginning of time—without even knowing it. The first foods and beverages were chosen to stay alive. Ancients ate meat and vegetation for sustenance and drank water for hydration. Little did they realize that the substances in meats and plants (proteins, fats and carbohydrates) are nutrients that are responsible for energy, strength and well-being.

Our ancestors ate foods raw—much like some people do today. Once fire was discovered, they cooked and baked foods to improve their flavor. Little did they realize that heat breaks down some foods into their components (amino acids, fatty acids and sugars) for digestion and absorption.

Grains, such as rice and wheat, were chewed by early people for taste and nourishment. Little did they realize that saliva breaks down carbohydrates into more digestible substances and that cooking has similar effects. Once the benefits of cooking grains were discovered, this improved their taste and texture further.

Milk from goats, sheep and cows was used to produce a variety of dairy products, including fermented milk, cheese and yogurt. Yogurt was accidentally discovered when milk soured after a long journey inside a pouch that resembled a cow's stomach. Little did shepherds realize that substances called enzymes are responsible for this transformation—and are still used today.

As time went on, raw ingredients changed in appearance, character, form and nature—thanks to nutrition, food science and the culinary arts. Meats, fowl and fish were sliced, chopped and ground into fillets, stews, patties, sausages and forms otherwise previously unknown. Grains were pulverized into flours and made into flat and leavened breads with the help of yeast and starters.

Foods functioned for enjoyment and as curatives. Vegetables and fruits, originally known for their medicinal qualities, were added to meat-based soups and stews and savory breads and transformed into an array of tasty side dishes. Herbs and spices, initially used for healing, enhanced recipes of all kinds. Fats and oils, valued for richness, also supplied satiety. Alcoholic beverages, frequently used in health and disease, etched their place in gastronomy.

Just like hundreds of years ago, nutrition, food science and the culinary arts are still inescapably linked. Advances in nutrition, food science and the culinary arts are now multifaceted, rapidly paced and transformational.

People no longer have to hunt and forage to meet their nutritional needs. Food science has created hearty, resistant foods that are available year-round from worldwide sources. The culinary arts have shaped foods into gustatory delights. And many foods and beverages are now enriched or fortified with nutrients that hardly resemble what our ancestors consumed or Mother Nature intended.

As a result, nutrition, food science and culinary professionals may find it harder than ever to sort out the good from the bad, the wrong from the right, and the healthy from the not-so-healthy. This is why it is so important to learn about nutrition, food science and the culinary arts in an interdisciplinary approach like the one this book presents.

HOW TO USE THIS BOOK

Culinary Nutrition: The Science and Practice of Healthy Cooking combines nutrition, food science and the culinary arts unlike other culinary nutrition texts. It translates the science of food and nutrition into the culinary arts by using a straightforward, comprehensible and palatable approach.

Each of the 12 chapters contains a menu of offerings: main courses, basics, tantalizing sides, hands-on approaches and useful takeaways. These items are accompanied by morsels of nutrition, food science and culinary knowhow that apply to many consumer and professional settings.

Recipe ideas are interspersed throughout the chapters. Full recipes, serving ideas and nutrition information are located in a *Recipe file* within the companion *Culinary Nutrition* website at www.culinarynutrition.elsevier. com. Photos of these recipes are located in the centerfold of the book. Short summaries and review questions are included at the end of each chapter to help digest the contents, with additional resources to tantalize tastes.

Finishing Touches include a *Word Pantry* that is filled with key terms from each chapter and references that reflect each chapter's contents. To whet appetites even further, the companion Culinary Nutrition website at www.culinarynutrition.elsevier.com. includes additional hands-on approaches In *Serve it Forth* and review questions in *Check Please*, as well as the *Recipe file*. A comprehensive *Index* completes the text for easy access.

CONTENTS OF THIS BOOK

Culinary Nutrition: The Science and Practice of Healthy Cooking contains 12 chapters that cover the topics that incorporate nutrition, food science and the culinary arts:

Chapter 1—Nutrition Basics: What Is Inside Food, How It Functions and Healthy Guidelines
The Nutrients in Foods and Beverages in Healthy Cooking and Baking
Chapter 2—Food Science Basics: Healthy Cooking and Baking Demystified
The Science behind Healthy Foods, Cooking and Baking
Chapter 3—Culinary Arts Basics: Healthy Cooking Fundamentals
The Culinary Competencies of Healthy Food Selection, Preparation and Food Service
Chapter 4—Carbohydrate Basics: Sugars, Starches and Fibers in Foods and Health
Healthy Carbohydrate Choices, Roles and Applications in Nutrition, Food Science and the Culinary Arts
Chapter 5—Protein Basics: Animal and Vegetable Proteins in Foods and Health
Healthy Protein Choices, Roles and Applications in Nutrition, Food Science and the Culinary Arts
Chapter 6—Lipid Basics: Fats and Oils in Foods and Health
Healthy Lipid Choices, Roles and Applications in Nutrition, Food Science and the Culinary Arts
Chapter 7—Vitamin and Mineral Basics: The ABCs of Healthy Foods and Beverages Including Phytonutrients and Functional Foods
Healthy Vitamin and Mineral Choices, Roles and Applications in Nutrition, Food Science and the Culinary Arts
Chapter 8—Fluid Basics: Healthfully Meeting Fluid Needs
Healthy Fluid Choices, Roles and Applications in Nutrition, Food Science and the Culinary Arts
Chapter 9—Diet and Disease: Healthy Choices for Disease Prevention and Diet Management
Practical Applications for Nutrition, Food Science and Culinary Professionals
Chapter 10—Weight Management: Finding the Healthy Balance
Practical Applications for Nutrition, Food Science and Culinary Professionals
Chapter 11—Life Cycle Nutrition: Healthy Eating throughout the Ages

Practical Applications for Nutrition, Food Science and Culinary Professionals
Chapter 12—Global Food and Nutrition: World Food, Health and the Environment
Practical Applications for Nutrition, Food Science and Culinary Professionals

CHAPTER MENUS

Each of the 12 chapters is arranged into a **Chapter menu** that functions as a table of contents and provides a taste of each topic.

- Objectives
- Introduction
- Main Courses
- Bite on This
- Serve it Forth
- What's Cooking?
- Morsels
- Food bytes
- Over Easy
- Check Please
- Hungry for More?
- Take Away
- Finishing Touches
- Word Pantry
- Website

CHAPTER MENU FEATURES

Objectives: *Learning objectives* state competencies and outcomes for each chapter.
Introduction: The *Introduction* provides an overview of the *Main Courses*, along with thought-provoking insights that are found in *Bite on This* and *Take Away*.
Main Courses: The "meat" or foundation of each chapter is found in the *Main Courses*. Each of the *Main Courses* is filled with relevant information to help to digest the science of food and nutrition and recognize its relevance to food science and the culinary arts.
Bite on This: In-depth explorations of important chapter topics in *Bite on This* are designed to modernize food and nutrition issues and inspire curiosities.
Serve it Forth: Hands-on, in-class and outside activities in *Serve it Forth* cover a variety of real-life nutrition, food science and culinary arts topics and underscore their significance. Additional activities are found in the *Culinary Nutrition* website at www.culinarynutrition.elsevier.com.
What's Cooking?: Hands-on, in-class experiments in *What's Cooking?* utilize food and nutrition tips and techniques and reveal their implications and applications.
Sidebars (Morsels and Food bytes): Plenty of useful nutrition, food science and culinary arts information appear in the *Sidebars*, which include *Morsels* and *Food bytes*. *Morsels* interject amusing, historic and paradoxical quotes about food and nutrition. *Food bytes* add in-depth quips and tips that enhance many of the *Main Courses* and *Bite on This* selections.
Over Easy: A summary of the *Chapter menu* is provided at the end of each chapter for emphasis and review.
Check please: Multiple-choice and essay questions appear in *Check Please* to assess knowledge and prepare for the upcoming chapters. Additional questions are found in the *Culinary Nutrition* website at www.culinarynutrition.elsevier.com.
Hungry for More?: *Hungry for More* presents additional resources such as books, organizations, websites, and more to keep current and resourceful.
Recipes, Recipe file and Photo file: To showcase the concepts presented in Chapters 4 to 12, recipes are noted throughout the text and are featured in a *Recipe file* located within the *Culinary Nutrition* website at www.culinarynutrition.elsevier.com. Full descriptions of each recipe include the category, cooking time, techniques, equipment, description, ingredients, instructions, yield and serving size, nutrient analysis,

nutrient modifications, substitute ingredients, optional ingredients and recipe variations. Many of the finished recipes appear in the *Photo file* within the centerfold of this book. These full-color photographs correspond to the recipes in Chapters 4 to 12 and are identified by a plate number for easy referencing. The list of plate numbers and accompanying photos are also found within the *Culinary Nutrition* website at www.culinarynutrition.elsevier.com. These recipes and photos help to illustrate that healthy and flavorful foods and beverages can be visually appealing, too.

Take Away: *Take Away* looks at ongoing topics in nutrition, food science and the culinary arts and offers food for thought.

Finishing Touches: The *Finishing Touches* are additional elements that enhance the chapter contents. These include the *Word Pantry* and the *Website*.

Word Pantry: The comprehensive *Word Pantry* supplies the definitions for the boldfaced and italicized words in each chapter. It contains both practical and scientific terminology.

Website: The student-instructor *Culinary Nutrition* website at www.culinarynutrition.elsevier.com, includes additional *Serve it Forth* activities, *Check Please* assessments and the *Recipe file*.

CHAPTER 1

Nutrition Basics: What Is Inside Food, How It Functions and Healthy Guidelines

The Nutrients in Foods and Beverages in Healthy Cooking and Baking

1

Culinary Nutrition. DOI: http://dx.doi.org/10.1016/B978-0-12-391882-6.00001-7

OBJECTIVES

1. Define the concepts of normal, under- and over-nutrition and the components of a healthy diet
2. Identify the benefits of a healthy diet
3. Relate the concepts of nutrition and the benefits of a healthy diet to food science and the culinary arts
4. Detail how ingredients, foods and beverages become nutrients
5. Explain how food science and cooking affect foods and beverages that become nutrients
6. Apply the factors that affect food choices to nutrition, food science and the culinary arts
7. Decipher food and nutrition labels
8. Calculate basic kitchen math
9. Link nutrition issues with societal and environmental concerns
10. Address food as medicine

INTRODUCTION: DIGESTING THE SCIENCE OF NUTRITION

Nutrition is more than just eating foods and drinking beverages. Nutrition is the science of how organisms take in and use food and drink for nourishment. This book centers on human nutrition, but nutrition really covers all organisms, including animals, fungi, microorganisms and plants.

The science of nutrition is explained and comes to life in this chapter and others through food science, cooking and baking. Food science is the study of the biological, chemical and physical properties of foods and their effects on the culinary, nutritional, sensory, storage and safety aspects of foods and beverages.

Cooking and baking are the processes of preparing foods and beverages for consumption by using various equipment, ingredients, methods and tools. Cooking and baking utilize food science to influence the appeal, digestibility and satisfaction of foods and beverages—which, in turn, affect their nutritional values.

Food scientists and culinary professionals require a good working knowledge of how nutrition, food science, cooking and baking interact. Foods and beverages must look good and taste great to be selected, consumed and utilized for good health.

To this end, this chapter examines foods and beverages "from the inside out." The molecules that comprise carbohydrates, lipids, proteins, vitamins, minerals and water are explored to see their effects on ingredient and food product formulations and cooking and baking practices.

Many foods and beverages are considered nutritious and fit into a healthy diet. Other foods and beverages are controversial. This chapter sorts out these disagreements. It highlights what is thought to be normal nutrition, undernutrition and overnutrition to establish what humans should consume for health and wellness.

The remarkable pathways that foods and beverages take during their consumption, digestion, absorption, metabolism, storage and use are featured in this chapter. It helps to "digest" the biochemistry of nutrients and translates nutritional science into understandable and practical applications.

Up-to-date nutrition guidelines for healthy eating from the US Department of Agriculture (USDA) and prominent health associations are covered, as well as how these guidelines translate into healthy cooking and baking methods and new product development.

Knowledge about why consumers select or avoid certain foods and beverages is also incorporated. There is information about which factors motivate consumers to make food choices, including food and nutrition labeling, marketing and media along with environmental, religious and societal concerns.

This is a lot to digest! This chapter breaks it down into bite-sized morsels. Whether you are a nutrition, food science or culinary student or professional, this chapter is fundamental to see the progression that foods and beverages take from the land or the laboratory to the kitchen, then on for human consumption, satisfaction and health.

What is nutrition, and why it is important in food science and culinary education?

MAIN COURSES
Nutrition, Nutritional Science and Nutrients

Nutrition is multifaceted. It is the sum of all of the processes in the consumption and utilization of foods and beverages. Nutritional science examines how organisms consume and process foods and beverages for nourishment. Nutrients, including carbohydrates, lipids, proteins, vitamins, minerals and water, are the essence of nutrition. They are also fundamental to ingredient and product development, cooking and baking. As we purchase, prepare and consume foods and beverages we should be cognizant that their nutrients contribute to our health and well-being.

There are hundreds of chemicals in the foods and beverages for human consumption. Many of these chemicals are affected by cooking and baking. In addition, cooking and baking add other chemicals to our food supply and manipulate their structures and functions.

The impact of these chemicals on human nutrition cannot be understated. Nutrition, food science and culinary professionals need to keep current about rapidly evolving nutrient research and guidelines to create the healthiest products, recipes and menus. Nutrients and their functions pave the way.

Essential, Energy-Yielding and Non-Energy-Yielding Nutrients

There are about 40 nutrients that are known to be essential for humans. Essential nutrients are those that the human body cannot make on its own and must be supplied by the diet through foods and beverages. Essential nutrients are considered to be indispensable to life. Nonessential nutrients can be made by the body, such as vitamin D synthesis when ultraviolet rays of sunlight strike the skin and vitamin K production from microorganisms that live in the digestive tract.

This book focuses on the energy-yielding nutrients, which are carbohydrates, protein and lipids (fats and oils), and the non-energy-yielding nutrients, which are vitamins, minerals and water. The main difference between energy-producing nutrients and non-energy-yielding nutrients is that energy-producing nutrients contain calories to create energy. These six nutrients are the basis of most food science and culinary chemical and physical reactions.

By the time this book is completed, many of the other 40 nutrients that accompany foods and beverages and affect nutrition and health will also be examined. Before we can see where each of these nutrients fits into the bigger picture of nutrition and health, we need to establish what is "normal" nutrition, undernutrition and overnutrition and what is considered to be a nutritious or healthy diet.

> **Morsel** "The greatest wealth is health."
> —Virgil (Roman poet, 70–19 BC)

Normal Nutrition, Undernutrition and Overnutrition, and Healthy Diets
NORMAL NUTRITION

Normal nutrition is identified by what most people eat and drink under normal or ordinary circumstances. It accounts for everyday activities and the ability to stay healthy under reasonable conditions.

Nutrition guidelines and recommendations have been designed to qualify and quantify normal nutrition, including the average number of calories and amount of nutrients that most people need daily to stay healthy and prevent disease. These are detailed in food and nutrition guidelines and recommendations later in this chapter.

3

UNDERNUTRITION

Undernutrition describes a condition whereby normal nutritional guidelines and recommendations are not met. It can result from inadequate food intake, poor absorption of nutrients or excessive loss of nutrients. Undernutrition may or may not be accompanied by malnutrition, a medical condition that may be caused by an improper or inadequate diet. Malnutrition may be the consequence of disease, infection or starvation.

While undernutrition and malnutrition are more common in Third World countries, both conditions are found in the United States and other developed countries as well. Poverty and food availability may lead to undernutrition and malnutrition. People who have access to food and choose not to eat it may become undernourished or malnourished, as in the case of eating disorders, discussed in Chapter 10.

OVERNUTRITION

Overnutrition is characterized by overeating or excessive intake of certain nutrients, such as carbohydrates and lipids. Overnutrition may be caused by consuming too many calories compared to expending or burning too few calories through everyday activities and exercise. Obesity is an example of overnutrition, as is consuming excessive nutritional supplements over dietary needs.

NUTRITION AND HEALTHY DIETS

The underlying factors of normal, under- and over-nutrition influence food and beverage choices. Nutrition, food science and culinary professionals can use these factors to help modify ingredients and techniques for healthier diets.

While normal nutrition is designed for most daily needs, many conditions affect normal consumption, such as business demands, busy lifestyles, illnesses, school, traveling and more. Any one of these conditions may alter normal nutrient requirements. Some of these conditions can benefit by special foods and/or beverages.

People who are undernourished may require foods and beverages that are higher in calories and nutrients, while people who are overnourished may need to reduce their caloric intake, particularly certain nutrients. Both conditions require unified approaches by nutritionists, food scientists and culinary specialists. The parameters of a healthy diet must first be established before the needs of normal, under- and overnutrition can be met.

What is considered a *healthy* diet? Babies intuitively know what to eat, and they tend to select the right amounts of food and beverages. But as they age and the selections of foods and beverages grow, it becomes increasingly challenging for them to select the healthiest foods in the right amounts. A host of factors, including education, family, finances, friends, technology and others, can interfere. What is a healthy diet, and how does one know if it is effective?

THE DEFINITION AND FUNCTIONS OF A HEALTHY DIET

Simply put, a healthy diet is one that supports a person's daily and long-term health and well-being. A healthy diet does the following:

- Fuels the body with energy (calories) and nutrients for everyday activities
- Provides additional energy and nutrients for recreational activities and sports
- Supplies nutrients for growth, repair and maintenance
- Fights disease
- Cushions the body, protects it from accidents, regulates body temperature and heals
- Sustains many different body systems as shown in Table 1-1
- Keeps these body systems functioning under many challenging circumstances throughout the life cycle

A look at what is inside foods and beverages will help show why many foods and beverages fit into a healthy diet. It will also indicate why some foods and beverages are considered healthier to consume than others.

TABLE 1-1 The Human Body Systems

Systems	Descriptions
Central nervous system	Brain, neurons, spinal cord and peripheral [sensory and motor] nervous system
Circulatory system	Heart, blood vessels [arteries, capillaries and veins] and lungs
Digestive system	Salivary glands, esophagus, stomach, liver, gallbladder, pancreas, and small and large intestines
Endocrine system	Adrenal glands, hypothalamus, pancreas, parathyroids, pineal gland, pituitary gland, sex organs and thyroid gland
Excretory system	Lungs, large intestine and kidneys
Immune system	Adenoids, cells, leukocytes, organs, proteins, spleen, thymus, tissues and tonsils
Integumentary system	Fat, hair, nails and skin
Lymphatic system	Lymph, nodes and vessels
Muscular system	Skeletal muscles
Reproductive system	Female reproductive organs: fallopian tubes, mammary glands, ovaries, uterus and vagina; male reproductive organs: prostate, seminal vesicles, testes and vas deferens
Respiratory system	Bronchi, diaphragm, larynx, lungs, nose, pharynx and trachea
Skeletal system	Bones, cartilage, ligaments and tendons
Urinary system	Bladder, kidneys, ureter and urethra

Sources: [1], [2], and [3].

What Is Inside Foods and Beverages

MACRONUTRIENTS, MICRONUTRIENTS AND NONNUTRIENTS

Foods and beverages are filled with countless substances, from macronutrients, including carbohydrates, fats and oils, proteins, lipids and water that are needed by the body in "macro" or relatively large quantities, and micronutrients, including vitamins and minerals, that are needed by the body in "micro" or relatively smaller quantities.

Foods and beverages are also filled with nonnutrients, substances that may have some biological effects on the body, such as dietary fiber and phytochemicals, plant compounds with reportedly healthful benefits. Foods and beverages also carry bacteria, microscopic organisms that can be either beneficial or harmful and potentially toxic substances that may find their way into our food supply.

Chemicals that are used in the growth, production, transport and preservation of foods and beverages, such as antibiotics, hormones and preservatives, may also leach into our food supply. While many are safe for human consumption, sometimes undesirable chemicals may circulate. The Food and Drug Administration (FDA), an agency of the US Department of Health and Human Services (HHS), is responsible for ensuring that the US food supply is safe, sanitary and wholesome.

ESSENTIAL AND NONESSENTIAL NUTRIENTS

Essential nutrients are nutrients that the body cannot make or produce in sufficient quantities. Essential nutrients must be obtained through the diet. They include the building blocks of carbohydrates, lipids and proteins, certain vitamins and minerals, and water.

Nonessential nutrients can be made by the body or obtained from sources other than foods and beverages. These include biotin that is produced by gastrointestinal bacteria, cholesterol that is produced by the liver, vitamin K that is produced by intestinal bacteria, and vitamin D that is produced by sunlight. If a person consumes a broad-range diet with a variety of foods and beverages, then he or she should be able to obtain most of the essential and nonessential nutrients they need. When people eliminate certain foods or food groups, restrict calories and/or skip meals on a regular basis, then they may run the risk of nutrient deficiencies. Nutrient knowhow may help to enlighten and guard against these deficiencies.

FOOD BYTE

The term *empty calories* is prevalent in food and nutrition. It is believed that Dr. Michael Jacobson, cofounder of the Center for Science in the Public Interest in Washington, DC, created the terms *empty calories* and *junk food*. The Center for Science in the Public Interest (CSPI) has been a strong advocate for nutrition and health, food safety, alcohol policy and sound science since 1971. The dual mission of CSPI is to conduct research and advocacy programs in health and nutrition and provide consumers with current and useful information about health and well-being.

NUTRIENTS AND CALORIES

Nutrients provide energy, function, protection and structure, among many other roles in the human body. The energy-producing nutrients are carbohydrates, lipids (more commonly known as fats and oils) and proteins. When these energy-producing nutrients are metabolized or "burned" by the human body, they release energy. Energy is the ability to do work—anything as simple as merely living or as complex as climbing mountains.

Energy is measured in *calories*. A *calorie* is a unit of energy that is often used when measuring the energy content of foods and beverages (dietary calories). A *calorie* is the amount of heat that is required to raise the temperature of 1 kilogram of water 1° Celsius (1.8 °Fahrenheit).

Calories are reported as small 1,000-calorie units called *kilocalories* (or *Calories* with an upper case "C"). Kilocalories are commonly abbreviated as *kcal*.

For example, 1 slice of whole-grain bread contains about 69 kilocalories (69 kcal or 69 Calories). Once consumed, 1 slice of whole-grain bread supplies about 69 kilocalories worth of energy for the body to do its work.

FOOD BYTE

In everyday use, the terms *calorie* and *kilocalorie* are often used interchangeably, but this is incorrect. The term "kilo" means 1,000. One kilocalorie contains about 1,000 calories. Conversely, 1 calorie is the equivalent of 1,000th of a kilocalorie. One kilocalorie is equal to 1 Calorie (dietary calorie). In the example of 1 slice of whole-grain bread that contains 69 kcal or 69 Calories, this is the equivalent of about 69,000 calories!

The term calorie (with a lower case "c") is used throughout this book since it is very commonly used in food and nutrition today. In precise science, the term kilocalories is more accurate.

A gram is a measure of weight. The number of calories per gram for each of the energy-producing nutrients (carbohydrates, lipids, protein and alcohol) is shown in Table 1-2. While alcohol is not a nutrient per se, it does produce energy (7 calories per gram). It is included in this table to show how caloric alcohol is compared to carbohydrates and proteins. Alcohol is discussed in Chapter 8.

WHY CALORIES MATTER

The calories per gram of carbohydrates, lipids and proteins are important to remember. They are used to calculate the number of calories per gram of foods and beverages. There are times, such as when reading food labels, that this information is helpful. Computerized programs that calculate calories and nutrients are shown in the section "Hungry for More?" later in this chapter.

TABLE 1-2 Energy-Producing Nutrients and Alcohol		
Energy-producing Nutrients	**Weight (in grams)**	**Calories (per gram)**
Carbohydrates	1 g	4 cal
Proteins	1 g	4 cal
Lipids	1 g	9 cal
Alcohol	1 g	7 cal

Few foods and beverages contain only one nutrient; many contain a combination of carbohydrates, lipids and/or proteins. For example, 1 slice of whole-grain bread is not purely carbohydrates; 1(8-ounce) glass of dairy skim milk is not purely proteins, and 1 tablespoon of butter is not purely lipids (fat), contrary to some popular notions.

In fact, 1 slice of whole-grain bread contains about 69 calories, of which about 44 calories are from carbohydrates, about 16 calories are from protein, and about 9 calories are from fats, as follows:

> 1 slice whole-grain bread = ~69 calories
> 11 grams carbohydrate × 4 calories per gram = 44 calories
> 4 grams protein × 4 calories per gram = 16 calories
> 1 gram fat × 9 calories per gram = 9 calories

One (8-ounce) glass of dairy skim milk contains about 84 calories, of which about 48 calories are from carbohydrates, about 32 calories are from proteins, and about 2 calories are from fats, as follows:

> 1 (8-ounce) glass dairy skim milk = ~84 calories
> 12 grams carbohydrate × 4 calories per gram = 48 calories
> 8 grams protein × 4 calories per gram = 32 calories
> .2 grams fat × 9 calories per gram = 2 calories

One tablespoon of butter contains about 99 to 103.5 calories, of which about .04 calories are from carbohydrates, about 0.48 calories are from proteins, and about 99 to 103.5 calories are from fat, as follows:

> 1 tablespoon butter = ~102 calories
> .01 grams carbohydrate × 4 calories per gram = 0.04 calories
> .01grams protein × 4 calories per gram = 0.48 calories
> 11–11.5 grams fat × 9 calories per gram = 99–103.5 calories

These figures demonstrate that whole wheat bread and dairy skim milk mostly consist of carbohydrates, butter mostly consists of fats, and dairy skim milk contains more protein than whole wheat bread or butter.

The nutrients and calories in whole wheat bread, dairy skim milk and butter may be changed by substituting or enhancing the ingredients. For example, high-gluten flour may be substituted for bread flour in whole-grain bread. (High-gluten flour has as much as 14 percent more protein than bread flour.) Dry-milk powder may be added to boost the protein content of dairy skim milk. (One-third cup contains 8 grams of protein.) The fat content of butter may be lowered by adding water in the manufacturing process (as in soft tub butter). This is how food scientists, nutritionists and chefs create new foods and beverages to maximize certain nutrients and reduce others.

Though this information about calories and nutrients is quite telling, people choose or reject foods and beverages for other reasons. The next section explains the complexity behind our food choices and rejections: what triggers us to eat or not to eat and why.

> **Morsel** "Whatever will satisfy hunger is good food." —Chinese proverb

How Food Works: Appetite, Hunger and Satiety (satisfaction)

APPETITE

Appetite is the psychological desire for foods or beverages. Many factors influence appetite, including sensory responses to the sights, sounds, smells and tastes of food. Other factors include behavioral and social issues that may affect these sensory responses. For example, the sight of food may tempt a person to eat, even if she is not hungry. Or if a diner is not hungry, he may be tempted to eat because others are eating. In each of these instances the sight of food is transferred through neurons to the brain, which registers a desire to eat. It may override the physical feelings of satisfaction from earlier meals.

HUNGER

Hunger includes a range of feelings that signal the need to eat. When hungry, a person may feel dizzy, headachy and irritable; have difficulty concentrating; or suffer stomach discomfort. Some people confuse

7

hunger with appetite and vice versa. This may be due to misinterpreting the psychological desire to eat with the physical signals of hunger. By consuming balanced meals that are spaced throughout the day to offset hunger, this may help to curb the psychological urge to eat.

SATIETY OR SATISFACTION

Satiety is the physical and psychological satisfaction that one acquires from consuming certain foods or beverages. Satiety may be immediate, such as thirst quenching, or it may be sustained and last a few hours between meals, such as a feeling of "fullness." Much depends on the nutrients in foods and/or beverages.

After drinking a sugary soft drink, a person may be satisfied for a brief time. This is because sugar, particularly if it is in liquid form, is digested and absorbed by the body rather quickly compared to other nutrients. If, however, the sugary soft drink is consumed with a protein-packed sandwich, such as lean beef or poultry, then satisfaction may be longer lasting. This is because it takes longer for the starch in the bread and the protein in the meat to be digested.

If a little fat, such as butter or mayonnaise, is spread on the bread, then satiety may be even longer lasting. This is because fat takes longer to be digested and absorbed than carbohydrates and protein.

Satiety is an important consideration in calorie intake and weight management. Highly satisfying foods and beverages will last longer before hunger develops. The key to weight management is to discover which foods and beverages and what amounts are satisfying without overburdening the body with excessive calories and nutrients.

Bite on This: the speculations behind food cravings

Food cravings are intense desires for food. They are different from hunger, which is driven by the physiological need to eat. Food cravings are more related to appetite, which is driven by the psychological need to eat.

Many speculations exist about food cravings. Food cravings may be triggered by hormones, such as serotonin or endorphins, which may prompt the need for sweet foods and pleasurable responses. Serotonin and endorphins are neurotransmitters—brain chemicals that are thought to contribute to feelings of well-being and happiness. Food cravings may also be triggered by the deprivation of certain foods, followed by their reward.

Food cravings may be specific, marked by desires for certain foods, such as french fries or chocolate. Food cravings may also be general, marked by desires for the specific sensory characteristics of foods, such as taste or texture.

The hypothalamus is a region of the brain that controls satiety, or satisfaction. There are two centers of the hypothalamus: one that controls feeding and one that controls satiety. They work together to maintain feeding and satiety in balance.

The amounts of nutrients in the bloodstream may affect both of these centers. When the nutrients in the bloodstream are low, then a person is cued through a complex system of neurological and hormonal responses to replace these nutrients. And when these nutrients are high, a person is cued to stop eating.

Chemicals, medical conditions and other factors may throw off this balance. A question of continued debate is whether or not food cravings are involved in this balance. The following examples show the power of food cravings and their psychological and physiological connections:

- When pregnant women crave pickles and ice cream, this may be caused by a multitude of chemicals that are activated by pregnancy. The sodium in salty foods helps to balance increased fluids that are needed during pregnancy.
- When people go on extreme weight reduction diets and severely limit calories, some may crave high-calorie foods because their diets are too limited.
- When women are premenstrual, their hormone levels fluctuate. Some women may crave chocolate before they menstruate. Chocolate has been linked to serotonin levels in the brain. Serotonin acts like a hormone with calming effects. Chocolate also contains theobromine and phenethylamine, substances that trigger mood-enhancing chemicals and neurotransmitters in the brain.

Three disorders may also prompt food cravings: seasonal affective disorder (SAD), taste addiction disorder (TAD) and pica. Seasonal affective disorder (SAD) is a mood disorder that may be related to serotonin, but this is disputed. Symptoms may range from little energy, too much sleep and/or depression. Those affected may seek certain foods to reduce their symptoms.

Taste addiction disorder (TAD) is a psychological condition with a biochemical basis. A person may develop an obsessive/compulsive relationship to a food, generally due to its sugar (specifically glucose) content. Sugar raises the level of dopamine, a brain neurotransmitter that is partially responsible for reward-driven learning. Nonfood factors may also increase dopamine, such as exercise.

Pica is a disorder that is characterized by unusual nonfood cravings for substances such as chalk or clay. Pica may be the result of acquired tastes, chemical imbalances, cultural traditions or neurological mechanisms that result in nutrient deficiencies, including iron deficiency or anemia.

As can be seen, the topic of food cravings is extremely complex and closely linked to our psychological and physiological needs to eat. Like other controversial topics in nutrition, it is best to examine all of the research about food cravings within the context in which they are experienced before any conclusions are reached.

FOOD CHOICES

Why do Eskimos eat certain foods, while Africans eat other types of foods? Why do people of certain religious beliefs restrict some foods and beverages? Why do food commercials tempt some people to eat, while others are not swayed? Why do some people repeatedly consume the same foods, while others eat more adventurously?

> **Morsel** "Don't dig your grave with your own knife and fork." —English proverb

People make several food and beverage choices every day, thanks to a large extent to our global food supply. Not all of them are healthy. Designing healthy foods, using healthy ingredients and preparation techniques, and communicating the benefits of healthy foods may not drive their selection. Following are some of the reasons people accept or reject certain foods and beverages.

Availability

We tend to eat food that is easily available to match our fast-paced lifestyles. In some places around the world, people still make daily shopping trips for local ingredients. As cities grow and it becomes more difficult to shop locally, people may purchase food that has been produced or manufactured on one side of the world and transported to another. While our global food supply provides us with a broad range of food choices and nutrients, some foods may not transport well or they may carry undesirable bacteria or viruses, which may affect their nutritional value and safety.

Eating locally and seasonally produced foods is becoming more popular. While this makes sense in more temperate climates, in other locations it may mean selecting different foods at different times of the year. For example, in late November, apples, Brussels sprouts, cabbage, carrots and potatoes may be plentiful in Oregon, while apples, bell peppers, cabbage, cucumbers, greens, pecans, sweet potatoes, tomatoes, Vidalia onions, yellow squash and zucchini are available in Georgia. Home and neighborhood gardens and food cooperatives (food coops) improve the accessibility of local and seasonal foods such as these [4].

Familiar Foods

We tend to choose familiar foods because they are comforting and/or safe. Familiar foods remind us of celebrations, family and traditions. We opt for familiar foods when we are sick to help us to feel better.

Consider a bowl of chicken noodle soup with its warmth, richness and saltiness. Chicken soup may be comforting for its warm memories—not to mention its anti-inflammatory and mucous-reducing effects. A hot dog that is loaded with condiments may be comforting at holiday and sporting events because it represents good times. The spicy, salty and sweet tastes are difficult to replicate. A favorite relative's home cooking

9

or baking, such as macaroni and cheese or chocolate chip cookies, is also difficult to substitute in both ingredients and memories.

Convenience

We live in a busy world that keeps getting busier. The concept of a "family meal," where family members gather to eat and discuss the day, is rapidly being replaced by eating on-the-run. Convenience and fast foods are fairly economical, handy and tasty. But foods and beverages such as these with instant taste gratification often come at a cost: more calories, fat, salt and sugar. While some cultures still place much value on the family meal, convenience and fast foods are creeping into their cuisines, too.

Customs

Some people eat raw foods because it is customary to their culture. Examples include sushi, a dietary staple in Japan, and steak tartare, a raw ground beef dish that is originally attributed to French cuisine.

Several population groups consume dried or preserved foods because they need to withstand long periods without fresh food. For example, beef jerky and salted, dried codfish are popular in northern Canada and Scandinavia where the winters are long and cold.

Many diners in Italy and Spain are known to eat dinner late at night, whereas Americans tend to eat earlier. After dinner, they often snack or do not eat anything until breakfast the next morning. As global borders continue to open and trade increases, customs and cuisines are blending.

Examples of these blended cuisines include Pan-Asian and Tex-Mex. Pan-Asian is a combination of Asian ingredients and flavors, and Tex-Mex blends the ingredients and spicy south-of-the-border flavors of the cuisines of Texas and Mexico. A number of cuisines and customs are harmonious, while others may clash.

Cost

As natural resources become scarcer and food production and transportation costs multiply, consumer food costs continue to rise. This may prohibit people from choosing the optimal diet for good health. An economical diet may be filled with too many calories from fats and sugars (overnutrition), or it may not supply enough calories to thrive (undernutrition).

Food and nutrition professionals need to collectively work toward economical ways to ensure that healthy diets are affordable and attainable for everyone. One example of such an ongoing collaboration is the one between Walmart and the USDA. In 2011, Walmart announced it would open as many as 300 stores in areas where affordable and healthful foods are needed the most and are difficult to obtain. This collaboration is expected to help build healthier families and stronger communities with access to an abundance of fresh foods at affordable prices [5].

Food Safety

The foods we eat contain both beneficial and harmful bacteria. Beneficial bacteria, such as those found in cultured yogurt, supply healthy microorganisms to aid digestion. Harmful bacteria, such as those that accidentally creep into our food supply, may be deadly, as demonstrated by past *E. coli* (*Escherichia coli*) outbreaks in strawberries and beef. Safe food production, transportation, preparation and storage are of critical importance for health and well-being. As more foreign foods appear on grocery shelves and restaurant menus, food safety monitoring is paramount.

People may choose or reject certain foods or beverages due to their reported contamination. Instead, they may choose organic foods, believing they are superior.

As a whole, organic foods are produced without food additives, genetically modified organisms, industrial solvents, irradiation, or synthetic fertilizers and pesticides. Still, organic foods may not always be better than foods that are grown or produced in nonorganic conditions. Much depends on safe food handling, production and storage—both in food service operations and in home kitchens [6].

Religion

People have selected or rejected foods and beverages for centuries because of their religious preferences. Some food practices are dictated by sacred writing and religious laws that instruct practitioners on which foods are healthy, religiously correct and/or safe.

Among other pious parameters, Jewish and Muslim religious-based dietary laws are based on food safety. Some non-Jewish or Muslim people choose Kosher or Halal (Arabic for "permissible" according to Islamic law) foods because they perceive that these foods are healthier to consume.

> **Morsel** *"Tell me what you eat, and I will tell you what you are."* —Anthelme Brillat-Savarin (French gastronome and lawyer, 1755–1826)

Bite on This: religion and food choices

The beliefs and practices of certain religions help to mold the food choices that their followers make. Food rituals are fundamental to some religions. They serve to demonstrate faith and disciplined behavior and to show respect for a higher being. Food rituals may include any or all of the following:

- Fasting and/or other cleansing rituals
- Food preparation
- Permitted and prohibited foods and beverages
- Rules of religious days
- Times to consume religious foods
- Utensil preparation and use

Buddhism, Christianity, Hinduism, Islam, Judaism and Seventh-Day Adventists each have certain food rituals or customs. These are merely cross-samplings of the many practices.

Buddhism started as an outgrowth of Hinduism. Buddhists abstain from harming living creatures, but some Buddhists will eat meat and fish. Other Buddhists fast, while some do not eat before noon.

In Christianity, practitioners traditionally abstained from meat on certain days, while eggs and dairy milk products were permitted. Historically, there were fast days, and specific foods were and still are avoided during Lent.

The life goals in Hinduism are enjoyment, liberation, prosperity and righteousness. Many devout Hindus are vegetarian because they respect life. This may be because some Hindus believe that their ancestors were animals. Forbidden foods include domesticated poultry, garlic, onions, mushrooms and salted pork. The coconut is considered sacred.

Islam follows the Koran, the sacred text with its dietary rules. Islam practitioners believe "to eat is to worship" and that food is sacred and must be shared. Dietary restrictions are similar to Kosher restrictions, since pork or carnivorous animals are restricted and slaughter is monitored. A major fast called Ramadan is held annually. It requires complete abstinence from food and drink for one month from sunrise to sunset, beginning with adolescence. Light meals may be consumed after sundown.

Orthodox and some Conservative Jewish people observe kashrut or Kosher dietary laws, which translate to "fit." Only those animals that have cloven hooves and chew their cud (cattle, deer, goats and sheep) may be consumed. Pigs are forbidden. Only meat from animals that are slaughtered under the supervision of a rabbi is permitted. Meat and dairy products may not be consumed at the same meal. There are a set number of hours that one must wait after meat-based meals before dairy foods or beverages can be consumed.

One group of Protestants, the Seventh-Day Adventists, are mainly lacto-ovo-vegetarians, which means that they abstain from meat, but consume dairy milk, dairy products and eggs. Some Seventh-Day Adventists avoid alcohol, coffee, tea and tobacco, too.

These religious-based food preferences should be factored into ingredient, food, meal and menu planning; kitchen design, tools and equipment; and in food preparation, cleanup and storage. As the world becomes more diverse, these challenges and responsibilities will continue to grow.

The Media

Food choices are shaped by the media, including books, the Internet, magazines, newspapers, radio, television and social media, both consciously and subconsciously. Even the products and promotions at supermarkets may persuade people to purchase foods and beverages.

Food manufacturers target certain media to reach a greater number of consumers. For example, women's magazines might target mothers to promote family meals, while children's television programs might target kids to promote snack foods and sweetened beverages. Information about the effects of the food environment on weight management and health is presented in Chapter 10.

NUTRITION, FOOD SCIENCE AND CULINARY PROFESSIONALS

Some food and nutrition organizations serve to educate their members about food choices, and other organizations also serve to educate the public. These organizations and their members are key authorities on nutrition, food science and the culinary arts, with the capabilities of greatly influencing food choices. They are able to exercise their authority through their large national and international memberships, government lobbying, and media spokespeople, among other initiatives.

- Registered dietitians (RDs) and dietetic technicians, registered (DTRs) have completed an Academy of Nutrition and Dietetics (AND) approved undergraduate program in nutrition, performed a clinical internship, and then passed national and state licensing examinations. They may have additional training in the culinary arts and/or food science, including certifications.
- Food and nutrition professionals may both become members of The Society for Nutrition Education and Behavior (SNEB), an international community that educates families, fellow professionals, individuals and students, and influences policy makers about food, nutrition and health promotion. SNEB members embody colleges, schools and universities; communications and public relations agencies; cooperative extensions; the food industry; government agencies; and service and voluntary organizations.
- Chefs may be certified by the American Culinary Federation (ACF). ACF requires a nutrition component for chef certification and continuing education. Some culinary schools also offer a nutrition degree in addition to chef education. Some culinary schools and colleges also prepare students for the RD certification.
- Chefs and food professionals with interests in nutrition and food science might also be members of the Research Chef's Association (RCA), which unites culinary skills and food science in such fields as food manufacturing, research and development. Its members pioneered the discipline of Culinology®, which is the blending of culinary arts and the science of food.
- The Institute of Food Technologists (IFT) is an international, nonprofit professional organization that is dedicated to the advancement of food science and technology. Long range, IFT seeks to ensure a safe and abundant food supply that contributes to healthy people all over the world. Food scientists and technologists, research chefs and registered dietitians may become members, as well as food manufacturers, food producers and other food science–related professions.

Food and Nutrition Agencies, Associations, Guidelines and Recommendations

The US Department of Agriculture (USDA) is the primary agency that establishes food and nutrition guidelines and recommendations for Americans. It provides leadership on agriculture, food and natural resources that is based on the best available science and sound public policy. The USDA has developed the guidelines and recommendations to help plan and/or execute healthy diets, food choices, products, menus and recipes.

The US Food and Drug Administration (FDA) is an agency within the US Department of Health and Human Services (HHS). The FDA investigates food and nutrition associations to monitor their effectiveness. In its role, the FDA closely monitors the ingredients, foods and beverages in our food supply and protects public health by ensuring that foods and dietary supplements are properly labeled and that food is safe, sanitary and wholesome. The FDA also helps the public to obtain accurate scientific-based information about foods for health enhancement [7].

The following guidelines, objectives, references and tools have been developed by the USDA, FDA, and other US government, medical, nutritional and scientific organizations to help educate and promote the health and well-being of Americans. They are useful to nutrition, food science and culinary professionals because they help qualify and quantify foods and beverages in normal nutrition for the US public.

- *US Dietary Guidelines for Americans, 2010*
- *Nutrition Objectives for the Nation: Healthy People 2010* and *2020*
- US Dietary Reference Intakes (DRIs)
- Basic food groups
- Food exchange system
- Food composition tables and databases
- USDA Food Guide Pyramid
- USDA MyPlate
- US food label and food labeling regulations
- Nutrition Facts Panel
- Daily Values (DVs)
- US FDA approved nutrient content claims
- US FDA approved health claims
- Structure/function claims

US DIETARY GUIDELINES FOR AMERICANS, 2010

In 2010, the USDA and HHS produced the seventh version of the *US Dietary Guidelines for Americans*. These guidelines are a set of dietary and other lifestyle recommendations for healthy people who are two years of age and older. They are updated every five years. The US Dietary Guidelines for Americans serve to promote adequate nutrition and health and reduce the risk of some major nutrition-related diseases, such as cardiovascular disease and alcoholism.

The *US Dietary Guidelines for Americans, 2010* recommendations cover two all-encompassing concepts:

1. Maintain caloric balance over time to achieve and sustain a healthy weight.
2. Focus on consuming nutrient-dense foods and beverages.

Maintain Caloric Balance over Time to Achieve and Sustain a Healthy Weight

By consuming the right amount of calories and nutrients to meet daily needs and by being physically active a person may attain and maintain a healthy weight. To accomplish this, decrease the calories that are consumed and increase the calories that are expended. In other words, calories "in" should equal calories "out." Key recommendations for balancing calories to manage weight as presented by the *US Dietary Guidelines for Americans, 2010* are shown in Table 1-3.

Focus on Consuming Nutrient-Dense Foods and Beverages

Americans consume too many calories from added sugars, refined grains and solid fats. Nutrient-dense foods and beverages are higher in nutrients. They include eggs, fish and seafood, fruits, lean meats and poultry, legumes (dried beans, lentils and peas), low-fat or nonfat dairy products or their equivalents, nuts and seeds, vegetables and whole grains.

TABLE 1-3 US Dietary Guidelines for Americans, 2010

Key recommendations for balancing calories to manage weight

- Prevent and/or reduce overweight and obesity through improved eating and physical activity behaviors.
- Control total calorie intake to manage body weight. For people who are overweight or obese, this will mean consuming fewer calories from foods and beverages.
- Increase physical activity and reduce time spent in sedentary behaviors.
- Maintain appropriate calorie balance during each stage of life—childhood, adolescence, adulthood, pregnancy and breastfeeding.

13

Key recommendations for foods and food components to reduce and foods and nutrients to increase as presented by the *US Dietary Guidelines for Americans, 2010* are shown in Table 1-4.

Recommendations for specific population groups and building healthy eating patterns as presented by the *US Dietary Guidelines for Americans, 2010* are shown in Table 1-5.

NUTRITION OBJECTIVES FOR THE NATION: HEALTHY PEOPLE 2010 AND 2020

In 2000, the HHS established ten-year objectives, which it outlined in the document *Nutrition Objectives for the Nation: Healthy People 2010* (see "Hungry for More?" later in this chapter).

This document includes objectives for disease, food safety and nutrition. Each objective targeted goals for improvement by 2010, which are shown in Table 1-6. This was the third generation of this initiative.

Nutrition Objectives for the Nation: Healthy People 2020 is the fourth generation of this initiative and document. It is committed to a society in which all people live long and healthy lives. *Healthy People 2020* emphasizes health equality; it addresses the social determinants of health and promotes health across all stages of life.

TABLE 1-4 US Dietary Guidelines for Americans, 2010

Foods and Nutrients to Reduce	Foods and Nutrients to Increase
Reduce daily sodium intake to less than 2,300 milligrams (mg), and further reduce intake to 1,500 mg among persons who are 51 and older and those of any age who are African American or have hypertension, diabetes, or chronic kidney disease. The 1,500 mg recommendation applies to about half of the US population, including children, and the majority of adults.	Increase vegetable and fruit intake.
Consume less than 10 percent of calories from saturated fatty acids by replacing them with monounsaturated and polyunsaturated fatty acids.	Eat a variety of vegetables, especially dark green and red and orange vegetables and beans and peas.
Consume less than 300 mg per day of dietary cholesterol.	Consume at least half of all grains as whole grains. Increase whole-grain intake by replacing refined grains with whole grains.
Keep *trans* fatty acid consumption as low as possible by limiting foods that contain synthetic sources of *trans* fats, such as partially hydrogenated oils, and by limiting other solid fats.	Increase intake of fat-free or low-fat dairy milk and dairy milk products, such as dairy milk, yogurt, cheese, or fortified soy beverages.
Reduce the intake of calories from solid fats and added sugars.	Choose a variety of protein foods, which include seafood, lean meat and poultry, eggs, beans and peas, soy products, and unsalted nuts and seeds.
Limit the consumption of foods that contain refined grains, especially refined grain foods that contain solid fats, added sugars, and sodium.	Increase the amount and variety of seafood consumed by choosing seafood in place of some meat and poultry.
If alcohol is consumed, it should be consumed in moderation—up to one drink per day for women and two drinks per day for men.	Replace protein foods that are higher in solid fats with choices that are lower in solid fats and calories and/or are sources of oils.
	Use oils to replace solid fats where possible.
	Choose foods that provide more potassium, dietary fiber, calcium, and vitamin D, which are nutrients of concern in American diets. These foods include vegetables, fruits, whole grains, and dairy milk and dairy milk products.

14

What distinguishes *Healthy People 2020* from earlier initiatives are 26 Leading Health Indicators (LHIs)—high-priority health issues that address the factors that promote healthy behaviors across the life cycle and the quality of life. These LHIs are intended to motivate national, state and local actions and highlight strategic opportunities.

The LHIs for nutrition, obesity and physical activity include total vegetable intake for persons 2 years of age and older; child, adolescent and adult obesity; and aerobic and muscle-strengthening activities [9].

Nutrition Objectives for the Nation: Healthy People 2020 provides a framework whereby food scientists, culinary professionals and registered dietitians can collectively improve our national health. Initiatives that encompass the LHIs for nutrition, obesity and physical fitness integrate each of these food and nutrition professions.

DIETARY REFERENCE INTAKES

The Institute of Medicine (IOM) is the health branch of the National Academy of Sciences (NAS). The IOM is an independent, nonprofit organization that provides authoritative and unbiased advice to decision makers and the public.

The IOM developed the Dietary Reference Intakes (DRIs), a set of several nutrient reference values that provide the scientific basis for the development of food guidelines in the United States and Canada. These nutrient reference values cover more than 40 nutrient substances that are classified according to age, gender and life stage.

The DRIs replaced the US Recommended Dietary Allowances (RDAs) that were established in the mid-1990s. (They also replaced the Recommended Nutrient Intake [RNIs] in Canada.) In 2010, the IOM released new DRIs for calcium and vitamin D.

If certain foods or beverages meet or exceed the "US RDA" or if a diet provides "Adequate Intake" of certain nutrients, it means that nutrient reference values exist for these comparisons. The DRIs appear throughout this book to guide in the decision making about which foods and beverages constitute a healthy diet and which should be consumed occasionally or not at all.

The DRIs and resources with the Estimated Average Requirement (EAR), Recommended Dietary Allowance (RDA), Adequate Intakes (AI), Tolerable Upper Intake (TUI), and Estimated Energy Requirement (EER) are shown in Table 1-7.

TABLE 1-5 Recommendations for Specific Population Groups	
Population Groups	**Recommendations[a]**
Women capable of becoming pregnant	Choose foods that supply heme iron, which is more readily absorbed by the body, additional iron sources, and enhancers of iron absorption such as vitamin C–rich foods.
	Consume 400 micrograms (mcg) per day of synthetic folic acid (from fortified foods and/or supplements) in addition to food forms of folate from a varied diet.
Women who are pregnant or breastfeeding	Consume 8 to 12 ounces of seafood per week from a variety of seafood types.
	Due to their high methyl mercury content, limit white (albacore) tuna to 6 ounces per week and do not eat the following four types of fish: tilefish, shark, swordfish, and king mackerel.
	If pregnant, take an iron supplement, as recommended by an obstetrician or other health care provider.
Individuals ages 50 years and older	Consume foods fortified with vitamin B12, such as fortified cereals, or dietary supplements.
Building healthy eating patterns	Select an eating pattern that meets nutrient needs over time at an appropriate calorie level.
	Account for all foods and beverages consumed and assess how they fit within a total healthy eating pattern.
	Follow food safety recommendations when preparing and eating foods to reduce the risk of foodborne illnesses.

Source: [8].
[a]*Specific information about meeting these key recommendations may be found throughout this book.*

TABLE 1-6 Nutrition Objectives for the Nation: *Healthy People 2010*

Disease-related	• Reduce the Rates of Heart Disease, Stroke, Hypertension, Diabetes, Osteoporosis, and Tooth Decay
Nutrition-related	• Reduce obesity, growth retardation, and iron deficiency. • Increase healthy weight, safe and effective weight loss, and sites for nutrition and weight management instruction. • Increase the number of people who consume the recommended amount of fat, sodium and calcium. • Increase the amount of fruit, vegetables and grains (especially whole) in the diet. • Increase the number of women who breastfeed, the number of children who have meals at school to improve their diet quality, and schools that offer nutrition.
Food safety-related	• Reduce food allergy–related deaths and improper food-safety techniques in retail food establishments. • Increase the number of people who practice food-safety behaviors.

TABLE 1-7 Dietary Reference Intakes and Resources

Reference Values	Descriptions
Adequate Intake (AI)	The recommended average nutrient intake level that is considered *adequate* for healthy people for each gender and life stage.
Estimated Average Requirement (EAR)	The *average* daily nutrient intake that is estimated to meet the nutritional requirements for *half* of the healthy individuals for each gender and life stage.
Estimated Energy Requirement (EER)	The *average* daily energy (calorie) intake of healthy people that is needed to *maintain* their body weight.
Recommended Dietary Allowance (RDA)	The *average* daily nutrient level that is needed to meet the needs of nearly all (97 to 98 percent) healthy people for each gender and life stage.
Tolerable Upper Intake (TUI)	The *highest* daily nutrient level that is likely to pose no risk of toxicity to almost all healthy individuals for each gender and life stage.

The basic food groups, USDA Food Guide Pyramid, and USDA MyPlate are resources that help to translate these DRI reference values into foods and beverages. They, too, have a scientific basis and are useful for food product, recipe and menu development and diet design.

BASIC FOOD GROUPS

The first classification by the USDA to organize foods and beverages for dietary recommendations was in 1894. Then in 1916, the first food guide, "Food for Young Children," was published. It divided food into five food groups: dairy milk and meats, cereals, fruit and vegetables, fats and fatty foods, and sugars and sugary foods.

In 1941, the USDA created the first set of Recommended Dietary Allowances (RDAs). Then in 1943, the USDA introduced the "Basic Seven" to help people manage their food rationing during World War II. These included green and yellow vegetables; oranges, tomatoes and grapefruit; potatoes and other vegetables and fruits; dairy milk and dairy milk products; meat, poultry, fish or eggs; breads, flour and cereals; and butter and fortified margarine.

The Basic Four Food Groups were introduced in 1956 to help classify foods based on their nutritional properties. These included the dairy milk, meats, fruits and vegetables, and grain groups. They were used as food guide standards for about a decade. Consumers were instructed to have two standard servings each from the dairy milk and meat groups and four standard servings each from the fruit and vegetables and grain groups. Standard serving sizes of representative foods and beverages are shown in Table 1-8. While fats and oils are not included in the Basic Four Food Groups, a standard serving is about 1 teaspoon.

In the 1970s, the USDA addressed unhealthy foods and health. They added a fifth category to the Basic Four Food Groups, which included fats, sweets and alcohol and recommended that if these substances are consumed, it should be in moderation. In 1988, a graphic that represented all of the food groups was introduced to convey moderation, proportionality and variety.

TABLE 1-8 Standard Serving Sizes of Foods and Beverages

Servings	Descriptions
1 standard grain serving	1 slice of bread, 1 cup of dry cereal, or ½ cup of cooked cereal or cooked grain, such as rice
1 standard dairy milk serving	1 (8-ounce) cup of dairy milk or yogurt, 2 cups of cottage cheese, 1½ ounces of natural cheese, or 2 ounces of processed cheese
1 standard meat serving	1 ounce of fish, poultry or meat; ¼ cup of cooked, dry beans, lentils or peas; 1 egg; 1 tablespoon of peanut butter; or ½ ounce of nuts or seeds
1 standard fruit serving	1 cup of fruit, ½ cup of fruit juice, or 2 tablespoons of dried fruit
1 standard vegetable serving	1 cup raw vegetables, ½ cup cooked vegetables or vegetable juice, or unlimited servings of leafy salad greens
1 standard grain serving	1 slice of bread, 1 cup of dry cereal, or ½ cup of cooked cereal or cooked grain, such as rice
1 standard dairy milk serving	1 (8-ounce) cup of dairy milk or yogurt, 2 cups of cottage cheese, 1½ ounces of natural cheese, or 2 ounces of processed cheese
1 standard meat serving	1 ounce of fish, poultry or meat; ¼ cup of cooked, dry beans, lentils or peas; 1 egg; 1 tablespoon of peanut butter; or ½ ounce of nuts or seeds

FOOD EXCHANGE SYSTEM

In the food exchange system, foods and beverages can be substituted for one another with similar nutrients. The food exchange system was originally designed to help people manage diabetes and weight. It is also a useful tool for anyone who is interested in food selection and meal planning.

The food exchange system consists of three main groups of foods that are based on three major nutrients: carbohydrates, fats and proteins (meat and meat substitutes). Each group of food has similar nutrient content (about the same amount of calories, carbohydrates, fats and protein) and serving sizes so they can be "exchanged" for one another.

For example, 1 small apple can be exchanged for 1 small orange. Three ounces of lean meat, such as ground beef or flank steak, can be exchanged for 3 ounces of fresh fish, such as halibut or tilapia, or 3 ounces of poultry without skin. One teaspoon of regular mayonnaise can be exchanged for 1 teaspoon of safflower oil.

One slice of whole-grain bread can be exchanged for 1 corn tortilla. One-half cup of cooked broccoli can be exchanged for ½ cup of cooked carrots, and so on. Some exchanges are even (such as these examples), while others may vary in serving size. It is the nutrients inside the foods that are being exchanged—and these are similar.

THE USDA FOOD COMPOSITION TABLES AND DATABASES

The USDA food composition databases (FCDBs) provide information about the nutritional composition of foods. Macronutrients, which are required in larger quantities and include carbohydrates, lipids and proteins, and micronutrients, which are required in smaller quantities and include vitamins and minerals, are provided. Some nonnutritive substances, such as plant cell compounds like carotenoids and polyphenols, are also included.

The data are available in food composition tables, or nutrient databases. The values are based on the chemical analyses of foods and beverages, or they are estimated from available data, including manufacturers' information.

A sample food (macaroni and cheese) and its nutrients as shown in a food composition table is featured in Table 1-9. Access to food composition tables is provided in "Hungry for More?" later in this chapter.

Nutrition, food science and culinary professionals can use food composition tables to discover the nutrients in foods for comparison and distinction. This is useful in developing new ingredients or foods and creating new recipes that are dependent on specific amounts of nutrients or feature certain nutrients.

TABLE 1-9 Sample Food and Nutrients from a Food Composition Table

Food	Serving Size	Weight (grams)	Water (grams)	Energy (calories)
Traditional macaroni and cheese	1 cup	200 g	122 g	393 cal

15g *Protein*; 40g *Carbohydrates*; 1g *Dietary Fiber*; 19g *Total Fat*; 8g *Saturated Fat*; 7g *Monounsaturated Fat*; 3g *Polyunsaturated Fat*; 0g *Trans Fat*; 22mg *Cholesterol*; 323mg *Calcium*; 2mg *Iron*; 42mg *Manganese*; 263mg *Potassium*; 800mg *Sodium*; 2mg *Zinc*; 327µg *Vitamin A*; 3mg *Thiamin*; 7mg *Vitamin E*; .4mg *Riboflavin*; 2mg *Niacin*; 1mg *Vitamin B6*; 12µg *Folate*; <1mg *Vitamin C*; <1µg *Vitamin B12*; --Sel(µg).

For example, it can be seen in Table 1-9 that there are 19 grams of total fat in a 1-cup serving of traditional macaroni and cheese. If a reduced-fat version of macaroni and cheese is called for, then food composition tables can be referenced and ingredient reductions, substitutions and/or eliminations made.

THE USDA FOOD GUIDE PYRAMID AND MYPYRAMID

The Food Guide Pyramid was a recognizable nutrition tool that was introduced by the USDA in 1992. It was shaped like a pyramid to suggest that a person should eat more foods from the bottom of the pyramid and fewer foods and beverages from the top of the pyramid.

The Food Guide Pyramid displayed proportionality and variety in each of five groups of foods and beverages, which ascended in horizontal layers starting from the base and moving upward toward the tip: breads, cereals, pasta and rice; fruits and vegetables; dairy products; eggs, fish, legumes, meat and poultry; plus alcohol, fats and sugars. The 1992 USDA Food Guide Pyramid is shown in Figure 1-1.

In 2005, the USDA introduced MyPyramid, an updated version of the Food Guide Pyramid. Food groups were depicted in ascending vertical bands that emphasized the right proportions of food groups. An image of a person walking up a flight of stairs flanked the pyramid to emphasize activity. Instead of servings, quantities were measured in cups and ounces. The 2005 USDA Food Guide Pyramid is shown in Figure 1-2.

Other food guide pyramids followed, including the Mediterranean and Asian. Each of the ethnic food guide pyramids added, deleted, or substituted culturally correct foods with those in the USDA Food Guide Pyramid. For example, yogurt and goat milk products appeared in the Mediterranean Food Guide Pyramid, since intolerance to dairy products from cows is prevalent in this region of the world. Likewise, the Asian Food Guide Pyramid included soy products to replace the nutrients that are normally found in dairy products.

Morsel "If we could give every individual the right amount of nourishment and exercise, not too little and not too much, we would have found the safest way to health."
—Hippocrates (Greek physician, 460 –c. 370 BC)

Additional food guide pyramids have been developed for children, seniors, vegetarians and a number of other groups to meet their specific nutritional needs. Yet, in 2011, after six years, the USDA replaced the Food Guide Pyramid with the nutrition guide MyPlate. Food guide pyramids are still used in other parts of the world and by some specialty groups.

USDA MYPLATE

MyPlate is the USDA nutrition guide that was released in 2011. It depicts a place setting with a plate and glass that represent the five food groups. The plate is split into four sections for fruits, vegetables, grains and protein. The image of a glass alongside is for dairy products. Figure 1-3 shows the USDA MyPlate.

At ChooseMyPlate.gov one can find Selected Consumer Messages; the SuperTracker; personalized nutrition and physical activity plan; and the Ten Tips Nutrition Education Series that includes "10 Tips to a Great Plate." Selected Consumer Messages include the following:

Balance calories
- ○ Enjoy food, but eat less.
- ○ Avoid oversized portions.

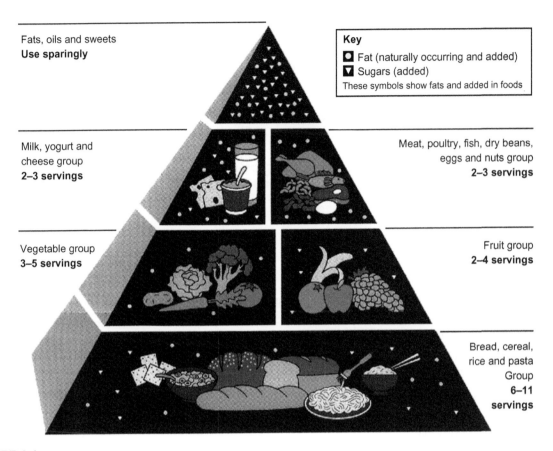

FIGURE 1-1

The 1992 USDA Food Guide Pyramid.

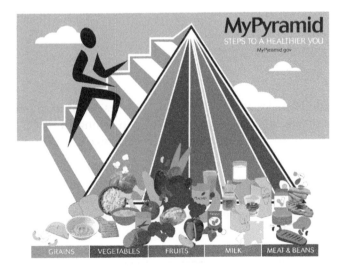

FIGURE 1-2

The 2005 USDA Food Guide Pyramid [10].

Foods to increase

- ○ Make half your plate fruits and vegetables.
- ○ Make at least half your grains whole grains.
- ○ Switch to fat-free or low-fat (1%) dairy milk.

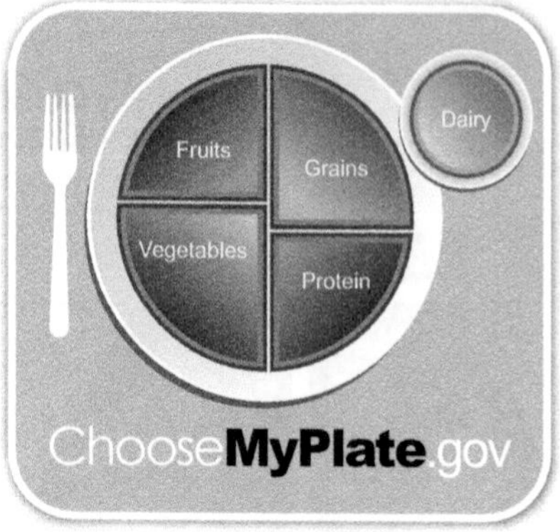

FIGURE 1-3
USDA MyPlate.

Foods to reduce
- Compare sodium in foods like soup, bread and frozen meals, and choose foods with lower numbers.
- Drink water instead of sugary drinks.

The "10 Tips to a Great Plate" are based on the *US Dietary Guidelines for Americans, 2010* and offer the following advice [11,12]:

1. Balance calories.
2. Enjoy your food, but eat less.
3. Avoid oversized portions.
4. Foods to eat more often
5. Make half your plate fruits and vegetables.
6. Switch to fat-free or low-fat (1%) dairy milk.
7. Make half your grains whole grains.
8. Foods to eat less often
9. Compare sodium in foods.
10. Drink water instead of sugary drinks.

FOOD EXCHANGE LISTS

The Academy of Nutrition and Dietetics and the American Diabetes Association have created food exchange lists for diabetes and weight management that can be accessed in "Hungry for More?" later in this chapter. Table 1-10 shows these exchange lists with nutrients in one serving.

> **Morsel** "Be moderate in order to taste the joys of life in abundance."
> —Epicurus (Greek philosopher 341–270 BC)

A sample meal with food exchanges, calories, carbohydrates, protein and fats is illustrated in Table 1-11. It shows the importance of the types and amounts of nutrients in meal planning. In this otherwise low-fat meal, one can see that the fat calories in butter are significant.

20

FOOD BYTE

Most people need no more than 3 to 4 ounces of meat in a serving (about the size of a deck of playing cards, or the size and thickness of the palm of the hand). Just two to three servings of protein a day suffice for the average adult. Yet, some fast-food sandwiches provide as much protein as what is needed in an entire day. One popular sandwich contains three flame-broiled beef patties and two slices of cheese and provides 71 grams of protein when the Daily Value (DV) for protein is just 50 grams. Extra protein over and beyond body needs may be converted into fat.

TABLE 1-10 Exchange Lists with Nutrients in One Serving

Food Groups	Calories (cal)	Carbohydrates (grams)	Protein (grams)	Fat (grams)
Carbohydrates				
Fruits	60 cal	15 g	0 g	0 g
Dairy milk				
Fat-free, low-fat, 1%	100	12	8	0–3
Reduced-fat, 2%	120	12	8	5
Whole	160	12	8	8
Nonstarchy vegetables	25	5	2	0
Starches (beans, lentils, peas, breads, cereals, grains, crackers, snacks, starchy vegetables)	80	15	0–3	0–1
Sweets, desserts	Variable	15	Variable	Variable
Meat/meat substitutes				
Lean	45	0	7	0–3
Medium-fat	75	0	7	4–7
High-fat	100	0	7	8+
Meat substitutes	Variable	Variable	7	Variable
Other				
Fats	45	0	0	5
Alcohol	100	Variable	0	0

Source: [13,14].

TABLE 1-11 Sample Meal with Food Exchanges

Amounts of Food and Beverages	Exchanges	Calories (cal)	Carbohydrates (grams)	Protein (grams)	Fat (grams)
3 ounces broiled fish	3 lean meat	135 cal	0 g	21 g	0–3 g
½ cup cooked pasta	1 starch	80	15	0–3	0–1
½ cup cooked carrots	1 nonstarchy vegetable	25	5	2	0
1 tablespoon butter (for fish, pasta and carrots)	3 fats	135	0	0	15
½ large grapefruit	1 fruit	60	15	0	0
1 cup fat-free dairy milk	1 fat-free milk	100	12	8	0

PORTION SIZES VERSUS SERVING SIZES

Often what people *should* eat is not what people actually eat. This is because sometimes our eyes estimate more food than what our stomach may tolerate. It is also the result of people taking portions that are too large and then eating everything on their plate.

A portion size is the amount of food that is consumed at one time, whether it is from a restaurant meal, can or package, or homemade recipe. In contrast, a serving size is the amount of food that is accounted for in the food exchange system and listed on a food label.

The average serving sizes per serving that are consistent with the exchange lists are shown in Table 1-12. While they are particularly useful for diabetes and weight management, they represent the portion sizes that people should consume.

Supersize was a trademark for the largest portion size available in meals offered by the fast-food giant McDonald's. A smaller meal portion could be made larger by "supersizing" the meal. Initially, the term had positive support, but it lost appeal due to its negative association with obesity and is no longer used.

TABLE 1-12 Average Serving Sizes Per Serving for Exchange List Planning

Food Groups	Average Serving Sizes Per one Serving
Vegetables	½ cup cooked vegetables or vegetable juice
	1 cup raw vegetables or salad greens
Fat-free/low-fat dairy milk	1 cup dairy milk or plain yogurt
Lean protein	1 ounce cheese, fish, poultry or meat
	1 egg
	½ cup cooked legumes or tofu
Fruit	½ cup fruit juice or canned fruit
	1 small whole piece of fruit
Starches	½ cup cooked grains or starchy vegetables (peas or corn)
	½ bagel or roll
	1 slice bread
Fats	1 teaspoon butter, margarine, mayonnaise or oil
	1 tablespoon salad dressing or cream cheese

Throughout culinary history, once recipes were recorded, the amounts of ingredients were roughly estimated by sight. Ingredients were given as "a leg of lamb," "a basketful of apples," "a cupful of beans," "a knob of butter," "a touch of salt," and so on.

Bite on This: kitchen math

Kitchen math is a collection of measurements, conversions and simple calculations that help nutrition, food science and culinary professionals to adjust the amounts and proportions of nutrients in foods and beverages and ingredients in recipes.

While some websites provide quick conversions (see "Hungry for More?" later in this chapter), kitchen math shows the step-by-step changes that are integral to nutrition, food science, cooking and baking. Many of these conversions are used throughout the chapters of this book.

The metric system is a system of measure that is used in almost every country of the world other than in the United States, where the English system is used almost exclusively. There are many compelling reasons why the metric system is preferable to the English system, especially the fact that all metric units are related by factors of 10, which facilitates ease and accuracy.

The metric system is largely the measurement system of choice in the laboratory and professional kitchen. The English system is primarily used by home cooks and consumers. Common metric system–to–English system equivalents are provided in Table 1-14.

Before there were measuring cups and spoons, people used their hands for measurements because they were portable and fairly uniform. Fingers, fists and palms were used to illustrate the amounts of food for purchase or trade. A person's hands are still very useful for estimating food portions today, as depicted in Figure 1-4. Table 1-13 also provides a handy portion guide.

Simple percentages are important calculations in kitchen math. Percentages are used to determine the amount of calories from carbohydrates, lipids and proteins in foods and beverages. They are also used to calculate the amounts of carbohydrates, lipids and proteins in diets as percentages of total calories.

This information aids nutrition, food science and culinary professionals who are involved in new ingredient and food product design and/or in recipe, menu and diet development. Knowing how to use percentages helps if an ingredient, recipe or diet requires a reduction in calories and nutrients. The following three examples explain how percentages are used in kitchen math.

A fist or cupped hand = 1 cup

Palm = 3 oz. of meat

A thumb = 1 oz. of cheese

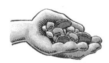

Thumb tip = 1 teaspoon

Handful = 1-2 oz. of snack food

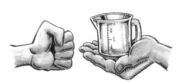

1 tennis ball = 1 serving of fruit

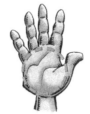

FIGURE 1-4
The use of hands and fingers for measuring.

23

TABLE 1-13 Handy Portion Guide		
Measures	**Hand Portions**	**Food Portions**
1 pat	Thumbnail	Smidgen of butter or chocolate
½ teaspoon	Tip of index finger	Swipe of guacamole or cookie dough
1 teaspoon	Tip of thumb to first joint	Scoop of peanut butter or mayonnaise
1 tablespoon	One thumb	Chunk (1-ounce) of cheese
2 tablespoons	Two thumbs	Salad dressing
½ ounce	One bent thumb	Smear of cheese spread or chicken wing
1 ounce	Space between outstretched thumb and forefinger	Hard cheese, small drumstick or fish stick
1 ounce	One handful	Nuts or small candies
1 ounce	Two handfuls	Chips or pretzels
½ cup	Small fist or cupped hand	Cottage cheese, cooked rice or pasta
1 cup	Large fist or cupped hand	Chopped leafy fresh greens or cold cereal
2 ounces	One-half palm	Two slices meat, poultry, fish or cheese
3 ounces	Full palm	Three slices meat, poultry, fish or cheese
4 ounces	Open palm plus thumb	Ice cream scoop
6 ounces	Two open palms	Whole chicken breast
8 ounces	Two open palms plus thumbs	Restaurant portion meat, poultry or fish
2 inches wide	Circle from tip of thumb to tip of index finger	Small biscuit, muffin, cookie or potato chip
5 inches wide	Circle from tip of thumbs to tips of index fingers	Large biscuit, muffin or cookie
3 inches long	Two fingers span	Small potato or piece of fruit
4 inches long	Three fingers span	Medium potato or piece of fruit
6 inches long	Four fingers span	Large potato or piece of fruit
8 inches long	Five fingers span	Extra-large potato or piece of fruit

TABLE 1-14 Common Metric System to English System Equivalents

Weight

1 gram (g)	.352739619 ounces, or about .35 ounce
1 ounce (oz)	28.35 grams, or about 30 grams
1 gram (g)	1,000 milligrams (mg)
1 milligram (mg)	1,000 micrograms (mcg)
1 kilogram (kg)	1,000 grams (g)
1 kilogram (kg)	2.2 pounds (lbs)
1 pound (lb)	about 454 grams

Volume

1 milliliter (ml)	⅛ teaspoon, or .034 fluid ounce
1 teaspoon (tsp)	5 milliliters
1 tablespoon (T)	15 milliliters
1 fluid ounce (fl oz)	30 milliliters, or 2 tablespoons
1 cup (c)	8 fluid ounces, or 16 tablespoons, or 240 milliliters
1 quart (qt)	32 fluid ounces, or 4 cups, or .95 liters
1 liter (L)	1.06 quarts, or 1,000 milliliters
1 gallon (gal)	16 cups, or 4 quarts, or 128 fluid ounces, or 3.79 liters

Weights and Measures

16 tablespoons	1 cup
12 tablespoons	¾ cup
10 tablespoons	⅔ cup *plus* 2 teaspoons
8 tablespoons	½ cup
6 tablespoons	⅜ cup
5 tablespoons	⅓ cup *plus* 1 teaspoon
4 tablespoons	¼ cup
2 tablespoons	⅛ cup
2 tablespoons	⅙ cup *plus* 2 teaspoons
1 tablespoons	1/16 cup
1 cup	48 teaspoons, or 16 tablespoons
½ cup	24 teaspoons, or 8 tablespoons
2 cups	1 pint
2 pints	1 quart
4 quarts	1 gallon

Source: [15].

Example #1 demonstrates how the percentage of total calories from fat on a food label can be used to calculate the number of calories from fat in a food or beverage.

Example #1:
1. Review the food label for the total number of calories and the percentage of total calories from fat.
   Total number of calories = 125 calories
   Percentage of total calories from fat = 30 percent
2. To determine how many calories of the food or beverage are from fat, multiply the total number of calories by the percentage of total calories from fat, expressed as a decimal.

Solution:

125 calories (total number of calories) × .30 total fat (30 × .01) = 37.5 total calories from fat

Example #2 demonstrates how to use a percentage to calculate the number of calories in a diet.

Example #2:
1. If a person consumes 2,000 calories daily and requires a diet that is 30 percent total fat, how many calories of fat should he consume daily?

Solution:

2,000 daily calories × .30 total fat (30 × .01) = 600 daily calories from fat

Both of these examples have many practical purposes. In the first example, the amount of fat in a recipe may be limited to no more than 30 percent total fat so it can be labeled reduced-fat. This may require a 30 percent reduction of most of the ingredients in the recipe. This information directs the food developer or chef to use one-third less fat.

In the second example, a daily diet may be limited to no more than 30 percent total fat for cardiovascular disease prevention. On an average 2,000–daily calorie diet, up to one-third of the calories may come from fats. This information shows health professionals that fat does not have to be eliminated on a restricted-fat diet.

Example #3 requires the information about the number of calories per gram of carbohydrates, lipids and proteins that were provided earlier in this chapter. First a brief review:

Energy-producing Nutrient	Weight in Grams	Number of Calories/Gram
Carbohydrates	1 gram	4 calories/gram
Protein	1 gram	4 calories/gram
Lipids	1 gram	9 calories/gram
Alcohol	1 gram	7 calories/gram

Example #3:
If 2,400 total calories are consumed daily and these calories contain 60 grams of total fat, then what is the percentage of total calories that is contributed by these grams of fat?

Solution:
60 grams of total fat × 9 calories/gram of total fat (lipids) = 540 calories from total fat

540 calories from total fat/2,400 daily calories × .01 (to convert into a percentage) =

22.5 percent total fat

Example #3 illustrates the importance of nutrient information such as this in ingredient, recipe, menu and diet development. Knowing how to calculate the percent of total fat is also useful in nutrition labeling. By becoming skillful with kitchen math, one may be able to compute decisive values and contribute missing links. There are additional exercises in the "Check please" section in this chapter that provide practice with kitchen math.

US FOOD LABEL AND FOOD LABELING REGULATIONS
The Nutrition Labeling and Education Act

In the United States, food packaging has been required to carry definitive labeling since 1990 with the passage of the Nutrition Labeling and Education Act (NLEA). The NLEA amended the Federal Food, Drug and Cosmetic Act (FFDCA) of 1938. These food labeling regulations are designed to be rigorously truthful, science based, and uniform.

The NLEA is implemented by the **US Food and Drug Association (FDA).** The FDA is an agency within the HHS, which is responsible for regulating the safety of most types of foods and dietary supplements.

The NLEA requires that a label appear on most foods, and it approves nutrient claims and FDA-approved claims on food labels. Some foods and substances that do not require food labels include bulk food, coffee, meat, poultry, spices, tea and food prepared on-site, such as in bakeries, cafeterias or delis.

One cannot understate the importance of food and nutrition labels to nutrition, food science and culinary professionals. Not only do they convey the ingredient content of US-produced foods and beverages, but they can be used to compare the nutrients among products and as a vehicle for diet and health messages [16].

US Food Labels

In 1994, food labeling legislation was introduced in the United States to comply with the NLEA and to help US consumers follow the Food Guide Pyramid. It was revised in 2008 and 2009. Food labeling legislation applies to US food manufacturers and foreign exporters of foods into the United States.

25

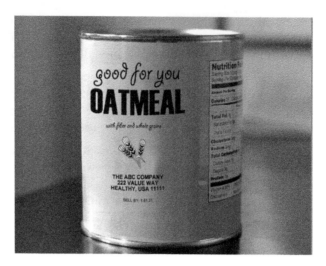

FIGURE 1-5
Front panel of typical US food label.

This legislation requires that most foods carry nutrition labeling and that food labels that carry nutrient content claims and certain health messages comply with specific requirements. Since regulations frequently change, it is the responsibility of the food industry to keep current with legal requirements.

In 2006, the *Food Allergen Labeling and Consumer Protection Act (FALCPA)* was introduced, which requires food labels to disclose any of eight major food allergens (eggs, fish, dairy milk, peanuts, shellfish, soybeans, tree nuts and wheat) within foods and beverages [17].

Some substances are exempt from certain food labeling, such as very small products like candy and those that have few nutrients, like soft drinks. The front panel of a typical US food label is shown in Figure 1-5. The following information is required on most US food labels [18]:

- Statement of identity (common name of the food or food product on the front of the package or on the principal display panel)
- Business information (name and address of the manufacturer)
- "Sell by" date
- Net contents or weight of the package or container
- Recommended serving size
- Number of servings in the package or container
- Ingredient statement (nutrients and subingredients; special rules apply to colorings, flavorings and spices)
- Ingredients listed in *descending order* of predominance by weight in the food or food product
- Nutrition labeling (see the "Nutrition Facts Panel" section that follows)
- Allergen declaration (for eight major allergens: eggs, fish, dairy milk, peanuts, shellfish, soybeans, tree nuts and wheat)

FOOD BYTE: SERVING SIZES VERSUS NUMBER OF SERVINGS

The first place to look at the Nutrition Facts Panel is the serving size and the number of servings in a package or container. Serving sizes are based on the amount of food that people *typically* eat. They are provided in *familiar* units, such as cups or pieces, followed by the *metric* amount, such as the number of grams or milligrams. When people open packages or containers, they may consume more than one serving—or the entire amount. One ounce of potato chips (about two handfuls) contains about 155 calories, and an entire 16-ounce bag may contain about 2,480 calories!

TABLE 1-15 Nutrition Facts Panel: Mandatory and Voluntary Nutrients	
Mandatory Nutrients	**Calories**
	Calories from fat
	Total fat
	Saturated fat
	Trans fat
	Cholesterol
	Sodium
	Total carbohydrates
	Dietary fiber
	Sugars
	Protein
	Vitamin A
	Vitamin C
	Calcium
Voluntary nutrients	Iron
	Calories from saturated fat
	Polyunsaturated fat
	Monounsaturated fat
	Potassium
	Soluble fiber
	Insoluble fiber
	Sugar alcohols
	Other carbohydrates
	Percent vitamin A as beta-carotene
	Other essential vitamins and minerals

Source: [19,20].

NUTRITION FACTS PANEL

The *Nutrition Facts Panel* has been required on all food labels of US manufactured foods and food products since 1994. It is under US FDA regulation. The Nutrition Facts Panel must display mandatory nutrients for one standard serving of food or a food product. The following nutrients are considered to be mandatory on the Nutrition Facts Panel and must appear in the order that is shown in Table 1-15.

Other nutrients do not have to appear if they are zero. Foods and food products that contain more than 5 grams are rounded to the nearest .5 gram. Foods and food products that are less than .5 gram are rounded to 0 grams. Foods and food products that claim to be classified as low-fat or high-fiber must be uniform with food and food products that bear similar labels. A sample Nutrition Facts Panel is shown in Figure 1-6.

The Daily Values

The Daily Values (DVs) are a set of reference values that quantify the nutrients that appear within the Nutrition Facts Panel of US produced foods and food products. The DVs assist consumers and food and nutrition professionals in interpreting the amounts of these nutrients and comparing their nutritional values with similar foods and food products.

The DVs are established for adults and children age 4 and over based on a caloric intake of 2,000 calories, for adults and children four or more years of age. The US FDA Daily Values are shown in Table 1-16.

The percentages of the Daily Values that appear on the Nutrition Facts Panel show what one serving of a food or food product supplies. Each nutrient is based on 100 percent of the daily requirements for that particular nutrient.

Figure 1-7 shows the Daily Values on a sample Nutrient Facts Panel. The nutrients are listed with their weights on the left-hand side and the percent Daily Value for each of these nutrients is listed on the right-hand side. For example, if one serving of food contains 470 milligrams of sodium and this amount is 20 percent

Nutrition Facts
Serving Size 1 cup (228g)
Servings Per Container about 2

Amount Per Serving

Calories 250	Calories from Fat 110

% Daily Value*

Total Fat 12g	**18%**
Saturated Fat 3g	15%
Trans Fat 3g	
Cholesterol 30mg	10%
Sodium 470mg	20%
Total Carbohydrate 31g	10%
Dietary Fiber 0g	0%
Sugars 5g	
Proteins 5g	
Vitamin A	4%
Vitamin C	2%
Calcium	20%
Iron	4%

*Percent Daily Values are based on a 2,000 colorie diet. Your daily values may be higher or lower depending on you calorie needs:

	Calories:	2,000	2,500
Total Fat	Less than	65g	80g
Saturated Fat	Less than	20g	25g
Cholesterol	Less than	300mg	300mg
Sodium	Less than	2,400mg	2,400mg
Total Carbohydrate		300g	375g
Dietary Fiber		25g	30g

For edicational purposes only. This label does not meet the labeling requirements described in 21 CFR 101.9.

28

FIGURE 1-6
Nutrition facts panel [21].

of the Daily Value for sodium, then one serving of this food supplies about one-fifth of the Daily Value (20 percent/100 percent = 1/5).

According to Table 1-16, the Daily Value for sodium is 2,400 milligrams, about five times the amount of sodium in one serving of this food. This example demonstrates how the Daily Value can be used for food selection and meal planning.

Bite on This: deciphering a food label

A typical food label from a can of tuna fish is depicted in Table 1-17. Key terms are listed along with their interpretations. The DVs and their interpretations follow. This depiction demonstrates the challenges and benefits in deciphering food labels.

The food label in Table 1-17 shows that one serving of canned tuna in water (just 2 ounces or ¼ cup) provides almost one-third of the DV for protein, with little fat and no carbohydrate. One-quarter cup of another food with appreciable protein, such as chicken, can be compared to see how its nutrients measure up to canned tuna fish in water.

US FDA Approved Nutrient Content Claims

Nutrient content claims are statements on the labels of foods, food products and dietary supplements that describe the amounts of nutrients or dietary substances in these products. The US FDA establishes the requirements and regulates the compliance of nutrient content claims.

TABLE 1-16 US Food and Drug Administration Daily Values, Based on a 2,000-Calorie Daily Diet

Food Components	Daily Values (DV)
Total fat	65 grams (g)
Saturated fat	20 g
Cholesterol	300 milligrams (mg)
Sodium	2,400 mg
Potassium	3,500 mg
Total carbohydrate	300 g
Dietary fiber	25 g
Protein	50 g
Vitamin A	5,000 International Units (IU)
Vitamin C	60 mg
Calcium	1,000 mg
Iron	18 mg
Vitamin D	400 IU
Vitamin E	30 IU
Vitamin K	80 micrograms µg
Thiamin	1.5 mg
Riboflavin	1.7 mg
Niacin	20 mg
Vitamin B6	2 mg
Folate	400 µg
Vitamin B12	6 µg
Biotin	300 µg
Pantothenic acid	10 mg
Phosphorus	1,000 mg
Iodine	150 µg
Magnesium	400 mg
Zinc	15 mg
Selenium	70 µg
Copper	2 mg
Manganese	2 mg
Chromium	120 µg
Molybdenum	75 µg
Chloride	3,400 mg

Source: [22].

29

Examples of nutrient content claims include such statements as *fat-free, fortified, excellent source, healthy, high potency, lean, light, low, made with, more, percent* and *reduced*. A list of US FDA approved nutrient content claims, definitions, and amounts per serving are shown in Table 1-18. Additional claim information for *antioxidant,* healthy and *high potency* can be found at www.fda.gov.

US FDA Approved Health Claims

Health claims are statements on the labels of foods, food products and dietary supplements that describe the relationship between the components of these products and the reduced risks of certain diseases or conditions. Like the nutrient content claims, the FDA has established specific language and guidelines for the use of health claims.

An example of a US FDA approved health claim is "Three grams of soluble fiber from oatmeal that is consumed daily in a low-saturated fat and cholesterol diet may reduce the risk of heart disease. This cereal has 3 grams of soluble fiber per serving."

Food manufacturers must use the words *may* or *might* in declaring the connections of certain nutrients with diseases. They must also phrase the relationship in very understandable consumer-friendly language and note the importance of other factors in disease prevention or reduction, such as exercise. Notice the words *may* or *might* in

```
Nutrition Facts
Serving Size 1 cup (228g)
Servings Per Container about 2

Amount Per Serving

Calories 250          Calories from Fat 110

                                    % Daily Value*

Total Fat 12g                            18%
    Saturated Fat 3g                     15%
    Trans Fat 3g
Cholesterol 30mg                         10%
Sodium 470mg                             20%
Total Carbohydrate 31g                   10%
    Dietary Fiber 0g                      0%
    Sugars 5g
Proteins 5g

Vitamin A                                 4%
Vitamin C                                 2%
Calcium                                  20%
Iron                                      4%

*Percent Daily Values are based on a 2,000 colorie
diet. Your daily values may be higher or lower
depending on you calorie needs:
                      Calories: 2,000      2,500
Total Fat             Less than  65g        80g
    Saturated Fat     Less than  20g        25g
Cholesterol           Less than  300mg      300mg
Sodium                Less than  2,400mg    2,400mg
Total Carbohydrate               300g       375g
    Dietary Fiber                25g         30g
```

For edicational purposes only. This label does not meet the labeling
requirements described in 21 CFR 101.9.

FIGURE 1-7
Daily values on a sample food label [21].

the example above. Also notice the importance of low saturated fat and cholesterol in heart disease risk reduction. US FDA approved health claims are shown in Table 1-19.

Structure/Function Claims

Structure/function claims are statements on the labels of foods, food products or dietary supplements that describe how a product may affect the body organs or systems. *Specific diseases cannot be mentioned.*

Structure/function claims do not require the approval of the FDA, but they must receive the text of the claim within 30 days of marketing the product from the manufacturer. The affixed label must include a disclaimer that reads, *"This statement has not been evaluated by the FDA. This product is not intended to diagnose, treat, cure, or prevent any disease."* An example of a structure/function claim is *"Calcium builds strong bones."* Some other examples of structure/function claims are shown in Table 1-20. Not all structure/function claims are provided.

Morsel "Eat to live and not to eat."
—Socrates (Roman philosopher, 469–399 BC)

What Is a Healthy Diet? The ABCs of Healthy Eating

Now that the foundation of nutrition and its importance in food science and culinary arts have been established, along with the nutrition goals and regulations as established by US government, medical and scientific associations, it is time to turn our attention to the ABCs of healthy eating: adequacy, balance, moderation, calorie control plus moderation, and variety. These simple principles help to put a healthy diet into perspective.

TABLE 1-17 What's Inside a Can of Tuna Fish?

If the Label Reads:	It Can Be Interpreted to Mean:
"Premium Tuna"	It informs the consumer that it is high quality.
"Solid white albacore" in water rather than oil	The product may be lower in calories and fat than tuna canned in oil.
Ingredients: White tuna, water, vegetable broth, salt, pyrophosphate added.	Tuna is listed first, so it is the main ingredient. Pyrophosphate is not normally present.
Contains: Tuna and soy	Soy is disclosed for people who have a soy allergy. There is probably a negligible amount.
Distributed by _____	Must be included. The distributor may be different from the manufacturer.
For Inquiries_____	Business information must be included.
Nutrition Facts Panel:	Must be included.
Serving Size: 2 oz. drained (56 g—about ¼ cup)	The serving size is only ¼ cup.
Servings: About 5	One can of tuna contains 5 (¼-cup) servings.

	Amount/one serving	Percent Daily Value (% DV[a])	Interpretation
Total fat	1.0 g	2	Low in total fat
Saturated fat	0 g	0	No saturated fat
Trans fat	0 g		No DV for trans fat
Cholesterol	25 mg	8	Low in cholesterol
Sodium	250 mg	11	About one-tenth DV for sodium
Total carbohydrate	0 g	0	No carbohydrate
Fiber	0 g	0	No fiber
Sugars	0 g		No DV for sugars
Protein	15 g	27	Almost one-third DV for protein
Vitamin A		0	No vitamin A
Vitamin C		0	No vitamin C
Calcium		0	No calcium
Iron		0	No iron
Niacin		25	One-quarter DV for niacin
Vitamin B6		10	One-tenth DV for vitamin B6
Vitamin B12		15	One-fifteenth DV for vitamin B12
Phosphorus		10	One-tenth DV for phosphorus

Source: [22].
[a]Percent Daily Values are based on a daily 2,000-calorie diet.

ADEQUACY

Adequacy is a measure of whether or not a diet meets the nutritional needs of generally healthy people according to the US DRIs. Adequacy is determined and categorized by age, gender and life stage. A diet for a child is not adequate for a teenager and a diet for a teenager is not adequate for a pregnant woman or a senior. Extenuating circumstances, such as accidents and disease, may also affect the adequacy of a diet.

An adequate daily diet offers 100 percent of the DVs. An adequate long-term diet also contributes to health and well being.

BALANCE

Balance is an even distribution of the foods in a meal or the nutrients in a diet. The human body seeks balance in many of its functions. For example, too little or too much protein is imbalanced and may lead to protein malnutrition or burden the kidneys. Similarly, a high-protein meal may be considered imbalanced if other nutrients are missing.

TABLE 1-18 US Food and Drug Administration Approved Nutrient Content Claims

Claims	Amounts per Serving
Calories	
Calorie-free	Fewer than 5 calories
Low-calorie	40 calories or fewer
Reduced or fewer calories	At least 25% fewer calories[a]
Light or lite	Calories reduced by at least 30% fewer calories (if food is less than 50% calories from fat)
Total fat	
Fat-free	Fewer than .5 gram fat
Low-fat	3 grams or fewer of fat and no more than 30% calories from fat
Reduced or less fat	At least 25% less fat[a]
Light or lite	Fat reduced 50% or more (if food is 50% or more calories from fat)
Cholesterol	
Cholesterol-free	Fewer than 2 milligrams cholesterol and 2 grams or fewer of saturated fat
Low cholesterol	20 milligrams or fewer per reference amount (and per 50 grams of food if the reference amount is small) and 2 grams or fewer saturated fat per reference amount
Reduced or less cholesterol	At least 25% less cholesterol and 2 grams or fewer saturated fat
Saturated fat	
Saturated fat-free	Fewer than .5 gram saturated fat and fewer than .5 gram trans fat
Low saturated fat	1 gram or fewer saturated fat and no more than 15% of calories from saturated fat
Reduced or less saturated fat	At least 25% less saturated fat
Sodium	
Sodium free	Fewer than 5 milligrams sodium
Very low sodium	35 milligrams or fewer sodium
Low sodium	140 milligrams or fewer sodium
Reduced or less sodium	At least 25% less sodium
Light in sodium	At least 50% less sodium than appropriate reference food
Sugar	
Sugar-free	Fewer than .5 gram sugars
Reduced sugar or less sugar	At least 25% less sugars[a]
No added sugar	No sugars added during processing or packing, including ingredients that contain sugars, such as juice or dry fruit
Fiber	
High fiber	5 grams or more
Good source of fiber	2.5 to 4.9 grams
More or added fiber	At least 2.5 grams more[a]
Other	
High, rich in, excellent source of	20% or more of % DV[a]
Good source, contains, provides	10% to 19% of % DV[a]
More, enriched, fortified, added	10% or more of % DV[a]
Lean[b]	Fewer than 10 grams fat, 4.5 grams or fewer saturated fat and fewer than 95 milligrams cholesterol
Extra lean[b]	Fewer than 5 grams fat, fewer than 2 grams saturated fat and fewer than 95 milligrams cholesterol

Source: [23].
[a]Compared to an appropriate reference food.
[b]Game meats, meat, poultry and seafood

32

TABLE 1-19 FDA Approved Health Claims

- Calcium, vitamin D and osteoporosis
- Dietary lipids (fat) and cancer
- Dietary saturated fat and cholesterol and risk of coronary heart disease
- Dietary noncariogenic carbohydrate sweeteners and dental caries
- Fiber-containing grain products, fruits and vegetables and cancer
- Folic acid and neural tube defects
- Fruits and vegetables and cancer
- Fruits, vegetables and grain products that contain fiber, particularly soluble fiber, and risk of coronary heart disease
- Sodium and hypertension
- Soluble fiber from certain foods and risk of coronary heart disease
- Soy protein and risk of coronary heart disease
- Stanols/sterols and risk of coronary heart disease

TABLE 1-20 Examples of Structure/Function Claims

Vitamins	Structures or Functions
Vitamin A	• May contribute to maintenance of healthy vision • May contribute to maintenance of healthy immune function • May contribute to bone health • May contribute to cell integrity
Vitamin C	• Functions as an antioxidant to neutralize free radicals • May contribute to healthy immune function • May contribute to maintenance of bone health
Vitamin D	• Helps regulate calcium and phosphorus • Helps contribute to bone health • May contribute to healthy immune function • Helps support cell growth
Vitamin E	• Functions as antioxidant to neutralize free radicals • May contribute to healthy immune function • May contribute to maintenance of heart health
Folate/folic acid	• Supports healthy brain and spinal cord development • May contribute to maintenance of heart health
Vitamin B12	• Helps regulate metabolism • Supports blood cell formation • May contribute to maintenance of mental function
Minerals	
Calcium	• Builds strong bones
Magnesium	• Contributes to bone health and healthy immune function
Potassium	• Helps maintain healthy blood pressure level in combination with low-sodium diet
Selenium	• Neutralizes free radicals and supports healthy immune system
Other	
Omega-3 fatty acids	• May contribute to maintenance of heart health • May contribute to maintenance of mental and visual function
Probiotics	• May improve gastrointestinal health and systemic immunity
Phytoestrogens	• May contribute to maintenance of bone health • May contribute to a healthy brain • May contribute to healthy immune function • For women, may contribute to maintenance of menopausal health

33

Source: [24].

A balanced meal contains the basic food groups in recommended portion sizes. A balanced diet provides a range of nutrients over time.

CALORIE CONTROL

If a person follows the ABCs of healthy eating, then she should consume the right amount of calories. This assumes that the calories she consumes equal the calories she expends. Sedentary activities and labor-saving devices have reduced the calories that we expend, so people should eat less and practice *calorie control* to compensate.

Instead, our collective caloric intake has increased. We barely find time to exercise, and our national "waistline" has suffered; our society is simply growing too large. We need to tighten our belts, eat less and exercise more, particularly as we age and our metabolism slows down. A calorie-controlled meal provides about one-third of daily calories. A calorie-controlled diet may lead to weight loss over time.

DISCRETIONARY CALORIES

Discretionary calories are the amount of calories that a person chooses whether or not to consume. If a person requires 2,000 calories daily but consumes only 1,800 calories and meets their nutritional needs, then 200 calories are considered "discretionary." A regular soft drink or small chocolate bar contains about 150 to 230 calories and may fit an otherwise healthy diet. On the other hand, eating fewer discretionary calories may benefit a person's diet and health over time.

EMPTY CALORIES

Empty calories refer to the calories in nutrient-poor foods and beverages, such as candy or soft drinks. Empty calories still contain calories, but they may be devoid of nutrients and other health-enhancing substances such as fiber, minerals, protein and vitamins. For example, 15 jelly beans contain 159 calories, the majority of which are from sugar. One-quarter cup of raisins contains 122 calories. While many of these calories are from sugar, raisins also contain fiber, vitamins and minerals. Consuming fewer empty calories is sensible for both weight and health.

NUTRIENT DENSITY

The concept of *nutrient density* is virtually the opposite of empty calories. A *nutrient-dense* food is rich in nutrients compared to a *calorie-dense* food that is higher in calories. For example, a 1-cup serving of fresh broccoli contains about 30 calories. Broccoli is filled with calcium and magnesium; vitamins A, C, and K; and other nutrients. A regular soft drink contains about 150 calories per 12 ounces, with sugar, water and chemicals. The broccoli is considered a nutrient-dense food, while the soft drink is considered a calorie-dense food. It is best to consume more nutrient-dense foods most of the time.

MODERATION

Moderation is restraint without excesses or limitations. Moderation means consuming what is "just right" so a person is neither too full nor too hungry. Moderation may be difficult to achieve if people do not know correct portion sizes—or stick to them. The hand portion guidelines in Table 1-13 and "Bite on This: food math" in this chapter illustrate correct portion sizes. By practicing moderation, a person may be able to consume an array of foods and beverages and still be within his or her daily calorie allotment.

A moderate daily diet is satisfying and leaves room for discretionary calories. A moderate long-term diet may also be health-promoting.

VARIETY

A diet with the same color, taste or texture may be *un*appealing. This is why some diets are more successful than others. They offer a *variety* of foods and beverages from which to choose. Diets that are rich in fruits and vegetables provide all of the basic tastes: bitter (cruciferous vegetables), salty (seaweeds), sour (citrus fruits), sweet (ripe stone fruits) and umami (mushrooms and other fungi). Whole grains taste earthy, lean proteins taste meaty or mild (depending on their sources), and healthy fats taste light. By selecting a variety of foods such as these, a diet may be pleasing and beneficial. A variety-filled diet brings a daily array of nutrients and appetite for life.

How Food Becomes Nutrients: Digestion, Absorption, and Metabolism

Good nutrition depends on the proper digestion of foods and beverages and the normal absorption and metabolism of their nutrients.

DIGESTION

Digestion is the process by which food and beverages are physically and chemically broken down into smaller components by the human body. These components are then absorbed and metabolized or stored for future use. Most foods and beverages undergo some form of digestion before they can be absorbed and used.

Each stage of the digestive process is designed to break down carbohydrates, lipids and proteins into smaller parts and move them along for absorption and metabolism. Much depends on the nutrients that are contained in foods and beverages. A beverage may be digested faster than a piece of whole-grain bread, which may be digested faster than a chicken breast, which may be digested faster than a pat of butter. The more difficult a food or beverage is to digest, the longer the digestive process may be. Digestion may take 24 to 72 hours depending on food composition.

Digestion really starts before a food or beverage ever comes close to the mouth. The appearance, aroma and sounds of foods and beverages arouse the senses and start the "digestive juices flowing." Very appealing foods and beverages stimulate the central nervous system to anticipate what may follow. The brain and stomach communicate the deliciousness of foods and beverages through a maze of chemical transmitters. This triggers salivation and readies the body for digestion.

Digestion then occurs in the mouth, stomach, and small and large intestines. Carbohydrates take the shortest amount of time before they are digested—sugars (especially liquids) as little as 30 minutes and starches around 2 to 3 hours. Protein takes longer—as much as 6 hours. Lipids take the longest—sometimes up to

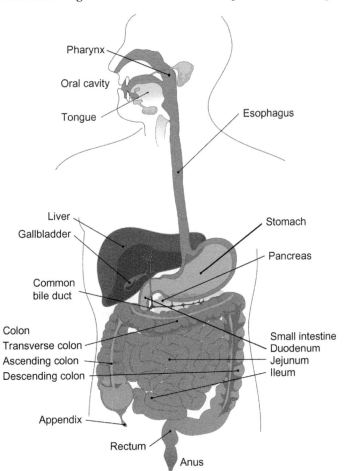

35

FIGURE 1-8
Digestion.

9 to 12 hours. In total, foods take 24 to 36 hours to fully pass through the gastrointestinal tract. This process is illustrated in Figure 1-8.

Digestion in the Mouth

The two types of digestion that take place in the mouth are *chemical digestion*, which occurs when enzymes are released by the salivary glands, and *physical digestion*, which occurs when food is chewed and moved to the back of the mouth with the help of the tongue. This is why it is important to chew food well and let it mix with saliva. People with eating and swallowing problems and those who do not produce sufficient saliva due to medical conditions might compromise the digestive process at this point.

The enzyme that breaks down foods and beverages inside of the mouth is called *salivary amylase.* (The suffix "-ase" indicates that it is an enzyme that is involved in a chemical reaction but stays intact.) Salivary amylase is then returned to its intact form to handle more foods and beverages.

As foods are chewed and mixed with saliva, they form a *bolus,* or ball, that is moved toward the back of the throat to be swallowed into the *esophagus.* There is a cartilage flap that controls the bolus's passage and prevents the bolus from entering the *trachea,* or the windpipe that leads to the lungs. It is called the *epiglottis.*

When people choke on foods or beverages, it may be due to food accidentally entering the trachea instead of the esophagus. This may be due to speaking or laughing while there is food in the mouth, putting too much food in the mouth at one time, or not chewing food well. Choking may require the *Heimlich maneuver,* a series of under-abdominal thrusts to remove food quickly and prevent choking.

Once the bolus is correctly swallowed, it is propelled by the esophagus, which is a short tube that leads to the stomach. Think of the esophagus as a band of strong muscles that pump and propel foods and beverages after they leave the mouth.

The esophagus is lined with saliva for moisture and protection. At the end of the esophagus is a muscle called the *diaphragm* that controls the movement of the bolus into the stomach and a valve, called the *cardiac sphincter,* which shuts the opening once the bolus has passed into the stomach. If the cardiac sphincter does not function properly, food from the stomach may move back into the esophagus. This is called *acid reflux,* which may be reduced by dietary changes, such as consuming smaller meals, medications or surgery.

FOOD BYTE

Digestive enzymes help to break down proteins. Some digestive enzymes are derived from papayas *(papain)* and pineapples *(bromelain)*, which are also found in supplement forms. Papain and bromelain are used in culinary applications as tenderizers. If they are overused, they can make protein foods too "mushy." Cooked or canned pineapple does not have a tenderizing effect, since bromelain is heat-sensitive. Other digestive enzymes can help break down lactose (milk sugar) into a more digestible form and decrease the flatulence created by legumes (dried beans and peas).

Digestion in the Stomach

Some, but not all, foods and beverages are digested in the *stomach,* a pouch at the end of the esophagus. The stomach is filled with *hydrochloric acid,* a strong acid that can digest protein foods and mucous and enzymes that break down other foods and beverages. These substances, along with muscular contractions, help to turn the bolus in the stomach into *chyme,* a semisolid mixture of partially digested food and gastric fluids, so it can be ready for its next passage.

The next route for digestion depends on whether foods or beverages are comprised of carbohydrate, lipids or proteins. The stomach does very little to digest carbohydrates. Carbohydrates mainly move into the small intestine for additional digestion.

Proteins are broken down by digestive fluids in the stomach, especially hydrochloric acid and the enzyme *gastric protease.* Little happens to lipids in the stomach. Instead, lipids head to the small intestine for additional digestion.

36

Digestion in the Small Intestine

The small intestine is not small; it is about 20 to 23 feet long and coiled inside the body. It is called the small intestine because its diameter is small. There are three sections in the small intestine: the *duodenum*, the *jejunum* and the *ileum*. The *liver*, *gallbladder* and *pancreas* are organs that secrete substances into the small intestine to further digest the chyme. By the time the chyme passes through the duodenum, jejunum and ileum, most of the nutrients are digested.

The Liver, Gallbladder and Pancreas

The *liver* is an essential organ for breaking down and processing nutrients. It is responsible for almost 500 critical functions in the human body. One of these functions is storage: the liver stores carbohydrates, lipids, minerals and vitamins. Because the liver processes alcohol and drugs, eliminates or transforms certain foreign substances that filter into our food supply, and restores new cells, it sustains a tremendous burden.

The liver also produces *bile*, a substance that helps to digest fat, which is stored in the gallbladder. Unquestionably, the liver is absolutely essential in handling all the foods and beverages that are consumed.

Unlike the liver, the *gallbladder* is a nonessential organ, which means that a person can live without it. The gallbladder serves to secrete bile into the small intestine for fat digestion.

Bile is comprised of *cholesterol,* a type of lipid, and other substances including bile salts, cholesterol, fats, inorganic salts, mucus, pigments and water. The formation of *gallstones*, which are made mostly of cholesterol, may prevent the normal functioning of the gallbladder. Both gallstones and the gallbladder can be removed by surgery. If the gallbladder is removed, then a person needs to reduce his intake of fat and cholesterol, since there is no longer a place to store bile for fat management. More information on cholesterol can be found in Chapter 6.

The *pancreas* is another vital organ in nutrient breakdown. Like the liver and gallbladder, the pancreas also secretes substances into the small intestine for digestion. The chyme that passes into the small intestine is acidic, thanks to the action of hydrochloric acid in the stomach. Secretions by the pancreas serve to neutralize this acid.

The pancreas also produces enzymes that further digest carbohydrates, lipids and proteins. One of these enzymes is *pancreatic amylase.* The pancreas also produces two important *hormones, insulin* and *glucagon,* that are critical in the management of carbohydrates by the body.

Insulin and glucagon help to maintain the level of blood glucose (sugar) in the body. Insulin is secreted by the beta cells of the pancreas in response to high blood glucose. In contrast, glucagon is secreted by the alpha cells of the pancreas when blood glucose is low (between meals and during exercise). There is more information about these hormones in Chapter 4.

Digestion in the Large Intestine

The large intestine is only five feet in length and larger in diameter than the small intestine. Like the small intestine, the large intestine has three sections: the *cecum*, the *colon* and the *rectum.* What is not absorbed by the small intestine passes into the large intestine and mixes with water and minerals. While the large intestine is essentially the holding and exiting site for foods, there also is some vitamin absorption from the bacteria that resides inside it. Strong muscles propel the release of the food residue.

ABSORPTION

Once food is digested, it is ready for *absorption.* Absorption is the movement of nutrients and other substances into the cells or tissues. Since most digestion is completed in the small intestine, the nutrients, which have already been digested into smaller substances, are now ready to move into the bloodstream and lymph throughout the body. *Lymph* carries body fluids that transport the by-products of fat digestion to the heart and back into the bloodstream. The other nutrients are carried by the *bloodstream.*

Absorption in the Small Intestine

Once carbohydrates are digested into their building blocks of simple sugars, lipids are digested into their building blocks of fatty acids, and proteins are digested into their building blocks of amino acids, they are ready to be absorbed. These building blocks of carbohydrates, lipids and proteins then join minerals, vitamins and water in the small intestine to move out and throughout the body. This movement is accomplished with the help of *villi*, little projectiles throughout the lining of the small intestine. Lined with muscles, these villi use wave-like motions to propel nutrients into the blood and lymph system.

Then the *portal system*, which includes the liver, takes over. The word *portal* means "port" or "entryway." Simple sugars, amino acids, water-soluble vitamins, and water are transported by the portal system. Fatty acids and fat-soluble vitamins are transported through the *lymphatic system.*

Lipid (fat) Absorption

Once dietary fats and oils, such as butter and olive oil, are digested into fatty acids, then the smallest fatty acids can pass into the cells that line the small intestine. They are fairly water soluble, so they can pass right into the bloodstream through the capillaries. These fatty acids then head to the liver, as does *glycerol*, a type of alcohol that is another product of lipid breakdown.

The larger fatty acids require their own means of transport. Since fat and water do not mix (think about vinegar and oil salad dressing), the fatty acids need a "package" to help them travel through the bloodstream (which is mostly water). Protein that is supplied by dietary proteins encapsulates the fatty acids. This package of lipids and protein is called a *lipoprotein.* The interior of the package also contains the lipids *cholesterol* and *triglycerides,* which are detailed in Chapter 6.

Lipoproteins are delivered to the cells as they require energy. Excess lipoproteins are sent to the liver, which breaks them down and reformulates them. Some of the lipoproteins carry more lipids; some carry more protein. The lipoproteins with more protein are called *high-density lipoprotein* or *HDL.* High-density lipoproteins tend to be better for cardiovascular health than the lipoproteins that carry more lipids, which are called *low-density lipoproteins* or *LDL.* More information about lipoproteins, diet and cardiovascular disease is provided in Chapters 6 and 9.

METABOLISM

Once the nutrients are sent to the cells, they need to be converted into energy for the many body functions. *Metabolism* is the sum of all of the physical and chemical processes by which energy is created and made available to the body. This energy can be used for such purposes as to build new body structures, including cells; heat the body; maintain or repair it; and provide energy for everyday activities and exercise.

Simple sugars, fatty acids and amino acids, the building blocks of carbohydrates, lipids, and proteins, may also be combined into bigger and different compounds for the body to use. This process is called *anabolism* (as in anabolic steroids that are used to build muscles). *Catabolism* is the opposite process—when compounds break down, as in severe muscle wasting that might occur during certain diseases or eating disorders.

Factors That Affect Metabolism

Many factors affect the rate at which the body uses carbohydrates, lipids, and, to a lesser extent, proteins for energy. Some factors that raise the metabolism include caffeine, fever, growth, height, lean body mass, male gender, nicotine and stress. When a person is young, her metabolism is high. Also, tall, muscular men tend to have higher metabolisms than shorter and rounder women.

The factors that lower the metabolism include age, fasting, hormones, sleep and starvation. As a person ages, his or her metabolism decreases. This is similar to what occurs during severe dieting. The hormones that are produced by the thyroid gland may either increase or decrease the metabolism if they are too high or too low. While sleep is important to good health, too much sleep means that the body is less active. More information about the factors that affect the metabolism and how they are important in determining daily caloric needs appears in Chapter 10.

Bite on This: healthy digestion

Healthy digestion begins with a healthy gastrointestinal tract. No matter how healthy foods and beverages are, various conditions, diseases, medications, stress and other factors may compromise normal digestion.

A number of digestive disorders occur from simple stomachaches to those that require hospitalization. Digestive disorders include ulcers, heartburn, irritable bowel syndrome (IBS), vomiting, constipation, diarrhea, lactose intolerance, gluten intolerance—even "growling" and "hiccups."

ULCERS AND HEARTBURN

The stomach and small intestine have protective linings that are filled with mucus and other substances. If hydrochloric acid eats away at the linings, then an *ulcer,* which is a small erosion or hole, may form. Ulcers may form in the esophagus, stomach or intestines.

The bacteria that are associated with some ulcers may further irritate the linings. Stomach acid may also back up into the esophagus and lead to *heartburn.* It is called heartburn because it occurs in an area that is close to the heart.

Although certain substances, such as acidic foods, alcohol, caffeine and fats have been implicated with heartburn, stress and frequent use of some medications, such as aspirin or ibuprofen, may also be to blame. Protective measures against heartburn include consuming small meals, increasing fiber in the diet and refraining from lying down after meals.

IRRITABLE BOWEL SYNDROME, DIARRHEA, CONSTIPATION AND VOMITING

In *irritable bowel syndrome (IBS)*, spasms and/or cramps occur in the large intestine. Common symptoms of irritable bowel syndrome may include bouts of diarrhea and/or constipation.

Generally a low-fat, higher-fiber diet is recommended. *Probiotics,* live microorganisms in plain yogurt or other cultured dairy products, may help to improve the intestinal microbial balance. Not all brands of yogurt contain "active" cultures, so check the food label. Some probiotics are added to cheese, breakfast cereals, protein and meal replacement bars and desserts.

Most cases of *diarrhea* are caused by bacteria or viruses from foods or beverages. Severe and long-lasting diarrhea may lead to nutrient disorders and/or dehydration, as can vomiting. While *vomiting* is nature's way of removing undesirable substances from the body, vomiting that is associated with illnesses or self-induced vomiting may have serious consequences.

Constipation may be caused by a fiber-poor diet, inadequate fluids, lack of exercise and other physical or psychological issues. Increased fiber from breakfast cereals and other whole grains depends on adequate fluids to maximize its effectiveness in relieving this disorder.

HICCUPS, GROWLING, AND FLATULENCE

Hiccups are caused by involuntary spasms of the diaphragm muscle. This action sucks air down the *trachea,* or windpipe, into the lungs; causes the vocal cords to close; and creates a "hic-like" sound. Eating or drinking while taking in too much air might be to blame.

If the stomach "growls," it may mean that gas bubbles are present. When the stomach is empty, then *growling* may be louder.

Flatulence is normal. It is frequently due to inadequate chewing, swallowing air while chewing, drinking beverages while chewing, or chewing gum. Other causes include consuming *too many* high-fiber foods, such as bran cereal or legumes; cruciferous vegetables, such as broccoli or cauliflower; foods high in *fructose* (fruit sugar) or *sugar alcohols* (such as sorbitol found in sugarless candy); or foods in the onion family, which require certain bacteria for breakdown.

OTHER INTESTINAL CONDITIONS

Lactose sensitivity or intolerance is provoked by the milk sugar lactose, and *gluten intolerance* is the inability to digest the protein in some grains. Both conditions are usually inherited and may require the avoidance of dairy products and certain grains. Look for more information about these carbohydrate-related diseases in Chapter 9.

While there are over-the-counter and prescribed medications to help ease some of these digestive disorders, identification and/or elimination of any suspected foods and beverages might first offer some relief. Be sure to check any symptoms with a health care provider to rule out any other serious conditions and to develop a coordinated care plan.

FOOD BYTE

Processed foods have been transformed from their natural states into other forms for availability, consistency, convenience, safety and taste. Processing includes such procedures as canning, dehydrating, freezing and refrigerating. Many processed foods are nutritious, such as dairy milk or bread. Dairy milk is pasteurized to destroy bacteria and homogenized to keep fats blended. Bread is processed from flour, leavening and water. A stigma exists about the inclusion of processed foods in a healthy diet, although many basic and common foods are processed, including baking powder and baking soda, honey (unless raw) and salt. The inclusion of processed foods in a healthy diet should be kept in perspective.

How Cooking Affects Nutrition

A food can be more or less digestible depending on the type of food, the temperature to which the food is heated, and the time it takes to cook the food. This is because cooking begins the digestive process by physically and chemically breaking down nutrients. Food processing may also influence the digestive process because it affects the bioavailability of certain nutrients. Some carbohydrate-containing foods, such as fruits and vegetables, can be consumed raw or they may only require partial cooking. More complex carbohydrates, such as the starches in grains and legumes, require longer cooking.

Like carbohydrates, some proteins may be consumed raw or partially cooked. Raw fish in sushi, an uncooked egg in a Caesar salad, and raw ground beef in steak tartare are examples of protein in raw forms. However, any time protein is consumed raw, there is a risk of foodborne illness. Sear the fish to caramelize the exterior, boil the egg for a few minutes, and cook the ground beef to medium to destroy any microorganisms. Additionally, the heat will cause the proteins to slightly break down, or *denature.*

Lipids are commonly consumed without cooking. Consider the fats that are contained inside avocadoes, olives or nuts, or the oils that dress fresh salads. When heat is applied to fats during cooking, this begins their lengthy breakdown. Overcooking fats may cause them to smoke or burn and create potentially harmful substances. More information about the healthy way to cook with fats and oils can be found in Chapter 6.

Vitamins and minerals may be destroyed from overcooking. This is why many fruits and vegetables are better consumed raw or lightly cooked. Healthy cooking and baking methods for preserving the vitamins and minerals in foods are provided in Chapter 7 and in the recipes throughout this book.

Food as Medicine

In Greek and Roman times, food was considered more than nourishment; it served as elixirs or aids to stay healthy and prevent and manage disease. Hippocrates, the Greek physician, connected the role of diet and disease. While some of his statements are not attributed to science, he did establish the possibilities of the nutrient-disease connection when he reportedly said, "Let food be thy medicine, and let medicine be thy food."

In some areas of the world, food is still considered Mother Nature's best medicine, and people choose diets according to their health-enhancing benefits. Think about the traditional Chinese diet, with its balance of *yin* (feminine) and *yang* (masculine) foods. According to the Chinese, an unbalanced diet could result in illness.

40

Supposedly, excessive yin foods found in vegetables can lead to weakness, and excessive yang foods found in meat can lead to restlessness.

Herbs and spices have long been recognized for their ability to prevent, manage, and even cure some diseases. For example, garlic and turmeric are used in some cultures to prevent some degenerative diseases and as remedies for others. *Phytochemicals* found in plant foods are associated with the prevention and management of certain diseases, such as beta-carotene in brightly colored orange and red fruits and vegetables. While not nutrients, phytochemicals have beneficial properties. They may ward off diseases, protect the eyes, and defend against the common cold, among other functions.

Functional foods have physical and psychological roles in the diet. Some serve as *antioxidants* and protect the body against damaging free radicals from sunlight and environment hazards. Other functional foods help protect the bones, heart, and stomach, while still others help to reduce blood pressure and cardiovascular disease. Some functional foods are also called *nutraceuticals*; they act as *pharmaceuticals*, with druglike effects on the body.

Finally, the emerging field of *nutrigenomics* or *personalized nutrition* offers immeasurable promise. *Nutrigenomics* applies the human *genome* (the entirety of an organism's hereditary information) to nutrition and health for individual dietary recommendations. It uses a person's unique genetic makeup and nutritional requirements to tailor-make recommendations for disease reduction and health optimization.

How can nutrition, food science and culinary professionals apply their skills to the rapidly growing interests in food as medicine? They must first have a solid foundation in nutrition, food science and the culinary arts. They should understand the complex roles that foods and beverages play in health and disease. And they should collaborate with allied health professionals to help translate the science behind medicinal foods into health-enhancing foods and beverages of the future. Chapters 7 and 9 provide additional information about the "food as medicine" connection.

SERVE IT FORTH   41

While many factors influence food choices, knowing what is inside foods and beverages may be quite motivational to make better choices. The following three examples compare two different breakfasts, lunches and dinners. They illustrate the nutrients in fast food and carry-out foods compared to home-prepared or restaurant "sit-down" meals.

After each example is reviewed, answer the questions that follow. Use nutrient data tables, such as the ones that can be found at http://nutritiondata.self.com/ or at http://www.livestrong.com/diet-analysis/. Record all of the information. Upon completion, these activities may help to direct wiser food and beverage selections.

1. **A doughnut and coffee fast-food breakfast**
   A plain doughnut mostly contains carbohydrates, with traces of protein and fat. Once it is fried in vegetable oil, the amount of fat increases. Coffee contains only a few calories per cup from traces of fat in the coffee beans. If cream and sugar are added, then fats and carbohydrates increase.
   ○ What are the amounts of calories, carbohydrates, fiber, **total fat, saturated fat**, cholesterol, protein and sodium in this meal?
   ○ Compare these amounts to the DVs in Table 1-16.
   ○ What conclusions can be made about this meal, especially about total fat and saturated fat?
2. **A fiber-rich cereal, low-fat dairy milk and banana home-prepared breakfast**
   Swap the doughnut and coffee breakfast to a homemade breakfast of fiber-rich cereal with low-fat dairy milk and a small banana and the nutrient profile changes. The cereal contributes carbohydrates, fiber and protein with only a small amount of fat. The low-fat dairy milk is filled with carbohydrates and protein and less fat and the banana is mostly carbohydrates.
   ○ What are the amounts of calories, carbohydrates, **fiber,** total fat, saturated fat, cholesterol, protein and sodium in this meal?
   ○ Compare these amounts to the DVs in Table 1-16.
   ○ What conclusions can be made about this meal, especially about fiber?
   ○ How does this home-prepared breakfast compare to the fast-food doughnut and coffee breakfast?

3. A fast-food hamburger, french fries, and soft drink fast-food lunch

The hamburger consists of a bun, which is the equivalent of two pieces of bread; a 4- to 10-ounce hamburger patty with lettuce, onions and tomatoes and often a special sauce; likely a mixture of catsup, mayonnaise and mustard. The bun, vegetables and sauce are mostly carbohydrates. The hamburger patty is mostly protein and fat, with a very small contribution of carbohydrates. The french fries are mostly carbohydrates and fat, with a small amount of protein. The soft drink is mostly sugar and water.

- ○ What are the amounts of calories, **carbohydrates**, fiber, total fat, saturated fat, cholesterol, protein and sodium in this meal if small sizes are selected? Large sizes?
- ○ Compare these amounts to the DVs in Table 1-16.
- ○ What conclusions can be made about this meal, especially about carbohydrates?
- ○ How does the small-sized meal compare to the large-sized meal?

Three additional activities can be found within the *Culinary Nutrition* website at www.culinarynutrition.elsevier.com.

WHAT'S COOKING?

The following experiments investigate how foods dissolve, supermarket strategies, healthy pizza, digestive enzymes and acids in action, sensible servings, and emulsions and the human bloodstream. They are designed to be conducted in or outside the classroom and have real-life implications and applications.

1. How foods dissolve

Objectives
- ○ To see how foods dissolve in liquids outside of the body
- ○ To understand how foods dissolve in fluids inside of the body

Materials: Water, measuring cup, three glasses, three pieces of dark-colored hard candy without filling, waxed paper, rolling pin

Procedure
1. Pour about ¼ cup of warm water into each of the three glasses.
2. Place one piece of candy between two sheets of waxed paper; using the rolling pin, break the candy into large pieces.
3. Place a second piece of candy between two fresh sheets of waxed paper; using the rolling pin, smash the candy into a fine powder.
4. Leave the third piece of candy whole.
5. Drop the whole piece of candy into the first glass with water, the broken pieces of candy into the second glass with water, and the powdered candy into the third glass with water.

Evaluation: Observe each solution after 10 to 15 minutes, again after 30 minutes, and again after 1 hour. Record this information on the Data Sheet like the one below.

- ○ Which form of candy dissolves faster?
- ○ Why do you think this happens?
- ○ What would happen if the water temperature is cold? Hot?
- ○ What does this exercise suggest about how foods dissolve inside the body during the process of digestion?
- ○ Support all of your comments.

Data Sheet

Type of Solution	Time of Observations		
	10 to 15 minutes	30 minutes	1 hour
Solution #1 with whole piece of candy			
Solution #2 with large pieces of candy			
Solution #3 with powdered candy			

2. Supermarket strategies

Objectives

○ To assess the displays of healthy foods and beverages in supermarkets or grocery stores

○ To see how food marketing may persuade people to make or not make healthy food choices

Materials: A supermarket or a grocery store

Procedures: Take a walk through a supermarket or grocery store. Note the locations where any healthy foods and beverages are found throughout the store.

Evaluation: Evaluate *each* department and answer the following questions:

○ Does the store showcase healthy foods and beverages, or does it make them difficult to find?

○ Which healthy foods and beverages are prominently marketed and why?

○ Which healthy foods and beverages need more prominence and why?

○ Do you think customers will be persuaded to make healthy food and beverage purchases based on what you have observed? Why or why not?

○ Support all of your comments.

3. Healthy pizza

Objectives

○ To evaluate a menu from a fast-food operation

○ To consider ingredients and preparation methods to help improve the nutritional values of the menu items

Materials: A take-out menu from a pizza restaurant

Procedure

1. Suppose this pizza restaurant wants to add some healthy items to its menu.

2. Also suppose that the management wants to know which ingredients and preparation methods to use to help make their items healthier.

Evaluation

○ Which ingredients should be added, reduced or eliminated to improve the nutritional values of the menu items?

○ What nutrition tools (i.e., guidelines, recommendations, etc.) from this chapter would you use in your decision making?

○ Support all of your comments.

4. Digestive acids and enzymes in action

Objective

○ To identify how different acids "digest" or break down protein

Materials: Raw or cooked fish, five glass or ceramic bowls, lemon juice, vinegar, cooking wine, pineapple juice, papaya juice, measuring spoon

Procedure

1. Place a small piece of fish into each of the five glass or ceramic bowls.

2. Be consistent and place the same-sized piece in each bowl.

3. Add 1 tablespoon of lemon juice over the piece of fish in the first glass bowl.

4. Repeat the process with each of the acidic ingredients, placing one uniform piece of fish and 1 tablespoon of the vinegar, cooking wine, pineapple juice or papaya juice into each glass or ceramic bowl.

Evaluation: Note your observations after 30 minutes, 1 hour and overnight on the Data Sheet like the one below.

○ Compare and contrast the enzymatic action of each of the acids on the fish.

○ What can be concluded about each of the acids at each observation?

○ Support all of your comments.

Data Sheet

Fish *plus* Acidic Ingredient	Time of Observations		
	30 minutes	1 hour	Overnight
Fish *plus* lemon juice			
Fish *plus* vinegar			
Fish *plus* cooking wine			
Fish *plus* pineapple juice			
Fish *plus* papaya juice			

43

5. Sensible servings
Objectives
- To select the correct types and portion sizes of foods in real life or mock settings
- To demonstrate adequacy, balance, moderation, variety and calorie control

Materials: Salad bar, salad and dinner plates, food photos of salad ingredients from magazines, paper plates

Procedure
1. If a salad bar is accessible, then assemble the ingredients on a salad plate.
2. Show adequacy, balance, moderation, variety and calorie control through food choices and portion sizes.
3. Repeat by using a dinner plate.
4. If a salad bar is not accessible, then select magazine photos of salad ingredients that convey adequacy, balance, moderation, variety and calorie control.
5. Arrange the photos on both a paper salad plate and paper dinner plate.

Evaluation
- Support the reasons why you chose the types and amounts of salad ingredients.
- Address adequacy, balance, moderation, variety, and calorie control.
- Compare and contrast the types and amounts of salad ingredients on the salad and dinner plates. What does this exercise relate about choosing the right types and portions foods when eating out?
- Support all of your comments.

6. Emulsions and the human bloodstream
Objectives
- To determine the type and amount of a substance that is needed to create a suspension
- To witness how long a suspension is held
- To see how emulsifiers bring nonreactive substances together
- To compare this reaction to the human bloodstream

Materials: Three glass jars with lids, ½ cup measure, vegetable oil, white vinegar, food coloring, eye dropper, 1 tablespoon, egg whites, water, egg yolk, liquid lecithin or lecithin granules, lemon juice

Procedure
1. Pour ½ cup of vegetable oil, ½ cup of white vinegar, and a few drops of food coloring into each of the glass jars.
2. Add 1 tablespoon of egg whites and 1 tablespoon of water to the mixture in the first jar.
3. Add 2 tablespoons of egg whites to the mixture in the second jar.
4. Add 2 tablespoons of water to the mixture in the third jar.
5. Secure the lids on each jar; shake each of the jars. Record the time that it takes for the division between the water and the vinegar to reappear (the food coloring makes it easier to see).
6. Clean out the jars and repeat the experiment, replacing lemon juice for the vinegar and egg yolks for the egg whites. Record the reactions and times.
7. Clean out the jars and repeat the experiment, using vinegar or lemon juice and 1 tablespoon of liquid lecithin or lecithin granules for the egg whites.

Evaluation
- Observe the consistency of each mixture after shaking the jars and the times that each of the mixtures takes for the oil and water and the acid to separate.
- Note your observations on the Data Sheet like the one below.
- What does this exercise tell you about suspensions, emulsifiers and duration (time)?
- How does this experiment compare to the bloodstream?
- Support all of your comments.

Data Sheet

Solutions	Observations	Time to Separate
Water *plus* vegetable oil *plus* vinegar *plus* 1 tablespoon egg whites		
Water *plus* vegetable oil *plus* vinegar *plus* 2 tablespoons egg whites		
Water *plus* vegetable oil *plus* vinegar *plus* water		

Other additions

Lemon juice

Egg yolk

Liquid lecithin

Lecithin granules

Culinary applications: How can the information from *each* of these six exercises be applied to new product or recipe development?

OVER EASY

This chapter covers the importance of nutrition in the context of food science and the culinary arts and the applications of nutrition in professional and consumer settings. Creating healthy ingredients, foods and beverages and making nutritious choices are complicated. A number of tools have been created by the US government and medical and scientific organizations to help guide these choices.

These include the *US Dietary Guidelines for Americans, 2010*; *Nutrition Objectives for the Nation: Healthy People 2010* and *2020*; US Dietary Reference Intakes (DRIs); food exchange systems and food composition tables and databases; basic food groups; USDA Food Guide Pyramid; USDA MyPlate; US food label and food labeling regulations, including the Nutrition Facts Panel, Daily Values (DVs), US FDA approved nutrition content claims, US FDA approved health claims, and structure/function claims, which are all featured in this chapter.

Equally important for making healthy food and beverage choices is an understanding of how foods and beverages are broken down into their components and used or stored by the human body. This is why the complex journeys that carbohydrates, lipids and proteins take throughout the body during digestion, absorption and metabolism are simplified.

Food science, cooking and baking impact the sensory qualities of foods and beverages, which affects digestion and absorption. The more appealing that foods and beverages are perceived, then the greater chances they will be consumed. Numerous other factors, including ethnicity, economics, lifestyle and religion, also impact dietary choices, nutrition and health.

Simple tools are presented that include the ABCs of healthy diets (adequacy, balance and calorie control), kitchen math, and how to decipher a food label, which pave the way for healthy eating.

Methods that raise eco-consciousness and promote "greener" food and beverage choices and fewer carbon footprints are highlighted, which influence personal and collective nutrition and health.

CHECK PLEASE

1. Most of the carbohydrates consumed are *digested* in the:
   a. stomach
   b. mouth
   c. liver
   d. small intestine
   e. large intestine
2. Most of the proteins consumed are digested in the:
   a. stomach
   b. mouth
   c. liver
   d. small intestine
   e. large intestine

3. Most of the lipids consumed are digested in the:
   a. large intestine
   b. small intestine
   c. liver
   d. mouth
   e. stomach

Essay Question

1. The principal of a middle school with a student population that represents over 40 different countries wants to hire a registered dietitian-chef team to plan and prepare nutritious meals. Discuss the considerations that this team must make. Support your answers.

For additional questions, please see the *Culinary Nutrition* website at www.culinarynutrition.elsevier.com

HUNGRY FOR MORE?

Academy of Nutrition and Dietetics (AND)   http://www.eatright.org
Center for Nutrition Policy and Promotion   http://www.cnpp.usda.gov
Center for Science in the Public Interest (Nutrition Action Newsletter)   http://www.cspinet.org
Food and Agriculture Organization of the United Nations   www.fao.org
Food and Nutrition Information Center (FNIC)
http://fnic.nal.usda.gov/nal_display/index.php?info_center=4&tax_level=1&tax_subject=244

Choose Your Foods

Exchange Lists for Diabetes and Choose Your Foods Exchange Lists for Weight Management
http://www.eatright.org/shop/product.aspx?id=4962
Healthy People 2010, 2020   http://www.healthypeople.gov/2020/default.aspx
International Food Information Council (FoodInsight)   http://www.foodinsight.org
Learning Seed (Kitchen Math)   http://www.kitchenmath.com
Nutrition Analysis Tool 2.0   http://www.myfoodrecord.com
Food Science and Human Nutrition Department at the University of Illinois
Society for Nutrition Education and Behavior (SNEB)   http://www.sne.org
USDA MyPlate and MyPyramid   http://www.choosemyplate.gov
US FDA Labeling and Nutrition   www.cfsan.fda.gov/label.html

> **FOOD BYTE**
>
> Few of the foods we eat today originated or were domesticated in the United States. Most of the foods we consume originated from Africa, Asia, Europe or South America. Some exceptions include blueberries, cranberries, Jerusalem artichokes and sunflowers. Certain food products or preparations are unique to the United States. These include New England clam chowder, New Orleans po-boy sandwich, San Francisco sourdough bread, Texas fajitas, Pennsylvania shoe fly pie and Smithfield ham. "American" foods belong to all of the Americas (North America, Central America and South America), not just the United States.

TAKE AWAY
A Century of Food and Nutrition

One hundred years ago, a homemade meal looked strikingly different than it does today. At the turn of the twentieth century, people primarily ate from the land. They grew, harvested, slaughtered and prepared a good deal of what they consumed daily.

Much of their food and nutrition was dependent on which foods were cultivated, where these foods were grown and their seasonality. Food choices were also contingent upon where people lived (rural or urban locations), how people lived (poverty or wealth), and what people practiced (ethnic and religious traditions).

Today, food availability, cultivation and seasonality are less important factors in food selection than they were in the 1900s due to modern transportation and our global food supply. Rural or urban settings, poverty or wealth, and ethnic and religious practices still determine what people eat and why.

Today, typical US meals are a fusion of processed foods and beverages, purchased on-the-run from mega-supermarkets, gas stations, vending machines, coffee shops and other nontraditional food settings. They bear little resemblance in form or function to the meals of yesteryear.

Following is an overview of the foods and beverages from each decade in the United States, starting with 1900 until today. This overview shows how our food and nutrition choices have developed throughout the years to what we now consider "the typical US diet."

In the 1900s . . . The daily menus reflected what was available during certain months and seasons and food preservation. The main meal shifted from midday to evening as it remains today. A typical breakfast consisted of melon, hash, broiled meats, fried vegetables and coffee. Lunch was based on broiled poultry, baked root vegetables, salads and dairy desserts. Supper included sliced meats, biscuits, baked fruits, cakes and tea.

In the 1910s . . . The United States was a melting pot of new immigrants who brought a variety of ethnic cuisines from coast to coast. During World War I, food was rationed for the soldiers, and civilians experienced scarcity and allotments. The middle class grew in size and expanded in their tastes; they aspired for the newer foods that technology afforded.

In the 1920s . . . Due to the continued influx of ethnicities, exotic foods became even more fashionable. Cities boasted expensive restaurants alongside meager kitchens in public housing. Social movements fostered the importance of food in ladies organizations and the popularity of home economics. Prohibition brought the exclusion of alcohol. Interest in vegetarian alternatives grew, thanks to experimentation with the lowly peanut.

In the 1930s . . . War bought extreme hardship and famine to some citizens, yet an ample and inexpensive food supply existed for others. People had the choice of cheaper grades and cuts of meats and dairy substitutes, such as vegetable spreads. There were private soup kitchens and government programs for residents with few resources.

In the 1940s . . . Foods were rationed again, and proteins were "stretched" to feed more with less. Sugarless cookies, eggless cakes and meatless meals extended food supplies (contrary to how these food "substitutes" are used today). Food was reserved for World War II soldiers, which created a shortage for civilians.

In the 1950s . . . Meals were very filling, partially due to increased meat consumption and the influx of prepackaged goods. (Both developments were a backlash from WWII rationing.) The American homemaker used convenience foods and time-saving appliances. New flavors and recipes were introduced by soldiers returning from foreign lands.

In the 1960s . . . Conventional foods were at odds with radically changing food choices. Traditional French cuisine converged with barbecues, drive-ins and increased interest in vegetarian cuisine. Soul food rose in popularity. Foods and beverages were aimed at baby boomers. Suburban families patronized family-style restaurant chains.

In the 1970s . . . Diners chose between classic and fresh innovative cuisines. Southwest cuisine entered the culinary landscape. Economic challenges of the 1970s forced consumers to make difficult food shopping choices. Local butcher shops transitioned into butcher counters in neighborhood supermarkets.

In the 1980s . . . Consumers devoured dishes from all across the United States as the economy flourished: blackened fish from the south, pasta dishes throughout metropolitan areas and growing ethnic cuisines, especially Asian from the coasts. More ethnic and specialty markets opened nationwide, reflecting broad diversities in food histories, experiences and tastes.

In the 1990s . . . US consumers clamored for baked snack foods, bottled beverages, butter substitutes, diet frozen entrees, frozen pizzas, low-carb breadstuffs and desserts, lean hamburgers and vegetable burgers. The concept of "healthy choices" morphed into a popular brand name.

In 2000 . . . US consumers ate foods with excess fats, sugars and sodium in super-sized portions. They had more food and beverage choices than ever before, but made nutrient-poor, calorie-dense selections that expanded the national waistline and nutrition-related disease rates.

47

In 2010 and beyond . . . US consumers are thinking green: local and sustainable to help save our planet and reduce our carbon footprint—which is the topic of the "Take away" section in this chapter [25].

The "Greening" of US Diets

The "typical US diet" is one of contradictions. On the one hand, obesity among children, teenagers and adults is growing in unprecedented numbers, concurrent with diet-related diseases. On the other hand, there is a growing segment of the US population that is concerned with *eco-consciousness, sustainability,* the *"green" movement* and *carbon footprints* to help protect individuals and the earth.

What do eco-consciousness, sustainability, the "green" movement and carbon footprints have to do with food, nutrition and health?

- *Eco-consciousness* is an awareness of the environment and its ecological (biological) systems. To be eco-conscious means that one is consciously aware of what they purchase, how they live (*including what they eat and drink*), and how these habits affect their lives and the earth.
- *Sustainability* is the ability to persist through the maintenance of diverse and productive *biological systems for human well-being*.
- The *"green" movement* is an organized effort for addressing the environmental issues that affect ecology, health and human rights through individual actions and public policies.
- *Carbon footprints* are greenhouse gas (GHG) emissions from events, organizations, people and/or products. GHG may be released through the *production and consumption of foods,* in addition to such activities as construction, fuel production, manufacturing and transportation.

Individuals can make eco-conscious, sustainable and green choices to reduce their carbon footprints and impact food, nutrition and health. By doing so, they may also contribute to the health and well-being of the general public. These are some eco-friendly food habits and kitchen habits that people may take:

FOOD HABITS

Buy . . .

- **Whole foods** from sources where farming is regulated and fertilizers and pesticides are minimized. Look for labels such as "USDA Organic." Whole fruits, vegetables and whole grains reduce processing costs and are diet-friendly.
- **Grains, legumes, nuts and seeds** in bulk to reduce packaging costs.
- **Grass-fed beef** with smaller carbon footprints than grain-fed beef. Grass-fed beef is also lower in total calories and saturated fat because it is leaner.
- **In-season fruits and vegetables** that offer decreased transportation costs, improved taste and nutrients at their peak. Watch out for pesticide residues.
- **Organic dairy milk** to help control the transfer of synthetic growth factors. Or use soy milk that produces less GHG.
- **Wild fish** from unpolluted waters that are sustainably harvested. Wild fish may be higher in heart-healthy omega-3 fatty acids than farm-raised fish.
- **Whole poultry**, which is more economical with less environmental impact than poultry parts. Look for USDA-certified organic-fed poultry.

Do . . .

- Consider a vegetarian or part vegetarian diet—with fewer GHG than a meat-based diet.
- Read labels when grocery shopping—look for the "USDA Organic" seal, which ensures no chemical pesticides, growth stimulators, radiation or synthetic fertilizers.
- Prepare only what is needed; stick to serving sizes instead of portion sizes to reduce food waste.
- Save food scraps and compost into nutrient-rich mulch instead of discarding.

KITCHEN HABITS

Use . . .

- **Energy-efficient cooking and baking pans**—use glass or ceramic pans for baking and copper-bottomed stainless steel or aluminum pots for stove-top cooking.
- **China plates and cups, stainless steel flatware**—for meals to reduce paper and plastic waste.
- **Reusable containers**—for storage, lunches and snacks to reduce container waste.
- **Cloth napkins and towels**—for meals and drying dishes to reduce paper waste.

Use wisely . . .

- **Oven**—keep the door closed to maintain temperature and be more efficient. Decrease baking times when possible.
- **Stove**—turn off the flame a few moments before some dishes are done; the residual heat will cook them a little longer.
- **Refrigerator**—fill so cold items insulate one another.
- **Dishwasher**—skip the prerinse cycle and fill to capacity.
- **Water**—do not run the tap when doing dishes. Use soapy water; then scrub, drain and rinse. Use less water when boiling pasta and other grains, but stir often.

Join . . . [26–28]

- *Community Supported Agriculture (CSA)*—memberships with farms where shares are purchased in exchange for a variety of seasonal fruits and vegetables. CSAs build relationships with farmers and support local agriculture.
- *Food cooperatives*—grocery stores that are commonly supported, community owned, and typically filled with local, organic foods and beverages that appeal to eco-conscious consumers.
- The *locavore movement*—collaborative effort that emphasizes that people eat locally, buy from farmer's markets and local farms, join CSAs and/or grow their own foods.

49

References

[1] InnerBody. <http://www.innerbody.com/htm/body.html/>; [accessed 01.03.08].

[2] University of Buffalo: Human organism—Body systems, Department of Biological Sciences. <http://www.biology.buffalo.edu/courses/bio531/lecture7.html/>; [accessed 01.03.08].

[3] City University of New York. Basic anatomy—tissues and organs. John Jay College of Criminal Justice. <http://web.jjay.cuny.edu/~acarpi/NSC/14-anatomy.htm/>; [accessed 01.03.08].

[4] Natural Resources Defense Council (NRDS). <http://www.nrdc.org/about/>; [accessed 01.03.08].

[5] Walmart Corporate. http://walmartstores.com/pressroom/news/10635.aspx/>; [accessed 01.0308].

[6] G.J. Allen, K. Albala, The business of food: encyclopedia of the food and drink industries. Greenwood Publishing Group, Santa Barbara, CA 2007.

[7] US Food and Drug Administration (FDA). <http://www.fda.gov/AboutFDA/Transparency/Basics/ucm194877.htm/>; [accessed 01.03.08].

[8] US Department of Agriculture (USDA). <http://www.cnpp.usda.gov/Publications/DietaryGuidelines/2010/PolicyDoc/ExecSumm.pdf/>; [accessed 01.03.08].

[9] HealthyPeople.gov. <http://www.healthypeople.gov/2020/default.aspx/>; [accessed 01.03.08].

[10] US Department of Agriculture (USDA). <http://www.choosemyplate.gov/print-materials-ordering/mypyramid-archive.html/>; [accessed 01.03.08].

[11] US States Department of Agriculture (USDA). <http://www.choosemyplate.gov/food-groups/downloads/TenTips/DGTipsheet1ChooseMyPlate.pdf/>; [accessed 01.03.08].

[12] US Department of Agriculture (USDA). <http://www.choosemyplate.gov/print-materials-ordering/selected-messages.html/>; [accessed 01.03.08].

[13] National Heart Lung and Blood Institute (NHLBI). <http://www.nhlbi.nih.gov/health/public/heart/obesity/lose_wt/fd_exch.htm/>; [accessed 01.03.08].

[14] Academy of Nutrition and Dietetics. <http://www.eatright.org/HealthProfessionals/content.aspx?id=101/>; [accessed 01.03.08].

[15] US Department of Agriculture (USDA). <http://www.nal.usda.gov/fnic/foodcomp/Bulletins/measurement_equivalents.html/>; [accessed 01.03.08]

[16] Philipson T. Government perspective: food labeling. Am J Clin Nutr 2005;82:262S–4S.

[17] US Food and Drug Administration (FDA). <http://www.fda.gov/food/labelingnutrition/default.htm/>; [accessed 01.03.08].

[18] US Food and Drug Administration (FDA). <http://www.fda.gov/Food/GuidanceComplianceRegulatoryInformation/Guidance Documents/FoodLabelingNutrition/ucm173838.htm/>; [accessed 01.03.08].

[19] J. Anderson, L. Young, S. Perryman, Understanding the food label. <http://www.ext.colostate.edu/pubs/foodnut/09365.html/>; [accessed 01.03.08].

[20] US Food and Drug Administration (FDA). Food labeling guide. <http://www.fda.gov/Food/GuidanceComplianceRegulatory Information/GuidanceDocuments/FoodLabelingNutrition/FoodLabelingGuide/default.htm/>; [accessed 01.03.08].

[21] US Food and Drug Administration (FDA). <http://www.fda.gov/Food/LabelingNutrition/PrintInformationMaterials/ucm114155. htm/>; [accessed 01.03.08].

[22] US Food and Drug Administration (FDA). <http://www.fda.gov/Food/GuidanceComplianceRegulatoryInformation/ GuidanceDocuments/FoodLabelingNutrition/FoodLabelingGuide/ucm064928.htm/>; [accessed 01.03.08].

[23] US Food and Drug Administration (FDA). <http://www.fda.gov/>; [accessed 01.03.08].

[24] International Food Information Council Foundation (IFIC). <www.foodinsight.org/>; [accessed 01.03.08].

[25] Food Timeline: FAQs: popular 20th-century American foods. <http://www.foodtimeline.org/fooddecades.html/>; [accessed 01.03.08].

[26] Ivanko J, Kirvirst L. In: Farmstead Chef. New Society Publishers; Gabriola Island, BC Canada 2011.

[27] Susko MK. In: The Locavore's Kitchen: a Cook's Guide to Seasonal Eating and Preserving. Athens, OH: Ohio University; 2011.

[28] Daly KA. 30 ways to green your plate. Shape 2011, November, pp. 168–175.

CHAPTER 2

Food Science Basics: Healthy Cooking and Baking Demystified

The Science behind Healthy Foods, Cooking and Baking

OBJECTIVES

1. Apply the basic concepts of food science to nutrition and the culinary arts
2. Describe the sensory process and how it affects food selection
3. Demonstrate the steps in flavor balancing
4. Detail the roles of carbohydrates, lipids, proteins and water in cooking and baking

Culinary Nutrition. DOI: http://dx.doi.org/10.1016/B978-0-12-391882-6.00002-9

5. Specify the roles of common ingredients and their functions in cooking

6. Explain the principles behind common cooking and baking reactions

7. Identify why some recipes succeed or fail

8. Describe the steps for fixing common mistakes in foods and recipes

9. Adjust certain ingredients to maximize nutrients

10. Apply food science basics to new food and beverage applications

INTRODUCTION: THE SCIENCE BEHIND FOOD AND COOKING

Chapter 1 covered the many intrinsic factors that compel and sustain food selection. Chapter 3 examines the art and science of cooking and how cooking techniques and ingredients drive consumers' preferences.

This chapter provides a segue between the nutrients that are required by the human body and the transformation of these nutrients into recipes that delight the senses and appetite. At the core is food science: the applied science that deals with the biochemical, biological, chemical, physical and physiochemical properties of foods.

Studied in their individual contexts, nutrition, the culinary arts and food science are exacting, demanding and exciting disciplines on their own. When viewed together as a comprehensive whole, the wonder and delight of foods and beverages and their nutrients make sense and their possibilities seem limitless.

In this chapter, the sensory considerations of food and beverage selection and how they drive flavor for enjoyment and health are explored. The basic principles of food science are presented with their explanations for why food behaves as it does. Carbohydrates, lipids, proteins and water are connected to common cooking and baking reactions. These include emulsions, enzymes, heat transfer, the Maillard reaction, temperature, time and texture. Ingredients like meats, dairy products, fruits and vegetables, legumes, grains and fats are explored to clarify their functions in healthy baking and cooking. You'll observe why some recipes succeed or fail, how they can be repaired, and methods for enhancement by the art of flavor balancing.

Finally, the organizations that intermesh food science, nutrition and the culinary arts—Culinology® and the Research Chefs Association (RCA) and the Institute of Food Technologists (IFT)—are showcased, and futuristic endeavors in molecular gastronomy and biotechnology are explored.

Morsel "The discovery of a new dish does more for human happiness than the discovery of a new star." —Anthelme Brillat-Savarin (French gastronome and lawyer, 1755–1826)

This chapter reveals how challenging it is to adjust ingredients, foods and beverages to help make healthy choices more appealing. It illustrates how the applications that integrate nutrition, the culinary arts and food science hold the most promise.

MAIN COURSES
Food Science Demystified

Food science is an interdisciplinary field of study that investigates and applies biology, engineering and the physical sciences. Food science explores the nature of foods—why some foods thrive and others deteriorate. It focuses on the technical aspects of food, from growing, harvesting or slaughtering through all aspects of food processing and preparation for consumer appeal. Food science helps determine why certain foods are consumed before others for enjoyment and nutrition.

Food scientists are involved with all aspects of foods, such as new food development and production, microbiological and chemical testing, food packaging, shelf-life issues and sensory evaluation. Some food scientists are also registered dietitians (RDs) or chefs, which helps them to view foods and beverages from multiple perspectives.

The fields of study within food science include *food chemistry*, which examines food molecules in chemical reactions; *food engineering*, which explores the development and manufacturing of new food products;

food microbiology, which studies the interactions among microorganisms and foods; *food packaging*, which looks at how food is packaged after processing to preserve maximum nutrients; *food preservation*, which studies the causes and prevention of food degradation or breakdown; *food safety*, which advances the causes, prevention and communication of foodborne illnesses; *food technology*, which examines the physical aspects of foods, such as flavor and texture; *molecular gastronomy*, which delves into gastronomical experiences; and *sensory analysis*, which investigates how food is perceived.

While these disciplines seem highly specialized for nutrition and culinary professionals, there is also a great deal of commonality. The material in Chapters 1, 2, and 3 demonstrates how nutrition, the culinary arts and food science are inextricably connected.

In Chapter 1, the digestion and metabolism of major nutrients are presented; these processes involve food chemistry. Also in Chapter 1, nutrition labeling and the USDA Nutrition Facts Panel are featured; these are essential elements in food packaging.

In Chapter 3, various ingredient manipulations in cooking and baking are explored; these are considered food chemistry. Also in Chapter 3, helpful and dangerous microorganisms are identified and debated; these practices include food microbiology, food preservation and food safety. In this chapter, the importance of taste and texture in food acceptance or rejection are emphasized; these practices engage sensory analysis, food technology and food engineering. This interchange helps to demonstrate why emerging food scientists should integrate nutrition and the culinary arts in their work—and why nutritionists and chefs are well served to incorporate food science in their endeavors.

This chapter helps to demystify some of the science behind food and reveals opportunities in the rapidly growing fields of food science for nutrition and culinary professionals. Mostly this chapter focuses on food chemistry, technology and the sensory aspects of food as they relate to nutrition and the culinary arts. It begins with the organizations that focus on these relationships: the *Research Chefs Association (RCA)* and the *Institute of Food Technologists (IFT)*.

53

Bite on This: Research Chefs Association and Institute of Food Technologists

The Research Chefs Association was formed in the late 1990s by food and culinary professionals with a common interest in the interactions between the culinary arts and food science. It is now one of the leading sources of culinary arts, food science and technological information.

Members of the RCA include chefs and other culinary specialists and food scientists, who work in such areas as academia, consulting, distribution, food product research and development, manufacturing, marketing, media and sales. RCA members also are employed at laboratories, ingredient supply houses, restaurants hotels, and other food service operations.

The Research Chefs Association is the primary association that advocates the principles of Culinology®. Culinology® merges the culinary arts with food science and technology. It uses the principles of the culinary arts and food science to drive product, recipe and menu development and planning. Culinology® professionals work in areas that blend the culinary arts with the scientific and technological aspects of food. These include experimental chefs, such as those involved in molecular gastronomy (see "Take away" at the end of this chapter); research chefs, such as those involved with the development of new food products and manufacturing; and chefs who are concerned with menu planning and fine dining—all who strive to bring the science of eating to the table.

The RCA offers certification programs for the Certified Research Chef (CRC) and Certified Culinary Scientist (CCS) designations. It publishes the magazine *CULINOLOGY®*; *Culinology Currents®*, a newsletter for food industry professionals; and *Food Product Design*, an online magazine that combines the culinary arts with technology in the design of ingredients and foods and includes practical information for the retail, food service and functional food markets.

The Institute of Food Technologists is an international, nonprofit professional organization for the advancement of food science and technology. Its publications include the monthly magazine *Food Technology* and the *Journal of Food Science (JFS)*.

IFT functions in four main roles: a steward for the food science profession and its community; research champion and innovation catalyst; influential advocate and trusted spokes organization; and global citizen and partner in the advancement of food science and technology.

The focus areas and core sciences within IFT include the following [1,2]:

- Food product development and ingredient innovations, including additives, encapsulation, nanotechnology, nonthermal processing, sodium reduction, sweetener blends and others
- Food health and nutrition, including foods that maintain and improve health for the prevention and management of bone and joint diseases, certain cancers, coronary heart disease, diabetes, nutrigenomics, weight management and others
- Food processing and packaging, including the efficiency, quality and sustainability of food processing and packaging and others
- Food safety and defense, including additive and ingredient safety, allergens, microbial and chemical contaminants, novel technologies and others
- Public policy and regulation, including food laws, public policy and regulations with consumer food safety, food industry and research implications that embrace defense, import/export requirements, labeling, marketing, safety and others
- Sustainability, including efforts in food production sufficiency throughout product lifecycles—from sustainable ingredient sourcing to product development, waste management and others

Morsel "The more you eat, the less flavor. The less you eat, the more flavor." —Chinese proverb

Sensory Basics: the Science and Application of Flavor for Pleasure and Health

Today's chefs, food scientists and nutritionists are creating foods and recipes that help to bring the latest innovations to our tables, cross cuisines, meet diet and health needs, and restore food memories. Their efforts help to enlighten consumers about improved or innovative foods and beverages and inspire their food choices—based in significant part by sensory science.

Sensory science is a cross-disciplinary field of study that addresses how our five senses (hearing, sight, sound, taste and touch) function—from stimulation and perception to cognition and behavior. Sensory science integrates research in quality perception, preferences, communication, and health and well-being to gain insights in the underlying factors of food choices and eating behaviors. It explores how our senses can be used in food quality control and product design.

Sensory science is young and complex. Sensory scientists are still unveiling and debating certain tastes and sensations. Still, nutrition, food science and culinary professionals need to understand the mechanisms that underlie sensory reactions in order to adjust the flavors in a recipe or meal for enjoyment and health.

A common saying among nutrition and culinary professionals is "No food is consumed unless it tastes good." Few foods look, smell and taste good without appealing sensory qualities. If a food looks appealing, sounds enticing, smells delicious, tastes great, feels right in temperature and texture, then it may be well perceived. This is because the sights, sounds, smells, tastes and textures of great food stir up specific responses by the body that makes it quite desirable.

Thanks to these sensory responses, once a person consumes a very appealing food, he may want to select this food over and over again. Food marketers know that the sensory attributes of food are keys for repeat purchases. Making healthy foods and beverages look good and taste great are important challenges for nutrition, food science and culinary professionals. This is embodied in another underlying saying: "No food is nutritious unless it is consumed." Sensory science helps to pave the way.

Morsel "Sweet, sour, bitter, pungent—all must be tasted." —Chinese proverb

THE FIVE SENSES

The sensory organs that process the sights, smells, sounds, tastes and textures of foods help to determine whether a food is perceived as good or bad, tasty or offensive, and nutritious or unhealthy. These organs are connected by an intricate network throughout the central nervous system to the brain, where they are translated and interpreted—and often acted upon.

The sense of *sight* translates visual messages about the foods on the plate or in a meal. The sense of *smell* transfers aromas from foods that are cooked or served. The sense of *taste* registers tastes throughout the entire mouth, not just on the tongue. The sense of *touch* identifies foods by their texture when held and inside the entire oral cavity. The sense of *sound* recognizes the noises that foods make when they are cooked or consumed. These five senses are elaborately linked to one another and to the brain for perception, identification and action.

THE FIVE BASIC TASTES

There are five basic tastes: *sweet*, *salty*, *sour*, *bitter* and *umami* (Japanese for "deliciousness"). In contrast, there are literally thousands of odors because there are so many combinations, and they are too numerous to test.

These five basic tastes correlate with primitive times. The sweet taste was instinctive for survival: the sign of calories to come from hunting or foraging for food. The salty taste drove food choices that replaced what was naturally lost in sweat. The sour taste suggested patience until a food turned riper and sweeter. The bitter taste warned that a food might be poisonous. The umami taste indicated that a food contained protein, which is fundamental for existence.

These five basic tastes have similar correlations today. Sweet-tasting foods provide energy; salty foods are necessary for fluid balance; sour (acidic) foods indicate readiness; bitter foods are sometimes detested; and foods with umami are primary to most Western diets.

The sweet taste is found in fruits and vegetables, but it is also found in protein foods, such as milk with the milk sugar *lactose* and *glycogen*—stored carbohydrate that is found in muscle tissue.

The salty taste is naturally present in some fruits and vegetables, such as tomatoes and deep leafy green vegetables, and protein foods, such as dairy products. Many salty ingredients are manmade and developed for preservation.

The sour taste is principally found in fruits and vegetables, such as citrus fruits and green apples, but it is also found in naturally sour dairy products, such as yogurt or cultured buttermilk.

The bitter taste is prominent in cruciferous vegetables—those that bear a cross at the root, such as Brussels sprouts, broccoli and cauliflower. It is also pronounced in coffee, tea and wine.

The umami taste is identifiable in aged cheese, fermented soy foods, savory steaks, seafood, mushrooms and tomato products. The umami taste can be boosted from flavor layering or synergy among ingredients, such as a Caesar salad with anchovies and Parmesan cheese or a roasted tomato sauce with porcini mushrooms.

Food scientists, chefs and nutritionists use these basic tastes to create delicious, harmonious and memorable flavors in product development, recipes and meals. Examples of foods that carry each of these basic tastes are shown in Table 2-1.

55

TABLE 2-1 Basic Tastes and Food Sources	
Basic Tastes	**Food Sources**
Sweet	Bananas, breadstuffs, carrots, corn, cream, dates, grapes, honey, onions, parsnips, peas, scallops, sugars
Salty	Anchovies, bacon, cheese, ham, oysters, sea salt, seaweed, soy sauce, Parmesan cheese, tomatoes
Sour	Buttermilk, citrus fruits (lemon, lime, orange), rhubarb, sorrel, sour cream, tamarind, vinegar, yogurt, wine
Bitter	Angostura bitters, beer, bitter oranges, chicory, coffee, dark chocolate, deep leafy greens, extra-virgin olive oil, rosemary, walnuts, watercress, wine
Umami	Aged cheese, aged meats, beer, fermented soy products (miso, soy sauce, tempeh), mushrooms, peas, Parmesan cheese, seafood, tomatoes, wine

FOOD FLAVOR

The term *taste* is often used synonymously for the term *flavor*. **Flavor** is the sensation that is created when a substance is taken into the mouth and stimulates receptors that register smell (olfaction), taste, tactile (touch) and temperature sensations, among others.

TEXTURE AND MOUTHFEEL

Texture is the appearance, consistency and/or feel of a surface or a substance. Texture also refers to the properties and sensations that are transmitted by the sense of touch to the brain for interpretation. Texture is a component of food flavor.

Mouthfeel is both the chemical and physical reactions of foods and beverages inside the entire oral cavity. The mouthfeel of foods and beverages is first determined by their presence inside the mouth, and then by mastication or chewing, mixing with saliva, moving around the oral cavity by the tongue, and finally by swallowing.

Some common terms that are used to describe texture include *bitter, chewy, creamy, crisp, crispy, crunchy, dry, fatty, firm, greasy, hard, juicy, mushy, oily, ripe, rough, runny, slippery, smooth, soft, solid, sticky, wet* and others.

Some common terms that are used to describe mouthfeel include *adhesiveness, bounce, chewiness, coarseness, coatability, cohesiveness, denseness, dryness, fracturability* (how foods crumble, crack or shatter), *graininess, gumminess, hardness, heaviness, moistness, roughness, slipperiness, smoothness, uniformity, viscosity* and others.

In wine tasting, mouthfeel explains the different types of sensations that wines create within the oral cavity. Descriptors include such terms as *big, chewy, sweet* or *tannic*, similar to descriptors that are used for taste or flavor.

By experimenting with different textures and mouthfeel of foods and beverages, food scientists, chefs and nutritionists are able to create and individualize foods, recipes and meals for a wide range of audiences. This may be of particular significance in designing foods for children, those with sensory issues and the elderly.

56

Flavor Balancing

While there are only five basic tastes, many taste combinations and sensations can be created with them, just like a painter uses an assortment of basic colors to create different pigments and variations.

Most foods contain more than one taste, and each taste affects our perception of other tastes. Consider a squeeze of lemon or lime on a ripe tropical fruit, such as guava or papaya. The acidity brings out the mild sweetness of the fruit. Top it with a few grains of sea salt and the sweetness is magnified even more. Another example is smoked salmon with a squeeze of lemon; the salty, smoky taste becomes more pronounced by the acidity of the lemon.

Some taste combinations are fundamental to cooking, such as the saltiness and bitterness of classic salt and pepper. Other taste combinations are less obvious; still, they demonstrate the interaction of food science and nutrition in action. These include foods that naturally combine the tastes or sensations of sweet and sour, sweet and bitter, salty and sour, salty and bitter, hot and bitter, and hot and pungent.

For example, in Szechuan hot and sour soup, the savory sourness helps to stimulate hunger, and in sugared espresso, the sweetened bitterness helps to satiate hunger. There are many more examples in global cuisines that have unknowingly been paired for centuries. Enhancing and negating tastes by flavor balancing holds a world of possibilities.

Examples of some taste combinations and sensations with the condiments, foods, herbs and spices that naturally achieve them are shown in Table 2-2. With some experimentation, other harmonious blends can be created.

Some herb and spice combinations inherently rely on these taste combinations and sensations with their naturally acidic, bitter, hot, pungent, salty, spicy, sweet and savory blends. Examples include **bouquet garni**, with bay, parsley and thyme; **Chinese five-spice powder**, with cinnamon, cloves, fagara, fennel and star anise;

TABLE 2-2 Taste Combinations and Sensations

Sensations	Taste Combinations/Sensations
Sweet and sour	Berries, green apples, kiwi fruit, oranges and pomegranates
Sweet and bitter	Bittersweet chocolate or cocoa, bitter-sweet-sour fruit jam or jelly (as cranberry, crab apple, damson plum or elderberry), caramel and caramelized sugar
Salty and sour	Pickled fish and vegetables, salsa, sorrel, sour cream or crème fraiche and tamarind
Salty, bitter and umami (savory)	Anchovies, blue cheese, capers, caviar, clams, marinated artichoke hearts, nuts, olives, Parmesan cheese, pickled gherkins, sardines, teriyaki sauce, smoked fish, tomato sauce and Worcestershire sauce
Pungent (strong)	Allspice, black and cayenne pepper, cumin, garlic, ginger, mustard, onions and turmeric
Hot	Cayenne pepper, chili pepper, curry powder, hot paprika, and wasabi
Hot and bitter	Cinnamon sticks, chicory, cloves, mustard or radish sprouts, and watercress

fines herbes, with chervil, chives, parsley and tarragon; *gremolata* with anchovies, garlic, lemon zest and parsley; *mirepoix*, with celery, carrots and onions; and *quatre epics*, with cloves, ginger, nutmeg and pepper.

> **Morsel** "The smell of cooking can evoke a whole civilization." —Fernand Brandel (French historian, 1902–1985)

Bite on This: other sensory considerations

When it comes to selecting or rejecting foods, appearance counts. Healthy foods and beverages, beautifully arranged in correct proportions with ethnically correct garnishes, cue our sense of sight and our desire to consume it. So does the quality of food. Food that is selected at its peak or cooked to preserve nutrients looks and smells fresh and enticing. While it is not always feasible to purchase food at its finest, it is practical to plant a window box, containers or backyard garden; frequent farmers markets or participate in a ***food cooperative***—either a cooperative grocery store or buying club.

Pleasant aromas also signal us to eat. Aromas may bring back good food memories, such as our favorite holiday meals. Unpleasant aromas from odorous foods, such as cooked legumes or spinach, might turn off our appetite, especially if these foods were forced upon us as children. With some ingenuity and culinary know-how, even foods with strong odors can be pleasantly masked and appeal.

Figure 2-1 shows how food interplays with our senses of sight, smell, taste, touch and sound to influence our food choices or rejections, health and well-being. It can be used to demonstrate the reactions to a hamburger by a carnivore and a vegetarian.

To a carnivore, a hamburger may look delicious, smell and taste great, and have multiple textures and a variety of sounds (crunchy lettuce, crisp onions and pickles, juicy ground meat, etc.). To a vegetarian, a hamburger may look, smell, taste, feel and sound unappealing. When sensorial factors interplay, they create a positive perception of a hamburger to a carnivore. They increase its desirability and satisfaction. As a result, a carnivore may prefer a hamburger to other options and select it more frequently. After a hamburger is consumed, its nutrients may contribute to the health and wellness of a carnivore—especially if the hamburger meat is lean.

A vegetarian may have totally different sensory reactions to a hamburger. The interplay of the senses may cause a vegetarian to reject it. Unless a suitable protein replacement is consumed, then the nutrition, health and well-being of a vegetarian may be compromised.

> **Morsel** "Dinner is and always was a great artistic opportunity." —Frank Lloyd Wright (American architect, educator, interior designer and writer, 1867–1959)

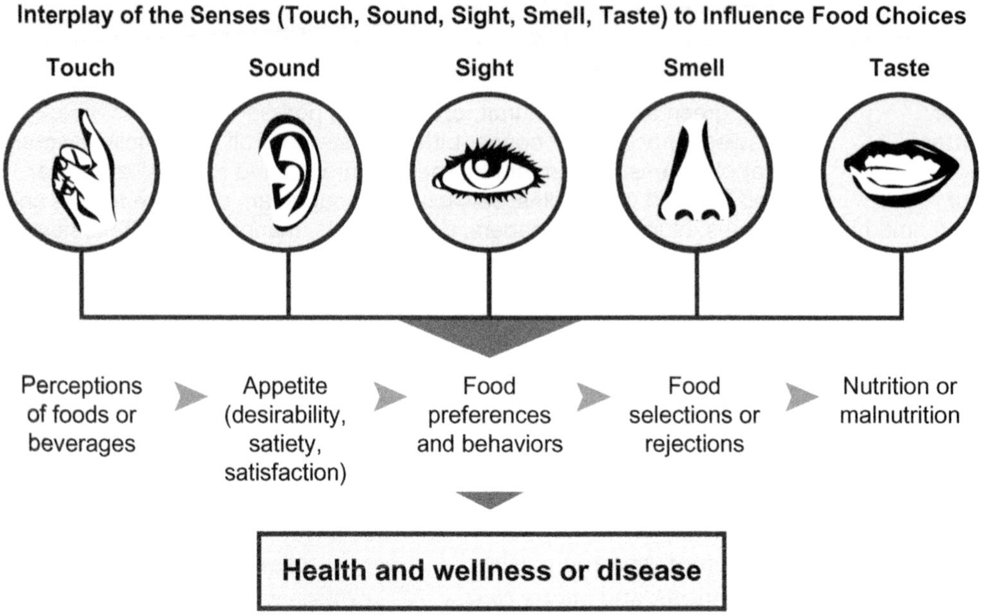

Interplay of the Senses (Touch, Sound, Sight, Smell, Taste) to Influence Food Choices

Touch	Sound	Sight	Smell	Taste

Perceptions of foods or beverages ➤ Appetite (desirability, satiety, satisfaction) ➤ Food preferences and behaviors ➤ Food selections or rejections ➤ Nutrition or malnutrition

Health and wellness or disease

FIGURE 2-1
Interplay of the Senses (touch, sound, sight, smell and taste) to Influence Food Choices.

Food scientists, chefs and nutritionists use these and other sensory considerations when creating new foods, recipes and menus. Nature has presented us with great-tasting ingredients: fruits, dairy products, healthy fats, herbs and spices, meats, nuts and seeds, vegetables and whole-grains for experimentation. But it really is the nutrients inside these foods—the building blocks of carbohydrates, lipids, proteins, vitamins and minerals, and water—that determine how different foods react with one another. Knowing their fascinating roles in food product development, cooking and baking helps to explain why carbohydrates, lipids, protein and water drive our food preferences, nutrition and health.

Morsel "A cook can never rise above his ingredients." —Anonymous

Why Food Behaves as It Does: Carbohydrates, Lipids, Protein and Water

In Chapter 1, the six major nutrients—carbohydrates, lipids (fats and oils), protein, vitamins, minerals and water—are presented with their sources and functions. Primarily carbohydrates, lipids, protein and water help to determine why food behaves as it does in product development, cooking and baking. While vitamin and mineral loss or gain occurs during cooking and baking and can be manipulated during product development, the other major nutrients rule.

CARBOHYDRATES

Carbohydrates, or sugars and starches, are found in the plant kingdom—primarily in fruits, grains, legumes (dried beans, lentils and peas) and vegetables—and in the animal kingdom—primarily in the muscle tissues of animal proteins. Carbohydrates serve to store chemical energy in plants and animals. When sugars and starches are consumed, then this chemical energy in the form of calories is released and used by the body for its many functions, or it is stored in the body for future needs.

The types of carbohydrates in plants are *sugars, starches, cellulose* (the main component of plant cell walls), and *pectin* (a gelatin-like substance) and *gums*. Besides contributing energy, sugars and starches help to supply the sweet taste in foods and beverages. Unlike sugars and starches, cellulose and pectin do not contain calories or supply energy. However, they do supply *fiber*, the noncaloric and nondigestible parts of plants that are associated with healthy digestion. The chemical and physical characteristics of sugar, starch and fiber help to provide important roles in product development, cooking and baking that are discussed throughout this chapter.

SUGARS

Sugars are *simple carbohydrates*. One simple sugar, *glucose*, is what the body utilizes for its many biological functions. Another is *fructose*, commonly found in berries, flowers, tree and vine fruits, honey and root vegetables. Fructose does not trigger the production of insulin by pancreatic cells like other sugars, so it is often recommended for diabetics. Granulated table sugar is *sucrose*, a combination of glucose and fructose.

Sucrose occurs naturally in every fruit and vegetable, but it is in greatest quantities in sugar cane and sugar beets. It is separated for commercial use and then processed through pressing, boiling, spinning, washing, filtering, crystallizing, drying and packaging.

There are many different types of granulated sugar that differ in crystal size. Each crystal size has unique functional characteristics. Some types of granulated sugar are preferred by the food industry and professional bakers. The food industry uses "extra-fine" or "fine" granulated sugar because its smaller crystals are superior for bulk handling and they are not prone to caking. Larger granulated sugar crystals are called for in most consumer recipes. The functions of sugars in cooking and baking include flavor, moisture retention and food preservation.

STARCHES

Starches are *complex carbohydrates*—long chains of glucose sugars that are stored in plants. When you eat a piece of bread (which is mostly starch), your body breaks down the starch into individual glucose sugars throughout the digestive process. This process is detailed in Chapter 1.

The functions of starch and carbohydrates in the cell walls of plants are mostly to provide bulk and texture in cooking. When starchy foods, such as potatoes, pasta or rice, are cooked with water or other fluids, the cooking water is absorbed by the starch granules, which cause these granules to swell. Once these starch granules cool, they mostly adhere to one another and cause foods to become sticky. These are important food science and cooking concepts that will be described in greater detail in this chapter.

GLYCOGEN

Long chains of sugars in animal tissues are called *glycogen*. While animal tissues are mostly protein, glycogen may have a small effect on the texture of meat. Additionally, the amount of glycogen in animal tissues at the time of slaughter affects the pH value of meat.

Before slaughtering, animal flesh has a pH value of about 7.1. After slaughtering, some of the glycogen converts into lactic acid and the pH value lowers. Beef reaches its lowest pH level of about 5.4 to 5.7 about 18 to 24 hours after slaughter. At a pH level of about 6.5, it starts to decompose. This is similar to the effect of an acidic ingredient, such as lemon juice or vinegar, in a marinade that softens the tough muscle fibers in fish, meat or poultry [3].

CELLULOSE

Cellulose is composed of glucose sugars. While the structure of cellulose is similar to starch, cellulose it is not affected by cooking the way starch absorbs the cooking liquid and swells. In fact, the opposite is true: cellulose is so durable that it is considered indigestible fiber. Cooking cellulose does not make it more digestible. However, as the cell structure weakens, it allows digestive enzymes to engulf the nutrients that are contained within the cells.

This is similar to the effect of baking soda when cooking vegetables. Baking soda preserves *chlorophyll*, the colorful green pigment in vegetables. However, it is an alkaline, and when it is added to cooking water, it makes vegetables soggy due to the breakdown of cellulose. Therefore, this practice is *not* recommended.

PECTIN

Pectin is a gelatin-like carbohydrate in the cell walls of plants. Pectin acts like a gel, sometimes referred to as a "fragile solid" in cooking. Pectin is semisoluble in liquids, which means that it is able to take up some liquid. This is especially important in cooking fruits and vegetables because it allows them to soften when cooked.

Pectin is extracted from apples and citrus fruits. Soluble pectin is capable of forming a gel once the correct concentrations of acid and sugar are reached. This is helpful to thicken syrups, such as those used to make jams and jellies.

GUMS

Gums are secretions of plants or trees that harden when they are released, but they are soluble in liquids. Gums function to create smoothness in candies and frozen confections, stabilize emulsions, and thicken and gel liquids.

Gums include *carrageenan*, used in desserts, ice cream, milk shakes and sauces; *gum arabic*, used in gummy candies, soft drinks and syrups; *guar gum*, used in baked goods and thickened dairy products such as yogurt; *locust bean gum*, used in cultured dairy products, cream cheese and frozen desserts; and *xanthan gum*, used in ingredients for gluten-free baking.

LIPIDS

Lipids are fats, oils, cholesterol, lecithin and other fatlike substances such as beta-carotene and vitamin E. Lipids are important in cooking and baking because they help to provide flavor, including mouthfeel, to recipes. Lipids also help to tenderize foods and allow foods to be heated to high enough temperatures in order to create crispness and convey richness. Despite all of these attributes, lipids are very concentrated in calories, so a little goes a long way.

When lipids are mixed with liquids, such as oil and water, by and large they do not mix. This is because water is composed of "polar molecules" and oils are composed of "nonpolar molecules." In polar molecules, the charge of one end of the molecule is attracted to the opposite end of another molecule. In nonpolar molecules, the charges are dispersed throughout the molecules. As a result, the liquid molecules can only bond with the oil molecules for short periods of time.

60

Oil and vinegar salad dressing is a good example of ingredients with polar and nonpolar molecules. Shake the salad dressing in a closed container vigorously and the molecules will stay together for varying degrees of time. Or use an *emulsifier*, such as an egg yolk, which acts as a liaison and stabilizes the ingredients. In an oil and vinegar salad dressing (vinaigrette), the molecules that make up salt and vinegar are also polar molecules, so they may be more easily dispersed throughout the mixture.

Some lipids mix with each other. For example, beta-carotene, the orangey-red pigment in fruits and vegetables, dissolves better in fat than in water. To increase the beta-carotene content of a recipe with brightly colored fruits or vegetables, add some fat. For example, use a little olive oil in a marinara sauce or tomato soup.

Lipids tend to float on water, which means they can be scooped up and discarded, as when visible fat is removed from the surface of soups or stews. After preparing soup, put it in the refrigerator to chill. The fat or oil will congeal on the surface and can be removed easily.

PROPERTIES OF FATS AND OILS

Fats are solid at room temperature. This is the reason why a stick of butter can be left out of the refrigerator and remain relatively solid. *Oils* are liquid at room temperature. If oils are refrigerated, they may become semisolid and cloudy.

Liquid oils and other vegetable fats are about 85 percent unsaturated fats. Generally, the more unsaturated the fats or oils, the healthier they are. In comparison, animal fats are about 50 percent saturated fat and 50 percent unsaturated fat. On the whole, the fat in beef and lamb is more saturated than the fat in poultry and pork.

An advantage of saturated fat in cooking is that it tends to be stable, which means that it is less likely to become *rancid* or *deteriorate* when it is exposed to metal, oxygen or water. Since poultry and pork have less saturated fat than beef and lamb, these two protein foods may deteriorate faster. Saturated and unsaturated fats are discussed in greater detail in Chapter 6.

A very important use of fats or oils in cooking and baking is in *emulsions*, the blending of dissimilar ingredients—often into creamy mixtures. In the example of the vinaigrette salad dressing just discussed, the egg yolk (a common emulsifying agent) helps to break down the oil into tiny droplets that are suspended throughout the vinegar, which yields a creamy consistency.

Other emulsions include butter, cream, ice cream, margarine and salad dressings. Bearnaise, hollandaise and mayonnaise are sauces that are created by emulsions. Other emulsifiers include *lecithin* in crystal or liquid form (in fact, egg yolks are about one-third lecithin), gelatin, mashed potatoes, meat extract, mustard, skim milk and starch "paste." The trouble with emulsions is that they tend to be unstable. If an emulsion separates, then a dressing or sauce may be whisked back into suspension. More information about emulsions and their essential roles in food product development, cooking and baking follow in this chapter.

Fats *melt* when exposed to heat, which means they slowly change from a solid to a liquid state over time. The fact that fats melt and do not instantly turn into liquids makes them versatile ingredients in food product development, cooking and baking. Some fats can eventually turn into gases, much like liquid evaporates into air, but it takes a considerable amount of heat for this to happen.

Fats can *decompose*, which is unlike deterioration. When fats decompose, they break down into noticeable gas. This is called the *smoke point* of fats. The smoke point varies among fats and oils; it is wise to select a fat or oil one with a high smoke point that is suitable for hot, sustained cooking to help prevent a change in food flavor.

Fats and oils with fewer free fatty acids tend to have higher smoke points. These include some vegetable oils, such as canola or safflower oils. Animal fats, fresh fats and refined oils tend to have more free fatty acids and thus lower smoke points. These include butter, coconut oil and lard. If a fat has impurities, the smoke point will be lower, which means it will smoke faster. The size of the pot or pan also makes a difference in the smoke point. A wider pot or pan with greater exposure to air lowers the smoke point, which means the fat or oil may decompose faster than one with less exposure. The approximate smoke points of common fats and oils are shown in Table 2-3.

TABLE 2-3 Smoke Points of Common Fats and Oils

Types of Fats and Oils	Smoke Points (°F[a])
Almond oil	430 °F
Avocado oil, refined	520
Butter	350
Canola oil, refined	400
Coconut oil	350
Corn oil, refined	450
Flaxseed oil, refined	225
Hazelnut oil	430
Grape seed oil	485
Lard	400
Olive oils, extra-virgin	410
Olive oils, virgin	420
Olive oils, pomace	460
Peanut oil, refined	450
Rapeseed oil	440
Safflower oil, refined	450
Safflower oil	510
Sesame oil, unrefined	350
Sesame oil, semirefined	450
Shortening, vegetable	370
Soy oil, refined	450
Sunflower oil, semirefined	450
Walnut oil, unrefined	320
Walnut oil, semirefined	400

Source: [4,5].
[a]Smoke points are approximate because oils differ within the same type of oil, such as olive (extra-virgin, pomace and virgin) and whether or not the oil is refined.

PROTEINS

Proteins assist in the *browning* of foods that occurs at high temperatures. They also contribute to the *overall flavor* of foods. Some proteins carry *distinctive tastes*, such as aged cheese like Parmesan or cured ham like prosciutto. These savory tastes are partially due to the fifth taste of umami that was described earlier in this chapter.

The *molecule structure* of protein is important in the cooking process. Some parts of the protein molecule attract water, while other parts attract fats or oils. Some parts are designed to form strong bonds, such as the connective tissues in meats. Other parts of the protein molecule offer some flexibility, such as the bonds in eggs and milk. The somewhat rigid but flexible egg white matrix is an important component in cakes and meringue-based desserts.

Another function of proteins is that they act as *enzymes*, which affect the rate at which chemical reactions take place. The enzymes that are responsible for the different stages of the digestive process are discussed in Chapter 1. These include *salivary amylase* that helps to break down starches into sugars in the oral cavity; *pepsin* that helps to break down proteins into smaller structures called peptides in the stomach; *lipase* that helps to break down lipids into fatty acids in the small intestine; and *pancreatic amylase* that helps to break down starches into sugars, also in the small intestine. The suffix "-ase" is indicative that these protein-based substances are enzymes.

In foods, *amylases* from fungi and other plants help to convert starches into sugars during food processing, such as in the production of high-fructose corn syrup. Amylases are also used in brewing to split polysaccharides and proteins during "malting," such as in the production of beer, malt vinegar and whisky.

Cellulases and *pectinases* are used to clarify fruit juice. *Lactases* are used to break down lactose into dairy products to glucose and galactose to aid digestion. *Lipases* are used in the production of Roquefort cheese to enhance ripening. *Proteases* are used to lower the protein content of certain flours. Many other types of enzymes with a variety of functions are used in food production.

Enzymes in plants and animals may alter the color, nutrients, taste and texture in foods. For example, enzymes may cause some vegetables to rot and fish to become mushy. Refrigeration helps delay spoilage caused by the destructive enzymatic action of some bacteria. Cooking helps speed up enzymatic action and food breakdown. A recipe might read to "heat quickly" to prevent enzyme activation and the ingredients from breaking down too soon.

When proteins break down either physically or chemically, this is called *denaturation*. Acid, agitation (disturbance) or heat may cause protein denaturation. If there is an acidic ingredient in a dish, such as citrus fruit or tomatoes; if the mixture is agitated, such as beaten or whipped; or if the recipe is cooked over high heat, such as in barbecuing or broiling, then the proteins might denature.

A classic example of denatured protein is overcooked egg whites, which are mostly egg albumin in water. If egg whites are overcooked over high heat, they typically become opaque and rubbery in an interconnected solidified mass.

Denatured proteins may *coagulate*, or become sticky. This might be fine to help set custard or quiche, but it is unacceptable for fragile white fish or scallops when only a little firmness is desired. If coagulation continues to a semisolid or solid state, then a dense custard or quiche or overcooked fish may result. This is why it is so important to follow the recommended cooking times of proteins in recipes.

WATER

As discussed in Chapter 1, water is one of the six essential nutrients. In fact, it could be argued that water is *the* most important nutrient. Two-thirds of the human body is water. Plants contain as much as 95 percent water, and raw meat contains as much as 75 percent water. When heat is applied to foods in cooking and baking, water is released. This action can add moisture to a dish in the form of *au jus* (French for "in its own juice"—usually in reference to meats) or a light sauce (often from fruits and vegetables). If foods are heated too long or at temperatures that are too high, then the ingredients may become overly dry.

As water is heated, it forms *steam* and the steam evaporates. This process is slow and has both advantages and disadvantages. For quick cooking, a hot pot or pan of oil will heat faster than water. Since the water will hold its temperature longer, it is a better medium for long, slow cooking. In Chapter 3, the moist-heat cooking techniques of braising, simmering and stewing are explored, which rely upon this ability of water to hold heat over time.

Steam is also responsible for quickly cooking foods at hot temperatures. It can be a healthy cooking technique to use for fragile vegetables, but it is also effective for sturdier vegetables to help preserve nutrients and prevent loss.

In *steaming*, foods are placed in a steamer basket over boiling water; then the boiling water evaporates and turns into steam. The steam rises and transfers the heat to cook the foods in a process called *convection*. The reason why a pot should be covered is that when the tiny water droplets of steam hit the lid, they drop onto the food with their moist heat.

Another feature of water is that it is a *weak acid* and a *weak base*. It may not taste very acidic like citrus juice or vinegar, but this characteristic may affect its cooking properties. Water can act as an acid or a base depending upon its chemical environment. It is important to note that nearly all foods are a slight bit acidic. This feature should be accounted for in food product development, cooking and baking.

Finally, water acts as a *solvent*, so a *solute*, such as food particles, can be suspended within it as a *solution* (such as sugar in brewed tea or prepared coffee).

Why Food Behaves as It Does: Common Cooking and Baking Reactions

EMULSIONS

As just explained, *emulsions* are mixtures of two or more liquids that are normally *immiscible* (unmixable), with an emulsifying agent that keeps the emulsion in suspension.

Most emulsions have three elements: an *emulsifier*, such as cream, egg yolk, lecithin or dairy milk; enough *liquid* to hold the emulsion in suspension; and *mechanical action*, such as whisking or rapid shaking that disperses the liquid into tiny droplets.

It may be difficult for an emulsion to hold its creamy consistency, even if careful attention is paid to each of these three features. This is where stabilizers may be effective. *Stabilizers* are thickeners and gelling agents that are used to give foods a firmer texture and in food preservation. They help to provide viscosity or thickness without too many extra calories, carbohydrates or fats.

Proteins (beans, seaweed such as agar-agar and seeds), starches (pectins and gums), and other plant tissues are used to stabilize emulsions in more permanent suspensions. Stabilizers are often used in such foods as dressings, frozen desserts, jellies, mousses, pickles, puddings, salad dressings, sauces and yogurt.

ENZYMES

Enzymes are a group of proteins that are important to food product development, cooking and nutrition because of their effects on the ingredients in a recipe. Enzymes are *catalysts*, which increase the rate of reactions and cause chemical and physical changes.

In Chapter 1 and earlier in this chapter you learned to identify an enzyme by the suffix "-ase," such as salivary amylase that helps to break down carbohydrates in the mouth and gastric lip*ase* that helps to break down protein in the stomach. Enzymes in the plants and animals that humans consume may affect the appearance, flavor, nutrients and texture in foods and beverages. Enzymes may be responsible for bacterial deterioration, dulling brightly hued colors and softening firmly textured foods. For example, a vegetable beyond its peak may look gray instead of green, smell foul, be limp, and have fewer vitamins and minerals due to enzymatic action.

As a whole, enzymes are not the cook's friend. The exceptions include the enzymes that are found in tougher cuts of meats (which become tender by their own enzymatic action); the enzymes in the fermentation of dairy, soy and other products (which help give cultured dairy foods, such as buttermilk and yogurt their characteristic flavor); the enzymes that process cornstarch into fructose syrup and glucose syrup.

The hot-cold technique of blanching vegetables before freezing freezes the biochemical enzymes in the vegetables that would normally cause color and flavor loss and deterioration. Cooking can denature or inactivate some enzymes and halt or slow their activity. When enzymes denature, their protein structure uncoils, which makes them less effective or sometimes fully inactive. For example, raw pineapple naturally contains the enzyme *bromelain*, which breaks down gelatin. If raw pineapple is used to prepare gelatin, it may interfere with gelling. However, when raw pineapple is cooked or processed during canning to denature the bromelain, the canned pineapple and gelatin should firm. This requires delicate treatment. In the process of denaturing the bromelain and other similar enzymes, they may rapidly do their damage before they denature.

To minimize the temperature range at which enzymes are most destructive, heat fruits and vegetables as quickly as possible. The activity of an enzyme or a system of enzymes can be destroyed at temperatures near 200°F.

When cooking tougher cuts of meats, the long, slow enzymatic action serves to soften their protein structure—particularly when paired with acidic ingredients. Freezing does not destroy enzymes; they retain some activity at temperatures as low as –100°F, although their reaction rates are extremely compromised.

HEAT TRANSFER

Heat is the process by which raw foods are transformed by heat energy into a fusion of cooked and baked creations. The roles of *heat transfer* in cooking and baking are of primary importance to the desirability, flavor and texture of foods. A detailed discussion of heat transfer through *conduction*, *convection* and *radiation* is found in Chapter 3.

THE MAILLARD REACTION

The *Maillard reaction*, also known as the *browning reaction*, is actually a series of complex chemical and physical reactions that produce sweet, brown compounds at *lower temperatures* than what are required to caramelize foods.

The Maillard reaction helps to explain why toast turns brown, fried foods become golden, and roasts develop a dark-brown coating. The difference between the Maillard reaction and caramelization is that the Maillard reaction involves proteins as well as carbohydrates. Carbon molecules in the sugars combine with amino acids in the proteins.

The Maillard reaction mostly entails the proteins in foods and beverages such as beer, bread, cocoa and meats and the reactions that these foods and beverages undergo when they are exposed to heat. It helps to give a brown color to beer and cocoa, convert bread into toast, and give meat a crusted exterior.

Many Maillard-type reactions occur at comparatively high temperatures that are achieved by dry-heat cooking methods, such as baking or grilling, as opposed to moist-heat cooking methods, such as braising or steaming. However, some moist-heat cooking methods may also produce Maillard-type aroma and color over extended periods of time, such as those that include reduction.

While caramelization and the Maillard reaction help to increase the deliciousness of food, browning foods beyond their crusty exteriors may cause some protein destruction and potentially become health hazards. For example, it is not wise to consume charred foods of any kind on a regular basis. This includes the burned crusts of bread or the blackened skin of poultry.

FOOD BYTE

Slow cookers, or crock pots, serve to cook food at low settings over a period of time by steady, moist heat. The advantages of slow cookers are that the cook does not have to be present and that less-tender cuts of protein can be cooked slowly with moisture to help tenderize them. Ground meats should be cooked thoroughly before adding to slow cookers to discourage bacterial growth. Dairy products should be added at the end of cooking to prevent curdling or toughening. Cooking fruits and vegetables with their skins increases fiber and helps to keep them intact in slow cookers.

TEMPERATURE AND TIME

Well-tested recipes often include the most optimal cooking or baking times and temperatures. The first time one attempts a recipe, it is best to follow whatever time and temperature are provided and note the results.

Beforehand, the oven must be calibrated to the right temperature. This is why the use of oven thermometers is essential in successful cooking and baking. It is equally important that the refrigerator and freezer temperatures are calibrated to the right temperatures in order to keep cold foods cold and frozen foods frozen.

An overview of the ranges of temperatures to heat, refrigerate and freeze food follow, with an additional section on the adjustments that must be made for high-altitude cooking and baking.

Oven Temperature

Recipe instructions often indicate oven temperature as "moderate" or "hot" and different degrees of doneness as "rare," "medium" or "well-done." This may be puzzling for novices. Oven temperature descriptions, degrees of doneness and oven settings are shown in Table 2-4, with ranges depending on the type of oven and its accuracy.

Other Temperatures

Sometimes recipes tell the reader to warm or cool foods, but they may not communicate how warm or how cool. Some common temperature descriptions and their temperature equivalents are shown in Table 2-5.

High-Altitude Cooking and Baking

At high altitudes (above 3,000 feet) preparation of food may require changes in time or temperature—or even an entire recipe. This is because there is a decrease in air pressure and air density at high altitudes.

TABLE 2-4 Oven Temperature Descriptions, Degrees of Doneness and Oven Settings	
If a Recipe Reads . . . **Temperatures**	*Set the Oven Temperature to . . .* Oven Settings (°F)
Very hot	475–500 °F
Hot	425–450
Moderately hot	400
Moderate	350–375
Very moderate	325
Warm	300–325
Cool	275–300
Very cool	225–250
Very slow/low	<225
Degree of doneness	
Well-done beef	160 *plus*
Medium-well beef	150–155
Medium beef	140–145
Medium-rare beef	130–135
Rare beef	120–125
Well-done Lamb	165 *plus*
Medium lamb	160
Medium-rare lamb	140–150
Rare lamb	135
Ground pork	160
Medium-rare pork	145
Pre-cooked ham (reheated)	140
Chicken	165–175
Turkey	165–175

Source: [6].

TABLE 2-5 Common Temperature Descriptions and Temperature Equivalents

Common Temperature Descriptions	Temperature Equivalents (°F)
In order to . . .	*Temperatures should be . . .*
Boil water	212 °F
Reheat cooked food	165
Maintain hot cooked food	140 or above
Food temperature danger zone	40–140
Hot liquid	120
Warm liquid	105–115
Warm to normal human body temperature	98.6
Warm liquid to lukewarm	95
Let bread rise at room temperature	80
Warm at room temperature	70–75
Cool at room temperature	65
Store in refrigerator	40 or below
Freeze water	32
Store in freezer	0 or below

Source: [6].

These factors affect cooking and baking because water will turn into steam quicker than at lower altitudes. This means that water and other liquids will evaporate faster and boil at a lower temperature; leavening gases in breads and cakes will expand more; and foods may require longer cooking times than what is specified in recipes. At high altitudes it is easy to overcook meat and poultry or scorch casseroles due to this moisture loss. A food thermometer is recommended.

Some general adjustments for high-altitude cooking include increasing the amount of water to cook pasta, rice, or other grains by 1 to 2 cups; simmering or boiling foods slightly longer than stated; and wrapping refrigerated and frozen items very carefully with extra layers to prevent drying.

Some general adjustments for high-altitude baking include increasing the oven temperature by 25 °F; adding 1 to 2 tablespoons of liquid to every cup of fluid; using slightly less sugar than called for (about 1 to 2 tablespoons less per cup); decreasing the leavening ingredients by one-fourth, and not overbeating egg whites to reduce the possibilities of quick rise and fall in baked goods.

Refrigerators

The recommended refrigerator temperature to slow bacterial growth and maintain food quality is 40 °F or lower. Since most foods will freeze at 32 °F, the refrigerator should be adjusted between 32 °F and 40 °F to prevent undesirable freezing, such as ice crystals in liquids.

FOOD BYTE

Freezing does not prevent bacterial, chemical or physical changes in foods; it delays them. To help decrease alterations in food quality, use freezer-designed wrap that is vapor- and moisture-proof; cool foods properly; remove as much air as possible before wrapping foods; and space foods well in the freezer to promote uniform freezing. Deterioration may appear as freezer burn, frost, change in color, or change in texture. Dry, toughened, lumpy and/or colorless frozen food has probably lost its culinary and nutritional attributes.

Freezers

The recommended freezer temperature is 0 °F or lower. At this temperature, bacterial growth should be reduced. Freezing does not kill all bacteria, nor does it stop flavor and texture changes, particularly if foods are not wrapped properly for the freezer. The longer foods are kept in the freezer, the more likely that texture and flavor changes may occur.

TABLE 2-6 Safe Storage Time Limits for Refrigeration and Freezing of Foods

Types of Foods	Refrigeration Time Limits (40°F or lower)	Freezer Time Limits (0°F or lower)
Mayonnaise-based salads (chicken, egg, ham, macaroni, tuna)	3–5 days	Do not freeze
Processed meats, hot dogs	3–7 days	1–2 months
Ground beef, chicken, lamb, turkey, veal *or* raw sausage (from beef, chicken, pork, turkey)	1–2 days	3–4 months 1–2 months
Fresh beef, lamb, pork, veal	3–5 days	4–12 months, *depending if* they are chops (4–6 months), steaks (6–12 months), or roasts (4–12 months)
Fresh poultry	1–2 days	9 months *if pieces* 1 year *if whole*
Soups/stews with meat or vegetables	3–4 days	2–3 months
Leftovers	3–4 days	1–6 months *if cooked*

The safe storage time limits for the refrigeration and freezing of foods are shown in Table 2-6. In general, unopened packages and whole cuts (as whole chickens, turkeys or roasts) will keep longer than opened packages or pieces [7].

When in doubt, throw it out. The appearance and aroma of foods are not guaranteed indicators of whether or not harmful bacteria have formed. Refrigerate perishable foods within two hours after preparation or eating. Never thaw or marinate foods on a kitchen counter. If a frozen food has exceeded these time limits, is poorly wrapped and/or shows signs of *freezer "burn"* (a state when frozen food has been damaged by dehydration and oxidation), it probably should be discarded

Ingredients and Functions

Food scientists, chefs and nutritionists have countless ingredients at their disposal to create new foods and recipes and to update old ones. In this section, ingredients are grouped according to their food groups: *meats* (including beef, eggs, fish, lamb, pork, poultry and seafood); *dairy milk and dairy products* (including cheese, cream, ice cream, dairy milk and yogurt); *legumes, grains, fruits, vegetables,* and *fats and oils.* Their characteristics, benefits and drawbacks in cooking and baking are discussed.

COOKING MEATS AND SEAFOOD

One of the challenges of cooking meats to the right degree of doneness is that different cuts of meat cook at different temperatures. For instance, the dark meat in poultry (the leg and thigh) must be cooked to an internal temperature of about 160°F to lose its raw taste and to melt its fat, while the white meat (the breast and wing) will be dry and tough over 150°F. When cooking a whole chicken, a fine balance must be achieved between the dark and white meats.

Meats are protein foods. When meat is cooked, the proteins in the muscles must first unwind, or denature. Then the proteins rejoin, and when this happens, the meat shrinks a bit and loses its natural juices. The result is that it becomes tougher and drier.

Under 120°F and the shrinkage is mostly in the diameter of the meat. Over 120°F and the shrinkage may also be in the length of the meat, with greater overall muscle loss. The best advice for cooking meats to the right degree of doneness is to follow the temperature guidelines that are provided in Table 2-5 and to use the hand "feel" method that is explained in the following section.

Beef

Raw beef has acidic, salty and savory tastes. Unlike raw beef, cooked beef is very aromatic, producing literally hundreds of compounds. This is because cooking deepens the natural aroma and taste of beef. When cooked beef is consumed, its fluids are released that bathe the inside of the oral cavity with the beef's aroma and taste. These fluids are the most flavorful when beef is just cooked, because this is the start of the breakdown of protein and fat.

As beef is cooked, the color and juices change from red to pink and then to brown. This change in color has to do with the pigment *myoglobin*, which is present in muscle tissue. Raw beef could still look brown, so it is better to depend on a meat thermometer to determine the accuracy of its doneness. Exposure to light and improper freezing may also affect the color of beef.

Before beef is cooked, the texture is soft and mushy. This is because about three-quarters of beef is moisture and the rest is composed of connective tissues, fiber and proteins. As beef is cooked, the softness disappears; it becomes firmer in texture and somewhat easier to chew. Additional cooking may dry the beef further, unless it is cooked with a liquid, such as in braising. Then the toughest cuts of beef may disintegrate or fall apart. This is because the connective tissue, or collagen, actually dissolves into gelatin. The beef may still seem stringy, but the gelatin works to thicken the fluids in which it is cooked and create a flavorful sauce. Beef stew from brisket, chuck, plate or rib relies on this cooking method for its succulence.

The texture of the degree of doneness of beef is similar to the feel of the fleshy part of the palm of the hand below the thumb. The more beef is cooked, the less flexible it becomes. The best way to experience this correlation is to first test it by hand, and then during cooking. Touch the thumb and forefinger together and press on the fleshy part below the thumb. It should feel soft to the touch with a little bounce. This is how a rare beef steak feels. Now, touch the thumb and middle finger together and press on the fleshy part below the thumb. There should be some give and spring to the touch. This is how a medium beef steak feels. Finally, touch the thumb and little finger together and press on the fleshy part below the thumb. There should be no give at all; it should be quite firm. This is how a well-done beef steak feels [8].

Poultry

Chicken and turkey are often browned by caramelization during the first step of their cooking process. Then a moist cooking method, such as braising or stewing, is often used. Other popular cooking methods include broiling, grilling, roasting, sauteing and stir-frying, and combining poultry with flavorful sauces in casseroles, soups, stews and preparing stock.

Poultry should be cooked until the meat is no longer pink near the bone, the juices run clear, or when the breastbone is opaque. The most accurate way to test for doneness in poultry is to use a meat thermometer. Insert it into the thickest part of the meat without touching the bone. The thigh should read 165° to 175°F, and the breast should read 150° to 160°F. A temperature of 160°F or higher complies with the US Food Safety and Inspection Service guidelines [9].

Fish and Shellfish

Very lean fish, such as cod or sole, have lean flesh that requires some moisture, fat or oil for cooking and flavor, since they are such delicate fish. Braising, frying, poaching, sauteing and seaming are the preferred cooking methods. Oily fish, such as salmon or tuna, can be cooked by the dry-heat cooking methods of baking, grilling or sauteing because their fats are released and bathe the fish during cooking.

The doneness in fish is signified by time—about 8 to 10 minutes per inch at the widest point of the fish. Flakiness and opaqueness are other indicators of doneness.

Shellfish react differently to cooking. Overcooking toughens shellfish. Mollusks, such as clams, mussels and oysters, are ready when their shells begin to open and the interiors begin to curl. Crustaceans, such as langoustines, lobsters and shrimp, turn red or bright pink. Sea scallops turn opaque and firm.

COOKING AND BAKING WITH DAIRY MILK AND DAIRY PRODUCTS
Dairy Milk

Dairy milk contributes body, flavor, moisture, sugar (for browning) and salts (for protein coagulation) in cooking and baking applications. It tolerates heat quite well, as does cream, because of the interaction between the milk proteins and fat globules. Both dairy milk and cream can be boiled and reduced. But dairy milk and cream crystallize when cold and their fat separates. Dairy milk *coagulates*, or forms a solid mass, and *curdles* when exposed to acids. The liquid that separates from the curds in this process is called *whey*, which is high in protein.

When dairy milk is cooked at low temperatures, the flavor may be slightly modified. Sulfur and/or green leaf aromas may be noted. With increased heat, other flavors may be distinguished, such as almond or vanilla. With prolonged heat, both browning and flavor changes may arise due to the Maillard reaction, leading to a butterscotch aroma. Dairy milk is highly perishable and may deteriorate due to exposure to air, light or age [10].

Bite on This: drawbacks of and remedies for cooking with dairy milk

Dairy milk is filled with carbohydrates, proteins and fats (depending on the type of milk). While these nutrients supply a number of physical and sensory attributes in cooking and baking, they may also contribute to some drawbacks. Following are some remedies.

Drawback #1:
Coagulation: In dishes where dairy milk is the main ingredient, such as cream soups, sauces or scalloped potatoes, or when milk is added to coffee, hot chocolate or tea, the milk proteins may coagulate and form surface skin on the top of the mixture. The skin is a web of casein (80 percent of the protein in dairy milk), calcium, whey (the watery part of dairy milk) proteins, and fat globules.

This happens because moisture evaporates from the surface of foods or beverages and the proteins concentrate. This is similar to what occurs when milk proteins coagulate on the bottom of pots and pans that are exposed to high heat.

Remedy:
To prevent evaporation from the surface of foods or beverages and skin formation, cover the pan or pot, use a layer of food wrap, or top the surface with foam.

Remedy:
To prevent scorching on the bottom of pots or pans, wet the bottom with water before dairy milk is added to reduce the proteins from adhering; use moderate and steady heat, or heat in a double boiler or microwave oven.

Drawback #2:
Curdling: Particles of ingredients may help the dairy milk proteins stick together and clump. Acidic ingredients in fruits and vegetables and astringent tannins in coffees, teas and potatoes may make proteins more susceptible to curdling.

Remedy:
To prevent curdling, use fresh dairy milk (with less bacteria that gradually sours milk) and moderate heat.

Drawback #3:
Boiling over: Like other liquids, as boiling milk bubbles, it can rise and spill over the pot or pan.

Remedy:
To prevent milk from boiling over, turn the heat down close to boiling, and leave the lid partly open so steam can escape.

Dairy Products

Some of the many types of dairy products that are widely available for consumption, cooking and baking follow.

- *Butter* is produced when cream is agitated and the milk fat separates. *Sweet cream butter* is made from pasteurized fresh cream. *Salted sweet cream butter* contains about 1 to 2 percent added salt. *Cultured cream butter* contains lactic acid bacteria, which causes it to be fuller in flavor. *Whipped butter* contains gas that is pumped into it to increase its spread. *Clarified butter* is devoid of milk solids and water, so it can withstand higher temperatures. It is known as *ghee* in Indian cuisine.

- *Buttermilk*, like *sour cream* and *crème fraiche*, is produced when a bacteria culture is added to dairy milk. *Cultured buttermilk* is made from skim milk that has been fermented. *True buttermilk* is made from churned whole milk. The curds have separated from the whey and then the whey is fermented. True buttermilk is not as acidic as cultured buttermilk and it has a fuller flavor.
- *Condensed or evaporated milk* contains less water than whole milk. It is creamy, a little brown in color and caramel in taste.
- *Evaporated dry milk* has 100 percent of the water removed, so it is shelf stable and relatively safe from microbes.
- *Ice cream* is a mixture of air, cream, ice crystals and sugar that are churned together to develop a creamy and sweet consistency. *Reduced-fat and nonfat ice cream products* use fat and carbohydrate substitutes to replicate the creaminess of ice cream. Corn syrup, dry milk and/or vegetable gums may be added to further mimic full-fat ice cream. *Soft-serve ice cream* is generally reduced in fat and contains more air than full-fat ice cream.
- *Reduced-fat milk* is thinner than whole milk because the fat is reduced. It may be fortified with vitamins A and D, which are normally found in fat and milk solids. This fortification might affect the flavor. *Lactose-free milk* is formulated for people who cannot tolerate the milk sugar lactose. In lactose-free milk, lactose is broken down into two simple sugars: galactose and glucose. These simple sugars are easily detected on the tongue. This is why lactose-free milk is sweet in taste.
- *Sweetened condensed milk* is reduced in consistency and sucrose, or table sugar is added during processing. It is milder, lighter, sweeter and thicker than condensed milk.
- *Yogurt* is fermented dairy milk that has thickened into a partial solid. It is useful in baked goods, dressings, drinks and soups for its creaminess and tanginess. The yogurt that is commonly consumed in the United States tends to be thinner and milder than the yogurt that is popular in Asia, Eastern Europe, India and North Africa. In these countries, plain yogurt is enjoyed just the way it is, or it is used to balance many of these hot cuisines.

70

Advantages of Dairy Products in Cooking and Baking

Dairy products provide body, carbohydrate (sugar, in the form of lactose), fat globules (depending on the fat content), flavor (aroma, taste and texture), milk protein, moisture and sodium in product development, cooking and baking applications. Dairy substitutes, such as soy milk and other plant-based products, may provide some but not all of these attributes. Sometimes their watery consistency, strong flavor, bitter aftertaste and/or astringency may be objectionable.

As a whole, dairy products are very versatile ingredients in savory and sweet recipes. The following are some of the *advantages* of using dairy products:

- Butter, with its rich flavor, is useful as a sauce and emulsifier. Butter can withstand a fair amount of heat; it is mostly saturated fats that hold together well.
- Cultured buttermilk and yogurt, with their mouthfeel, tanginess and tenderness, are useful in muffins, pancakes, scones and waffles where the major leavener is baking soda.
- Dairy milk adds rich and mellow flavor (depending on fat content).
- Dairy milk and cream, with their mouthfeel and richness, remain intact in milk and cream-enriched sauces, since both can withstand heat.
- Reduced-fat dairy milk, with its concentrated protein, is good for foaming (although the foam tends to be fragile and is not long lasting).
- Sweetened and condensed milk, with their concentrated protein and sugars, is useful for quick, caramel-flavored sauces.

As a whole, dairy products are not recommended for lactose-intolerant people or for those who are sensitive to casein, the major protein in dairy milk. The following are some general *drawbacks* of using some dairy products:

- Butter has a low smoke point and should not be heated to high temperatures.
- Butter is slightly more difficult to work with than shortening when preparing pastry and other doughs because it is harder.

- Butter is only about 80 percent fat; it contributes additional water to a mixture that could affect the outcome of a recipe.
- Cultured milk products are very susceptible to curdling when exposed to acid, heat, salt or stirring.
- Deterioration of dairy milk and some dairy products may affect their aroma and taste.
- Evaporated, aseptically packed, shelf-stable and some powdered milk may have a slight caramelized flavor and be less desirable in delicate desserts, such as cream pie filling, custard or pudding.
- Intense heat may cause dairy milk and some dairy products to brown and develop a caramelized flavor. This is usually due to their natural sugars.

Cheese

There are countless varieties of cheese availability for cooking and baking, with varying degrees of taste, meltability and texture. When cheese melts, the milk fat breaks down first and then the protein breaks down, releasing moisture. As moisture is lost, the melted cheese may toughen. This might be fine for cold pizza, but it may not be so desirable for a cheese sauce.

Some types of cheese can withstand heat and stay intact during cooking: fresh goat cheese, Italian ricotta, Indian paneer and Latin American queso blanco. Their textures are distinct, and they tend to take on the flavors of other ingredients in recipes.

Stringy cheese, such as mozzarella or Mexican Oaxaca, or crumbly cheese, such as English Cheshire or Roquefort, are well suited for dishes with characteristic stringiness or crumbliness, such as a topping for soups (as baked onion) or a sprinkling for salads. Parmesan and Asiago are suitable for grating because they disperse quite well when they are added to warm dishes, such as pasta, polenta or risotto.

Stringiness is not a desirable characteristic in some sauces or soups that depend on creaminess for desirability and satisfaction. It is best to use a moist cheese, such as such as Colby or Gruyère, that tends to blend well. Finely grating a cheese first may help to break it up more uniformly. Apply as little heat as possible and do not agitate the cheese while cooking. A little acid (such as lemon juice) might reduce some stringiness, as long as the final recipe will tolerate this acidity.

Eating raw cheese has been implicated in some pathogen-related outbreaks. Since 1949, the FDA has employed standards of identity [11] that prevent the manufacture of any cheese that is made from unpasteurized milk—unless the cheese has been aged at least 60 days at temperatures not less than 35°F. Since 1951, this legislation also includes raw-milk cheese imports. Raw cheese is still legal in some European countries.

People with fragile immune systems, such as children, the elderly, pregnant women, and those with chronic illnesses should probably avoid raw dairy milk and raw milk cheese. They should first check with their health care providers [12].

Reduced, Low-Fat and Nonfat Cheese

With the popularity of reduced-fat products in the marketplace, there are now numerous types of reduced, low-fat and nonfat cheese products from which to choose. In these products, fat is primarily replaced by protein or carbohydrate substitutes that act like fats.

Some reduced, low-fat and nonfat cheese products tend not to melt but first soften and then harden. If these cheese substitutes are used to reduce calories, cholesterol, saturated or total fat in recipes, they should probably be used in dishes where they will have less chance of drying out.

Processed Cheese Food

Processed cheese is a mixture of partially ripened and fully ripened cheeses, plus a number of sodium-containing chemicals, colors and flavors for aroma, taste and texture. Processed cheese foods can be moist and tasty, thanks to their chemical mixtures. Since they melt easily when cooked and are relatively inexpensive compared to natural cheeses, they are popular to eat out-of-hand, in cooked dishes and as dips.

The word *processed* means to alter something from its natural state by chemical or physical procedures for convenience, safety or both. Methods of processing include aseptic processing, canning, dehydration, freezing, refrigeration and others.

Dairy milk is a processed food that has been pasteurized to destroy bacteria. Processed cheese often incorporates pasteurized milk. Processing may add saturated fats, trans fats, sodium and sugar. When evaluating the many types of processed cheese and their uses, it is good to keep all of these issues in mind.

COOKING AND BAKING WITH EGGS

Eggs are nutritious and versatile foods in most diets. Whole eggs are often used in custards and creams in dishes like crème anglaise, creme caramel, crème brulee, flan, pastry cream and quiche. Egg white foams are useful for making meringues, mousses, soufflés, zabaglione and sabayon.

Eggs are also important for the flavor, structure and texture in cooked items and baked goods. Eggs firm up with acid, agitation (beating), heat and salt. Too much of any one of these factors and eggs may transform from a moist, semisolid state to a congealed and rubbery muddle.

Safe Egg Handling

The FDA requires that eggs be refrigerated at 45°F or lower. Once cold eggs are exposed to room temperature, they may "sweat," which facilitates the growth of bacteria and may increase the risks of contamination. Refrigerated eggs should not be left at room temperature for more than two hours.

In general, egg whites coagulate between 144° and 149°F. Egg yolks coagulate between 149° and 158°F, and whole eggs coagulate between 144° and 158°F. If eggs are used in recipes with other ingredients, then the egg mixture should be cooked at 160°F to ward off any harmful bacteria. Length of time may vary depending on the added ingredients [13].

Other Ingredients with Eggs

If eggs are cooked with fluid ingredients, they may take longer to cook. The same holds true if eggs are cooked with sugar. Egg recipes that combine fluid ingredients *and* sugar may require higher temperatures for the eggs to set.

Both acids and salt help eggs to set (assuming that these ingredients are compatible with the recipe). If a little salt and lemon juice or vinegar is added during the cooking process, then eggs may develop a creamy tenderness at lower temperatures.

Hot ingredients should slowly be added to cold ingredients; otherwise, eggs may be heated too quickly before they set. A little starch, such as cornstarch or flour, may slow down the egg protein from coagulating too quickly.

When egg whites are whipped into foams, such as in whipped toppings, their proteins link together. With further agitation, the foams usually inflate in size. If the foams separate and lose volume, this may be due to the tools that are used, or any acid, salt, sugar or water that is utilized in preparation.

Whipping egg whites in clean copper or steel bowls promotes tight bonds among the proteins and helps to create glossy foams. The presence of any trace of fat or detergent may interfere with these intricate protein bonds and successful foams.

If an acid, such as lemon juice or cream of tartar, is added to the egg whites, it helps to stabilize foams. Salt will increase the whipping time and decrease the strength of foams. While sugar may delay foaming, it contributes to the stability of foams. Water will make foams lighter, but they may separate.

The odorous nature of cooked eggs may be caused by the exposure of egg whites to high temperatures, especially if the eggs are old. It may also be a reflection of a hen's diet and if it is caged or free-range. A little acid, such as lemon juice or vinegar, in the preparation of eggs may help to reduce this odor.

COOKING FRUITS AND VEGETABLES

The composition of fruits and vegetables is mostly carbohydrates, as opposed to proteins in meats. Some fruits and vegetables have very firm cell walls and can withstand long heating. Others are more sensitive to heat and chemicals, and their color, flavor and nutrients may suffer.

FOOD BYTE

Acidulated water is water that contains an acid, such as citrus juice, vinegar, or white wine. The acid helps to prevent cut fruits and vegetables from turning brown when in contact with air. The amount of water to acid varies depending on the acid. It is best to experiment to see and taste what amount works to help prevent discoloration without affecting the flavor. Cut-up apples, artichokes, avocadoes and potatoes may benefit from acidulated water, as long as taste permits. Adding salt to water may also help to prevent discoloration in fruits and vegetables, but it increases sodium.

Color Changes

When plants lose their color in boiling liquid, it may be due to an acidic or alkaline environment or the escape of gases or heat. It is common for bright green vegetables to lose their hue during cooking. To help retain their colorful pigmentation, a little baking soda (which is alkaline) is often added to the cooking liquid. But this practice may cause vegetables to turn soggy.

In order to preserve the color of vegetables, it is better to shorten the cooking time; use tap water, which is a little alkaline; plunge the vegetables into ice water to halt the cooking process and then reheat briefly; or add a little protective seal of fat or oil right after cooking. This may be a bit of olive oil or butter. The use of an acidic ingredient in a sauce or dressing should be withheld until the very last minute, since the acid may further break down the cell walls.

Flavonoids (polyphenols) are plant pigments that give vegetables and other plants their vibrant colors. *Anthocyanins* are the most plentiful flavonoids; they are responsible for the blue, maroon or purple colors that are present in blackberries, beets, blueberries, cherries and grapes.

During cooking, these fruits and vegetables may lose their deep colors because these pigments are water-soluble. The cooking water may change or become colored as their anthocyanins leach into the boiling water.

Carotenoids are one of the most prevalent naturally occurring plant pigments. Brightly colored red and orange fruits and vegetables, such as apricots, sweet bell peppers and tomatoes, are fairly stable in water, but they are fat-soluble. If a little fat is added to recipes that contain these ruddy fruits and vegetables, then their vibrant colors may dissipate. Trace metals, such as iron from cooking tools or equipment, may also cause some fruits and/or vegetables to appear murky.

Texture Changes

The texture of fruits and vegetables may suffer from cooking. This is because their cell walls break down with heat and release water. At first, fruits and vegetables might lose their crunchiness but still be difficult to chew. With additional heating, their cell walls usually break down further and they become more tender.

Fruits and vegetables may be mushy and unappealing if they are cooked beyond their optimal cooking times. A range of cooking times for cooking vegetables is shown in Table 2-7.

Healthy Cooking Methods

Other healthy methods for cooking fruits and vegetables include microwaving, pressure cooking and stir-frying. Even these methods may be damaging or cause nutrient loss if they are misused. Use the following guidelines to help reduce nutrient losses in fruits and vegetables:

- Avoid presoaking.
- Cook in the least amount of water.

73

TABLE 2-7 Cooking Times for Common Vegetables

Vegetables (steaming)	Cooking Times (steaming in minutes)	Cooking Times (microwaving in minutes)	Cooking Times (other methods in minutes)
Artichokes (whole)	30–60 min	4–5 min each	60 min baked at 425°F
Asparagus	8–10	4–6	5 stir-fried pieces
Beets (whole)	40–60	14–18	60 baked at 350°F
Bell peppers	2–4	2–4	2–3 stir-fried
Broccoli (florets)	5–6	4–5	3–4 stir-fry
Brussels sprouts	6–12	7–8	3–4 stir-fry halves
Cabbage (wedges)	6–9	10–12	2–3 stir-fried shreds
Carrots (sliced)	4–5	4–7	3–4 stir-fried
Cauliflower (florets)	6–10	3–4	3–4 stir-fried
Corn (kernels)	4–6	2 per cup	3–4 stir-fried
Eggplant (diced)	5–6	5–6	10–15 baked at 325°F
Green beans	5–10	6–12	3–4
Greens (beet, kale, spinach)	5–6	3–4	3–4
Mushrooms	4–5	3–4	4–5
Onions (whole)	20–25	6–10	60 baked at 400°F
Potatoes (diced)	10–12	8–10	25–30 baked at 400°F
Squash (sliced)	5–10	3–6	20–30 baked at 350°F
Tomatoes (halves)	2–3	3–4	8–15 baked at 400°F

Source: [14].

- Minimize the contact time with water.
- Balance the amount of heat and water. (Think high heat, minimal water; low heat, more water.)
- Never boil over high heat too long.
- Preserve colors (use the recommendations in the preceding section on color changes).
- Aim for tenderness "to the tooth" rather than softness "to the touch."

COOKING LEGUMES

Dried legumes, such as black beans, kidney and lima, are filled with starchy carbohydrates. They require lengthy cooking times in water to soften, hydrate and expand. Split peas and lentils cook in shorter times.

Legumes may be presoaked in warm water with salt or baking soda to help to break down their cell coats and reduce their cooking time. But this practice has downsides. Salt adds sodium to the cooked legumes (and to the diet). Baking soda may affect both the taste and the mouthfeel of cooked legumes. It also contains sodium (sodium bicarbonate).

As heat and water break down the cell walls of legumes, pectin, the "glue" that holds the cells together, softens and dissolves. This also helps to tenderize the legumes. Too much rapidly boiling water may cause the legumes to disintegrate. To keep the bean coats intact, add an acidic ingredient and one that contains sugar, such as cabbage or tomatoes, and cook the beans at a slow, low temperature. Both the acid and the sugar react with the surface of the beans and prevent hot water from entering the cell walls and cooking the starch. Table 2-8 shows the amount of fluid required, cooking time and yield for common legumes.

COOKING GRAINS

When grains are exposed to heat and liquid, the membrane covering becomes porous, making it possible for water to enter the grains. This causes the starch granules inside the grains to absorb water and form gels, which softens the grains and makes them more palatable.

To cook grains correctly, first rinse them in warm water. The warm water removes residual starch and stickiness, starts the water absorption process, and speeds cooking. In general, use twice as much water or other liquids as the amount of grains.

TABLE 2-8 Cooking Times and Yields for Common Legumes

Legumes (1 cup dry)	Amounts of Fluid (cups)	Cooking Times (minutes/hour)	Yields (cups)
Black beans	4 cups	1–1½ hours	2 cups
Black-eyed peas	3	1 hour	2
Fava beans	3	45 minutes–1 hour	1–2
Garbanzo beans (chick peas)	4	1–3 hours	2
Great Northern beans	3	1½ hours	2–3
Green and yellow split peas	3	45 minutes	2
Kidney beans	3	1 hour	2¼
Lentils	2	30–45 minutes	2½
Lima beans	4	45 minutes–1 hour	2–3
Navy beans	3	45 minutes–1 hour	2–3
Pinto beans	3	1½ hours	2–3

Source: [15].

Bring the ingredients to a boil; then cover the pan tightly, reduce the heat and simmer until the grains are tender. Drain if desired; then return the grains back to the heat and shake the pot or pan for a few seconds over low heat to fluff the grains and to distribute any excess liquid.

Baking with Grains

Some grains contain protein in the form of *gluten,* a natural flour protein. When gluten mixes with water (as in bread baking), it adheres and forms a network. This protein network is one of the elements that cause bread to rise. Another factor is yeast.

Yeast is a microorganism that ferments sugar and produces carbon dioxide gas bubbles. These bubbles become trapped in the protein network of bread dough. They cause gluten to stretch and create structure for the bread dough to rise. The bread dough may double or triple in size.

If the bread dough is punched down, the carbon dioxide bubbles dissipate. The bread dough can be shaped and left to rise again (or can rise during baking). Once the larger gas bubbles are broken up, the bread should have an even and fine texture.

The trouble with gluten is that some people are sensitive to these gluten proteins and must avoid them. There is more information about how to make ingredient substitutions for gluten in Chapter 4 and other information on cooking and baking with grains.

Grains with Soluble Fibers: Barley, Oats and Rye

The stickiness in grains, such as barley, oats and rye, is due to soluble fibers. Soluble fibers are thought to help reduce cholesterol. More information about why this occurs and its effects on coronary heart disease can be found in Chapter 9.

The soluble fibers in barley, oats and rye may also help people feel full because they tend to swell in the stomach, much like they do when these grains are cooked. This feature may have important implications with weight management.

Some other characteristics of barley, oats and rye are that barley can absorb twice the amount of water than wheat; oats swell into a smooth mass, which contributes to their tenderizing effects in baked goods; and rye does not harden after cooking and cooling but lends a soft and moist texture and longer shelf life to some breads.

Rice and Corn

After wheat, rice is the mainstay for much of the world's population. Aromatic rice such as basmati; brown rice; glutinous or "sticky" rice; short-grain, medium-grain and long-grain white rice; parboiled or converted rice; pigmented rice; quick cooking rice; and wild rice are only some of the many rice varieties.

TABLE 2-9 Cooking Times and Yields for Common Grains			
Grains (1 cup dry)	**Amounts of Fluid (cups)**	**Cooking Times (minutes/hour)**	**Yields (cups)**
Hulled barley	3 c	1 hour *plus* 15 minutes	3½
Pearl barley	3	1 hour	3½
Buckwheat groats (kasha)	2	15 minutes	2½
Bulgur wheat	2	15 minutes	2½
Cornmeal (polenta)	3	30 minutes	2–3
Couscous	1–1½	5-10 minutes	1–2
Millet	3	45 minutes	3½
Whole oats	2	45 minutes–1 hour	2–3
Rolled oats	3	30 minutes	3–4
Quinoa	3	15 minutes	3½
Brown rice	2	30–45 minutes	3
Wild rice	3	45 minutes–1 hour	4
Rye	3	45 minutes–1 hour	4

Source: [15].

Since most rice is "milled" to remove the bran (outer coat) and the germ (seed), some consider rice a processed food. Brown rice is unmilled; it generally takes longer to cook, and it has a shorter shelf life due to the intact kernels that may become rancid.

Like rice and wheat, corn is a widely consumed food crop for humans and animals. It has a distinctive color, aroma, taste and texture. Corn can be used in a variety of food ingredients and products and cooking and baking applications.

Cornstarch is a product of corn processing. It is used as a thickener in cake fillings, casseroles, glazes, gravies, pies, puddings, sauces, soups and stews. When cornstarch is mixed with flour in cakes, cookies and pastries, it tenderizes these baked goods. Cornstarch is also used to lightly coat foods before frying and in batters. Table 2-9 shows the amount of fluid required, cooking time and yield for common grains.

COOKING WITH FATS AND OILS

Fats and oils have a range of cooking and baking applications, many of which are discussed in Chapters 3 and 6. First and foremost, fats and oils provide flavor. They contain certain compounds that impart specific flavors and coat the tongue, which permits flavors to linger and interact with other flavors. In the absence of fats and oils (as in some reduced-fat products), flavor may be lacking.

Fats and oils affect appearance. They can make foods look moist and shiny, milk look opaque and baked goods look golden. This is because milk fat refracts light and fats and oils aid in the browning process.

Fats and oils improve texture. They add their own richness and improve mouthfeel. Fats and oils help to tenderize baked goods by hindering gluten formation, which leads to flakier and more tender products. They create emulsions, which contribute to the creaminess of dressings, frozen desserts and sauces. Fats and oils also help to provide crispiness at high temperatures. They accomplish this by drying out food surfaces while retaining moistness.

Morsel "Anybody can make you enjoy the first bite of a dish, but only a real chef can make you enjoy the last." —François Minot (*Guide Michelin* editor)

Despite their essential functions in cooking and baking, fats and oils are concentrated sources of calories. They contain twice the calories per gram of carbohydrates or proteins (9 calories per gram in fats and oils compared to 4 calories per gram in carbohydrates or protein). One may still be able to achieve the benefits of fats and oils in cooking and baking by lightening up and using less.

Useful Ingredients and Functions

Some of these ingredients can make or break the chemical and physical reactions in foods and recipes. Think of them as the missing links that lead to a formula's or recipe's success or failure. This list of useful ingredients is hardly conclusive. Perhaps others will be discovered as new food products or recipes are designed or conventional ones are overhauled.

ALCOHOL

Alcohol has its own flavor and also lends flavor to foods and beverages. It tastes slightly sweet and pungent and unleashes its umami taste in dishes. At lower concentrations, alcohol may help to boost aromas. This is why adding a little alcohol to a dish when it is cooking may help to enhance its flavor. High concentrations of alcohol may bind both aroma and taste.

> **FOOD BYTE**
>
> Acidic foods, such as onions, lemons, or tomatoes, should not come into contact with aluminum foil. The acids can "digest" the foil. Instead, use a nonreactive cover for acidic foods such as parchment or waxed paper. Parchment paper is moisture and grease-resistant, and it stays intact at high oven temperatures. Waxed paper has a protective wax coating that is microwave safe, but it does not withstand high oven temperatures.

Acids, Alkalis and pH Measure

The term *pH* is a measure of the acid or alkali (base) content of a solution. A pH level of 7 is considered to be neutral. This is the pH measure of distilled water.

A pH measure under 7 indicates that a substance is acidic. Foods and beverages such as black coffee, citrus fruits and juices, milk, tea, tomatoes, vinegar, yogurt and wine fall into this category. Milk has a pH measure of 6.2–7.3; black coffee 5.2–6.9; tea 4.9–5.5; tomato juice 4.1–4.6; plain yogurt 4.0–4.1; orange juice 3.3–4.2; wine 3.0–3.5; lemon juice 2–2.6 and vinegar 2.0–3.4. There are considerable variations among growing conditions, processing and varieties. In comparison, gastric acid has a pH measure of 1.

Most of the foods we consume are acidic, especially condiments, fruits, pickled vegetables, vinegars and yogurt. Acids affect both color and texture in cooking and baking. In addition, the pH measure of a food or beverage may have significant effects on the types of processing that are required to safely preserve it.

A pH measure over 7 indicates that a substance is alkaline. Baking soda dissolved in water is alkaline with a pH measure of 9. Most cheese, meats, poultry and vegetables are low acidic and more alkaline. Fresh eggs have a pH measure of 7.6–8.0; shrimp 6.8–7.0; broccoli 6.3–6.9; asparagus 6–6.7; Brussels sprouts 6–6.3 and soybeans 6–6.0. Once again, there are considerable variations among growing conditions, processing and varieties.

Alkaline substances act to neutralize acids in cooking and baking and to break down proteins. This attribute makes them effective in leavening and tenderizing [16,17].

Arrowroot

Arrowroot is a root starch. It does not thin out as much as potato starch or tapioca starch, so arrowroot is useful in thickening. Arrowroot is often used to replace cornstarch or flour in puddings and sauces, without the chalkiness that is sometimes characteristic of these starches. Arrowroot lends a beautiful sheen to finished dishes. However, arrowroot does not hold up to reheating.

Agar (agar agar)

Agar (agar agar) is a gelatinous substance that is extracted from seaweed and processed into flakes, powders and sheets. It is commonly used in Asian cuisines and as a flavorless vegan substitute for gelatin. Agar helps gel, stabilize, texturize and thicken beverages, baked goods, confectioneries, dairy products, dressings, meat products and sauces.

Agar gels at low concentrations; the gel is opaque in color and chewy in texture, making it versatile in both cold and hot dishes. A general rule of thumb is to use 1 tablespoon of agar flakes or 1 teaspoon of agar powder to thicken 1 cup of liquid.

Baking Powder

Baking powder is a chemical leavening agent. It is integral to the rise of various batters during baking. When ingredients are creamed together, baking powder helps to enlarge the bubbles that contribute to leavening. It contains both acidic and alkaline substances: baking soda, one or more acid salts such as cream of tartar or sodium aluminum sulfate, and cornstarch to absorb any moisture.

Double-acting baking powder reacts to the liquid in a batter and heat in two stages. During the first stage, when double-acting baking powder is added to the liquid in a batter, the baking soda reacts with one of the acid salts, and a set of gas bubbles are released. During the second stage, another set of gas bubbles are released when the batter is exposed to the heat of the oven. These gas bubbles cause the batter to rise during baking. If too much baking powder is used in a recipe, then the color and flavor may be affected and browning may be intensified.

Baking Soda

Baking soda is an alkaline or basic ingredient. If dough contains an acidic ingredient, such as buttermilk, citrus fruit juice, sourdough starter or yogurt, baking soda will react with it to produce leavening. Like baking powder, baking soda may negatively affect the color and flavor of finished products and result in a very acidic or bitter taste.

If a recipe contains both baking soda and baking powder, then the baking powder will probably be responsible for the majority of the leavening. The baking soda will likely function more to neutralize any acids in the recipe and add tenderness.

Cocoa and Chocolate

Cocoa is a ground powder that is made from cocoa beans once the cocoa butter has been extracted. Cocoa powder provides color and flavor in biscuits, dairy beverages, cakes and ice cream and in coatings for confections and frozen desserts. By nature, cocoa powder is both acidic and bitter.

Dutch or alkalized cocoa is treated with an alkalizing agent. As a result, its taste is more balanced and milder than cocoa; the color is darker and it is more soluble. However, it cannot be used in recipes that use baking soda as a leavening agent, since it is not acidic like cocoa.

Dutch cocoa is primarily used in recipes that rely on baking powder for leavening, unless there are other acidic ingredients that are present in sufficient quantities. Dutch cocoa easily dissolves in liquids, such as in hot chocolate. Its delicate flavor makes it an ideal complement for some subtly flavored European cakes and pastries. Instant cocoa generally has an emulsifier such as lecithin and sugar added to it for quick dissolving and sweet taste.

Chocolate is a substance that is produced from the seeds of the tropical cacao tree. These seeds are fermented, roasted, shelled, ground and often combined with a flavoring agent and sweetener into a paste, powder or extract.

Chocolate functions as a food (because it is a confection), flavor and ingredient. The many types of chocolate include baking, bitter, bittersweet, chocolate chips, cocoa powder, *couverture* (very high-quality chocolate with extra cocoa butter), dark, milk, plain, semisweet, sweet, unsweetened and white chocolate (which is not really chocolate because it does not contain chocolate liqueur). The sugar and fat content varies in each type of chocolate, which makes them very difficult to substitute in recipes.

Chocolate lends its taste and texture to both savory and sweet applications in cooking and baking. It also provides moistness, richness, structure and thickness in recipes, depending on its composition.

Coconut

Coconut is the fruit of a tropical palm plant. It has a hard shell, edible white flesh and clear liquid, sometimes referred to as "water," which is often used as a beverage. *Coconut flesh* or "meat" is aromatic, chewy in texture and rich in taste.

Coconut milk is the liquid that is obtained by pressing coconut flesh with hot water. Its color and rich taste are attributed to its high oil content. *Coconut oil* is an edible oil that is extracted from a mixture of coconut milk and coconut water. Coconut milk helps to thicken sauces and soups. Coconut oil has a smoke point that is similar to butter, so it may not be useful at higher temperatures. It is often used in blended oils and shortenings.

Desiccated coconut is coconut flesh or meat that has been flaked or shredded and dried. It is available in sweetened and unsweetened versions. It is fibrous and swells slightly when it is exposed to moisture, such as in the batters of brownies, cakes, cookies and pies, and in recipes with savory sauces, including curries and other tropical dishes. Reduced-fat coconut milk is available in some markets, but because there is less fat, this may affect the consistency and flavor of a food or recipe.

Coffee and Tea

Coffee and *tea* are mixtures of acidity, astringency and bitterness, depending on the levels of aromatic compounds, body, caffeine and processing. Both coffee and tea are versatile ingredients in cooking and baking. Coffee and tea brews, extracts and powders may be added to dry or wet ingredients.

Coffee is a brewed beverage that is made from the roasted seeds (which are commonly called beans) of coffee plants and hot water. When black, coffee has a dark color and acidic and bitter flavors, depending on processing.

Coffee is an ingredient in breads, cakes, custards, dessert sauces, frostings, ice creams, pan gravies, stews and sauces. It marries particularly well with chocolate and cocoa, nuts and rum.

Tea is a steeped beverage that is made from the cured leaves of tea shrubs and hot water. When plain, tea has a range of green to dark-brown colors and has slightly bitter and astringent flavors, depending on processing. The four basic types of tea are oolong, black, green and white. *Herbal tea* usually refers to the infusions of fruit or herbs.

Tea is used as an aromatic, edible leaf, marinade, oil, spice rub and tenderizer and in desserts (cookies, ganache with chocolate and cream, muffins and sorbet).

Cream of Tartar

Cream of tartar is a white, powdery substance that is actually a by-product of wine making. It is mostly used to stabilize egg whites because it helps them to whip and hold their foam. Cream of tartar is also used in candy making because it prevents sugar from crystallizing. Plus, cream of tartar provides white, fine crumbs and height in angel food cake and creaminess in frostings.

Flaxseeds and Flaxseed Oil

Flaxseeds and *flaxseed oil* are the seeds and oil of the flax plant that are high in dietary fiber, lignans (estrogen-like chemicals that also act as antioxidants), and omega-3 fatty acids. These health-enhancing substances may help to lower serum cholesterol and benefit certain cancers, as described in Chapters 6 and 9. About one-third of flaxseed is composed of dietary fiber.

It is best to grind flaxseeds before using so fluid may access the gums in the seed coats. These gums produce a thick gel when they are mixed with fluid and act as emulsifiers and stabilizers.

A small amount (about one-fifth) of the flour in some baked goods may be replaced with ground flaxseeds to enhance their nutrient content. Flaxseeds may be used in cookies, muffins and pancakes when eggs are omitted because they perform similar functions. About 1 tablespoon of ground flaxseeds mixed with 3 tablespoons of water may be substituted for 1 whole egg. Baked goods that are made with ground flaxseeds may be slightly chewier than normal, with decreased volume.

Flaxseeds may substitute for oil or shortening in recipes because of their high oil content. Baked goods that are made with ground flaxseed may brown quickly, which may necessitate slight adjustments in time and/or temperature.

Flaxseed oil may be used as a dressing for salads or vegetables or to replace butter on popcorn, potatoes or rice. It should not be used in cooking applications that require heat.

Lard

Lard is pork fat from the back and kidneys, as opposed to *tallow*, which is beef fat. The culinary applications of lard depend on the part of the pig from which it is taken and how the lard is processed. Lard is not as high in saturated fatty acids as once thought.

Due to its relatively large fat crystals, lard is used in baking (especially in pies). It contributes flaky texture and rich taste. Lard is often combined with butter in pastries for its shortening properties. It is also used as a spread, like butter. Because lard has a high smoke point, it can be used for quick frying.

Margarine

Margarine is a butter substitute that is made from vegetable oils that have been solidified by a process called *hydrogenation*. Depending on the type of margarine, the process can be *fully hydrogenated*, causing the oils to solidify, or *partially hydrogenated*, causing the semisolid oils to be lighter and more spreadable with more water, carbohydrate and protein stabilizers. Colorings, flavorings, milk solids and salt are often added.

Trans fats that form during hydrogenation have been connected to cardiovascular disease. In 2003, the FDA issued a regulation that required food manufacturers to list trans fat content on the Nutrition Facts Panel of foods and in some dietary supplements. Due to growing concerns, trans fats have been removed from many ingredients and foods. Solid and partially solid margarines are now made by other formulations [18].

Stick margarine can be used as butter in many cooking and baking applications—but without the same aroma, taste and mouthfeel. Reduced-fat margarines have too much water and stabilizers for use in cooking and baking. As a result, they do not melt, and they often burn. They cannot replace butter in some recipes, such as butter cookies, pie crusts and puff pastries that require specific ratios of fat and moisture.

Mushrooms and Truffles

Mushrooms are *fungi*, like molds and yeast. They have meaty flavors and textures. Their meatiness is due to the natural presence of glutamate, which is also the foundation of the fifth basic taste of umami. When mushrooms are slowly cooked, their amino acids, aromas and sugars concentrate and their textures solidify. Since they are mostly water, mushrooms will release this water upon cooking; then they will reabsorb it and solidify. Salt will accelerate this moisture loss and will concentrate as the mushrooms solidify.

While mushrooms live off plants and plant remains and take on their neighboring flavors, *truffles* grow underground and develop musky aromas. Black truffles benefit by slow cooking, while white truffles are best sliced raw into dishes right before service.

Seaweed

Seaweed is derived from large sea plants, particularly those that occupy Asian and British waters. There are thousands of varieties of seaweed. Most seaweed is in shades of mild-brown to deep-red. They are sulfur-like to spicy in flavor, due to their protein, mineral and vitamin contents. The distinctive colors, flavors and textures of seaweed help to determine their uses in recipes.

Most seaweed only requires soaking and quick cooking. The longer seaweed cooks, the more pronounced their fishy flavors become. More information about cooking seaweed can be found in Chapter 5.

Shortening

Shortening is a solid vegetable fat that is typically made by hydrogenating, or solidifying vegetable oils. Trans-free shortenings are now available. Shortening is used in baking to help make products crumbly, flaky and tender. It is 100 percent fat as opposed to butter and lard, which are about 80 percent fat, so shortening results in especially tender cakes, cookies and pie crusts.

Shortening achieves these attributes by cutting through or "shortening" the dough, which helps it to bake into separate pastry layers. But shortening does not have the flavor of butter. For this reason, shortening is sometimes butter flavored.

Soy Milk and Soy Foods

Soy milk and soy foods are rich in carbohydrates, fats, minerals, proteins, vitamins and other nutrients. Soy milk may be added to recipes in a one-to-one ratio in place of dairy milk, but it does not have the same aroma, color, taste and other characteristics as dairy milk. Plus, brands of soy milk vary.

Soy milk that is in aseptic packages tends to be sweet and is best used in desserts. In savory dishes, some soy milks may taste "beany" and interfere with other flavors. Soy milk may also curdle when boiled. To avoid curdling, use soy milk in recipes with few to no acids and/or add it at the end of cooking.

Soy cheese, soy creamer, soy ice cream, soy milk (full and reduced-fat) and soy yogurt are a few of the many soy foods that are available as dairy substitutes. These substitutions are discussed in greater detail in Chapter 5.

Starters

Starters are portions of fermented dough or batter and fresh or wild yeast. They function as natural leaveners when added to flour and water mixtures in bread making. A starter is sometimes referred to as the "Mother Starter" or "Madre."

Starters are used to speed fermentation time and add distinct aroma, taste and texture. Sourdough starter with acid-forming bacteria is a popular ingredient that flavors the sourdough breads that bear its name.

Vinegar

Vinegar is a sour liquid that is made by fermenting substances that contain sugar, such as fruit or wine. It is used as a condiment to add flavor or as a preservative, as in pickling. Vinegar contributes acidic notes to foods, both in aroma and taste. It also "cooks" foods with its acidity by breaking down their structures and softening their textures.

The many types of vinegar include balsamic, cider, distilled white, malt, rice and sherry, which all have different flavor notes. Some of their flavors are quite acerbic and assertive. Their uses in cooking and baking depend on their flavor profiles and other compatible (and incompatible) ingredients.

Wheat Bran and Wheat Germ

Wheat bran is the outer hull of the wheat kernel, which is typically removed during processing. Wheat bran is rich in fiber and other noncalorie nutrients. *Wheat germ* is the embryo of the wheat kernel, much like an egg yolk is the "kernel" of a whole egg. Since the germ contains fats that can decompose, it is removed in the refining of whole wheat flour into white flour.

Wheat bran and wheat germ are intact in whole-grain flour. When wheat bran is present in a recipe, it may look less refined in texture and smell and taste earthier. Cooking and/or baking time may be affected. The fat in wheat germ has its own flavor, and it carries other flavors. Eliminating the wheat germ in a recipe may reduce its taste and texture.

Wine

Wine is the naturally fermented juice of grapes. It is also an alcoholic beverage that is created from fruits and even vegetables. Grape varieties, with their characteristic body, color and flavor, will influence the compatibility of wine with other ingredients and foods.

Wine is an acidic ingredient that contains both citric and tartaric acids in varying amounts. Depending on the amount of acid, wine may also taste sweet or sweet and sour.

The flavor notes of wine are important to cooking and baking and may affect the final outcomes of recipes. Wine is a useful source of sourness, particularly when it is reduced. It helps to balance the umami taste in recipes, such as in a reduced stock or stew. While doing so, wine helps to enhance the sweet taste in a recipe.

For example, wine balances the beefiness in beef bourguignon (beef braised in red wine, traditionally red Burgundy, and beef broth with pearl onions and mushrooms). It also brings out the sweetness in the vegetables. In stewed fruits, wine helps to bring out sweetness, temper earthiness and add tanginess.

Yeast and Brewer's yeast

Yeast is a class of fungi that requires a warm and moist environment and a food source (such as honey, molasses or white sugar) to grow. In baking, yeast functions as a dough developer, flavor binder and leavener. Yeast helps to produce the carbon dioxide gas that functions as a leavening agent.

Morsel "In cooking, as in all arts, simplicity is a sign of perfection."— Maurice Edmund Sailland Curnonsky (French writer and Prince of French Gastronomes, 1872–1956)

Brewer's yeast is used for brewing beer and wine. It converts sugar to alcohol and carbon dioxide during fermentation. Brewer's yeast also helps to determine the flavor of beer. In beer production, the carbon dioxide gas bubbles break away from the fermenting liquid and alcohol is collected. In baking, the carbon dioxide bubbles are contained by the dough and then released during baking, which causes the batter to rise.

WHY RECIPES SUCCEED OR FAIL

A recipe is an experiment in execution. Yet, some recipes are poorly written. Other recipes have gaps or take ingredients and instructions for granted. One of the most important factors in whether or not a recipe succeeds is the preparation.

Just like in an experiment, the ingredients should all be prepped, measured, "in their place" and ready for use. All of the necessary tools and equipment should also be close at hand. The oven should be calibrated and preheated to the proper temperature, and ingredients should be at room temperature, hot or cold as required. Finally, one should have a good working knowledge of the recipe. In French, this procedure is called *mise en place*, which helps to ensure that a recipe produces the anticipated results.

Even with excellent preparation, recipes may still fail. One must adhere to the given ingredients—at least during the first execution. In this chapter, the ingredients, foods and beverages that contain or support carbohydrates, lipids, proteins and water are featured, including how each of these functions in recipes. Stray too far from these ingredients, foods and beverages, and the aroma, taste, texture and/or other sensory components of recipes may suffer.

The right cooking and baking equipment and tools should be used as instructed. They, too, could make big differences between recipes that work and ones that fail. For example, if a recipe calls for pasta to be cooked in a stockpot and a deep fry pan is used instead, the fry pan has more surface water that is exposed to the air than a stockpot. This may cause rapid evaporation of the cooking water, which is not desirable, since there may be less water to cook the pasta. Recommended basic cooking and baking equipment and tools are provided in Chapter 3.

The right techniques should be followed to correctly prepare recipes. For example, if a recipe calls for lightly spooning flour from a bag or canister into a cup, then leveling the cup with a knife or spatula, this technique should be precisely executed. If the flour is scooped into the cup, it may become compacted and throw off the exact measurement of flour. This is a common mistake that may result in more flour than what is called for in a recipe. It is a subtle difference that may make a big impact on a recipe's success.

Finally, it is wise to review the entire recipe from start to finish before beginning to cook or bake. Well-written recipes will list the amounts and descriptions of each ingredient, guide every step in logical order, and prepare the chef or cook for what to expect and alternative courses of action to take. Misread or circumvent any of these steps and the ingredients, temperatures, timing and/or other factors may be overlooked, which may cause recipes to fail.

For example, preheat the oven *at the start* of the recipe to the *right temperature; lower the heat* as the recipe reads; measure the dry ingredients *separately* from the liquid ingredients; sift the dry ingredients and *then combine* with the liquid ingredients; and so forth. Either fast or inaccurate review of recipes may miss these specific directives.

All said and done, mistakes do happen. Following are some common mistakes in the execution of recipes, along with some of their remedies.

> **Morsel** *"A meal without salt is no meal."* —Hebrew proverb

COMMON MISTAKES IN RECIPE EXECUTION

- *Too much or too little salt:* Using too much salt can make the finished dish look brackish. Too little salt can make it flavorless. This is because salt both acts as an ingredient and interacts with other ingredients—boosting some tastes and diminishing others.

  Too much or too little salt is often the result of not measuring correctly or measuring right over a bowl or pot. The natural sodium content of the other ingredients in a recipe must also be considered. For example, recipes with celery, olives and/or tomatoes (especially canned tomato products) may already be high in sodium without additional salt.

  Salty ingredients should first be added in small quantities and then adjusted throughout recipes, unless indicated otherwise. Salt may be added right before serving to boost saltiness and round out flavor. Try to find the balance without oversalting.

  Sweetness appears to lessen saltiness, while bitterness and umami tend to increase its perception. For example, if soups or stews seem too salty, then add some sweet ingredients, such as carrots or onions, to counterbalance the saltiness. If broccoli with its bitter taste or mushrooms with their umami are already present, then the saltiness may be amplified.

  A little sourness may emphasize saltiness—for example, a splash of vinegar on french fries or cooked greens. The exception is when an ingredient is salty-sweet, in which case a little sourness enhances the sweetness. For example, if a little lemon juice is squeezed over salty-sweet fish and rice, such as smoked salmon risotto, then less of the salty-smoky taste of the salmon may be perceived and more of the sweetness from both the salmon and the rice.

- *Too much or too little fat:* A little fat or oil is invaluable for flavor and essential to the outcome of some recipes—even in reduced-fat cooking and baking. The functions and features of fats and oils in cooking and baking are shown in Table 2-10.

  Fats and oils help to supply the rich and intense flavors that are derived from caramelization and the Maillard reaction. They are **viscous**, or thick and sticky, and they help to provide moisture in recipes. If too little fat or oil is used, the foods may be dry, flavorless, thin and/or nontextured. Consumer acceptance may be poor. Fat substitutes may help to rectify some of these problems.

TABLE 2-10 Functions and Features of Fats and Oils in Cooking and Baking

Functions	Features
Appearance	*Adds* color, smoothness and shininess
Emulsification	*Emusifies* cream soups, gravies, mayonnaise, puddings, salad dressings and sauces
Flavor/mouthfeel	*Contributes* aroma, coolness, lubrication, taste, texture and thickness
Heat transfer	*Supports* frying and sautéing
Nutrients	*Contains* calories, lipids, minerals and vitamins
Melting point	*Softens* candies
Plasticity	*Shapes* confections, icings and pastries
Satiety	*Provides* satisfaction
Shortening	*"Cuts"* biscuits, cakes, cookies and pastries
Solubility	*Resists* water; *dissolves* in fats
Texture	*Creates* creaminess, ease in slicing, elasticity, flakiness, tenderness and viscosity

Source: [19].

83

If there is too much fat or the wrong proportions of fat to liquid in recipes, they may fail. Emulsions may not work or they may break down. Fats may overmelt and cause foods to be greasy or oily. Too much softened fat may squeeze out of pastries. Too much firm fat may tear dough. A higher proportion of fat in ice cream production may turn into butter. Too much fat in braises, soups and stews may require cooling, congealing and discarding; the same is true when cooking protein foods, such as fish, meats and poultry with too much fat, or rendering too much fat. They may also require chilling and disposing of the congealed fat.

- *Too much starch or sugar:* The fact that cooking causes starches to absorb cooking liquid, soften and swell presents both promise and problems in cooking and baking. These features provide promise because they help starches to gel and develop gelling properties. A whole host of ingredients, food products and foods and beverages may ensue.

These features present problems because once starches cool, they may *retrograde*, or solidify. If there is too much starch, the mixtures may become too gummy, and then too firm. The flip side is also true: too little starch and the starch granules may not be sufficient in number to take up fluids and coagulate. An example of **retrogradation** is risotto (a creamy rice dish) that solidifies upon chilling. It is difficult to restore risotto to its warm creaminess.

Like salt, sugar has its own taste. In addition to sweetening foods, sugar enhances other tastes. A little salt intensifies sweetness and helps to make dishes satisfying (think salted butter and honey on toast). Umami intensifies sweetness, too (think shrimp stir-fried with soy sauce).

Sourness minimizes sweetness (think sour cream in pea soup). Bitterness also lessens sweetness (think semisweet chocolate sprinkles over frosted cupcakes).

Sweetness should be reduced in recipes that taste sickly sweet in order to conserve carbohydrate calories. Conversely, sweetness should be enhanced in recipes that taste too subtle because their flavors may be uninspiring.

Too little sugar and baked goods may become dry; candy and cookies may disintegrate; dried fruits may decompose; frozen confections may solidify; and glazes may be hazy rather than glossy.

- *Too much or too little liquid:* Recipes call for a certain amount of liquid for a reason. For instance, different grains require varying amounts of liquid for absorption and swelling. This amount of liquid that is required is dependent on the strength of the cell walls to break down upon heating and their ability to take up liquid. Use too much or too little liquid and the cooked grains may become too soggy or too firm.

The amounts of water that are used to cook pasta are specified in recipes and should be followed. This is to promote absorption, dilute the starches and separate the noodles.

The proportion of liquid in fresh pasta dough may affect its consistency. If there is too much liquid, it may be sticky and difficult to knead or mix. If there is too little liquid, the dough may become dense, dry and/or firm. The right amount of liquid produces dough that is airy, elastic and soft.

Being a food scientist in the kitchen may help to rectify these issues and others. By viewing each recipe as a food science experiment, one may discover why a recipe succeeds or fails. Some solutions for repairing foods and recipes follow.

84

FOOD BYTE

The term **nonreactive** means that substances or materials do not act in response to other substances. In regards to cooking utensils and equipment, nonreactive means that materials do not react with the foods that are prepared or cooked within them. Reactive metals, such as aluminum, unseasoned cast iron and/or copper, can produce a metallic taste and off-color. This is the reason why cooking equipment is often clad, or lined, with a nonreactive material, such as stainless steel.

How to Repair Ingredients, Foods and Recipes

Despite taking painstaking care, sometimes ingredients, foods and recipes fail. Rather than start anew, food scientists use their knowledge in biology, chemistry and nutrition to forge ahead, armed with information about what went wrong and how it may be fixed. Some ingredient and technique problems follow, along with some suggested solutions.

SUGARS: CARAMELIZING PROBLEMS AND REDUCING OPTIONS

Sucrose, or granulated white table sugar, melts at very high temperatures—over 300°F; then it begins to caramelize. *Caramelize* means "to brown," but it also indicates that sucrose has begun to decompose, or break down into other sugars. Some of these sugars then recombine. Liquid sugar is first clear, then it changes to brown, and finally it becomes a dark caramel color. There may be over 100 sugars that form between these clear and caramelized states.

Certain conditions or factors are required for foods to brown at temperatures that are lower than 300°F. These include a nonacidic environment and the presence of protein and sugar. Acids such as citrus juice, vinegar or wine may prevent browning. However, certain proteins and sugars may still be able to overcome the interference of these acids.

Reducing sugars are sugars with specific shapes, as detected under a microscope. They contain a reactive aldehyde (CHO) group and may donate their ions to other molecules. Thermal processing may cause reactions between the reactive group of reducing sugars and the amino group of proteins. These reactions are called the Maillard reaction, which is responsible for altered flavors and browning. (The Maillard reaction is discussed earlier in this chapter.) Very high heat with little water may cause caramelization and also result in browning.

Corn syrup, with its simple sugar glucose, is a reducing sugar. When corn syrup is used in ingredients, foods and recipes, it assists in browning at lower temperatures. If 1 tablespoon of corn syrup is substituted for 1 tablespoon of granulated white sugar (as in some cookie recipes), a browner and crispier product may result.

Another example of the browning and crispiness that corn syrup may provide is when it is used to baste protein foods, such as poultry. The ever-popular use of barbecue sauce to baste grilled chicken is an example. The label of commercial barbecue sauce will probably list corn syrup as an ingredient.

When poultry is grilled, juices are released that contain fats, natural sugars and residual proteins. The sugars in poultry are stored in the muscle meat as glycogen. More information about sugar and glycogen is presented in Chapter 4.

The glucose in the corn syrup and fats, proteins and sugars in the poultry unite and create browning. With the intense heat of grilling, browning occurs rapidly. The heat can be controlled by moving the poultry around the grill and away from the heat source. The poultry should be basted infrequently to prevent overcaramelizing or burning.

STARCHES: GELLING PROBLEMS

The process of *gelatinization*—when starches take up liquid and swell upon heating—was discussed earlier in this chapter. Starches include arrowroot, cornstarch, potato starch, rice starch, tapioca starch and flour, and liquids include fruit juice, stock, vegetable juice, water, wine or some combination of these liquids.

Different starches become thicker at different points with the application of heat. Sometimes it takes a gentle boil, and other times it requires a full boil. It is best to watch this process very carefully and be patient before more starch is added to thicken the solution.

Once starch has gelatinized, or set, it should not be stirred or the gel may be broken. Starches such as cornstarch and/or flour tend to create a thick, clear gel when hot; then they cool to cloudy, and they may separate upon freezing. Arrowroot and tapioca gels are clearer no matter what the temperature, and they freeze better than cornstarch and flour-based gels.

FOOD BYTE

All-purpose (AP) flour is actually a blend of high-gluten hard wheat flour and low-gluten soft wheat flour. It is mainly the endosperm of the wheat kernel. The bran and germ are removed in processing. AP flour is available in both bleached and unbleached varieties. Unbleached AP flour is thought to have less chemicals and processing. AP flour has multipurposes for all kinds of baking, including biscuits, cakes, cookies, muffins and quick and yeast breads. Cake flour, with its fine grain and lower protein, can be substituted for AP flour in some recipes. Substitute 1 cup plus 2 tablespoons of cake flour for 1 cup of AP flour and evaluate the results.

STARCHES: GLUTEN PROBLEMS

Flours differ in the amount of gluten or protein they contain. High-gluten flours provide protein and structure to baked goods. They trap tiny carbon dioxide gas bubbles that are given off by yeast and help to expand the dough.

High-gluten flours are essential for good rise in breads and breadstuffs with firm textures. They produce stretchy but strong dough with firm texture for pasta and strudel, limit cookies from spreading too much, and expand pastries with the help of steam. If gluten is overdeveloped from too much mixing, it could toughen the finished products. Too much sugar destroys gluten and is one of the causes of dense bread loaves.

Low-gluten flours are preferred in recipes that contain leaveners (baking powder or baking soda), since too much gluten may interfere with their rise. A lower-protein flour, such as cake, pastry or soft flour, may be better for biscuits, muffins, pies and quick breads that incorporate leaveners. They will be more tender with a softer crumb.

STARCHES: STALING AND RETROGRADING PROBLEMS

Staling is both a chemical and physical process that reduces palatability. Freshly made bread should be stored at room temperature if it going to be quickly consumed, or it should be frozen to prevent staling. Bread stales rapidly at temperatures that are just above freezing. Moisture moves out of the starch granules, which degelatinizes the starch and leads to hard and leathery texture. Preservatives and emulsifiers, such as cinnamon, egg yolks or pureed prunes, may help to prevent staling.

Retrogradation occurs when long-grain rice and other grains are cooked and then cooled. Some of the starch molecules bond together and may cause the rice to harden. Retrogradation may be reduced by fats, emulsifiers or glucose. For example, vinegar and oil–type salad dressing may be added to rice while it is still hot, or shorter-grain rice with less surface area may be substituted to help reduce this state.

FRUITS: DETERIORATION AND RIPENING PROBLEMS

Fragile vegetables, such as some lettuces and greens, easily rot and turn slimy. This may be due to surface water and bacteria. First, soak fragile vegetables in cold water to fill their cells as much as possible. Then dry them between paper towels or a clean towel. Carefully squeeze out the air and refrigerate in a vegetable towel or bag. This process may delay (but not prevent) rotting. The idea is to reduce both water and oxygen, two promoters of deterioration.

The ethylene gas that is given off by some fruits, such as ripe apples and bananas, helps to quicken the *ripening* process. To hasten the ripening of underripe fruits and vegetables, place an apple or very ripe banana nearby or in a brown paper bag.

Berries, citrus fruits, cherries, dates and grapes should be picked when they are ripe and ready to eat, as they will not ripen any further. This is because the plants contain the ripening substances and sugars. When ripe, these fruits should be aromatic, juicy and plump for the best taste. They should be carefully stored and consumed within a few days.

Other fruits ripen only after they are picked, such as avocadoes. As avocadoes ripen, their color changes from green to black and their irregular skin slightly yields to the touch.

Apples, bananas, melons, peaches, persimmons, plums and tropical fruits continue to ripen and improve in sweetness after they are picked. Figs, kiwi fruit, mangoes and papayas will ripen in color, juiciness and texture once they are picked, but their aromas may not be as pronounced as when they are still on the trees. This is because the trees contain the aromatic compounds. Look for even color and slightly yielding texture as indicators of ripeness in these fruits [20,21].

VEGETABLES: COLOR PROBLEMS

Attention is given to color loss in vegetable cooking earlier in this chapter. There is additional information in Chapters 3 and 7. In summary, heat may cause bright green vegetables to lose their color during cooking.

Quick cooking and the least exposure to water or other fluids are recommended. Furthermore, acidic ingredients, such as citrus juice, tomatoes and vinegar, should be withheld during the very last minutes to help avert color loss.

The firm cellular structures of some vegetables are vulnerable to both heat and acids. Raw green vegetables are less affected than cooked vegetables because their protective cell walls have not been exposed to heat. If green vegetables are cut into small pieces to facilitate faster cooking, this may help retain the phytochemical *chlorophyll*, the source of their bright green color.

Potatoes and onions may turn a brownish-yellow when cooked with alkaline ingredients, such as egg whites, or in certain metal pots, such as aluminum or iron. This reaction may be due to the *flavonoids* in potatoes and onions, plant substances with antioxidant properties. More information about flavonoids is found in Chapter 7. An acidic ingredient, such as cream of tartar, lemon juice or vinegar, may be added to help neutralize the alkaline environment in which these vegetables are cooked and prevent discoloration. Acidic tomatoes, chili peppers and/or onions may also help to prevent avocadoes from turning brown in guacamole.

Other colorful *photochemicals*, or plant compounds that undergo the effects of cooking, include *anthocyanins*, *betalains* and *carotenoids*:

- Anthocyanins, found in ruddy cherries, red and purple grapes, red cabbage, walnuts and wine, tend to lose their color rapidly during cooking. Like bright green vegetables with chlorophyll, fruits and vegetables with anthocyanins should be quickly cooked with little exposure to water or other fluids.

    Red cabbage loses its color and turns green in some sauces because of two chemical reactions: one that produces a blue pigment and one that produces a yellow pigment. When these two pigments combine, they produce a blue-green color. To prevent this reaction, a little acidic lemon juice or vinegar may be added to the cabbage. Likewise, a little acidic buttermilk or yogurt may be added to cherries or walnuts during baking to help prevent their discoloration.
- Betalains, found in purple-red beets, rapidly stain other ingredients. To prevent staining, once beets are cooked, they should be carefully dried and added last to other ingredients.

    If beets are marinated in an acidic ingredient, such as lemon juice or vinegar, it may darken their color. The reverse is true with grapes: the longer grapes are immersed in a sauce or dressing, the greater the chance that they will lose their color.
- Carotenoids, found in brightly colored orange and red fruits and vegetables, such as carrots, tomatoes, pumpkins and sweet potatoes, generally retain their color unless they are overcooked.

FATS: CURDLING AND SEPARATING PROBLEMS

One of the features of fats is that they can hold dissimilar ingredients in a suspension or emulsion. To understand this notable feat, one must first recognize a solution. A *solution* is a uniform mixture of two or more substances: a *dissolving agent* and a *solvent*, such as water (dissolving agent) and sugar (solvent). The components of a solution are microscopic atoms, ions and/or molecules.

In a *suspension*, the solvent components are larger than the microscopic components of a solution. They may be evenly distributed by mechanical means, such as agitation, but the solvent components may eventually settle out.

An *emulsion* is a mixture of two or more liquids that normally do not mix, such as vinegar and oil in a vinaigrette. Emulsions usually require an emulsifier or they may separate. *Hollandaise sauce*, a classic emulsified sauce, will curdle or separate if it is not made "just right." Suspensions and emulsions are explained in greater detail earlier in this chapter and in Chapter 6.

If an emulsified sauce begins to curdle, remove the saucepan from the heat source. Lower the temperature by swirling an ice cube into the sauce. Discard the ice cube before it fully melts and vigorously beat (agitate) the sauce to bring it back to a suspension. While the sauce may be restored, it may still not be stable. If this does not bring the sauce back to suspension at all, one may need to redo the emulsifying process with dry, clean equipment.

If the sauce is not served immediately, keep it lukewarm (about 110°–120°F) by placing it in a hot water "bath" that is another pot of hot water (about 150°F); then whisk it before using. If the sauce is refrigerated, it must first be brought to room temperature before it is gently warmed by using a hot water bath.

SERVE IT FORTH

Sensory science plays a very important role in what we choose to eat and drink. In fact, there are institutions throughout the world that study its interdisciplinary relationship with food and nutrition in matters of disease, health, pollution, safety and security.

The Monell Chemical Senses Center, established in 1968 in Philadelphia, Pennsylvania, is one such nonprofit, independent, scientific institution. It conducts interdisciplinary research on taste, smell, chemical-sensory (chemosensory) irritation, and flavor.

The six major areas of research at Monell are sensation and perception, neuroscience and molecular biology, environmental and occupational health, nutrition and appetite, chemical ecology and communications, and health and well-being.

- Research in sensation and perception shows how humans recognize, distinguish and respond to chemical irritants, odors and tastes in our environment. It also demonstrates how age, experience, the environment, gender and genetics influence our senses.
- Research at the molecular level provides information about the chemicals in odors and tastes. These chemicals trigger electrical signals that are used by the central nervous system, including the brain.
- Research on environmental and occupational health explores the effects of chemicals in the environment, our home and work on our well-being.
- Research in nutrition and appetite investigates food and flavor throughout the human life cycle. It looks at how the chemicals in odors and tastes affect appetite, diabetes, digestion, metabolism and obesity.
- Research in chemical ecology and communications assesses the roles of chemical signals in human reproduction and communication. It also studies birds and reptiles to help protect endangered species and to minimize crop damage.
- Research in health and well-being examines sensory dysfunction and its effects on human lives.

Anyone who is "cooking up" new aromas, flavors, tastes and textures needs to be aware of the Monell Chemical Senses Center and other institutions throughout the world where similar research is performed. Nutrition, food science and culinary professionals can then translate this research into ingredients, products, foods and beverages that are not only pleasing to the senses but healthy and tasteful, too.

The following three activities are designed to explore potential research at the Monell Chemical Senses Center. While they are fictitious, they demonstrate the many possibilities that could materialize.

Three additional activities can be found within the *Culinary Nutrition* website at www.culinarynutrition. elsevier.com.

1. *Sensation and perception:* It has been said that "no food is consumed unless it tastes good, and no food is nutritious unless it is consumed." You have been asked to design a new food with sensory appeal for children who are picky eaters. It should appeal to each of the five basic senses. Which food will you design and why? How will this food be tested for sensory satisfaction? Which elements of food science, nutrition and the culinary arts will be incorporated in testing?
2. *Neuroscience and molecular biology:* The brain is a communications network that operates through chemical messengers. This is where smell and taste are registered and identified. You have been charged with the responsibility of developing a new beverage that appeals to teenage senses of smell and taste. It should appeal to each of the five tastes. There are many scents, and they are difficult to categorize like tastes. Which beverage will you design and why? How will this beverage be tested for smell and taste? Which elements of food science, nutrition and the culinary arts are incorporated in this design?
3. *Environmental and occupational health:* Chemicals in our environment, home and work may have both short- and long-term effects on our well-being. You have been given the task of developing guidelines

for cooking and storing foods to minimize food waste (which is a burden on our environment). Which guidelines in this chapter would you include? Which elements of food science, nutrition and the culinary arts are integrated in these guidelines?

WHAT'S COOKING?

1. Acids in foods and food colors

Objectives
○ To test foods for acidity
○ To see how acidity affects the color of food

Materials
One half of one red cabbage, saucepan, hot water, clean pitcher, sieve, three ceramic or glass jars or bowls, measuring spoons, lemon juice, plain yogurt, white vinegar

Procedure
1. Tear the cabbage into small pieces.
2. Put the pieces into the saucepan.
3. Pour enough boiling water to cover.
4. Let the mixture cool for about one hour.
5. Pour the cabbage water through a sieve into a clean pitcher. (The cabbage can be discarded.)
6. Note the color of the cabbage water on the Data Sheet like the one that follows.
7. Divide and pour the cabbage water equally into the three ceramic or glass bowls.
8. Add 2 tablespoons of lemon juice to one of the bowls. Note the color on the Data Sheet.
9. Add 2 tablespoons of plain yogurt to the second bowl. Note the color on the Data Sheet.
10. Add 2 tablespoons of white vinegar to the third bowl. Note the color on the Data Sheet.

Evaluation
○ Why are ceramic or glass bowls or jars used?
○ Compare and contrast the colors of the three solutions.
○ Why were each of these substances used?
○ What does this exercise demonstrate about the acids in foods and food colors, particularly the red color of the cabbage?

Culinary applications
What guidelines should be followed when experimenting with acids in food product or recipe production? (Consider equipment, ingredients and techniques.)

Data Sheet

Contents of Ceramic or Glass Bowl or Jar	Color
#1: Cabbage water *plus* lemon juice	
#2: Cabbage water *plus* yogurt	
#3: Cabbage water *plus* white vinegar	

2. Alkalis in foods and food colors

Objectives
○ To test foods for alkalis
○ To see how alkalinity affects the color of food

Materials
One-half of one red cabbage, saucepan, boiling water, sieve, clean pitcher, four ceramic or glass jars or bowls, measuring spoons, cooking water from boiled vegetables, liquids from canned vegetables, cream of tartar, egg white

Procedure
1. Tear the cabbage into small pieces.
2. Put the pieces into the saucepan.
3. Pour enough boiling water to cover.
4. Let the mixture cool for about one hour.

89

5. Pour the cabbage water through a sieve into a clean pitcher. (The cabbage can be discarded.)
6. Note the color of the cabbage water on the Data Sheet like the one that follows.
7. Divide the cabbage water among the four ceramic or glass jars or bowls.
8. Add 2 tablespoons of boiled vegetable liquid to one of the jars or bowls.
9. Note the color on the Data Sheet.
10. Add 2 tablespoons of canned vegetable liquid to the second jar or bowl.
11. Note the color on the Data Sheet.
12. Add 1 tablespoon of cream of tartar to the third jar or bowl.
13. Note the color on the Data Sheet.
14. Add one egg white to the fourth bowl.
15. Note the color on the Data Sheet.

Evaluation
○ Why are ceramic or glass bowls or jars used?
○ Compare and contrast the colors of the four solutions.
○ Why were each of these particular substances used?
○ What does this exercise demonstrate about alkalis in foods and food colors, particularly the red color of the cabbage?

Culinary applications
What guidelines should be followed when experimenting with alkalis in food product or recipe production? (Consider equipment, ingredients and techniques.)

Data Sheet

Contents of Ceramic or Glass Bowl or Jar	Color
Cabbage water *plus* boiled vegetable liquid	
Cabbage water *plus* canned vegetable liquid	
Cabbage water *plus* cream of tartar	
Cabbage water *plus* egg white	

3. **Taste tests: the five basic tastes**
   Objective
   ○ To determine the way that foods taste on the tongue and inside the mouth
   Materials
   Powdered sugar, powdered coffee, powdered lemon candy (crushed with a rolling pin between two sheets of waxed paper or in a food processor), fine salt, powdered dry mushrooms (available in the herb and spice section of a supermarket or pulverize dry mushrooms in a food processor), water
   Procedure
   1. Wash your hands.
   2. Dip one finger into one of the powders and dab it on your tongue, the roof of your mouth, and the inside of your cheeks.
   3. Note the taste or lack of taste on the Data Sheet like the one that follows.
   4. Rinse your hands and mouth with water.
   5. Repeat the procedure with each of the remaining powders, rinsing your hands and mouth with water between each tasting. *Only put your finger once into each powder.* Record each of your observations on the Data Sheet.
   Evaluation
   ○ Identify each of the basic tastes and where you perceive them inside of your mouth. (You may not taste some of the powders at all.)
   ○ Compare the intensity of the tastes at different points throughout your mouth.
   ○ What does this exercise demonstrate about the basic tastes?
   Culinary applications
   What guidelines should be followed when experimenting with basic tastes in food product or recipe production? (Consider equipment, ingredients and techniques.)

Data Sheet

Substances	Basic Tastes	Taste on Tongue	Taste on Roof of Mouth	Taste on Inside of Cheeks
Powdered sugar				
Powdered coffee				
Powdered lemon candy				
Fine salt				
Powdered/pulverized dry mushrooms				

4. **Taste tests: sugar and sugar substitutes**

Note: Do not do this exercise if you have sensitivity to sugar substitutes.

Objective

○ To determine how sugar and sugar substitutes taste on the tongue and inside the mouth.

Materials

Powdered sugar, variety of powdered sugar substitutes (at least 3), water

Procedure

1. Wash your hands.
2. Dip one finger into one of the powdered sugar substitutes and dab it on your tongue, the roof of your mouth, and the inside of your cheeks.
3. Note the taste or lack of taste and any other effects on the Data Sheet like the one that follows.
4. Rinse your hands and mouth with water.
5. Repeat the procedure with each of the remaining powdered sugar substitutes, rinsing your hands and mouth with water between each tasting. *Only put your finger once into each powdered sugar substitute.* Record each of your observations on the Data Sheet.

Evaluation

○ Try to identify each of the tastes and where you taste them inside of your mouth. (You may not taste some of these powdered sugar substitutes at all. If not, then why?)
○ Compare the intensity of each of their tastes at different points throughout your mouth.
○ What does this exercise show about the basic taste of sugar compared to each of these powdered sugar substitutes?

Culinary applications

What guidelines should be followed when experimenting with powdered sugar substitutes in food product or recipe production? (Consider equipment, ingredients and techniques.)

Data Sheet

Substances	Basic Tastes	Taste on Tongue	Taste on Roof of Mouth	Taste on Inside of Cheeks
Sugar substitute #1				
Sugar substitute #2				
Sugar substitute #3				
Others . . .				

5. **Smell tests: jelly beans**

Objective

○ To test the recognition of odor and flavor with and without the help of the nose

Materials

Three different colored and flavored jelly beans, water

Procedure

1. Wash your hands.
2. Place the three jelly beans on a table or counter in front of you.
3. Pinch your nose shut with one hand.
4. Put one jelly bean into your mouth; chew it well and swallow it. (Do not take your fingers off your nose.)

5. Release your fingers. Note the taste or lack thereof on the Data Sheet like the one that follows.
6. Rinse your mouth with water.
7. Pinch your nose shut with one hand.
8. Place the second jelly bean into your mouth.
9. When the jelly bean is partially chewed, remove your finger from your right nostril; continue to hold your left nostril shut.
10. Reverse nostrils; hold your right nostril shut and open your left nostril. Continue to chew the jelly bean.
11. When the jelly bean is well chewed, swallow it. Note the taste or lack thereof on the Data Sheet.
12. Rinse your mouth with water.
13. Pinch your nose shut with one hand
14. Begin to chew the third jelly bean. When it is partially chewed, remove your fingers from both nostrils.
15. Continue to chew the jelly bean and swallow it. Note the taste or lack thereof on the Data Sheet like the one that follows.

Evaluation
○ What is the flavor (or lack of flavor) after eating the first jelly bean?
○ Does the flavor change as you alternate nostrils while you are chewing the second jelly bean?
○ If so, which nostril is more dominant? *This may indicate if you are right- or left-handed.*
○ Notice if the flavor changes when you release both fingers from your nose while you eat the third jelly bean.
○ What does this exercise show you about the interaction between taste and smell for each of these procedures?

Culinary applications
What guidelines should be followed when experimenting with taste and smell in food product or recipe production? (Consider equipment, ingredients and techniques.)

Data Sheet

Taste after Chewing	Taste after Opening Right Nostril	Taste After Opening Left Nostril	Taste After Opening Both Nostrils
Jelly bean #1			
Jelly bean #2			
Jelly bean #3			

6. **Appearance, smell and taste tests: white fruits and vegetables**
   Objective
   ○ To determine how important the sense of sight is in taste perception
   Materials
   White potato, apple, turnip, knife, peeler, cutting board, small cup, water
   Procedure
   1. Wash your hands.
   2. Peel the potato, apple and turnip; then cut them into the same-sized cubes.
   3. Place one of each of the cubes in a small cup. (It is fine if the cubes are mixed inside the cup.)[1]
   4. Repeat Exercise #5 above, including your observations and evaluations on the Data Sheet like the one that follows. Use the cut-up fruit and vegetables instead of the jelly beans.
   Evaluation
   ○ Complete the evaluations as in Exercise #5 above.
   ○ Now that color has been removed as a sensory factor and the fruit and vegetables are all white, what does this exercise tell you about the interactions among appearance, smell and taste?
   Culinary applications
   What guidelines should be followed when experimenting with appearance in food product or recipe production? (Consider equipment, ingredients and techniques.)

---

[1] Note: *It is safe to taste the raw potato and turnip. If you have never tasted either of these vegetables, then you should taste them before you proceed so you will know what tastes to expect.*

OVER EASY

This chapter featured the significance of food science and its applications to nutrition and the culinary arts. If foods and beverages are studied at their basic levels—molecules of carbohydrates, lipids, proteins and water—this information can be applied to the techniques and principles of cooking and baking. This chapter on food science basics and the chapters on nutrition basics and culinary arts basics illustrate the interdisciplinary nature of these disciplines.

Paramount to foods looking, smelling and tasting great is the field of sensory science. When a person remarks that something "tastes" good, they are usually referring to its flavors. These may be combinations of appearance, smell, taste, texture and other considerations. Flavors may be masked, heightened or decreased by manipulating these factors.

Carbohydrates, lipids, proteins and water behave in certain ways in cooking and baking, depending on the configuration of their molecules. These unique designs must be taken into account in food product and recipe development.

For instance, carbohydrates with their starches, sugars and fibers serve to bulk, gel, provide texture and thicken. Lipids, including fats and oils, are immiscible in water unless they are aided by emulsifiers. Lipids also decompose and melt in different environments. Proteins with their amino acids help to brown foods and create distinct tastes. They also act as enzymes, coagulate and denature, which affects their performance in certain foods and beverages. Water acts as a solvent and a weak acid and base, and it is also inherent to steaming.

Foods and beverages also react as they do under a variety of circumstances. They form emulsions and participate in enzymatic reactions and the Maillard reaction, transfer heat and are affected or affect temperature, time and texture.

Meats, dairy products, fruits and vegetables, legumes, grains and fats react differently, depending on their chemical compositions. Recipes are contingent upon their reactions and may succeed or fail.

Once ingredients or techniques are used incorrectly and/or perform poorly, then some recipes may fail. Other recipes may be repaired. Too much or too little salt, fat, sugar or liquid may be to blame. Appearance, caramelization, color dissipation, curdling, deterioration, filming, gelling, gluten formation, overcooking, reduction, retrogradation, ripening, separation and staling may also be responsible—and often fixable.

This chapter concludes with different scenarios that depict a fictitious day in the life of a food scientist and thought-provoking reviews of molecular gastronomy and biotechnology. In summary, this chapter unites the essence of food science and technology with the creativity of the culinary arts as they relate to nutrition and health. It lays the groundwork for what may come.

CHECK PLEASE

1. Beer, coffee, deep leafy greens, rosemary, walnuts, and wine are characteristic of the _____ taste in foods.
   a. umami
   b. salty
   c. sweet
   d. acidic
   e. bitter
2. A mixture of celery, carrots, and onions that is fundamental to cooking flavor is called:
   a. bouquet garni
   b. fine herbs
   c. mirepoix
   d. quatre epices
   e. gremolata

93

3. The carbohydrate-like substance that is extracted from apples and citrus fruits to help thicken syrups is called:

a. gum
b. jelly
c. starch
d. pectin
e. sugar

ESSAY QUESTION

1. A cream sauce has curdled. Why did this happen? Can it be fixed? If so, how? What can be done to help prevent other sauces from curdling?

For additional questions, please see the *Culinary Nutrition* website at www.culinarynutrition.elsevier.com

HUNGRY FOR MORE?

American Chemical Society   http://portal.acs.org/portal/acs/corg/content
Institute of Food Technology   http://www.ift.org
Monell Chemical Senses Center   http://www.monell.org
Research Chefs Association   http://www.culinology.com
Brown A, Stewart, Tabori, et al. *Good Eats: The Early Years (2009), the Middle Years (2010) and the Later Years (2011)*.
Corriher SO. *BakeWise: The Hows and Whys of Successful Baking with Over 200 Magnificent Recipes*. New York: Scribner, 2008.
Corriher SO. *Cookwise: The Hows and Whys of Successful Cooking with Over 230 Great-Tasting Recipes*. New York: William Morrow and Company, 1997.
Hillman H. *Kitchen Science: A Guide to Knowing the How's and Why's for Fun and Success in the Kitchen*. Boston: Houghton Mifflin, 1989.
Kapoor S. *Taste. A New Way to Cook*. British Columbia, Canada: Whitehead, 2003.
Kunz G, Kaminsky P. *The Elements of Taste*. Boston: Little Brown, 2001.
McGee H. *On Food and Cooking: The Science and Lore of the Kitchen*. New York: Scribner, 2004.
Wolke R. *What Einstein Told His Cook*. New York: WW Norton, 2002.
Wolke R. *What Einstein Told His Cook 2. The Sequel*. New York: WW Norton, 2005.

TAKE AWAY
Molecular Gastronomy

The term *molecular gastronomy* is credited to Hungarian physicist Nicholas Kurti and French chemist Hervé This. They applied food science to explain and solve culinary issues. Old kitchen tales and cooking tips were collected and tested to support their principles. As a result of their curiosities, a new area of discussion, practice and study emerged: molecular gastronomy.

Molecular gastronomy, or progressive cuisine, is a movement that incorporates science and new techniques in the preparation, transformation and artistic presentation of food. It is the study of molecules as they relate to the chemical and physical processes of cooking. By discovering the food science behind cooking, molecular gastronomy is able to explain why some recipes fail and others succeed and which ingredients and techniques are optimal.

Morsel "The qualities of an exceptional cook are akin to those of a successful tightrope walker: an abiding passion for taste, courage to go out on a limb, and an impeccable sense of balance."—Bryan Miller (cookbook author, food writer and former *New York Times* restaurant critic)

Molecular gastronomy is sometimes referred to as *culinary alchemy*—a precursor of food chemistry but with fewer scientific roots. The concept of using food chemistry techniques to study food and cooking is far from modern; it dates back to the eighteenth century. Marie-Antoine Carême, a famous French chef, was an early molecular gastronomer who wrote carefully detailed essays about culinary pleasures, fusions of ingredients and functional techniques. It was not until the close of the twenty-first century and the years that followed that the integration of food technology with the culinary arts became a justifiable field of study in its own right.

Throughout the years, chefs, food scientists and nutritionists have grappled with the issues that surround and integrate the culinary arts, food science and nutrition. Some prominent food scientists and authorities on the chemistry of food and the art of cooking include Harold McGee, renowned author of *On Food and Cooking: The Science and Lore of the Kitchen* (Scribner, 2004); research biochemist and food writer Shirley Corriher, author of *CookWise: The Hows and Whys of Successful Cooking* (Morrow, 2007) and *BakeWise: The Hows and Whys of Successful Baking* (Scribner, 2008); and Hervé This, the French physical chemist who devised the idea of molecular gastronomy and authored *Molecular Gastronomy: Exploring the Science of Flavor* and *Kitchen Mysteries: Revealing the Science of Cooking* (Columbia University Press, 2007).

Modern investigators and experimenters of molecular gastronomy include chefs such as Ferran Adrià and Heston Blumenthal. Ferran Adrià was the celebrated executive chef of El Bulli restaurant in Roses, Spain, on the Costa Brava. Heston Blumenthal was the chef/owner of The Fat Duck in the village of Bray in Berkshire, England. (Both restaurants have since closed.) Their innovative culinary practices and high regard for food science were distinguished in their equally innovative cooking. They examined how cooking methods, the environmental context of a meal, ingredients, and the senses powerfully impact the dining experience.

Today's notable chefs of molecular gastronomy include Wylie Dufresne, the chef/owner of wd~50 restaurant in New York City, and chef/restaurateur Grant Achatz of Alinea and Next restaurants in Chicago, Illinois.

Some techniques of modern molecular gastronomy include flash-freezing, froth, meat glue and spherification. Flash-freezing is a process by which the exteriors of foods are quickly frozen with the help of liquid nitrogen. It sometimes leaves liquefied centers. Froth was once a sauce that was converted into foam by the use of a whipped cream canister. Sometimes lecithin acts as a stabilizer. Meat glue is transglutaminase, a substance that binds different proteins together. Spherification is achieved when liquidized foods are mixed with sodium alginate and then bathed in calcium chloride, which creates multiple spheres with liquid centers.

What's next for molecular gastronomy? As budding food science, nutrition and culinary arts professionals, it may be yours for the calling.

This chapter serves as a foundation for molecular gastronomy, similar to the way Chapter 1 serves as a foundation for nutrition and Chapter 3 serves as a foundation for the culinary arts.

You have seen how different foods and beverages are prepared; how various ingredients alter the chemical, physical and sensory qualities of foods; and how the artistic and social aspects of consumption interact to achieve the overall satisfaction of a meal. All this and more had its roots in the old kitchen tales and cooking tips that Nicholas Kurti and Hervé This first explored.

Biotechnology

Biotechnology, or *genetic engineering*, is a discipline that addresses the relationship between biology and technology. It explores biological concepts and their technical applications in order to create or modify products and processes.

Biotechnology includes such subjects as biochemistry, cellular biology, chemical engineering, embryology, genetics, information technology, molecular biology and robotics. While the early focus of biotechnology was on food processing and agriculture, a portion of the focus of biotechnology today is on DNA and gene transfer and their applications in food production.

Where do nutrition, food science and culinary professionals fit into the biotechnology picture? It is in a collaborative manner, through collective knowledge and decision making.

95

The most practical use of biotechnology today is the cultivation of plants to produce food that is not only suitable but is superior for human consumption. Because biotechnology seeks to engineer or modify organisms for humankind, biotechnology may have major impacts on plants and food crops, including food availability, food choices and human consumption.

The justification for the use of biotechnology includes potential for the enhanced appearance of foods, decreased resistance to environmental stresses, heightened taste and textures, increased formulations of innovative substances, boosted crops and yields, improved nutritional values and reduced reliance on fertilizers and pesticides. Two historic examples of biotechnology in action are the Flavr Savr™ tomato and *golden rice.*

THE FLAVR SAVR™ TOMATO

The *Flavr Savr*™ tomato was the first commercially grown, genetically modified food that was licensed for human consumption. It was produced in the early 1990s by Calgene Inc., a biotechnology company based out of Davis, California. Calgene developed genetically engineered plants and plant products for the food, oleo and seed chemical industries. The company was later acquired by the Monsanto Company. After evaluating the Flavr Savr™ tomato in 1992, the FDA concluded that processing the Flavr Savr™ tomato was as safe as a tomato that was conventionally bred.

The benefit of the Flavr Savr™ tomato was its resistance to rotting. This was achieved by modifying the tomato with a gene that blocked the production of an enzyme that caused the tomato to rot. This enzyme was responsible for the softening of the tomato's cell wall during ripening.

The Flavr Savr™ tomato replaced artificially ripened tomatoes that used ethylene gas for ripening. Ethylene gas acts as a plant hormone. Flavr Savr™ tomatoes could ripen on the vine, which improved their flavor, and they had a longer shelf life without rotting. Special labeling was not warranted because its features resembled nongenetically modified tomatoes, including their nutritional values. There appeared to be no evidence for health risks.

Concerns that were raised were not necessarily about the safety of *eating* the Flavr Savr™ tomatoes but more about the risks of *mass cultivation* of gene-carrying materials and other public safety issues.

Unfortunately, the Flavr Savr™ tomato failed. Its failure was attributed more to inexperience in the growing and shipping of Flavr Savr™ tomatoes than these public health concerns.

Flavr Savr™ tomato production was 25 to 50 percent that of other tomato growers; ripe Flavr Savr™ tomatoes were more delicate to process and ship than unripe fruits and vegetables, and Flavr Savr™ tomatoes were undersized to command premium prices. A newer, conventionally bred long shelf life (LSL) tomato ultimately led to Flavr Savr's™ demise [24].

GOLDEN RICE™

Golden rice™ was developed in the 1990s in Europe through the combined research of the Swiss Federal Institute of Technology and the University of Freiburg in Germany. Like the Flavr Savr™ tomato, golden rice was a major advancement in biotechnology.

Golden rice™ was designed to produce beta-carotene, an antioxidant and the precursor or originator of vitamin A. Beta-carotene is a pigment in the carotenoid family of plant chemicals that is responsible for the yellow-orange-red colors in foods, particularly fruits and vegetables. Vitamin A is responsible for eyesight and normal growth and development, among its other vital functions.

Over half of the world's population is dependent on rice as its mainstay, but the endosperm of white rice is mostly carbohydrate. The fact that golden rice could naturally produce beta-carotene with the help of genetic modification meant that many areas of the world could benefit by its consumption.

Like Flavr Savr™ tomatoes, golden rice is no longer available. Although it was initially developed as a product to help humanity, it met with significant resistance from antibiotechnological, antiglobal and environmental activists.

While biotechnology may seem like a universal remedy for the issues that face food production and distribution in the twenty-first century, critics of bioengineering continue to think otherwise. It is imperative that nutrition, food science and culinary professionals consider all aspects that influence ingredients and foods and apply safe and sound judgment about their use in products, recipes and meals.

References

[1] Research Chefs Association. <http://www.culinology.com/>; [accessed 23.02.08].

[2] Institute of Food Technologists (IFT). <http://www.ift.org/>; [accessed 23.02.08].

[3] Eutech Instruments. Measuring the pH value of meat. <http://www.eutechinst.com/techtips/tech-tips35.htm/>; [accessed 23.02.08].

[4] Good Eats Fan Page. Cooking oil smoke points. <http://www.goodeatsfanpage.com/CollectedInfo/OilSmokePoints.htm/>; [accessed 23.02.08]

[5] Chu M. Smoke points of various fats. Cooking for engineers. <http://www.cookingforengineers.com/article/50/Smoke-Points-of-Various-Fats/>; [accessed 23.02.08].

[6] Goodbody M, Miller C, Tran T. In: Williams-Sonoma kitchen companion: the A to Z guide to everyday cooking equipment & ingredients. San Francisco: Time-Life; 2000.

[7] FoodSafety.gov. Storage times for the refrigerator and freezer. <http://www.foodsafety.gov/keep/charts/storagetimes.html/>; [accessed 23.02.08].

[8] The accidental scientist: finger test for doneness. Science of Cooking. <http://www.exploratorium.edu/cooking/meat/activity-fingertest.html/>; [accessed 23.02.08].

[9] US Department of Agriculture (USDA). Food safety and inspection service. <http://www.fsis.usda.gov/>; [accessed 23.02.08].

[10] McGee H. On food and cooking: the science and lore of the kitchen. New York, NY: Simon and Schuster; 2004.

[11] USFDA 821 C.F.R. §133; 1949.

[12] Knoll L.P. Origins of the regulation of raw milk cheeses in the United States. Harvard Law School. <http://leda.law.harvard.edu/leda/data/702/Knoll05.pdf/>; [accessed 23.02.08].

[13] Egg Safety Center. Egg food safety frequently asked questions. <http://www.eggsafety.org/consumers/consumer-faqs#STRUCTURE6/>; [accessed 23.02.08].

[14] The Learning Channel. How to cook vegetables. <http://recipes.howstuffworks.com/tools-and-techniques/how-to-cook-vegetables24.htm/printable/>; [accessed 23.02.08].

[15] Vegetarians in paradise: cooking beans and grains. <http://www.vegparadise.com/charts.html/>; [accessed 23.02.08].

[16] University of Wisconsin-Madison. pH values of common foods and ingredients. Food Safety & Health. <http://www.foodsafety.wisc.edu/business_food/files/Approximate_pH.pdf/>; [accessed 23.02.08].

[17] The engineering toolbox: food and foodstuff-pH values. <http://www.engineeringtoolbox.com/food-ph-d_403.html/>; [accessed 23.02.08].

[18] Regulation: 21 CFR 101.9 (c)(2)(ii). Food and Drug Administration (2003-07-11). "21 CFR Part 101. Food labeling; trans fatty acids in nutrition labeling; consumer research to consider nutrient content and health claims and possible footnote or disclosure statements; final rule and proposed rule" (PDF). National Archives and Records Administration. Archived from the original on January 3, 2007. United States Food and Drug Administration (FDA): Food labeling; trans fatty acids in nutrition labeling; consumer research to consider nutrient content and health claims and possible footnote or disclosure statements; final rule and proposed rule. <http://www.fda.gov/food/labelingnutrition/labelclaims/nutrientcontentclaims/ucm110179.htm/>; [accessed 23.02.08].

[19] Eastern Illinois University. Fats and oils. <http://castle.eiu.edu/~srippy/FCS1120-Lecture/notes/Fats%20&%20Oils.pdf/>; [accessed 23.02.08].

[20] Fruitsinfo.com. Storage of fruits. <http://www.fruitsinfo.com/storage-fruits.htm/>; [accessed 23.02.08].

[21] wiseGEEK. How can I tell when fruit is ripe? <http://www.wisegeek.com/how-can-i-tell-when-fruit-is-ripe.htm/>; [accessed 23.02.08].

[22] Monell Center. <http://www.monell.org/>; [accessed 23.02.08].

[23] Geschwind DH. Advances in autism. Annu Rev Med 2009;60:367–80.

[24] Martineau B. In: First fruit: the creation of the Flavr Savr tomato and the birth of biotech food. McGraw-Hill; 2001.

CHAPTER 3

Culinary Arts Basics: Healthy Cooking Fundamentals

The Culinary Competencies of Healthy Food Selection, Preparation and Food Service

99

Culinary Nutrition. DOI: http://dx.doi.org/10.1016/B978-0-12-391882-6.00003-0

OBJECTIVES

1. Identify the components of healthy kitchens, including equipment, tools and ingredients
2. Identify the components of healthy meals, including meal plans, composition, recipes and layout
3. Adapt standard cooking and baking methods and techniques to healthful standards
4. Demonstrate how to convert recipes by reducing, substituting and/or replacing ingredients
5. Create new, healthy recipes based on current nutrition recommendations
6. Adapt common recipes for specialized dietary needs
7. Describe how to retain and build flavor with less fat, sugar and sodium
8. Choose economical healthy food and beverages choices
9. Use the principles of basic food safety in food handling and production
10. Compare slow food to fast food and its effect on diet, health and the environment

INTRODUCTION: HEALTHY CHOICES IN FOODS AND FOOD SERVICE

Restaurants, school and hospital cafeterias, catering and food service operations in businesses, and institutions and companies provide billions of meals and snacks annually. Having healthy options on menus can be beneficial for the food service industry in sales and customer satisfaction and for customers who want and need healthy food and beverage choices.

Morsel "Cooking is, for me, the perfect balance of art and science. There's that creative endeavor within you that can think out the seasons and the flavor profiles. Then there's the scientific part—what is actually going on with the whisk? If I'm blanching broccoli, why is it turning brown in the pan? As you study that, you learn that sometimes if you cook a lot of vegetables in the same water, an acid will develop. And if you cook a green vegetable in that acidic water, it's going to turn army brown. So these are things you start to learn through science."
—Gary Danko (James Beard Foundation award-winning chef and restaurateur)

The food service industry is an industry of choice, which means that most menus are influenced by consumer demand. To cater to increasingly health-conscious diners, food service operations are adding nutritious options to fit individual dietary needs and preferences.

Nutrition, food science and culinary professionals need to be equipped with the knowledge, techniques and tools to address the rapidly changing nutrition and health interests of the dining public. Nutritional science produces the research that helps drive nutrition recommendations. Food science creates the ingredients to help meet these recommendations.

The culinary arts utilize nutrition recommendations and ingredients to create nutritious recipes and healthy menus. By working together, these three disciplines can meet the rapidly changing nutrition and health needs of the consuming public.

Some food service establishments already meet consumer nutrition and health needs and preferences by customizing their menus and offering salad dressings or sauces on the side; cooking in vegetable oils rather than butter; and substituting starchy side dishes, such as potatoes or rice, with vegetables or fruit.

An increasing number of food service establishments already provide nutrition information on menus, posters, table tents, brochures and websites to promote nutritious and healthy restaurant-branded lifestyle programs.

Other food service institutions may be slow to change due to economics, location, size, tradition and a host of other factors. Still, they may be challenged by consumer demand for healthy and great tasting foods and beverages.

This chapter provides the rationale and resources that are needed, along with convincing hands-on exercises in healthy recipe conversions, menu development and flavor enhancement, plus kitchen makeovers, food economics and food safety.

MAIN COURSES
The Healthy Kitchen

If it is true that "you are what you eat," then a professional or home kitchen should reflect one's eating style. Deep fryers, meat slicers, ice cream machines, large roasting pans, gravy separators, candy thermometers, soda dispensers and other equipment of this nature may have fewer purposes in a healthy kitchen.

A healthy kitchen should be stocked with basic cooking and baking equipment (as described later in this chapter), plus other equipment and tools that make healthy cooking easier. These include such items as a cast-iron skillet, food mill, juicer, nonstick pots and pans, portion scoop, salad spinner, silicone baking sheets and wok.

Healthy cooking techniques, such as baking, broiling, reducing, searing, steaming and sweating are slowly replacing boiling, braising, char-grilling, creaming, deep and shallow frying and stewing, which tend to add fat and calories and decrease vital nutrients. However, some of these techniques can be adapted for healthier results.

Consumers "want to have their cake and eat it, too." While consumers are increasingly concerned about health, they still enjoy the pleasures that desserts and baked goods provide. Obesity, cardiovascular disease and diabetes restrict some people from enjoying traditional desserts and breadstuffs. Healthy desserts and baked items provide new tastes and textures and may be equally satisfying.

Food allergies and sensitivities to dairy products, eggs, certain flours and tree nuts may also prevent consumers from enjoying their favorite savory and sweet foods and beverages. Recipes and menus designed especially for allergic consumers can be found in Chapter 9.

In the process of making savory and sweet foods healthier, some ingredient adjustments, eliminations or substitutions may be essential. However, cooking and baking are exacting exercises in food science. Ingredients such as fat, salt and sugar have specific functions in recipes. Reducing or eliminating any one of these ingredients may cause a recipe to fail. A solid understanding of ingredient functions and reactions is essential before recipes can be adapted to make them healthier. The characteristics of some basic ingredients are featured in this chapter, with applications for healthy cooking and baking.

Making a recipe or meal healthier does not guarantee that consumers will choose to eat or enjoy it. Taste rules! This chapter addresses how to make foods that are "good for you" good to eat, too. The sensory aspects of foods and beverages and flavor enhancement address these issues.

There is also information about how to stock a healthy pantry, refrigerator and freezer and the proportion of foods and beverages that constitute a healthy plate and a healthy meal. Creating a healthy kitchen requires a new mindset: a fresh way of looking at how the nutrients in foods and beverages can be maximized for good health. This chapter provides the initiative.

Healthy Food

Foods should not be labeled good or bad, nutritious or unhealthy. Most foods and beverages can be occasionally consumed in a healthy diet because it is the overall effects of the diet that count. Some foods and beverages are considered more nutritious and health-enhancing, as determined by the US government and various health associations (see Chapter 1).

Table 3-1 defines the word "healthy" and how it can be used on food packaging. When these nutritious foods and beverages provide the backbone of a meal, there may be room for some "discretionary foods": foods with more calories, fat, sugar or sodium than desired. All foods can fit; it is simply a matter of proportion, which will soon be evident.

101

TABLE 3-1 The US Food and Drug Administration Implied Nutrient Content Claim for Healthy

According to the FDA, the term *healthy* and related terms *(health, healthful, healthfully, healthfulness, healthier, healthiest, healthily* and *healthiness)* are considered Implied Nutrient Content Claims and may be used on food packing *if* the food meets the following requirements:

- Low-fat: <5 grams total fat/serving or per 100 grams
- Low saturated fat: <2 grams saturated fat/serving or per 100 grams
- ≤480 milligrams sodium/serving or per 50 grams if serving size is small
- ≤95 milligrams cholesterol per serving or per 100 grams
- At least 10% of the Daily Value for vitamins A, C, calcium, iron, protein or fiber
- Fortification according to FDA guidelines

Source: [1].

> **Morsel** "A cook can never rise above his ingredients."
> —Anonymous

The Healthy Pantry, Refrigerator and Freezer

The number of healthy foods and beverages continues to grow. In 2012, the food industry confirmed that healthy eating is a critically important consumer "driver" and that it has considerable influence over company strategies.

According to food and beverage trends, although US consumers want foods to be healthy, they often do not purchase healthy foods or are unwilling to pay the prices for healthy foods. Some consumers do not even know what the term *healthy* really means [2]. This is due, in part, to increased interest in nutrition and healthy diets across many socioeconomic levels; the organic food movement; more local and regional growers; and the availability of global ingredients. Healthy foods and beverages now appear on many local grocers' shelves, as well as those in national giant supermarket chains.

This section provides an overview of the ingredients, foods and beverages that are considered to be *healthy* according to the above criteria. In addition, they are nutrient-dense compared to calorie-dense, which means that they contain a large amount of nutrients relative to calories in one serving. Some of these ingredients, foods and beverages are also high in disease-fighting nutrients, including antioxidants and phytonutrients. Brand names are not included.

THE HEALTHY PANTRY

A *pantry* is a storeroom for nonperishable items, such as bottled, canned and packaged goods. A healthy pantry contains the items that can help to transform ordinary-tasting dish into gratifying ones. Pantry items include baking supplies, beverages, condiments, fruits, grains, herb, spices and extracts, legumes, nuts and seeds, oils, protein, soups, vegetables and shelf-stable beverages, such as those that follow.

Baking Supplies

Some of these baking supplies help to thicken foods and beverages, although some can naturally thicken on their own from reduction, evaporation, pureeing and other processes. Others are important for leavening in various savory and sweet applications.

- Arrowroot
- Baking powder
- Baking soda
- Cream of tartar
- Sourdough starter
- Starches: arrowroot, corn, potato, tapioca
- Quick-rising yeast

Beverages

Coffee, tea and some alcoholic beverages, especially wine and beer, contain different degrees of antioxidants for their health-promoting abilities. Beer, wine and spirits can be used with discretion as a flavor enhancer in marinades, flambes and fondues and for leavening.

- Coffee: regular, decaffeinated and espresso beans and powder
- Tea: black, green and herbal
- Beer: ale, lager
- Spirits: brandy, gin, rum, tequila, vodka, whiskey
- Wine: red and white (drinking wine preferred, since cooking wine contains sodium)

FOOD BYTE

The French chef Auguste Escoffier (1846-1935) speaks of *condiments* in three classifications: fatty, hot and pungent. According to Escoffier, fatty condiments include a range of vegetable and animal fats, including avocadoes, butter, margarine, nuts, oils and olives. Hot condiments include chilies, hot sauce, mustard and wasabi. Pungent condiments include garlic, horseradish and onions. Condiments were and still are flavor enhancers; they still give food character and improve desirability—even in small amounts.

Condiments

Though often low in calories, condiments tend to be higher in sodium or sugar. They should be used sparingly for flavor enhancement. If they are required in a recipe, then the reduced versions should be used.

- Catsup: natural or reduced-sugar
- Chocolate: cocoa powder, bittersweet chocolate
- Horseradish: wasabi, white
- Mayonnaise: nonfat and reduced-fat
- Mustard: Dijon, honey-mustard, reduced-sodium
- Pepper: black, cayenne, green
- Salt: kosher, sea salt
- Sauces: hot sauce, reduced-sodium soy sauce or tamari, salsa
- Sweeteners: honey, light brown sugar, maple syrup, molasses, raw sugar (demerara or turbinado)
- Vinegars: apple cider, balsamic, distilled white, red and white wine, rice

Fruits

While fresh is usually best, canned and packaged fruits are a good source of vitamins and minerals and offer versatility in recipes. They provide taste and texture and can often be used to replace or reduce sugar and as a fat substitute.

- Applesauce: natural or reduced-sugar
- Canned fruit in 100 percent fruit juice
- Dried fruits: apricots, cranberries, currants, dates, figs, prunes, peaches, raisins
- Fruit spreads
- Olives
- 100 percent fruit juice
- Pureed prunes

Grains

It is wise to refrigerate whole grains once they are opened, since they quickly become rancid. Store whole grains in clearly labeled containers because many look similar, and store in a cool, dark location.

- Breadcrumbs: whole grain reduced-sodium and Japanese panko
- Breadstuffs: whole-grain bread sticks, crackers, croutons
- Cereals: whole-grain cold and hot cereals; oats and multigrain
- Grains and flours: whole-grain amaranth, barley, bulgur, cracked wheat, couscous, faro, yellow corn meal, job's tears, kamut, millet, oats, oat bran, quinoa, spelt, teff, triticale, unbleached all-purpose (AP), wheat berries, wheat bran, whole wheat and pastry flour

- Pasta: buckwheat noodles, gluten-free pasta, protein-fortified pasta, orzo, rice noodles, ramen noodles, 100 percent whole-grain, mixed whole-grain and durum wheat pasta
- Rice: brown, short and long grain white, wild, long cooking, and enriched and converted

Herbs, Spices and Extracts

Flavor enhancement depends on judicious use of salt, pepper, herbs, spices and extracts. A little bit of salt can make or break a dish that has been reduced in calories, fat and sugar. Tightly cover herbs and spices in a cool, dark location to retain their flavor (also see Chapter 9).

- Salt: kosher or sea
- Pepper: coarsely ground and pepper blends
- Dried herbs and spices including allspice, basil, cayenne pepper, chili powder, chives, cinnamon, crushed red pepper, cumin, dill, garlic, ginger, Italian seasoning blend, mustard, nutmeg, oregano, paprika, rosemary, tarragon leaves, thyme
- Flavor extracts including almond, anise, cherry, cinnamon, lemon, orange, peppermint and vanilla

Legumes

Dried beans, split peas and lentils and shelf-stable soy foods provide a wealth of inexpensive, nonperishable protein options. Legumes should be stored in airtight, clear containers to distinguish their varieties. Peanuts and peanut butter should be refrigerated once opened.

- Dry, packaged beans, split peas, lentils
- Canned beans in water: black, garbanzos, kidneys, lentils, limas, pinto and soy, among others
- Peanuts and peanut butter: reduced-fat and reduced-sodium
- Soy foods: shelf-stable tofu, tempeh, miso, soy "nuts," texturized vegetable protein (TVP)

Nuts and Seeds

While higher in total fat, nuts and seeds are rich in monounsaturated fatty acids. They are meant to be used in moderation for taste, texture and garnish. Due to their fat content, nuts and seeds should be stored unopened in their original packaging or in tightly closed containers if in bulk, preferably refrigerated or frozen.

- Almonds, cashews, English walnuts, hazelnuts, macadamia nuts
- Pumpkin, poppy, sesame, sunflower seeds
- Nut and seed butters: almond, cashew, macadamia, tahini
- Reduced-fat coconut milk

Oils

Since oils are pure liquid fat, they should be tightly covered and stored in opaque containers in a cool, dark location to prevent rancidity. Once opened, oils can be refrigerated, but they may cloud and thicken. They should return to normal viscosity once at room temperature.

- Cooking sprays or pumps: nonfat canola, olive
- Neutral-tasting oils: canola or safflower
- Flavorful oils: extra-virgin olive, olive or peanut
- Oils with high smoke point: canola or peanut
- Finishing oils: sesame or walnut

Protein

Like legumes, some canned and packaged protein makes healthy additions to mostly vegetable dishes. Though some are higher in fat and sodium, others are packaged in water or tomato sauce. The little bones are high in calcium. Some dried beef or poultry may need reconstituting before use.

- Canned anchovies, sardines, tuna, salmon, minced clams; preferably in water
- Dried beef, poultry

Soups

Generally, canned and packaged soups are higher in sodium. There are products that contain 20 to 30 percent less sodium. Freshly made or frozen stock is ideal, but these reduced products provide a base that herbs and spices can enhance.

- Reduced-fat and reduced-sodium broth and bouillon
- Dried soup mixes

Vegetables

Mushrooms have an umami taste and meatlike texture that transforms many vegetable-based dishes. Store in individual portions in airtight contains with tightly fitting lids in a cool, dark and dry location. If they get damp, they will mildew or rot. Tomatoes are naturally high in sodium, and sodium is used in processing, so select reduced-sodium varieties.

- Mushrooms: all varieties of dried, especially black trumpet, chanterelle, morel, shiitake, porcini and portabella
- 100 percent reduced-sodium vegetable juice
- Tomato based: reduced-sodium whole and diced tomatoes, sun-dried tomatoes, tomato paste, tomato puree, tomato sauce

Shelf-Stable Dairy, Soy and Rice Beverages

Shelf-stable dairy, soy and grain beverages provide the capability to add a creamlike consistency to sauces and dressings. Look for the nonfat varieties for the least fat with the most protein. Once opened, these beverages should be refrigerated.

- Canned evaporated nonfat milk
- Evaporated nonfat dry milk
- Shelf-stable reduced-fat soy milk
- Shelf-stable rice milk

THE HEALTHY REFRIGERATOR AND FREEZER

A refrigerator does not prevent food and beverage deterioration; rather, it delays it. A freezer is designed to stop bacterial action, since frozen bacteria should be inactivated. If packaged for refrigeration or freezing, most food should suffer minimal effects on taste or texture. Some frozen foods can be higher in nutrients than fresh foods.

Breads

The reason to refrigerate or freeze whole-grain breadstuffs is to prevent rancidity in the germ of the whole grains. Original bread wrappers are not adequately moisture-vapor resistant to be used for freezing. A freezer-weight polyethylene bag should be used instead.

- Whole-grain bagels, breads, English muffins, muffins, rolls, tortillas and others

Eggs

Eggs need to be refrigerated at a constant temperature in their original carton to protect them from absorbing flavors and odors. Raw foods should be separated from eggs. Raw eggs can be frozen whole, beaten and tightly sealed, as can egg whites. Egg yolks will likely gel or thicken unless they have salt or sugar added.

- Whole eggs, egg whites

Dairy Products

Dairy milk and other dairy products should be stored in their original sealed container in the coldest part of the refrigerator. At 38° to 40°F, this low temperature will slow bacterial growth, and the sealed container will help to prevent contamination and the absorption of flavors from other foods. Choose nonfat and reduced-fat products most often.

- Skim or reduced-fat dairy milk
- Frozen nonfat or low-fat yogurt
- Nonfat and reduced-fat cream and half-and-half
- Nonfat or low-fat ice cream
- Part-skim ricotta or Neufchatel cheese
- Plain, nonfat or low-fat yogurt, sour cream or buttermilk
- Reduced-fat cheeses

Meat, Poultry, Fish and Seafood

Protein foods, unless dehydrated or canned, are very perishable. Protein foods should be refrigerated at 40°F or below soon after purchasing and placed on a tray or inside a storage container to ensure that their juices do not leak. Meat and poultry should be wrapped individually for freezing with freezer paper or freezer-proof plastic bags. These cuts are some of the leanest:

- Beef: Well-trimmed top bottom round, eye of round, sirloin tip, top round, top sirloin
- Fish: Most fish are lower in fat, especially saturated fat. Mackerel, salmon, sardines and trout are good sources of omega-3 fatty acids.
- Lamb: Arm, leg, loin
- Pork: Fresh center-cut ham, tenderloin, loin
- Poultry: Skinless white meat chicken and turkey
- Shellfish: Most shellfish are lower in fat. Some shellfish, such as lobster and shrimp, are higher in cholesterol.

Vegetables

106

Vegetables should be at their peak before refrigerating. Do not refrigerate garlic, onions, potatoes, pumpkins, squash or sweet potatoes, as this can affect their flavor.

Leafy green vegetables need refrigeration for cool temperature and high humidity; otherwise they may shrivel and lose their nutritional value. If the temperature is too high, they will freeze due to their high water content.

Sturdier vegetables should be blanched (steamed or boiled to destroy the enzymes that destroy flavor and nutritional value) before freezing. These vegetables are grouped according to their botanical families:

- Allium: chives, garlic, leeks, onions
- Cruciferous: broccoli, cauliflower, Brussels sprouts, cabbage
- Flowering green and yellow: artichokes, asparagus, beans, cucumber, okra, peas, squash
- Leafy greens: spinach, collards, beet, kale, spinach, Swiss chard, turnip
- Nightshade: tomatoes, peppers, eggplants
- Root: beets, carrots, celery root, jicama, parsnips, radishes, rutabagas, salsify, sweet potatoes, turnips, yams
- Squash: acorn, butternut, Hubbard, pumpkin, spaghetti squash
- Frozen vegetables: carrots, corn, onions, peas, mixed vegetables, spinach
- Other: mushrooms

Fruits

Like vegetables, allow fruit to fully ripen before refrigerating. Do not refrigerate avocadoes, bananas, mangos, papayas, pineapple or tomatoes, as this will affect their flavor. Sturdier fruits should be pared, pitted and seeded and treated with ascorbic acid (such as lemon juice) to prevent browning before freezing. These fruits are also grouped according to their botanical families:

- Berry: blackberries, blueberries, cranberries, currants, gooseberries, grapes, huckleberries, raspberries, strawberries

- Citrus: clementines, grapefruit, kumquats, lemons, limes, oranges, tangelos, tangerines
- Melon: cantaloupe, casaba, Crenshaw, honeydew, watermelon
- Pome: apples, avocadoes, pears
- Stone: apricots, cherries, nectarines, peaches, plums
- Tropical: bananas, guava, figs, kiwi, lychee, mangoes, papaya, persimmons, pineapple, star fruit
- 100 percent pure fruit juice
- 100 percent pure fruit sorbet
- Frozen fruits: berries, melons, stone fruits

Soy Foods

Fresh soy foods require refrigeration to preserve their protein and fat content. Soy dairy-free products should be handled like perishable dairy products. Follow the "use by" dates on containers. Freezing tofu makes it chewier with a meatier texture, but it may also become spongy and turn a yellowish hue if not properly wrapped.

- Miso, soy cheese, soy milk, soy yogurt, tempeh, tofu, texturized vegetable protein (TVP)

Bite on This: healthy choices of meat, poultry and fish

Healthy entrees should begin with the healthiest choices of meat, poultry and fish. These are the cuts with the lowest amount of calories, total fat, saturated fat and cholesterol that offer the highest amount of protein, minerals, vitamins and flavor.

High-fat meats contain about 100 calories, 8 or more grams of total fat, and 7 grams of protein per 1 ounce. Some poultry may be considered high-fat if its nutrients fall within these categories. High-fat meats include the following choices with 8 grams or more of total fat per 1 ounce. Some of these products are also made with less total fat, so check the Nutrition Facts Panel.

- Bacon: pork and turkey
- Hot dogs: beef, pork or combination; chicken or turkey
- Pork: ground, sausages or spareribs
- Processed sandwich meats: bologna, hard salami, pastrami
- Sausages: bratwurst, chorizo, Italian, knockwurst, Polish, smoked, summer

High-fat meats need not be excluded from one's diet. While they may raise blood cholesterol levels if they are consumed on a regular basic, they have room in a healthy diet if they are consumed in moderation. What is moderation? It is infrequent and with restraint in recommended portion sizes—not the center of the meal.

Medium-fat meats contain about 75 calories, 4 to 7 grams of total fat, and 7 grams of protein per 1 ounce. Medium-fat meats include the following choices. Like high-fat meats, they should be consumed in moderation.

- Beef: ground beef, corned beef, meatloaf, prime grades trimmed of fat such as prime rib, short ribs and tongue
- Fish: fried fish
- Lamb: ground lamb and rib roast
- Pork: cutlet and shoulder roast
- Poultry: chicken or turkey with skin, dove, fried chicken, pheasant, some ground turkey and wild duck or goose
- Sausages (with 4 to 7 grams of total fat per 1 ounce)
- Veal: cutlet (without breading)

Lean meats contain about 45 calories, 0 to 3 grams of total fat, and 7 grams of protein per 1 ounce. Lean meats include the following choices. Whenever possible, choose lean meats or lean meat substitutes from plant-based proteins (described in Chapter 5).

- Beef: select or choice grades trimmed of fat: ground round, roast (chuck, rib and rump), round, sirloin, steak (cubed, flank, porterhouse and T-bone) and tenderloin

- Fish
  - Fresh or frozen: catfish, cod, flounder, haddock, halibut, orange roughy, salmon, tilapia, trout and tuna
  - Canned: salmon or sardines
  - Smoked: herring or salmon (lox)
- Game: buffalo, ostrich, rabbit and venison
- Lamb: lamb chops, leg and roast
- Poultry without skin: chicken, Cornish hen, domestic duck or goose (well drained of fat) and turkey
- Pork: Canadian bacon, ham, rib or loin chop/roast and tenderloin
- Processed meats, hot dogs and sausages (with 3 grams or fewer of total fat per ounce)
- Shellfish: clams, crab, imitation shellfish, lobster, scallops and shrimp
- Veal: veal loin chop or roast

Healthy choices of meat, poultry and fish and their best cooking methods are shown in Table 3-2. These dry and moist heat cooking methods are described in the section "What heat is, what it does and how it applies to healthy cooking and baking," later in this chapter.

Dry heat cooking methods include baking, broiling, deep-frying, grilling, pan-frying, roasting and sauteing. Moist heat cooking methods include boiling, poaching, simmering and steaming. Cooking in too much fat or liquid is generally discouraged due to added fat and/or nutrient loss.

TABLE 3-2 Healthy Choices of Meat, Poultry, Fish and Shellfish and Best Cooking Methods

Healthy Choices of Beef	Best Cooking Methods
Beef: flank steak, shank, inside (top round), outside (bottom round), round (eye of round), rump, sirloin tip, top sirloin butt **Ground beef:** low-fat ground beef (90 to 95% lean)	**Dry heat:** flank, ground round or sirloin, sirloin, tenderloin, top loin **Moist heat:** bottom round, eye of round, round tip, tenderloin, top round
Healthy choices of lamb and pork	
Lamb: chops (rack of lamb), shank, sirloin **Pork:** boneless rib roast, chops (sirloin, top loin and loin), lean or extra-lean ground pork, pork tenderloin, sirloin roast	**Dry heat:** boneless ham, boneless rib roast, boneless sirloin chop, boneless top loin roast, loin chop, loin strips, rib chop, tenderloin **Moist heat:** boneless rib roast, boneless sirloin chop, loin chop, rib chop
Healthy choices of poultry	
Poultry: skinless chicken and turkey breast, cutlets, ground chicken or turkey (90 to 95% lean or fat-free)	**Dry heat:** Cornish game hen, whole chicken, whole turkey (if whole poultry), breast, cutlet. (To retain taste, remove skin after cooking, or remove skin and baste with little neutral oil.) **Moist heat:** Cornish game hen, whole chicken, whole turkey (if whole poultry), breast, cutlet. (To decrease fat, remove skin before cooking, or cool and remove condensed fat.)
Healthy choices of fish and shellfish	
Fish: most fish and shellfish. Cod, flounder, halibut, orange roughy and shrimp are low in calories and fat. Tuna, herring, mackerel, sablefish, salmon, sardines, shad, trout and whitefish are higher in omega-3 fatty acids.	**Dry or moist heat:** most fish and shellfish can be cooked by dry or moist heat cooking methods. Those that are lower in fat will dry quicker with dry heat. Baste with a little neutral oil to preserve moistness with few calories and fat.

The Healthy Plate
SENSORY QUALITIES

Figuratively speaking, we "eat with our eyes" because our eyes tell us if foods and beverages are appealing or if we should select something else. Healthy food needs to look great on a plate if people are to choose it. *Appearance* drives healthy food selection.

Plated food should not only look great but should *communicate healthful ingredients*: an array of very colorful fruits and vegetables, textural whole grains, translucent fish, lightly marbled meats, pearly dairy products and lightly glistening fats (if at all) inform the consumer of good taste and health to come.

The *colors* of plated food should be harmonious. First and foremost, color conveys the quality of food, whether it is fresh, and how it has been cooked (or overcooked). Whole grains should look earthy, not drab; fruits and vegetables should look brilliant, not washed out; protein should be cooked to perfection, depending on the cut; and once combined on a plate, all of their colors should be harmonious and complement one another.

The *shapes* of plated food should be varied but in agreement. Classically cut vegetables show precision, while unpeeled heirloom vegetables convey homespun informality. Interesting shapes may detract from smaller portion sizes. For example, fanning a 3-ounce portion of lean steak or poultry may give the illusion of a larger portion.

The *textures* of plated food should be varied and interesting. Consider using a combination of harmonious textures, including soft, smooth, coarse and solid. These could translate into reduced-fat mashed potatoes, cream-style coleslaw, crunchy corn on the cob, and chewy skinless barbecued chicken. Even people with eating problems or dietary restrictions still need some texture for interest and appeal.

PHYSICAL ASPECTS

The average dinner plate has grown in size, which allows more food to fit on it. A portion of food on a plate will look smaller on a large plate. A healthy plate should highlight the portions; the portions should not take over the plate.

Plain white plates convey simplicity and serenity and are often matched by simply prepared and plated food. Angular plates look edgy and trendy and may be matched by equally unique and plated food. Either may work as long as they have flow and the three principles of balance, unity, and height prevail:

Plated food should have *flow*, which is achieved through a combination of *balance, unity* and *height or focus*. Our eyes tend to move from left to right and then inward toward the main ingredients when looking at plated food. Placing too much at the exterior of the plate or all over the plate can be confusing or overwhelming.

Balance and unity are achieved through a balance of foods with harmonious colors, shapes and textures. Height or focus communicates the importance of ingredients, such as a piece of lightly poached codfish atop a mound of steamed spinach or a spiral of carrot coins that mound to a stack of lean lamb chops.

A low-fat sauce or flavored oil can be dribbled around the rim of the plate, or a few drops can be sprinkled over the contents to communicate that the dish is inviting and will be satisfying, without excessive fat calories.

Garnishes should be ethnically appropriate, like a fresh chili on a plate of enchiladas or a pile of ginger that is grouped with fresh sushi.

According to the USDA MyPlate recommendations in Chapter 1, about one-half of the entree plate should be filled with vegetables and/or fruits; about one-quarter should contain grains (with one-half of them whole grains); and about one-quarter should contain lean protein. Balanced and united healthy plate suggestions with approximate portion sizes for appetizers, salads, entrees and dessert plates and soup bowls are shown in Table 3-3.

109

TABLE 3-3 Healthy Appetizer, Salad, Soup Bowl, Entree and Dessert Plates

The healthy appetizer plate

- 2 ounces lean protein (lean meat [select or choice], white meat skinless poultry, most fish and shellfish)
- 2 to 3 ounces vegetables and whole or fortified grains
- 1 to 2 ounces reduced- or low-fat sauce or dressing (if used)
- Garnish only: avocado, cheese, nuts, olives, seeds

The healthy salad plate

- 1 to 2 cups leafy salad greens and fresh vegetables
- 2 to 3 ounces whole grains, legumes, fruit or lean protein for entree salad
- 1 to 2 tablespoons oil and vinegar–type salad dressing
- Garnish only: avocado, cheese, croutons, nuts, olives, seeds

The healthy soup bowl

- 6 to 7 ounces defatted, lower-sodium chicken, beef or fish stock
- Greater proportion vegetables, legumes or whole or enriched grains to animal protein (if used)
- Vegetable or legume puree, cornstarch or arrowroot for thickening
- Herbs, spices, citrus juice or flavored vinegar for flavoring
- Reduced- or low-fat dairy products for creaming
- Garnish only: avocado, cheese, croutons, flavored oil, reduced- or low-fat sour cream, seeds

The healthy entree plate

- 3 to 4 ounces or less lean protein (lean meat [select or choice], white meat skinless poultry, most fish and shellfish)[a]
- 3 to 4 ounces or more vegetables and whole or fortified grains[a]
- 1 to 2 ounces reduced- or low-fat sauce (if needed)
- Garnish only: avocado, cheese, flavored oil, olives, nuts, reduced- or low-fat sour cream, seeds

The healthy dessert plate

- 3- to 4-ounce portion
- Fresh fruit emphasis
- Whole grains such as cornmeal, oats or rice
- Reduced- or low-fat frozen dairy or plant-based (rice, soy, etc.) confections
- Cornstarch or arrowroot for thickening
- Lower-fat dairy products for creaming
- Garnish only: chocolate, coconut, 100% fruit spreads, nuts, seeds

Source: [3].

[a]Follow the USDA MyPlate recommendations: make ½ of the plate vegetables and/or fruits; ¼ whole or fortified grains and ¼ lean protein.
[b]Portions are approximate.

110

> **Morsel** "Cooking should be a carefully balanced reflection of all the good things of the earth." —Pierre and Jean Troisgros (French chef and saucier, *Michelin Guide* 3-star recipients since 1968)

The Healthy Meal

A healthy meal has balance and proportion and represents most of the basic food groups that are described in Chapter 1. People with specialized dietary needs, such as vegetarians, some ethnic groups and those with food allergies, may not be able to consume certain groups of foods. Foods and beverages that meet their specialized needs will be addressed throughout this book.

A healthy meal should satisfy diners, not overwhelm them. Not all of the courses that are shown in Table 3-3 need to be served at one meal. A heartier appetizer with a greater proportion of ingredients should be followed by a lighter salad or entree. Likewise, a lighter soup makes way for a heartier entree, and an entree salad may only need a lighter dessert to follow.

Sample menus with serving sizes that are based on the USDA MyPlate recommendations can be found at http://www.choosemyplate.gov/food-groups/downloads/Sample_Menus-2000Cals-DG2010.pdf

Creating Healthy Recipes and Menus

Now the concepts of healthy food, healthy plates and healthy menus have been established, this information can be applied to recipe and menu development. It will be beneficial in revising traditional recipes and menus and in developing new ingredients, foods, recipes and menus for today's health-conscious consumers.

Recipes and menus can be adjusted to reduce calories, total fat, certain types of fat, sugar and sodium, and increase nutrients such as vitamins, minerals and fiber. However, it is not just a matter of reducing or eliminating ingredients to make a dish healthier. This is because these ingredients may also be important in the structure, function and flavor of a dish.

Reducing, substituting and eliminating ingredients in recipes are part science, part art, and part trial and error. It may take a series of ingredients to find the best ones to use in the right amounts. If one ingredient is reduced, then other ingredients may become more pronounced.

For example, a touch of sugar will temper, or soften, the natural sodium in tomatoes and bring out their sweetness. But add too much sugar, and the tomatoes may taste like jam.

Reducing the fat in a recipe might cause the final product to become too dry and unpalatable. Besides imparting moisture, fat carries flavor. The other flavors in a recipe may be lost or unbalanced without a little fat to unite them. The converse is also true: add too much fat or oil (even heart-healthy extra-virgin olive oil), and the final product may be unpalatable.

Basic Guidelines for Adapting Recipes

These are three basic guidelines for adapting recipes to make them healthier:

1. Change the cooking techniques and/or method of preparation
2. Reduce, remove, or replace ingredients
3. Rebuild flavor

CHANGE COOKING TECHNIQUES AND/OR PREPARATION METHODS

Fundamental cooking techniques form the basis of culinary education. The teachings of Antonin Carême, Auguste Escoffier and Jean Anthelme Brillat-Savarin, all great nineteenth-century chefs and food experts, have stood the test of time and will continue to do so. Like other disciplines, the culinary arts are in the process of integrating the old with the new.

Boiling, braising, char-grilling, creaming, deep and shallow frying, and stewing still have their place, but with some healthier upgrades. Instead of deep or shallow frying, consider sauteing with less fat and calories. Rather than braising, try roasting so the fat can drip off and be discarded. Searing, sweating and reducing can seal, release and concentrate ingredients and flavors.

Use stock, broth, juice or wine instead of basting meat, poultry or fish in their own fat. Nonstick pans and/or nonstick cooking sprays can further reduce the dependence on fat in cooking calories. The purpose behind changing preparation methods is to capture flavor and retain nutrients without excessive fat, sugar, sodium or calories.

REDUCE, REMOVE OR REPLACE INGREDIENTS

One ingredient at a time can be reduced, removed or replaced to note the effects that its reduction, removal or replacement has on the recipe. If too many ingredients are changed at once, one may not know which ingredient manipulation was effective.

With many recipes—but not all—the amount of fat, sugar, sodium and calories can be cut back without substantially losing too much flavor. The following are some of the ways to reduce or replace fat, sugar and sodium in recipes. Substitutes are discussed later in this chapter and throughout the book.

- *Fat reduction:* Think of fat reduction as baby steps, not giant ones. Start by cutting back on the amount of fat and oil in recipes by a tablespoon or two at a time and then noting the results. This is particularly important in sauces and mixtures that are dependent on fat and in baking. You'll learn more techniques about fat reduction and fat substitutes in Chapter 6.
- *Fat replacement:* Consider replacing fats with some of the following, often healthier, ingredients. Make sure that their flavors and textures are compatible. Many of these ingredients are quite flavorful, so less may be required.
  - ○ Bacon—Canadian, soy or turkey bacon; smoked lean meat such as Italian prosciutto or Spanish Iberian ham
  - ○ Butter—whipped butter; trans-free and nonhydrogenated margarine or shortening; vegetable oil; applesauce or prune puree in baking

111

- ○ Cream cheese—reduced, low- or nonfat cream cheese, French Neufchatel or mild goat cheese; pureed cottage cheese
- ○ Cream sauce or cream soup—dairy milk-based sauces or soups; evaporated skim milk; pureed vegetables such as potatoes or cauliflower; silken tofu or thickened soy milk; thickened rice milk
- ○ Eggs—egg substitutes; egg whites; smooth tofu
- ○ Ground beef—lean or extra-lean ground beef; ground turkey or chicken (both beef and poultry 90 to 95 percent lean or fat-free)
- ○ Mayonnaise—reduced, low- or nonfat mayonnaise or salad dressing; olive oil mayonnaise; soy mayonnaise
- ○ Dairy milk—reduced, low-fat or nonfat dairy milk; evaporated skim milk; soy or rice milk
- ○ Oil-based dressing—acidic fruit juice, such as lemon or orange; broth; flavored vinegar, wine
- ○ Sour cream—reduced, low-fat or nonfat sour cream; plain dairy or soy yogurt

- *Sugar reduction:* Like fat reduction, sugar reduction should also be carefully executed. Sugar reduction can be more aggressive in some syrupy dressings or sticky sauces. The goal is to retain a sweet but not overbearing taste and rounded texture.

  But sugar is a critical ingredient in appearance, flavor, moisture retention, sweetness, texture and volume in some recipes. Reducing too much sugar may adversely affect their outcome. Sugar reduction guidelines and sugar substitutes are discussed in Chapter 4.

- *Sugar replacement:* Sometimes nothing can replace the taste and texture of sugar. This is especially true in some recipes for baking. In other recipes, the imaginative use of some of these ingredients, alone or in combination, may help replace sugar.
  - ○ Artificial flavorings—sweet spices, such as allspice, cinnamon, cloves, ginger or nutmeg; sweet extracts, such as almond or vanilla, and sweet/fat flavorings, such as butter or nut, boost sweetness, intensity and uplift flavors and create aroma of "fattening" sweetness; zest, such as lemon or orange, bring out freshness and fruitiness
  - ○ Chocolate—cocoa powder plus strong coffee or espresso in concentrated liquid or powder forms to enhance the chocolate flavor
  - ○ Candied fruits—chopped dried fruits to distribute flavor and sweetness
  - ○ Fruits canned in heavy syrup—fresh fruits; fresh-frozen fruits; fruits canned in 100 percent fruit juice
  - ○ Fruit-flavored yogurt—plain low- or nonfat yogurt with fresh or dried fruits
  - ○ Fruit drink or "ade"—100 percent fruit juice
  - ○ Jams or jellies—fruit juice concentrates or fruit juices (concentrated to one-third volume)
  - ○ Sugar frosting—spice and brown sugar mixture or 100 percent fruit spreads
  - ○ Sugar syrup—reduced-sugar syrup; a lesser amount of honey, maple syrup or molasses; pureed fruit

- *Salt reduction:* Similar to sugar and fat, salt has other roles in cooking and baking besides flavor. Salt provides its own briny taste, and it functions as a flavor enhancer to bring out the other four basic tastes of acidic, bitter, sweet and umami. Salt also suppresses bitterness, slows yeast fermentation, and helps to preserve food. Salt reductions should be tiny at first, especially in baking. Suggestions for salt and sodium reductions can be found in Chapters 7 and 9.

- *Salt replacement:* Similar to fat and sugar, it may be almost impossible to replace the omnipresent taste of salt or sodium in some recipes. This may be due to its indispensible need in some cooking and baking preparations and its habitual uses and expectations.

  The following are some suggested salt/sodium replacements. However, they may not work in all recipes, so experiment with them for the best possible taste acceptance.
  - ○ Bottled and packaged salad dressings—oil, vinegar, herbs and spices
  - ○ Seasoned salt—herb and spice blends
  - ○ Canned bouillon, broths, soups, sauces and/or mixes—reduced-sodium varieties
  - ○ Canned vegetables—reduced sodium varieties; drain and rinse some canned vegetables
  - ○ Condiments—reduced-sodium sauces, such as catsup and mustard; rinsed garnishes, such as olives and pickles
  - ○ Food additives and preservatives (such as sodium citrate and sodium phosphate)—use fresh ingredients
  - ○ Processed meats and cheeses—freshly cooked or unprocessed meats and cheeses
  - ○ Salted cooking water—reduce salt or eliminate

○ Seasoning mixes—salt or sodium-free herb and spice blends
○ Soy sauce—reduced-sodium soy sauce or tamari
○ Table salt—herb and spice blends; course sea salt or kosher salt (less can be used because the crystals are large)
○ Tomato products—reduced sodium tomato products or fresh tomatoes

REBUILD FLAVOR

Healthy cooking is more than doing without certain ingredients or foods. It is also a matter of *rebuilding flavor* or *developing new flavors* through the inspired use of flavorful ingredients including chutneys, coulees, extracts, flavored oils and vinegars, herbs and spices, infusions, juices, marinades, purees, reductions, relishes, rubs and pastes, salsas, sauces, stocks and broths, wines and spirits and more.

- *Chutney:* Originally from India, **chutney** actually refers to a group of sweet and spicy condiments. Chutney is similar to relish or salsa. It usually contains fresh, chopped vegetables or fruits and a range of herbs and spices, from spicy and savory to sweet and tart.
- *Coulis:* A **coulis** is a thick sauce that is made from pureed and strained vegetables or fruits. A vegetable coulis is generally served warm with meats or vegetables, or it can serve as a base for soups and other sauces. A fruit coulis can be used cold or warm in desserts, but it can also be served with meats or vegetables. The flavor and color of a coulis are often that of the main ingredients.
- *Extracts:* An **extract** is made by extracting the aromatics from fruits, herbs, nuts and spices with a solvent, such as ethanol or water. Extracts can be sweet or savory. Sweet extracts include almond, cinnamon, cloves, ginger, lemon, nutmeg, orange, peppermint, pistachio, rose, spearmint, vanilla, violet and wintergreen. Savory extracts are generally concentrated reductions of meats or poultry. Both types of extracts function as intense flavor enhancers.
- *Flavored oils:* **Flavored oils** are oils that carry a distinct flavor and often aroma. They can be dribbled over food to add flavor or around the rim of a dish for color and a hint of richness. Flavored oils include basil, garlic or truffle-flavored oils and oils that are infused with citrus juice or zest, herbs or spices, among other ingredients. Flavored oils may appear in or on lower-fat dishes, such as soups, salads, grains or vegetables to lend flavor and richness.
- *Oils:* **Oils** are lipids that are liquid at room temperature. They can be relatively odorless and tasteless, such as canola or safflower, so they do not interfere with the flavor of a dish. Or they can be very aromatic and flavorful, such as extra-virgin olive oil or nutty walnut, hazelnut or sesame oils, which impart distinct flavors that should be accounted for in finished dishes.
- *Vinegars:* **Vinegars** are acidic liquids that are produced from the fermentation of ethanol. They are basically made from fermented wine. Vinegars add acidic taste to foods, sometimes color and help to balance flavor. Generally, the more aged the vinegar, the deeper the flavor.

   Vinegars include apple cider, balsamic, champagne, distilled white, malt, rice and wine (red and white), among others. **Flavored vinegars** can be savory or fruit-flavored. They are infused with fruits, herbs (such as basil or tarragon), grains, spices, vegetables (such as chilies or onions), wine and other ingredients. Just a few drops are usually enough to impart taste and color to dishes.
- *Herbs and spices:* **Culinary herbs** are aromatic plants. Their leaves, stems and flowers are used in cooking to impart flavor. **Medicinal herbs** are used for treating disease. Mostly all parts of the plant are used. **Spices** are strongly scented seeds, bark, roots, and fruits that are used to add flavor and aroma to dishes.

113

Bite on This: general guidelines for cooking with culinary herbs and spices

Herbs and spices have been used in culinary and medicinal applications since antiquity. Preserving their freshness, flavor and quality is essential. Spices do not spoil, but they lose their strength. Whole spices keep the longest, since their flavors are contained. Ground spices have a shorter shelf life. Herbs are more fragile; they may lose their aroma, color and intensity sooner. Place herbs and spices in airtight containers and store in cool dry places. Do not shake them directly from their containers while cooking because this may introduce moisture.

To determine whether or not herbs and spices are still useful, gently shake the closed containers. Then smell the contents to determine if their aroma is still present. You can also test their aroma by crushing a small amount in your hand.

Here are some general guidelines for the use of culinary herbs and spices:

- Use herbs or spices to enhance nutritious foods—not to disguise poor quality foods.
- Use only enough herbs and spices so the taste and aroma of the ingredients in a dish are enhanced and not masked.
- Generally add dried herbs and spices at the beginning of the cooking process so they can impart their flavors and soften over time, and fresh herbs toward the end of the cooking process to retain both color and flavor.
- Because their flavor is concentrated, use less dried herbs than fresh herbs. Each herb is slightly different. A general rule for using dried and fresh herbs is *about ¼ teaspoon of powdered dried herbs equals ¾ to 1 teaspoon of crumbled dried herbs, which equals about 2 to 4 teaspoons of fresh herbs.*
- *Herbes de Provence* are a mixture of dried herbs of the Provence region of France. They generally contain basil, fennel, lavender, savory and thyme, and can be used like other dried herb mixtures in longer cooking dishes or infused in oil.
- To clean fresh herbs, gently rinse them under cold water. Shake the herbs to remove excess water, or gently spin them in a salad spinner. Place the herbs in a slightly dampened paper towel and refrigerate in the vegetable drawer or cooler for short-term storage.
- Fresh herbs should be finely minced because more of the volatile oils will be released. *Fines herbes,* a Mediterranean minced herb combination with chervil, chives, parsley and tarragon, can be used as a garnish (it is also available dried). Fines herbes are particularly tasteful on lighter dishes, such as fish, poultry or vegetables.
- Fresh herbs, such as parsley, thyme and bay leaves, can be tied with string into a bundle, or a *bouquet garni,* and used to prepare soups, stocks or stews and then discarded.
- Other than the herb bundle, fresh herbs should be added close to the end of cooking hot dishes or just before serving to retain their aroma and flavor. Delicate herbs, such as basil, cilantro or dill, should be added during the last few minutes of cooking. Sturdier herbs, such as rosemary or thyme, may be added a little earlier.
- For cold dishes, such as dips, cheeses, vegetables or dressings, add minced fresh herbs; then refrigerate for several hours or overnight and bring to room temperature before serving. The exception is fresh basil, which may become bitter.
- Try mixing mild and strong dried and fresh herbs together to complement, such as milder basil, cilantro, lemon thyme or marjoram with more robust oregano, rosemary, sage or winter savory.

Some culinary uses of herbs, herb blends and spices are shown in Table 3-4. Some of their medicinal uses are provided in Chapter 9.

TABLE 3-4 Culinary Uses of Herbs, Herb Blends and Spices

Herbs, Herb Blends, Spices and Spice Blends	Culinary uses
Angelica	Cakes, chartreuse (French liqueur), gin
Basil	Minestrone, pesto, tomatoes
Bay	Braises, sauces, soups, stews
Borage	Salads, soups, stews, vegetables
Caraway	Akvavit (Scandinavian flavored spirit), cheeses, rye bread, sauerkraut
Chervil	Carrots, poultry, salads, seafood
Chives	Eggs, salads, soups, stews
Cilantro	Caribbean, Chinese, Indian, Mexican, Thailand and Vietnamese cuisines
Dill	Baked vegetables, pickles, savory pastries
Epazote	Indian and Mexican cuisines

(Continued)

TABLE 3-4 (continued)

Herbs, Herb Blends, Spices and Spice Blends	Culinary uses
Fennel	Eggs, lamb, pickling, sausages, sauces, stews
Garlic chives	Eggs, fish, poultry, potatoes, shellfish
Horseradish	Cocktail sauce, Japanese wasabi
Hyssop	Meats, salads, soups
Lavender	Infused syrups, lamb, poultry
Lemon balm	Eggs, fresh fruits, salads, soups
Lemon verbena	Custards, fruits, herbal teas, South American cuisine
Lovage	Southern European cuisines
Marjoram	Beans, eggplant, poultry, seafood, tomatoes
Mint	Dessert and beverage garnishes, lamb, poultry, vegetables
Oregano	Tomatoes, Greek, Italian and Mexican cuisines
Parsley	Most foods except desserts, garnishes
Rosemary	Chicken, lamb, seafood, vegetables
Sage	Fresh or cured pork, poultry, vegetables
Salad burnet	Dressing, salads
Sorrel	Pureed soups, sauces
Summer savory	Beans, stews, meat dishes, vinegar infusions
Tarragon	Eggs, chicken, fish, salads, vegetables
Thyme	Poultry, root vegetables
Winter savory	Beans, lentils, meats, poultry, tomatoes
Herb blends	
Bouquet garni	Sauces, soups, stews
Fines herbes	Cheeses, eggs, fish, game, meats, salads, sauces, soups, stews, vegetables
Herbes de Provence	Fresh vegetables, fish, game meats, soups, stews
Spices	
Allspice	Breads, braised meats, cakes, cookies, marinades, pickled foods, stewed fruits, tomato-based sauces
Anise	Italian breads and cookies
Annatto	Meat, rice, Indian, Spanish and Mexican cuisines
Capers	Fish, game, sauces
Caraway	Breads, casseroles, poultry, meat
Cardamom	Baked goods, curries, fruit dishes
Celery seed	Cole slaw, potato salad, pickling
Chiles	Indian, Indonesian, Korean, Mexican, Szechuan, Tex-Mex and Thai cuisines
Cinnamon	Cookies, pie, rolls, Greek, Indian and Moroccan cuisines
Cloves	Hams, pickling, sauerkraut, spice cake
Coriander	Baked goods, stews, Indian, Scandinavian and Middle Eastern cuisines
Cumin	Indian, Latin American and Moroccan cuisines
Fennel	Bouillabaisse (Mediterranean fish and shellfish stew), pork stew, roasts, sausages
Fenugreek	Ethiopian, Indian and Moroccan cuisines
Ginger	Asian and British cuisines
Juniper	Boar, lamb, sauerbraten, sauerkraut, venison
Mustard	Dressings, marinades, pickling, sauces
Nutmeg	Breads, cookies, custards, eggnog, squash, spice cakes
Paprika	Creamed sauces, deviled eggs, fish, salads, sausages
Pepper	Universal use as salt
Poppy seeds	Cakes, cookies, noodle dishes, strudels, yeast breads

115

(Continued)

TABLE 3-4 (continued)

Herbs, Herb Blends, Spices and Spice Blends	Culinary uses
Saffron	Breads, rice, chicken
Sesame seeds	Breads, crackers, Asian and Mediterranean cuisines
Star Anise	Baked goods, Asian cuisine
Turmeric	Curries, stews, Asian cuisine
Vanilla	Baked goods, ice cream, sauces
Spice blends	
Chinese five-spice powder *(Chinese five-spice mixture of cloves, cinnamon, fennel, Sichuan pepper and star anise)*	Chinese and Vietnamese cuisines
Curry powder *(South Asian mixture of coriander, cumin, fenugreek, red pepper and turmeric)*	Indian, Pakistani, Bangladeshi, Sri Lankan, Nepali, Indonesian, Malaysian, Thai, Chinese and other South Asian and Southeast Asian cuisines
Pickling spice *(Regional mixture of allspice, bay leaves, cardamom, cinnamon, cloves, coriander, ginger, mustard seeds and peppercorns)*	Pickling
Quatre-epices *(French four-spice mixture of cloves, ginger, nutmeg and white pepper)*	French charcuterie (patés, sausages, terrines), stews

Source: [4].

116

- **Infusions:** *Infusions* are extractions of flavors from foods at temperatures under boiling. Oils and vinegars can be infused with savory or sweet flavors, including basil, chili, chives or garlic and blueberry, fig, lemon, orange or raspberry. Infused oils and vinegars can be used on their own or in recipes for dressings, marinades, salads, sauces, soups and more.

- **Juices:** *Juices* are liquid extractions from plant tissues. Fresh juices, especially citrus, can be dribbled over foods to impart a sweet, tart or sweet/tart flavor and to balance flavor. Squirt fresh lemon juice over broccoli or fish: it balances both the bitterness of the broccoli and the sweetness of the fish and brightens the dish overall.

  Juices can be reduced to achieve both a syrupy consistency and concentrated flavor. Sweeter fruit juices, such as apple or white grape juice, work especially well. Herb and vegetable juices can also be reduced and then used to flavor stocks, sauces or glazes. Keep in mind that the colors of fruit and vegetable juice reductions will also concentrate in intensity or dullness.

- **Marinades:** *Marinades* are seasoned liquids that help to flavor and moisten food. They are generally used before cooking, and they frequently contain an acidic ingredient, such as citrus juice (citric acid), vinegar (acetic acid), wine (malic and tartaric acid) or yogurt (lactic acid). Marinades also serve to partially digest tougher cuts of protein (similar to the effects of hydrochloric acid on protein in the stomach during digestion).

  The advantage of using a marinade is that additional fat may not have to be added during cooking. To help prevent drying, the marinade could be used for basting. Most marinades only contribute a modest amount of fat calories.

- **Purees:** *Purees* are a general term for fruits, legumes or vegetables that have been passed through a sieve and formed into a soft paste or thick liquid. Purees can be used to thicken sauces or soups, as dips or spreads, or as side dishes.

- **Reductions:** *Reductions* are liquids that have been reduced in quantity by evaporation. Reduction concentrates flavors and thickens liquids, such as sauces (see *juices*).

- **Relishes:** *Relishes* are cooked or pickled sauces, typically made with chopped vegetables or fruits. Relishes can be chunky or smooth, savory or sweet, and hot or mild. *Chutneys* are a type of relish. Relish is normally made with vegetables, while chutney is mostly made with fruits.

- **Rubs:** *Rubs* are a type of marinade, but they are dry, not wet. Rubs are blends of herbs, spices and other ingredients, such as coffee or cocoa, that are rubbed onto the exterior of meat, poultry or fish. They serve to add flavor, seal in flavor, and protect the natural juices from leaking and drying out the meats. By using rubs, little additional fats or oils need to be used. Wet rubs, or **pastes**, can be mixed with mustard, oil, vinegar, water or other flavorful liquid, such as broth or stock, to produce a flavorful crust--also on meats.

- **Salsas:** *Salsas* are various cold vegetable–based sauces, generally of Italian, Latin American or Spanish origins. Some are thin or pureed, while others are chopped or chunky. Chilies, fruits, herbs and/or spices can be added to the vegetable mixtures. Roasting or toasting some of the ingredients will help to caramelize them and add a depth of flavor. Salsas can be used as sauces for many protein dishes, or they can be served on their own as dips.

- **Sauces:** *Sauces* are liquids or semisolid liquids with a thickening agent, such as arrowroot, cornstarch, or flour and seasonings. Sauces can also be prepared by reduction (see **juices** and **reductions**). Sauces can be used to moisten food and add flavor.

  In the nineteenth century, French chef Antonin Carême gave the name "Mother Sauces" to four sauces because they are the basis for all other sauces. These are bechamel (white), espagnole (brown), tomat (red) and veloute (roux or liason, as egg yolk or cream). Then in the twentieth century, Auguste Escoffier named hollandaise (butter) the fifth Mother Sauce, with its classical emulsions, including mayonnaise.

  Gravy, mayonnaise, simple pan sauces, tomato, vinaigrette and sweet sauces, such as caramel, chocolate, custard, fruit and sabayon, are useful to enhance the flavor of simple foods. But easy does it: use the least amount of any sauce to impart the most taste. Many of these sauces can also be slimmed down in calories, fat and sugar.

- **Stocks:** *Stocks* are the backbone of classic and modern dishes. Stocks are flavorful liquids made with a combination of ingredients that include a combination of bones (beef, fish or poultry), water, herbs and spices, and a **mirepoix.** Mirepoix is French for "mixture," and it generally includes a combination of 50 percent onions, 25 percent carrots and 25 percent celery (fennel, leeks or tomatoes can also be added). Besides flavorful, stocks are filled with gelatin, extracted from the bones, that provides structure and body and gels when it is chilled.

  The color and flavor of a stock are determining factors in how a final dish both looks and tastes. A brown stock is made by caramelizing the bones and vegetables before they are added to the water. It is hearty, and it is usually used in meat-based dishes. In contrast, a white stock tends to be delicate and is useful in equally delicate fish dishes.

  A vegetable stock can be made without bones. To create a depth of flavor, a variety of vegetables, herbs and spices may be used. Vegetables such as mushrooms, peas and tomatoes contribute a meaty quality. Very aromatic vegetables, such as broccoli or cauliflower, may offset the flavor of the finished dish. A splash of soy sauce adds a meatlike or umami quality.

- **Broth:** *Broth* is a thin liquid that is made by straining and reducing the cooking liquid in which foods are cooked. Broth is sometimes referred to as **au jus, essence, nage** or **tea.** It is sometimes served in a small pool underneath the main ingredient or entree. Vegetable or fruit juice can also be used in this manner. Canned beef or chicken stock is sometime referred to as broth. Reduced-fat and sodium versions may be versatile in some recipes.

- **Wine, beer and spirits:** *Wine, beer and spirits,* distilled from almost any food that contains sugar (such as barley, corn or grapes), can be used to enhance flavor without contributing too many calories. If added during cooking, the alcohol will probably burn off and the flavor should have time to mingle with the other ingredients. If added at the end of cooking, the alcoholic taste may dominate the finished dish. Thoughtful use is prudent.

117

Healthy Recipe Makeovers

New and/or improved cooking techniques and preparation; reduced, removed or replaced ingredients; and rebuilt flavors are the hallmarks of healthy recipe and menu makeovers. Two recipes will be examined to improve the techniques, change the ingredients, and rebuild the flavor. These suggestions can be employed to make over familiar recipes or to develop new ones.

RECIPES MAKEOVERS: INGREDIENT REDUCTIONS, SUBSTITUTIONS, ELIMINATIONS, AND TECHNIQUE CHANGES

BROCCOLI WITH MUSTARD SAUCE *(BEFORE MAKEOVER)*

Ingredients

1½ pounds fresh broccoli, washed and trimmed
¼ cup butter
½ cup mayonnaise
1 tablespoon Dijon mustard

Directions

- Cut broccoli into 3-inch pieces, including stalks and florets.
- Place broccoli into boiling water; cook about 7 minutes.
- Remove to platter; keep warm.
- Combine mayonnaise with butter and mustard; spoon sauce over broccoli.

Yield: 6 servings

Calories per serving: 233 calories

Percentage of calories from fat: 83%

BROCCOLI WITH MUSTARD SAUCE *(AFTER MAKEOVER)*

Ingredients

1½ pounds fresh broccoli, washed and trimmed
¾ cup reduced-fat mayonnaise
½ tablespoon Dijon mustard
1 teaspoon sugar
Dash reduced-sodium soy sauce
Reduced-fat dairy milk (to thin sauce)

Directions

1. Cut broccoli into 3-inch pieces, including stalks and florets.
2. Steam broccoli for about 7 minutes, or until fork-tender. Remove to platter; keep warm.
3. Combine reduced-fat mayonnaise with mustard, sugar and soy sauce.
4. Whisk milk into sauce to thin; spoon over broccoli.

Yield: 6 servings

Calories per serving: 64 calories

Percentage of calories from fat: 19%

- *Changed techniques:* Boiling to steaming (reduces nutrient loss).
- *New and improved techniques:* Whisked sauce to incorporate milk and thin (adds nutrients; decreases calories).
- *Reduced, removed or replaced ingredients:* Replaced mayonnaise with reduced-fat mayonnaise; reduced Dijon mustard (reduces fat, sodium).
- *Rebuilt flavor:* Added sugar (for balance), reduced-sodium soy sauce (for umami taste).

FRUIT NUT MUFFINS *(BEFORE MAKEOVER)*

Ingredients

Vegetable shortening
2 cups all-purpose (AP) flour
1½ cups white granulated sugar
2 teaspoons baking soda
1 teaspoon ground cinnamon
½ teaspoon salt
3 large eggs
1 cup vegetable oil
½ cup shredded coconut
1 teaspoon vanilla extract
2 cups apples, peeled and grated
½ cup raisins
½ cup carrots, peeled and grated
½ cup walnuts, chopped

Directions

1. Preheat oven to 350°F.
2. Grease well with vegetable shortening two (12-cup) muffin tins.
3. Sift dry ingredients together into large bowl; set aside.
4. Combine carrots, raisins, walnuts, apples and coconut in large bowl.
5. Whisk eggs, oil and vanilla together in medium bowl.
6. Gently stir carrot mixture into dry ingredients; coat to cover.
7. Add liquid ingredients; stir just to combine.
8. Spoon mixture into greased muffin tins.
9. Bake about 25 minutes.

Yield: 18 large muffins

Calories per muffin: 520 calories

Percentage of calories from fat: 47%

FRUIT NUT MUFFINS *(AFTER MAKEOVER)*

Ingredients

Nonfat cooking spray
1 cup all-purpose (AP) flour *plus* 1 cup whole wheat flour (OR ½ cup whole wheat flour *plus* ½ cup whole wheat pastry flour)
¾ cup white granulated sugar
2 teaspoons baking soda
1 teaspoon ground cinnamon *plus* ½ teaspoon each ground nutmeg and allspice
¼ teaspoon salt
2 large eggs *plus* 2 egg whites
½ cup vegetable oil *plus* ½ cup unsweetened applesauce
2 teaspoons vanilla extract
2 cups unpeeled apples, grated
½ cup raisins
¾ cup unpeeled carrots, grated
2 tablespoons walnuts, chopped

Directions

1. Preheat oven to 350°F.
2. Prepare muffin tins with nonfat cooking spray.
3. Sift dry ingredients together into large bowl; set aside.
4. Combine carrots, raisins, walnuts and apples in large bowl.
5. Vigorously whisk egg whites in medium bowl.
6. Whisk eggs, oil and vanilla together in medium bowl.
7. Gently stir carrot mixture into dry ingredients; coat just to cover.
8. Add liquid ingredients; stir just to combine.
9. Spoon mixture into prepared muffin tins.
10. Bake in nonstick muffin tins about 22 to 25 minutes.

Yield: 18 large muffins

Calories per muffin: 410 calories

Percentage of calories from fat: 40%

- *Changed techniques:* Left skin on apples and carrots (improves fiber).
- *New and improved techniques:* Whisked egg whites (increases rise); used nonfat cooking spray; baked in nonstick muffin tin (reduces fat, calories).
- *Reduced, removed or replaced ingredients:* Used one-half whole wheat flour and one-half white AP flour (improves fiber, nutrients); decreased salt and walnuts (decreases sodium and fat); substituted two egg whites for one whole egg (decreases cholesterol); substituted ½ cup unsweetened applesauce for ½ cup vegetable oil (decreases fat).
- *Rebuilt flavor:* Added nutmeg and allspice, one additional teaspoon vanilla, ¼ cup carrots.

120

Bite on This: healthy alternatives for fat in cooking and baking

The reason to cut back on fat as an ingredient in cooking and baking is that fat is calorie-dense and it contributes to obesity. Moreover, total fat and saturated fat are implicated in degenerative diseases such as certain cancers, coronary heart disease, diabetes and hypertension. While some fat is essential to the diet, these healthful alternatives will help to trim excess fat in cooking and baking.

FRIED FOODS

Fried foods are concentrated sources of calories, fats and carbohydrates. While breading lends a crunchy texture to fried chicken, tempura and fish and chips, healthier versions can be prepared. A little coating can be flavorful without overloading the palate. Try a light nut coating (if allergies are not an issue), chestnut flour, cornstarch, oatmeal, Japanese bread crumbs (panko) or rice flour to help lighten fat and calories. Use clean, hot oil and shorten the frying time to help decrease oil absorption.

CREAMY FOODS

Creamy foods, such creamed spinach or roux-based soups (often referred to as cream soups) are quite rich in fat and high in calories. A *roux* is a classically cooked combination of fat and flour in equal parts by weight. Rather than use cream or a roux, puree cooked bland vegetables, such as cauliflower or potatoes, or add instant mashed potato flakes to thicken. A reduced-fat dairy product may also be incorporated, but there might not be enough fat to hold the ingredients together.

BUTTER OR MARGARINE

A stick of butter can be replaced by a stick of margarine in some recipes, but oil is different. This is because oil is 100 percent fat, while butter, margarine and solid shortening are actually lower in fat than oil on a per volume basis. Use ⅞ cup of oil for 1 cup of butter, margarine or solid shortening.

In baking, substitutions of this nature can be even more problematic. Solid fats are creamed with air when they are whipped with sugar and eggs, but oil is more compact—and oily. Oil can make cakes, cookie and pastries greasy and dense.

If necessary, substitute about 3 parts oil for every 4 parts solid fat (or about ¾ cup oil to 1 cup solid fat). It may require a few trials to determine the exact amount that works. Diet, fat-free, light, lower-fat, reduced-fat, reduced-calorie and vegetable oil spreads are generally not successful substitutes in baking, since these products are higher in water and lower in fat.

CHEESE

Reduced-fat cheese has different melting characteristics than regular cheese. It takes longer to melt and it may be tougher. To compensate, finely shred, and let it melt over very low heat while stirring constantly. Before adding reduced-fat cheese to sauces, sprinkle with a little starch or flour, such as arrowroot, cornstarch, potato starch or rice flour, for uniform melting. Do not use reduced-fat or low-fat cheese on the top of a pizza, casserole or sandwich because it may become too dry and difficult to chew.

MEAT

About ¼ to ½ of the amount of ground meat in a recipe may be replaced with cooked grains or legumes, such as brown rice, couscous, millet, oats or soybeans. This substitution decreases fat and calories and adds fiber and nutrients. However, the finished product may be chewy or dry. Broth, stock or vegetable juice can be added during preparation to increase moisture. The cooking time may need to be decreased.

To retain moisture and flavor when cooking larger, lower-fat cuts of meat, marinate the meat; coat the meat with a flavorful rub; sear the meat before longer cooking, or cover the meat during roasting.

POULTRY

To prevent poultry from drying out, cook it with the skin on when baking or roasting. A dollop of fat (a tiny spoonful) can be mixed with herbs and spices and inserted under the skin; then the skin can be removed before serving. Despite these techniques, fat and calories may actually decrease once the skin is removed; plus, the finished dish will be moist and flavorful.

CAKES, COOKIES AND QUICK BREADS

While fat is an important ingredient in baking for taste and texture, some reductions may be made. One to 2 tablespoons of fat for each 1 cup of flour may be enough fat in biscuits, muffins or quick breads, and no more than 2 tablespoons of fat for each 1 cup of flour may be enough fat in cakes or soft-drop cookies. Chocolate, coconut, nuts, seeds and other higher-fat ingredients may be reduced by ¼ to ½ of the amount that is called for in some recipes.

Bite on This: healthy alternatives for sodium in cooking and baking

There is a compelling reason for using less sodium in cooking and baking: We consume far too much sodium in ingredients, foods and beverages in the United States, which is directly related to hypertension, or high blood pressure. By limiting sodium in cooking, and to a lesser degree baking, we may be able to retrain our taste buds to desire less.

While most people may benefit from sodium reduction, some people may need to be especially careful about all of the sodium that they consume. Options for cutting back sodium include the use of kosher salt, sea salt, finishing salt and salt substitutes. More ways to reduce sodium are covered in Chapters 7 and 9.

KOSHER SALT

Kosher salt is also called *koshering salt* because it is used in the process of koshering meats by removing surface blood. It has a much larger and more porous grain size than common table salt. Kosher salt contains sodium chloride, but it typically does not contain the mineral iodine, so it is not considered iodized salt. Some kosher salt contains anticlumping agents in small amounts.

Kosher salt may be useful in sodium reduction. One teaspoon of kosher salt contains about 1,120 milligrams of sodium. In comparison, 1 teaspoon of table salt contains about 2,325 milligrams of sodium.

Total sodium should be limited to less than 2,300 milligrams daily; and 1,500 milligrams for people aged 51 or older, African Americans or people with existing chronic kidney disease, diabetes or hypertension.

Kosher salt can be used in most cooking applications. Some chefs prefer Kosher salt to table salt for its purity. However, Kosher salt is generally not recommended for baking applications—especially recipes that contain a small amount of liquid ingredients, since it may not thoroughly dissolve.

In recipes that contain more liquid, use up to twice as much kosher salt (by volume) to replace table salt (because kosher salt grains are larger and occupy more volume for equal weight). Since the size of kosher salt grains vary, check each type of kosher salt for specific conversion guidelines.

Kosher salt may be used as a finishing salt for cooked and baked goods to give the illusion that an item is saltier. However, its porous grains help to remove moisture, so other finishing salts may be superior to retain moisture and infuse a mineral-like taste.

SEA SALT

Sea salt is produced through the evaporation of seawater. Sea salt usually undergoes little processing, so depending on its water source, some trace minerals may remain. These minerals may contribute both color and flavor in cooking and baking.

Coarse sea salt with its large crystals contains, on the average, about 1,872 milligrams of sodium per teaspoon compared to 1 teaspoon of table salt at 2,315 milligrams. By weight, sea salt (like kosher salt) and table salt contain about the same amount of sodium chloride.

Finer-grained sea salt is shaped like little hollow and flaky pyramids. This shape allows the grains to better adhere to food than table salt and also to dissolve better. As a result, less may be needed. Some varieties of sea salt may be better for baking than table salt because their trace minerals may help in the development of gluten. Like kosher salt, sea salt may be used as a finishing salt to communicate a briny taste.

FINISHING SALT

A *finishing salt* can be both the first introduction to a food and the last lingering taste. Strategically sprinkled finishing salt transmits salty and sometimes mineral tastes, combines and increases food flavors, provides flavor complexity, and lends texture and sometimes aroma.

Similar to sea salt, most finishing salts come from the sea. They include Black Diamond from the Mediterranean, Fleur de Sel from Guatemala, Maldon from England, and Molokai Red and Kauai Guava from Hawaii.

SALT SUBSTITUTES

The use of "lite," "low-sodium" and "salt-free" salt substitutes is discussed in Chapters 7 and 9. In general, do not use salt substitutes where sodium is a vital ingredient in the success of a dish or baked item. A higher ratio of sodium chloride to potassium chloride moderates some of the bitterness, but then it is not a sodium-free product.

Some salt substitutes that contain part sodium chloride may be used successfully in baking, and this may reduce the total amount of sodium in recipes. Salt substitutes that only contain potassium chloride are not recommended for baking. The flavor and texture of baked goods will not be the same quality as those that are made with sodium chloride (table salt).

Bite on This: healthy alternatives for sugar in cooking and baking

Sugar substitutes are designed for people who want to reduce their carbohydrate consumption due to weight control or diabetes restrictions. Others may choose sugar substitutes for their alleged health properties. For a complete discussion of sugar and sugar substitutes in health and disease, see Chapters 4 and 9.

Healthy alternatives for granulated white sugar in cooking and baking include the following:

- *Fructose* (fruit sugar) is about 2½ times sweeter than white sugar (sucrose). About ½ cup of granulated fructose can be substituted for about 1 cup of white sugar. Fruit sugar has a slightly finer and more uniform crystal than white sugar. For this reason, it is used in dry mixes such as gelatin, powdered drinks and puddings. The uniformity of its crystal size prevents separation or settling of larger crystals, which is an important quality in dry mixes.
- *Date Sugar* is not really sugar but is made from ground, dehydrated dates. It is about 60 to 80 percent sugar. About 1 cup of date sugar can be substituted for about 1 cup of white sugar in some cakes, muffins and quick breads, but adjust to taste. Date sugar can replace the brown sugar in crumb toppings for fruit crisps or pies.
- *Honey* is 20 to 60 percent sweeter than white sugar. About ¾ cup honey can be substituted for about 1 cup of white sugar. For every 1 cup of honey, reduce the amount of other liquids in a recipe by ¼ cup and add ¼ teaspoon of baking soda. This is because honey is naturally acidic and baking soda helps to balance its acidity. Lower the oven temperature about 25° to prevent baked goods that contain honey from overbrowning.
- *Raw sugar* is sugar at the point before the molasses is removed in the processing of sugar cane. Different types of raw sugar include demerara from Guyana, finely textured Barbados, and light, molasses-flavored turbinado. Their sweetening properties are similar to white sugar. Varying degrees of brown color and flavor may affect the final products in both cooking and baking.
- *Sucanat* resembles raw sugar, but it is actually the evaporated juice of sugar cane. Sucanat is less refined than white sugar and it tends to have a strong aftertaste. It contains 12 calories per teaspoon—about 25 percent fewer calories than white sugar at 16 calories per teaspoon. Substitute an equal quantity of sucanat for white sugar and add ¼ teaspoon of baking soda to balance the acidity.
- *Stevia* is a South American herb that is 150 to 400 times sweeter than white sugar. The sweet taste of stevia has a slower onset than white sugar, but it lasts longer. The benefit of stevia is that it does not significantly alter blood sugar, so it can safely be consumed by diabetics. At high concentrations, stevia can have a bitter, licorice off-taste. Substitute one pinch to ¹⁄₁₆ of a teaspoon of stevia for 1 teaspoon of white sugar.
- **Other:** Other substitutions for one cup of white sugar include the following ingredients. Their tastes vary considerably, which may affect the outcome of recipes, so choose carefully.
  - ⅓ cup agave nectar
  - ½ cup fruit juice concentrate
  - ½ cup molasses
  - ⅔ cup maple sugar
  - ⅔ cup rice syrup
  - 1 cup malted barley

123

FOOD BYTE

Cookware with nonstick surfaces has improved since DuPont, a science-based products and services company, trademarked Teflon, the nonstick coating that affects the ability of cookware to conduct heat, in 1945. Today's nonstick cookware has better heat conduction, plus it is durable and easy to maintain. But nonstick cookware does not caramelize protein as well as metal cookware. Its main purpose is the reduction of fat in cooking.

Basic and Specialized Cooking Tools and Equipment

A chef's tools and equipment are like an artist's brushes, paints and canvases. To create appealing recipes and meals, certain basic and specialized tools and pieces of equipment are essential, which are shown in Table 3-5.

TABLE 3-5 Basic and Specialized Tools and Equipment for Cooking
Cooking Tools

High-carbon stainless steel knives
2- to 4-inch paring knife for cutting fruits and vegetables[a]
4- to 6-inch butcher knife for cutting raw meat
8- to 14-inch all-purpose French or chef's knife for chopping, slicing and mincing[a]
6- to 8-inch utility knife for cutting fruits and vegetables[a]
Serrated bread knife[a]
Slicer
Sharpening stone
Chef's fork
Measuring cups and spoons
3-cup glass measuring cup with spout
Set of measuring cups: ¼ cup, ⅓ cup, ½ cup and 1 cup
Set of measuring spoons: ¼ teaspoon, ½ teaspoon, 1 teaspoon and 1 tablespoon
Spatulas
Angled handle spatula
Small and standard-sized rubber scraper spatulas
Straight spatula
Metal grill spatula[a]
Spoons
Large metal spoon
Stainless-steel slotted spoon[a]
Sturdy metal spoons
Wooden spoons
Strainers
3-inch-diameter wire mesh strainer[a]
7-inch-diameter wire-mesh strainer[a]
China cap for removing seeds, coarse matter from liquids and soft foods[a]
Chinois for straining custards, purees, sauces and soups[a]
Spider skimmer[a]
Whisks
8-inch wire whisk[a]
Balloon whisk
Rigid whisk
Miscellaneous tools
Bottle opener
Cheese cloth[a]
Chopping boards (plastic and wooden)[a]
Colander[a]
Corer[a]
Corkscrew
Egg beater
Flour sifter
Food mill for pureeing and straining food[a]
Hand can opener
Hand grater[a]
Hand citrus juicer[a]
Instant-read thermometer[a]

(Continued)

TABLE 3-5 (continued)

Cooking Tools

Kitchen scale[a]
Kitchen shears[a]
Kitchen timer[a]
Meat mallet
Meat thermometer
Mixing bowls
Molds
Portion scoop[a]
Potato masher[a]
Ricer for extruding food[a]
Rolling pin
Salad spinner[a]
Sieves[a]
Sifter
Soup ladle[a]
Straight tongs
Vegetable peeler[a]
Zester[a]

Cooking equipment

Pots and pans

2-cup, 2-quart and 6-quart saucepots with lids
8-cup ovenproof casserole
8-inch frying pan with lid
10- or 12-inch saute pan with lip[a]
12×17-inch roasting pan
Cast-iron skillet[a]
Hotel pans
Pasta pot[a]
Sautoir pan with straight sides for reductions[a]
Wok with lid[a]

Miscellaneous equipment

Blender[a]
Grill[a]
Food processor[a]
Hand-held electric mixer[a]
Juicer[a]
Mandoline for slicing[a]
Stand mixer with attachments[a]

[a]Tools and equipment especially suited for healthy cooking—often for lower-fat and/or nutrient retention.

FOOD BYTE

Cast-iron cookware heats slowly and holds heat well. It is good for searing and frying food. While cast iron may impart a metallic taste and react with acidic foods, some of the iron particles may be passed on to the food that is being cooked. This may be beneficial for women who tend to have iron deficiencies. Another benefit of cast-iron cookware is its longevity. A good cleansing, scrubbing and drying should clean old cast-iron cookware and prepare it for contemporary use.

What Heat Is, What Heat Does and How Heat Applies to Healthy Cooking and Baking

The process of digestion bears so much resemblance to heat and cooking. Heat helps to physically break down food and move it around a cooking or baking vessel for further processing. Our teeth physically break down food inside the mouth; then our tongue moves the food to the back of the mouth to be swallowed and digested.

Heat also prepares foods for chemical reactions, which are similar to what occurs inside the mouth when food is mixed with saliva. The following sections explore what heat is, what it does, and how it applies to healthy cooking and compares it to the remarkable process of human digestion.

HEAT IS ENERGY

Heat is transferred to foods by three basic methods: *conduction, convection* and *radiation*. **Conduction** is the direct-contact transfer of heat, such as when a pot or pan is placed on a flame or coil. In conduction, heat is moved from the flame or coil to the food to be cooked, thereby transferring heat, or energy.

A good example of conduction is the searing (or browning) of meat. Searing is quick, as is the transfer of heat from the flame or coil to the pan and then to the meat. As the meat is exposed to heat for a longer period of time, the heat is then transferred from the seared exterior to the interior of the meat.

Heat is also transferred through **convection** through fluids. Picture a pot of soup that is just beginning to warm. As the flame or coil heats the pot through conduction, the liquid on the bottom of the pot heats and rises, and the cooler liquid from the top of the pot descends into the pot to warm the remaining liquid.

Unlike conduction and convection, **radiation** does not require contact with a heat source. Rather, radiation relies upon an element that gives off radiant heat, such as a broiler or a toaster oven.

Microwave cooking uses a combination of conduction and radiation heat. In microwave cooking, radiation is created inside the oven, which stir ups molecules and creates heat. Then the heat spreads throughout the foods and beverages through conduction and convection, depending on whether the food is solid, liquid or both. Microwave cooking generally does not brown food.

All three methods of heat transfer can be healthy *if* foods are not overheated or overcooked, liquids are not overboiled and there are no major changes in nutrient retention.

WHAT HEAT DOES

Anytime heat is applied to food it can change a food's characteristics and nutrients. It is very important to be mindful of its effects when considering the finished products. This is especially true with protein.

> **FOOD BYTE**
>
> Sometimes the "feel" of food is the best judge of readiness or doneness. To determine **doneness in meat,** use your fingers. Gently press the center of the meat with perfectly clean fingers to determine the degree of resistance. Very rare meat will feel like raw meat and offer little resistance. Rare meat will feel springy; medium meat will feel slightly firm but yield to the touch, and well-done meat will feel firm to the touch. Make sure to wash your hands before touching other foods.

The Effect of Heat on Protein

Heat causes proteins to *coagulate,* or firm up. Examples of coagulated protein include egg whites that turn from clear to white when heated and bread dough that rises and forms into loaves when baked.

Protein transforms into different degrees of **doneness,** depending on how much heat is transferred over time. For example, a 1-inch steak that is cooked for 3 minutes and is soft in the center is considered rare. If it is cooked for 5 minutes and firm in the center, it is considered well done.

Too much heat may cause protein to toughen or lose its functionality. This is called **denaturation**. Examples of protein denaturation from too much heat include rubbery egg whites and hardened cheese pizza. Other causes of protein denaturation include overwhipping, acids, bases or a high salt concentration.

Gastric acid in the stomach is also responsible for protein denaturation. The acid helps to break down the protein and prepares it for further digestion.

126

The Effect of Heat on Carbohydrates

Heat also causes carbohydrates to change in structure. When grains are cooked with a fluid, such as water or stock, heat causes the grains to absorb, or take up the liquid and swell. This process is called *gelatinization*, and it is said that the grains *gelatinize*. The mixture becomes gruel-like, and if it continues to cook, it becomes even more solidified. Gelatinization occurs both in cooking and baking. Acceptability and nutrients may be compromised.

In addition, the building blocks of carbohydrates, or sugars, are affected by heat. They *caramelize*, which means they brown in color and change flavor. Some caramelizing is desirable because of the unique flavors and colors that develop. Bread crust becomes golden with a toasted taste, and *caramelized sugar* becomes lightly browned with a pleasant earthy taste. Sometimes a food that is overcaramelized can have a burnt taste and flavor.

The Effect of Heat on Fats and Oils

Upon heating, fats first *melt* if they are solid, but they do not evaporate like water. Fats and oils have different *melting points*—the temperature range at which they change from a solid state to a liquid state.

Fats and oils may be heated too high, which may cause them to break down and form unhealthy substances and undesirable flavors. This depends on their *smoke point*—the temperature at which fats and oils start to smoke. Oils with high smoke points include canola oil, corn oil, refined peanut oil and vegetable oil. Butter and olive oil have lower smoke points. There is more discussion about the smoke point of fats and oils in Chapter 6.

FOOD BYTE

Broiling is advantageous in healthy cooking, since fat drops away from food and can be discarded. When broiling, make sure to preheat the broiler and the broiler pan. This will ensure that the food to be broiled is well seared by the flame or element and that the natural juices are retained. Do not use a fork to turn the food; a tong or metal spatula is preferred. These tools protect foods from being pierced, the juices from leaking out, and the food from drying out. An instant-read thermometer is good to keep handy.

HEAT APPLICATIONS IN HEALTHY COOKING

Healthy methods of cooking include both *dry- and moist-heat cooking methods.* Explanations of dry- and moist-heat cooking methods follow, along with their healthier adaptations.

Dry-Heat Cooking Methods: Baking, Broiling, Deep-frying, Grilling, Pan-frying, Roasting and Sauteing

Dry-heat cooking methods generally rely on air or fat to cook food. While some fat helps to impart and carry flavor, too much fat can overpower dishes or cause them to fail, contribute too many calories and lead to health problems. The following methods can decrease the amount of fat in dry-heat cooking:

- *Baking: Baking* is a dry-heat cooking method by which food is surrounded by hot, dry air. Baking cooks food first by convection, then by conduction, and finally by caramelization. Baking is used to cook fruits, proteins, starches and vegetables and both savory and sweet baked goods.
- *Broiling: Broiling* is a dry-heat cooking method that uses radiant heat from a source above the food that is to be cooked. If the food is placed on a grate over a broiler pan, then the fat can drip away and be discarded. The advantages of broiling are that food can be quickly broiled to doneness, and caramelization intensifies taste. A disadvantage of broiling is that more expensive (and richer) cuts of meat may be used, which may not retain heat well during service or at a buffet.
- *Deep-frying: Deep-frying* is a dry-heat cooking method that transfers heat by convection through flame or coil to a pot, and then by conduction to the foods that are submerged in hot fat. Foods are typically

first coated in batter or breading. While deep-frying is not synonymous with healthy cooking, in some Mediterranean countries deep-frying is done with little coating and at very high temperatures. Foods cook rapidly and absorb little fat.

- **Grilling:** *Grilling* is a fast and hot dry-heat cooking method where foods are cooked directly over a source of dry heat, such as a charcoal or gas grill, or on a stovetop grill pan. Foods are typically placed on a grate, thus allowing fat to drip away and be discarded. **Barbecuing** is a type of grilling. A disadvantage of grilling and barbecuing is that foods can be charred. This blackening can produce potentially cancer-causing substances. There is more information about this connection in Chapter 9.

- **Pan-frying:** *Pan-frying* is a dry-heat cooking method that is similar to both sauteing and deep-frying, but only a moderate amount of fat or oil is used. The heat is transferred by conduction to the pan and then by convection to foods by hot fat or oil. Like deep-frying, foods are usually first usually coated in batter or breading. In order for pan-frying to be considered a healthy technique, a minimal amount of fat, oil, batter or breading should be used.

- **Roasting:** *Roasting*, like baking, is a dry-heat cooking method that depends on dry heat in a closed environment, such as an oven. Meats and poultry are usually roasted, as opposed to vegetables, fruits, grains and savory and sweet desserts, which are typically baked (with some exceptions). Roasting also uses the heat transfer processes of convection, conduction and caramelization for more depth of flavor. Roasting is a healthy cooking method for larger cuts of meat. The advantage of roasting is that foods are usually cooked on a rack so that fat can drip away and be discarded. The disadvantage of roasting is that more expensive cuts of meat with sufficient marbling are generally used; other cuts of meat may dry when roasted.

- **Sauteing:** *Sauteing* is a dry-heat cooking method that uses a small amount of fat or oil to cook food over high temperature by conduction. **Dry-sauteing** is generally done in a very hot pan in order to sear foods, such as fish, poultry or meat. Both sauteing and dry-sauteing are considered healthy cooking techniques because only a small amount of fat is used at hot temperatures. The advantages of dry sauteing are that additional fat is not used and that food is caramelized for depth of flavor. The disadvantage of dry-sauteing is that more expensive (and richer) cuts of meat may be used, which may not retain heat well during service or on a buffet.

- **Stir-frying:** *Stir-frying* is a dry-heat cooking method that is similar to sauteing. What distinguishes stir-frying from sauteing is that it relies on the use of a pan with sloped sides or a Chinese wok to circulate the heat and to ready the food for gentle tossing. The advantage of stir-frying is that very little fat or oil is used, like sauteing.

- **Sweating:** *Sweating* is a dry-heat cooking method that cooks food in a pan without browning or caramelizing, typically by conduction over low heat. The purpose of sweating is to help foods release their natural liquids and flavors and slightly soften. An advantage of sweating is that no additional fat or oil may be needed. Another advantage is that delicate foods, such as fruits and vegetables, can be cooked in this manner and their nutrients can be preserved.

FOOD BYTE

The secret of cooking vegetables to the correct degree of doneness begins with cutting the vegetables into same-sized pieces so they can transfer heat and cook evenly. Cooking time should be as short as possible to maximize their nutrients and preserve their color and texture. Typically vegetables are done when they are fork-tender, unless they are to be added to other ingredients for additional cooking. Vegetables can also be **shocked**—plunged into ice water directly after blanching to halt the cooking process and preserve color.

MOIST-HEAT COOKING METHODS: BOILING, POACHING, SIMMERING AND STEAMING

Moist-heat cooking methods generally use water, stock, broth or steam into which foods are submerged. They are generally considered to be healthy cooking methods, with some exceptions as noted:

- **Boiling:** One of the most common moist-heat cooking methods that uses convection heat is *boiling*. First, heat is transferred by conduction from a flame or coil to a pot. Then heat is transferred by convection to the liquid that is contained within the pot. The high heat and rapidly boiling water cook foods quicker than poaching or simmering. The disadvantage of boiling foods is that if they are boiled too long, they can lose nutrients, especially if the cooking water is discarded.

- *Poaching*: Like boiling, *Poaching* is a moist-heat cooking method that uses conduction heat from a flame or coil to heat a pot or pan, then convection heat through a poaching liquid to heat food. The poaching liquid can be broth, juice, stock, water, wine or some combination. The advantages of poaching is that tender foods, such as eggs, fish and vegetables, may be poached for short cooking times and that additional fat is not required. When cooked to the right degree of doneness, poaching can produce tasty and nutritious foods that absorb the flavor of the cooking liquid. The disadvantages of poaching include the flavor of food may not be deep, since there is no caramelization; once removed from the poaching liquid, foods may dry out; and overpoaching may lead to stringy or toughened fish, poultry and meats and overcooked fruits or vegetables.

- *Simmering*: Similar to boiling and poaching, *simmering* **is** a moist-heat cooking method that uses convection heat that has been first been transferred by conduction from a flame or coil to a pot or pan, then convection heat through a simmering liquid to heat food. In simmering, the temperature of the cooking liquid is higher than in poaching, and the liquid is more agitated. Simmering is usually used for tougher cuts of protein or foods that need more time to cook than poaching. Like poaching, the flavor of the simmered food may be affected by the cooking liquid. The disadvantages of simmering are that the temperature is higher and the time is longer than poaching. Both have the potential of causing nutrient loss.

- *Steaming*: *Steaming* is a moist-heat cooking method that also uses heat transfer by convection and conduction, like boiling, poaching and simmering. In steaming, foods are placed in a steamer basket or colander and then lowered over steam that is produced by boiling liquid. A lid that is placed over the pot or pan can speed the steaming process. The advantage of steaming is that foods can be steamed until just "fork tender," which helps retain the nutrients that may filter into the cooking water, such as minerals, phytonutrients and vitamins.

COMBINATIONS OF COOKING METHODS

A combination of cooking methods can be used to first brown grains, protein or vegetables by convection, and then continue to cook these foods in liquid by conduction. A combination of cooking methods is often used for less-tender cuts of meats and/or fibrous vegetables that may take a longer time to cook.

- *Braising* and *stewing* normally use a combination of dry- and moist-heat cooking methods. As long as fat can be removed or reduced, they can be considered healthy cooking methods.
  - *Braising*: Braising uses dry- and moist-heat cooking methods. First, less-tender cuts of meats are browned in fat or oil at a high temperature. Then vegetables and seasonings are added with a liquid or sauce. The heat is then reduced and the pan is covered.
  Foods are then cooked by simmering in the liquid or sauce and by steaming from steam that is released by the simmering liquid and captured by the lid. The process is long and slow until the foods are tender. To make a braised dish healthier, it should be cooked in advance and then cooled. Then the fat should be removed before the dish is reheated for serving.
  - *Stewing*: Stewing also uses dry- and moist-heat cooking methods. The differences between stewing and braising are smaller pieces of foods are used in stewing and the pieces are blanched, or cooked quickly in a boiling liquid, fat or oil. Like braising, a flavorful liquid or sauce is then added, and then the foods simmer in the liquid or sauce until tender.
      The advantage of stewing is that the cooking time is shorter than in braising due to the smaller pieces of food, which facilitate faster heat transfer. Like braising, to help make the stewing process healthier, the stew should be cooled and the fat should be removed. Then the dish should be reheated before serving.

- *Slow cooking*: *Slow cooking* deconstructs tougher cuts of meat, fruits grains, legumes and vegetables. An acidic ingredient, such as citrus or tomato juice, vinegar or wine, helps to break down the protein and rounds out the flavor. The advantages of slow-cooking are that leaner cuts of meat can be used at lower temperatures and no additional fat needs to be added. The food and ingredients create their own sauce and nutrients are retained.

Healthy Baking Equipment and Tools

Careful, correct and safe baking requires some essential tools and equipment—similar to the basic cooking tools and equipment that are required for healthy cooking. Specialized equipment can be quite expensive with limited functions. Basic baking tools and equipment and those with the most versatile uses in healthy baking are highlighted in Table 3-6.

TABLE 3-6 Basic and Specialized Tools and Equipment for Baking
Baking Tools
High-carbon stainless steel knives
2- to 4-inch paring knife for cutting fruits and vegetables[a]
6- to 8-inch utility knife for cutting fruits and vegetables[a]
8- to 14-inch all-purpose French or chef's knife for chopping, slicing and mincing[a]
Serrated bread knife
Slicer
Sharpening stone
Cutters
Aspic
Corer
Doughnut
Melon ball[a]
Round biscuit
Rolling (pastry wheel)
2-inch cookie
Decorating and finishing tools
Cake combs
Cake-decorating turntable
Dispensing tips
Pastry bags
Graters
Flat metal[a]
Four-side box[a]
Rotary[a]
Measuring cups and spoons
3-cup glass measuring cup with spout
Set of measuring cups: ¼ cup, ⅓ cup, ½ cup and 1 cup
Set of measuring spoons: ¼ teaspoon, ½ teaspoon, 1 teaspoon and 1 tablespoon
Spatulas
Angled-handle spatula
Metal cake
Small and standard-sized rubber scraper spatulas
Straight spatula
Racks
Cake
Wire
Rolling pins
Hard wooden
Marble
Teflon-coated
Sifters
Flour sifter,
Drum sieve (tamis) for grating, straining or as a food mill
Spoons
Perforated[a]
Plain
Slotted[a]

(Continued)

TABLE 3-6 (continued)

Baking Tools

Strainers
3-inch-diameter wire mesh strainer[a]
7-inch-diameter wire-mesh strainer[a]
China cap for removing seeds, coarse matter from liquids and soft foods[a]
Chinois for straining custards, purees, sauces and soups[a]
Spider skimmer[a]

Whisks
8-inch wire whisk[a]
Balloon whisk[a]
Rigid whisk[a]

Miscellaneous tools
Can opener
Cheesecloth[a]
Food mill[a]
Instant-read thermometer[a]
Pastry brushes
Portable timer[a]
Portion scoop[a]
Straight tongs
Vegetable peeler[a]
Zester[a]

Baking equipment

Baking pans, baking dishes and tins
8-inch and 9-inch round cake pans
8×8×2-inch cake pan or baking dish
9-inch pie pan
9-inch square cake pan
9-inch springform pan
9×5-inch loaf pan
9×13×2-inch baking pan
12-cup muffin tin
Flan pan
Full and half size heavy-gauge aluminum pans[b]
Hotel pans

Baking sheets, trays and racks
Cooling racks
Full- and half-size sheet trays and baking sheets (including nonstick and rimmed)[b]
Silicone baking sheets or mats[a]

Bowls and cups
1-quart stainless, ceramic or glass mixing bowl
3-quart glass mixing bowl
8 small glass cups

Molds, ramekins, cups and tarts
Molds
¾ cup ramekins or custard cups[a]
Tart pans

Pots and pans
2-cup, 2-quart and 6-quart saucepots with lids
8-inch frying pan with lid
10- or 12-inch saute pan with lid[a]
Randeau/brazier (medium to large pot, more shallow than saucepot)

Miscellaneous
Baker's scale[a]
Blender[a]

131

(Continued)

TABLE 3-6 (continued)

Baking Tools

Food processor[a]
Immersion blender[a]
Juicer[a]
Kitchen scale[a]
Mandolin[a]
Mixer[a]
Slicer[a]

[a]Tools and equipment especially suited for healthy baking—often for lower-fat and/or nutrient retention.
[b]Size dependent on home or restaurant use.

Healthy Baking Ingredients and Techniques

Special dietary and health needs, including certain cancers, diabetes, food allergies, gastrointestinal disorders, heart disease and hypertension, may require changes in baking ingredients and/or techniques. As in cooking, some baking ingredients may be *reduced*, *substituted* or *eliminated*. Baking techniques may also need adaptations. Since baking is such an exacting process, care and respect must be taken for the finished products.

Certain ingredients can be reduced in some recipes, such as sugar in fruit filling or butter in frosting. However, these ingredients may be critical to other recipes, such as sugar in meringues or fat in pie crusts.

Some ingredients may be substituted, such as oil for butter or honey for sugar, but this will not work in all recipes. When fat or sugar is eliminated in a recipe, this may cause the recipe to fail. But sometimes this is essential, such as the elimination of gluten or nuts for allergic consumers.

Bite on This: healthy baking reductions, substitutions and eliminations

Certain foods and beverages have specific roles in baking—just like in cooking. A thorough knowledge of these roles is fundamental before any ingredient can be successfully reduced, substituted or eliminated.

Dairy products, eggs, fat and oils, gluten, nuts and seeds, salt, soy and sugar are reviewed here for their purpose and use in baking, as well as the effects of reducing, substituting or eliminating these ingredients.

Dairy Products
- **Purpose:** Contributes appearance, flavor, structure and texture
- **Use:** Creates body, contributes sweet flavor (from lactose, or milk sugar), promotes browning (from caramelization)
- **Reduction:** Replace liquid dairy products with an equal amount of other liquids, such as water, juice or nut milk, depending on recipe.
- **Substitution:**
    - ○ Reduced-fat dairy milk for whole dairy milk
    - ○ Nut milk, rice milk, soy milk, reduced-fat coconut milk, unsweetened fruit juice or water for whole dairy milk
    - ○ Light cream, half-and-half or soy "creamer" for cream
    - ○ Reduced, low-fat or soy-based sour cream, cottage cheese, yogurt or ice cream for full-fat varieties
    - ○ Clarified butter (with milk solids removed), oil, soy margarine or **tahini** (sesame seed paste) for butter

TABLE 3-7 Egg Substitutes for One Whole Egg

Serving sizes	Products
¼	cup silken tofu[a] or soy yogurt,[b] blended
1	tablespoon ground flaxseed[c] *plus* 1½ fluid ounces (2 to 3 tablespoons) warm water
1	medium banana, pureed[d]
1	tablespoon soy flour *plus* 1 tablespoon cornstarch *plus* 2 tablespoons water
1	tablespoon soy flour *plus* 2 tablespoons water (less thickening)
2	tablespoons arrowroot starch
2	tablespoons cornstarch
2	tablespoons potato starch
2	tablespoons water *plus* 1 tablespoon vegetable oil *plus* ½ teaspoon baking soda

[a]***Silken tofu*** *can be used in dense cakes or brownies, but it may make cookies cakey. One teaspoon of arrowroot or cornstarch can be added to a recipe to help compensate for this change in texture.*
[b]***Soy yogurt*** *functions the same way as silken tofu. It works best in quick breads and muffins.*
[c]***Flax*** *is very earthy in taste and smell and works best in equally earthy whole-grain recipes. The taste and gelling effect of flax can be overpowering if too much is used. It is best to first experiment with less.*
[d]***Pureed bananas*** *hold the air bubbles in batter fairly well. They help to impart moisture, flavor and browning due to their natural sugars. Pureed bananas work well in quick breads, muffins, cakes and pancakes.*

- **Elimination (for food allergies, vegetarians and some ethnic diets):** To eliminate dairy products altogether, look for butter, buttermilk, casein, cheese, cream, ice cream, lacto-albumin, dairy milk in all forms, and yogurt in recipes and on food labels.

  Caution: When dairy products are substituted with any of the above ingredients, the final product may be less tender with less structure. Also, some fat-reduced dairy products contain ingredients that may interfere with a recipe's success. For example, gelatin is a protein that is sometimes used in reduced-fat yogurt; it may cause baked products to become spongy.

Eggs
- **Purpose:** Contributes appearance, flavor, structure and texture
- **Use:** Captures air, binds ingredients, creates structure, helps achieve browning (from caramelization), imparts richness
- **Reduction:** Reduce the number of whole eggs in a recipe by replacing one whole egg with two egg whites. If fat and cholesterol are not issues, one egg yolk can be added to the egg whites.
- **Substitution:** A number of commercial egg-substitute products are available for whole eggs. Most are a combination of egg whites with ingredients that add color and flavor. Some egg substitutes use flaxseed or other starches or gums to provide body, but they may not achieve the same richness or caramelization that whole eggs provide. Egg substitutes are best used in recipes that require only a few eggs, such as cookies, because they can produce a dense product. Different egg substitutes are shown in Table 3-7.
- **Elimination (for food allergies, vegetarians and some ethnic diets):** If eggs are totally eliminated, then the appearance, flavor, texture and structure of baked goods may suffer.

  Caution: Baking with egg substitutes requires a great deal of trial and error. The egg substitutes that are shown in Table 3-7 have great variability, based upon flour and other ingredients, heat and baking time.

Fat: butter, oil and lard
- **Purpose:** Contributes appearance, consistency, flavor, texture and structure
- **Use:** Adds moisture and richness, assists leavening, extends shelf life, produces tender products, provides flavor and color, shortens gluten strands

  Caution: Butter helps to make cakes light and delicate; it holds the air bubbles that are produced by leaveners such as baking powder or baking soda, and it makes cakes tender by coating the protein in the flour. Reduce, substitute or eliminate butter and a cake recipe may fail.
- **Reduction (for calorie and fat reduction):** Total fat can be reduced as much as 30 percent in some recipes. As an ingredient, fat can be reduced to a ratio of 1 ounce of fat to 4 ounces of flour in some quick breads. To help compensate for reduced fat and maintain tenderness, some bread flour can be exchanged by cake flour in some recipes.

133

Caution: Cookies that are made with butter tend to spread and thin during baking. Less butter means less spread. To reduce the amount of butter and to preserve crispness, a little corn syrup may be added to the dough.

- **Substitution (for calorie and fat reduction):** Fat substitutes include reduced-fat butter, buttermilk, cream cheese, sour cream and yogurt and pureed fruits and vegetables. General guidelines for using these fat substitutes are provided in Table 3-8. Other information on fat substitutes can be found in Chapter 6.
- **Elimination:** Eliminating fats altogether may affect the appearance, flavor, structure and texture of baked items.

Caution: While it might be possible to make light, moist and tender baked items using some of these fat substitutes, replicating the delicious, rich taste of butter is challenging. In the process of reducing fat, you may end up with higher-calorie, tasteless products. Instead of using fat substitutes, smaller-sized cookies, loaves and muffins can be made. This is another way to reduce fat.

Gluten
- **Purpose:** Contributes appearance, structure, texture, volume
- **Use:** Creates elasticity: changes shape with pressure and resumes shape when pressure is removed

---

TABLE 3-8 General Guidelines for the Use of Fat Substitutes

- Some recipes are easier to substitute fats than others. Prepare a recipe a few times to determine what works best.
- In general, quick breads and muffins adapt fairly successfully to fat substitutes, as do carrot, chocolate and coffee cakes with denser textures. It may be more difficult to substitute fat in cakes with very light and tender texture because they depend on fat. You may still be able to eliminate ½ to ¾ of the total fat and retain some fat for texture.
- Substituting oil in place of butter or other solid fat may not achieve the same final product in some recipes. In recipes that require liquid fat (as melted butter), this substitution may work.
- Cakes that are made with butter or solid shortening develop volume from air when fat is creamed with sugar. When fat is eliminated, they may become more compacted. This may be partially solved by whipping egg whites and gently folding them into the cake batter or by adding a fat substitute with the liquid ingredients.
- Look for logical blends of ingredients that make sense with recipes. For example, fruit and vegetable purees, such as applesauce, cooked squash or pureed bananas pair nicely with aromatic spices (allspice, cinnamon or nutmeg) in quick breads and muffins. Milder-tasting yogurt or buttermilk may be better matched with delicate biscuits or scones.
- Many fruits and vegetables contain pectin, a carbohydrate that acts like fat and "shortens" or tenderizes baked goods. Fruit and vegetable purees, reduced-fat buttermilk and yogurt may be able to replace about ½ of the fat in some cookie recipes, unless the recipes contain quite a bit of liquid. Then they may become cakey, chewy, fudgy, rubbery or sticky.
- Use nut milk in place of whole dairy milk, made by pulverizing ¼ cup of blanched almonds, cashews, macadamia nuts or others, and blending this pulp with 1 to 2 cups of water until it is creamy.

  Caution: Nut butters may contain as much fat as dairy milk, but it is mostly unsaturated fat, which is considered healthier than saturated fat in animal products.

- Use coconut sparingly in order to retain the intended flavor of the recipe. Substitute reduced-fat coconut milk for whole fat milk; add coconut-flavored extract to the batter, or sprinkle fresh coconut over the top and edges of baked goods to give the illusion of a rich taste.
- Prune puree may be able to replace as much as all of the fat in some recipes. It works well in chocolate recipes, while applesauce works better in muffins and quick breads because the flavor is more neutral.
- If the final baked product is too dry, add about 1 to 2 tablespoons of lecithin granules to the recipe for the next testing. Lecithin is a by-product of soy oil refining that can greatly improve the texture of baked goods

  Caution: Lecithin is not a low-fat product. One tablespoon of lecithin granules provides about 6 grams of fat; 1 tablespoon of liquid lecithin provides about 12 grams of fat.

- Try some dried butter granules in the batter to mimic the flavor of butter.
- Use a butter-flavored vegetable oil spray to coat the baking pans or sheets.

134

Caution: While not a fat substitute per se, a change in gluten may affect the appearance, structure, texture or volume of a baked product in the same way fat does. When fat is reduced in baking, the exact type and precise measurement of flour are critical. Low-gluten (soft wheat) cake flour can be substituted for all-purpose (hard wheat) flour, which should create a tender product with a soft crumb, like chiffon cake.

- **Reduction:** Gluten is reduced in low-gluten products (see above). It is eliminated for those who are gluten-intolerant (see Chapter 4).
- **Substitution**
  - Tolerated grains include buckwheat, corn, millet, montina quinoa, and rice. Tolerated starches include arrowroot, garfava, potato, soy and other legumes, and tapioca.
  - A combination of tolerated flours and starches is best to replace gluten in recipes. Possible combinations include buckwheat, millet, rice or sorghum with at least 30 percent starch, such as corn, potato or tapioca. For example, 1 cup of bread flour (with gluten) could be replaced with ⅔ cup of rice flour plus at least ⅓ cup of potato starch.
  - Some of the protein and elasticity of gluten can be replaced with **gums**—especially **xanthan, guar** or **locust bean**. Add 1 teaspoon of gum per cup of tolerated flour for pastries and 2 teaspoons of gum per cup of tolerated flour for breads.
- **Elimination (for food allergies):** All traces of these grains must be eliminated on a gluten-free diet: barley, bulgur, oats, rye and wheat (couscous, durum, triticale, kamut, semolina and spelt).

Caution: Gluten-free products are increasing in number as gluten intolerance rises in the United States. Besides grains and flours, gluten lurks in processed foods, such as egg substitutes and frozen yogurt. It is very important to read the ingredient lists on food labels to make sure that they are gluten-free, since gluten is not destroyed in cooking and baking.

Nuts and Seeds

- **Purpose:** Supplies fiber, some fats and oils, texture
- **Use:** Contributes depth of flavor earthiness and texture, especially if toasted
- **Reduction:** Nuts and seeds are not entirely necessary in some recipes, except for recipes that depend on them for particular taste or texture, such as pecan pie or sunflower seed bread. For this reason, nuts and seeds can be easily reduced in some recipes, but dry ingredients and fat may need to be adjusted.
- **Substitution:** Crunchy ingredients, such as bran, flaxseeds, granola or toasted oats may be substituted for nuts and seeds in some recipes. Lightly dust these ingredients with flour before using; this way they can evenly distribute throughout the batter.
- **Elimination (for allergies):** Nuts and seeds may need to be eliminated altogether due to food allergies or digestive problems, such as diverticulosis (outpocketings in the walls of the colon).

Caution: Like gluten, nut and seed allergies are growing in the United States. Peanuts and soy "nuts" are not nuts but legumes. While they may be used as nut substitutes in some recipes, people may also be allergic to peanuts and soy. More information about food allergies can be found in Chapter 5.

Salt

- **Purpose:** Imparts and enhances flavor and sweetness
- **Use:** Slows yeast fermentation for richer, fuller flavor; helps strengthen gluten structure for density, tenderness and crumb; thickens egg yolks
- **Reduction (for hypertension):** The amount of salt in a bread recipe may be decreased from 1 teaspoon to ½ teaspoon per loaf. However, reducing or eliminating salt may cause the dough to rise too quickly and adversely affect the shape and flavor of baked goods. The dough should be prepared with cool water; care should be taken so it doesn't overferment, and it should be left to rise at room temperature.
- **Substitution (for hypertension):** Commercial, sodium-free leavening agents, including baking soda and baking powder, produce variable results. Salt substitutes can impart a bitter off-taste. The amount of sodium varies in these products, so check the labels carefully.
- **Elimination (for hypertension):** If salt is eliminated altogether in bread recipes, knead the dough very well to develop the gluten as much as possible and keep the dough on the stiff side. Do not let the shaped loaves rise too high in the bread pans. Place the bread pans in the oven a little before they are fully risen; otherwise the breads may collapse.

Caution: Breads made without salt may never rise as high as breads that are made with salt, and they may not have as much flavor. An alternative is to use the bread dough for rolls, because the increased amount of crust may produce more flavor.

Soy

- **Purpose:** Contributes color, fine texture, flavor, moistness and protein. Toast soy flour to enhance its nutty flavor.
- **Use:** Supplies dairy-free, ethnic and vegetarian options; inexpensive and cholesterol-free egg substitute (see Table 3-7); gluten-free

  Caution: Baked products that contain soy flour tend to brown more quickly; shorten the baking time or slightly lower the temperature.
- **Reduction:** Soy flour reduces the amount of fat that is absorbed by the dough in fried foods.
- **Substitution:** Since soy flour is gluten-free, it cannot replace all of the rye or wheat flour in bread recipes. Use about 15 percent soy flour (about 2 tablespoons of soy flour per 1 cup of all-purpose or other flour) to produce a dense, moist and nutty-flavored bread. Up to ¼ of the total amount of flour in a recipe may be replaced with soy flour in baked goods that are not yeast-raised. Stir soy flour before measuring to prevent packing.
- **Elimination (for food allergies):** Soy must be omitted in recipes because of soy (or legume) allergies. Soy flour can be used in combination with tolerated flours for those who are gluten-intolerant. To replace 1 cup of wheat flour in recipes, the suggested ratio is about ¼ cup of soy flour to ¾ cup of tolerated flour (see the preceding section on gluten).

  Caution: Soy flour has a higher proportion of fat than some other flours, so it can become rancid and develop an off-flavor unless it is refrigerated.

Sugar

- **Purpose:** Adds caramelization, flavor, moisture, structure, texture and volume
- **Use:** Acts as a creaming agent, assists with leavening, serves as a preservative, supplies food for yeast, tenderizes (prevents gluten formation)
- **Reduction:** Products made with less sugar may be dry, light in color and have a shortened shelf life.
- **Substitution (for calorie and diabetic management):** The following ingredients may be substituted for all or part of the *sucrose*, or white table sugar in some recipes. The success of these substitutions may vary depending on the other ingredients in a recipe, pan size, oven temperature and time. Other sugar substitutes, including artificial sweeteners, are discussed in Chapter 4.
  - ○ **Fructose,** or fruit sugar, is 2½ times sweeter than sucrose. About ½ cup granulated fructose may be substituted for about 1 cup of white sugar in some recipes.
  - ○ **Honey** is 20 to 60 percent sweeter than sucrose. About ½ to ⅔ cup of honey may be substituted for about 1 cup of white sugar. For every 1 cup of honey in a recipe, reduce the amount of other liquids by about ¼ cup, and add ¼ teaspoon of baking soda. This is because honey is naturally acidic and baking soda helps to temper the acidity. Also, lower the oven temperature about 25°F to prevent overbrowning.
  - ○ **Sweet spices,** such as allspice, anise, cardamom, cinnamon, cloves, fennel, ginger or nutmeg, are not too sweet by themselves, but they lend a sweet flavor, particularly when combined.
  - ○ **Elimination:** Elimination of sugar may affect caramelization, flavor, moisture, structure, texture and volume.

  Caution: With obesity and diabetes mounting in the United States, sugar and calorie reduction are critical. But sugar substitutes may fall short of expectations in baking. The finished products may taste too bland, too sweet or too artificial. It may be better to reduce the portion sizes of baked items and decrease the sugar in frostings, glazes or sauces to cut sugar calories.

136

Basic Food Safety in the Kitchen

Food safety is of growing global concern because of resistant microorganisms, questionable food safety practices and our rapidly expanding food supply. The knowledge and ability for handling food safely helps to ensure that food is fit for human consumption. What follows is just an overview of basic food safety in the kitchen. For more information, see "Hungry for More?" at the end of this chapter.

Microorganisms are bacteria, fungi, parasites and viruses. Some microorganisms are friendly and some can be deadly. Some friendly bacteria are located inside the gastrointestinal tract and assist in digesting foods and beverages. Potentially deadly bacteria are called *pathogens.*

When bacteria produce *toxins*, or poisons, these bacteria can kill by ingestion or by intoxication, such as in *botulism. Salmonella* is an example of a bacterial infection in which the bacteria, not the toxin, causes the disease. *Clostridium* is a bacterium that causes a *toxin-mediated infection*, which means that both the toxin and the bacteria may cause illness. Cooking at high temperatures may destroy salmonella, but it may not prevent the dangers of botulism or clostridium.

Factors that breed bacterial infections include the aerobic (oxygen) or anaerobic (lack of oxygen) conditions, the degree of moisture, the degree of temperature, the time of exposure, the type of food and whether the food is in an acid or base environment.

High-protein foods, such as eggs, dairy products, fish and shellfish, meats, poultry and some grains and vegetables, are subject to bacterial infections. Generally high temperatures destroy some of the bacteria in these foods and beverages, but not all. Very low temperatures, such as in refrigeration or freezing, may only prolong bacteria growth.

The *temperature danger zone*, between 40° and 140 °F (4° to 60°C), increases bacteria growth, as does time of exposure. The least amount of time that food is exposed to the temperature danger zone is best. Hot food should remain hot and cold foods should remain cold. Any moisture can foster bacteria growth. This is why dry foods are less risky of bacterial growth.

Bacteria prefer a neutral environment; neither too acidic nor too basic. Adding an acid, such as lemon juice, vinegar or wine, to foods will acidify the food, but it will not necessarily destroy the bacteria. Certain bacteria thrive well in oxygen; others prefer a lack of oxygen, such as in canned foods. These tend to be the most deadly bacteria.

Other microorganisms that spread diseases are *parasites,* of which *trichinosis* is the most common. Trichinosis is caused by consuming undercooked pork or game that has been exposed to the parasite. Originally it was thought that pork needed to be cooked to at least 170°F (77°C), but this caused pork to toughen. Since most of the trichinosis in pork has been eliminated through testing, the current FDA recommendation is that pork should be cooked until 145°F (63°C) with a 3-minute rest time [5].

While the virus hepatitis A may be transferred through fish and shellfish, viruses may be carried by any food, not just proteins. Many viruses enter our food supply through poor food handling and *cross-contamination.* This is when microorganisms are carried from an object to another object, from an object to a person, or from a person to a person. Foods may be cross-contaminated if food service employees do not wash their hands before they come in contact with food or if uncooked and cooked foods interface at any step in the cooking or baking process.

Cross-contamination guidelines emphasize the following:

- Keep dishes and equipment clean and sanitary.
- Practice personal cleanliness in the kitchen.
- Wash hands frequently in hot water.

Though gloves may be worn, they do not guarantee hygiene. Similarly, just because an item looks clean, it may not be sanitary. *Clean* means that visible dirt and food residue have been removed. *Sanitary* means that microorganisms have been destroyed.

Fungi, molds and yeasts may also cause foodborne illness, and in some instances death, such as when poisonous mushrooms or toxin-carrying molds are consumed. These organisms can also affect the taste and quality of foods.

Some chemicals may filter into foods during growth, handling and production. Other chemicals may enter the food supply through the water or soil in which food is grown. Still other chemicals may enter through food processing. This is why it is important to rinse fresh foods before cooking—especially fruits and vegetables.

137

The *Hazard Analysis Critical Control Points (HACCP)* is a method for managing sanitary conditions in food service operations. A summary can be found in "Hungry for More?," along with additional food safety guidelines.

Bite on This: the costs of healthy eating

Buying healthy foods and beverages can be pricey. Calorie per calorie, junk foods and beverages frequently cost less than fresh fruits and vegetables. As food costs soar, how can healthy food and beverage choices be affordable and available for *all* people?

Arguments have been made that the poor can only afford cheap food and that healthy foods and beverages are neither available nor convenient. This may help explain why the highest rates of obesity are seen among people in the lowest-income groups. Impoverished people may compromise the quality of their diet because they *think* it is too expensive to eat healthfully. This is called **food insecurity**—the inability to acquire or consume an adequate quantity or quality of food in a socially acceptable manner.

The notion that healthy eating costs more is well founded. Fresh fruits and vegetables are vulnerable to environmental factors, as are grasses and grains for feeding livestock; thus, they are more likely to increase in price compared to junk food. When people have to economize, they may opt for trimming from the top of the food chain—expensive cuts of meats, cheese and pricier fruits and vegetables. Calorie-dense, lower-nutrient foods and beverages frequently cost less and are perceived as better bargains.

These relatively inexpensive foods and beverages generally contain more fats, sugar and other refined carbohydrates and sodium—substances that plague the US food supply and imply health consequences. Can our society afford these trade-offs? With obesity and diseases of overconsumption (coronary heart disease, diabetes, hypertension and some cancers) on the rise, the answer is "not with good conscience." We must encourage healthy food consumption among the most needy and create ways to make healthy food more affordable and convenient for them.

As nutrition, food science and culinary professionals, we can collaborate in our efforts to inform consumers that "less is more." By decreasing the portion sizes of lean protein, lower-fat dairy products and fresh fruits and vegetables, lower-income consumers may be able to make healthier choices. (The average sizes of some of these foods are two to three times what is recommended by the US government and health associations.)

Two ways to create cost savings and pass these gains on to these consumers are by making seasonal and locally grown foods more available that do not have to bear transportation costs and by cutting back the excessive sugar and fat calories in jumbo soft drinks and oversized fried foods. These savings may be then applied to healthier options.

Just a few years ago, a thrifty food plan to feed a family of four cost about $130 per week; a low-cost food plan cost $6 a day more than the thrifty food plan, or about $170 per week; a moderate-cost food plan cost $11 a day more than the thrifty food plan, or about $210 per week; and a liberal-cost food plan cost $18.50 a day more than the thrifty food plan, or about $260 per week—almost double that of the thrifty food plan [6].

A thrifty food plan is generally just that: frugal, with costlier and more nutritious fruits and vegetables noticeably absent. The US Healthy Eating Index (last revised in 2006) confirms that both fruits and vegetable consumption in the United States is down from 10 years earlier—particularly in impoverished communities [7].

Over 20 million Americans are said to live in "food deserts"—areas across the country with little to no easy access to fresh food. The US government has pledged to eradicate these food deserts by 2017 to help curtail the country's diet-related disease and obesity epidemics and to create new jobs in these communities [14,15].

In 2010, the US government announced a joint plan by Walmart, Walgreens, SuperValu and three regional chains to open 1,500 new stores in food deserts across the United States. Whether or not these actions will help to achieve its goals is left to be seen.

If the United States is to overcome food insecurity as a nation, it must focus on making healthy food appealing, available and economical. Only then will it begin to close the gap between those who have and those who have not and to reduce the explosion of obesity- and diet-related diseases that inflict the poorest inhabitants [8].

SERVE IT FORTH

The following activities are designed to integrate concepts in nutrition and food science with contents from this chapter on culinary arts basics. The goals are to demonstrate hypothetical situations that have real-life applications.

> **Morsel** "Cooking is one of the oldest arts and one which has rendered us the most important service in civic life." —Jean-Anthelme Brillat-Savarin (French epicure, gastronome, lawyer and politician, 1755-1826)

Making a Difference in Culinary Education

A number of associations serve to meet the needs of chefs and other culinary specialists. Some provide specialized education in culinary nutrition and/or include nutritionists in their membership. Still others offer student memberships. Affiliations in these associations and others provide opportunities for continuing education, competitions, employment, networking and scholarships. For the purpose of these activities, assume the following:

You have a new healthy dining program that you want to promote among culinary associations. It contains healthy recipes, menus, techniques and procedures that reduce calories, fat, sodium and sugar. You are seeking to make a difference in the nutrition and culinary education of their members. You are willing to take the necessary steps to market this program among these memberships, but you are not a member of any of these associations. Answer the following questions regarding *each* association:

- Which aspects of the association will/will not make it receptive to a healthy dining program?
- Describe the strategies you would take to market your healthy dining program to the association membership.

1. The American Culinary Federation (ACF) is the largest professional chefs' organization in North America. It was established in 1929 through the unified visions of three chefs' associations in New York: the Chef de Cuisine Association of America, the Societe Culinair Philanthropique, and the Vatel Club. ACF seeks to make a positive difference for culinarians through apprenticeship, education and certification. Nutrition education is required for ACF certification.
   Junior members of ACF enrolled in a postsecondary or apprenticeship program but with less than three years of field experience are entitled to all ACF resources and to compete in regional and national events.
2. The American Personal and Private Chef Association (APPCA) is a young organization that was created in response to interest in personal and private chefs across the United States. Its mission is to promote education and advancement of its members in the personal chef industry and to help better the personal chef industry as a whole. It offers opportunities for business support, education, idea exchange and standards of excellence.
   Student members of APPCA qualify for this membership designation by being enrolled in a training program of an accredited institution or program.
3. The International Association of Culinary Professionals (IACP) is a nonprofit association that is dedicated to continuing professional education and career development for its members in culinary education, communications and the preparation of food and drink. IACP seeks to be an international forum for the professional worldwide food community. Its mission is to assist its members in ethical, responsible and professional means of achieving success in food-related careers.

Three additional activities can be found within the *Culinary Nutrition* website at www.culinarynutrition. elsevier.com.

WHAT'S COOKING?

The following experiments integrate nutrition, food science and the culinary arts into observable and practical applications. Flavor in recipes, sensory interactions, acidity in dairy milk, color and food perception, plate presentation and proportionality all serve to illuminate the concepts in this chapter to show their usefulness in many food service and consumer settings.

1. **Flavor in recipes**

   Objectives
   ○ To demonstrate the perception of flavor in recipes
   ○ To determine how basic tastes affect the overall flavor in recipes

   Materials: Recipe; ingredients, tools and equipment for preparation of recipe

   Procedure
   1. Find a cooking or baking recipe that you consider to be flavorful.
   2. Fully explain your choice.
   3. Note which of the basic tastes are represented by each of the ingredients. (If an ingredient does not lend a taste, explain what it does in conjunction with other ingredients.)
   4. Prepare the recipe as written.

   Evaluation
   ○ Use a Data Sheet like the one that follows to rate each of the basic tastes in the recipe. Note if they are/ are not apparent.
   ○ Rate the overall flavor of the recipe.
   ○ Which of the ingredients would you adjust, and how would it/they affect the overall flavor of this recipe based on the information in this chapter?

   Data Sheet

Basic taste	Apparent (yes/no)	Too little	Too much	Just right
Salty				
Acidic				
Bitter				
Sweet				
Umami				
Overall flavor before adjustment:				
Ingredient adjustment:				
Overall flavor after adjustment:				

   Culinary applications
   How can this exercise be applied to new product and recipe development?

2. **Sensory interactions**

   Objective
   ○ To demonstrate the importance of sight and smell in taste perception

   Materials
   Plated protein entree with starch and vegetables, such as chicken, mashed potatoes and cooked carrots (This food can be prepared at home or obtained from a school cafeteria or restaurant.)
   Scarf or blindfold

Procedure
1. Seat a volunteer behind a table that is set with a place setting.
2. Cover the volunteer's eyes with a scarf or blindfold.
3. Place a dish before the volunteer that contains the plated entree, starch and vegetables at the right temperature for serving.
4. First, instruct the volunteer to take deep sniffs of the aroma and describe his/her reactions; record on the Data Sheet like the one that follows.
5. Then instruct the volunteer to eat the meal and describe his/her reactions; record on the Data Sheet. (This step may require some help!)
6. Remove the scarf or blindfold; have the volunteer react to the appearance of the food; record on the Data Sheet.

Evaluation
○ Based on your recordings, how would you assess the sense of smell in meal perception?
○ Based on your recordings, how would you assess the sense of taste in meal perception?
○ Based on your recordings, how would you assess the sense of sight in meal perception?

Data Sheet

Basic Taste	Apparent (yes/no)	Too little	Too much	Just right
Reactions to aroma				
Reactions to taste				
Reactions to appearance				

Culinary applications
Based on the sensory information in this chapter, what would you do to modify cooking techniques or preparation for people with reduced smell, taste, vision or multiple sensory issues?

3. **Acidity in dairy milk**
   Objective
   ○ To determine if the amount of fat in dairy milk affects flavor perception
   Materials: Three small glasses, skim, 2% milk and whole milk; eye dropper; vanilla extract
   Procedure
   1. Pour milk into three small glasses of milk, using skim milk, 2% milk and whole milk.
   2. Using an eye dropper, place exactly 3 drops of vanilla extract into each of the glasses of milk.
   3. Taste each of the contents. (You can cleanse your palate with a sip of water between tasting each type of milk and vanilla solution.)
   Evaluation
   ○ Note the way each of the milk solutions look on the sample Data Sheet like the one that follows.
   ○ Note the way each of the milk solutions smells; record on the Data Sheet.
   ○ Now compare the taste of each of the milk solutions; record on the Data Sheet.
   ○ Which milk solution has the strongest taste of vanilla? The weakest?
   ○ Why do you think this has happened based on the information that you have learned about fat in this chapter?

141

   Data Sheet

Type of Milk (with vanilla)	Appearance	Aroma	Taste
Skim milk			
2% milk			
Whole milk			

   Culinary applications
   If a recipe calls for higher-fat dairy products, fat or oil and vanilla, and you are to make the recipe more heart-healthy, how should these ingredients be adjusted, if at all?

4. **Color and food perception**
   Objectives
   ○ To witness how the sense of sight affects food perception
   ○ To identify how past experiences affect food perception
   Materials: Package lemon Jell-O, eye dropper, red food coloring
   Procedure
   1. Prepare package of lemon Jell-O according to package directions.
   2. Add 2 to 3 drops of red food coloring to Jell-O liquid while still warm
   3. Stir thoroughly before cooling to evenly distribute red coloring.
   4. Refrigerate until congealed.

Evaluation

○ After the Jell-O has solidified, serve a small portion to a group or class.
○ Before the Jell-O is tasted, ask the tasters to describe what they see and what flavor they think the Jell-O is.
○ Keep a tally of the replies on the Data Sheet like the one that follows.
○ Let the tasters taste the Jell-O; ask for their reactions and tally their responses. Record on the Data Sheet.
○ What can you conclude by the tasters' responses? Are they fooled by the red color? Do they expect cherry or strawberry Jell-O? What happens when the Jell-O tastes lemony?

Culinary application

Which sensation is one of the most important in food perception? How can this information be applied to new food product development? Food presentation?

Data Sheet

Sensory Qualities	Responses	Totals
Appearance of Jell-O		
Suspected taste of Jell-O		
Taste of Jello-O		

5. Plate Presentation

Objective

○ To observe the importance of appearance, color, flow, garnish, height and shape in plate presentation

Materials: A meal that is similar to the meal in Exercise #2 (protein entree, starch and vegetables); lunch and dinner plates; garnishes such as citrus fruit or herbs, flavorful sauces, oils or vinegars

Procedure

1. Using the concepts of appearance, color, flow, garnish, height and shape as described in this chapter, plate a meal that is similar to the meal in Exercise #2 (protein entree, starch and vegetables) on a lunch plate.
2. Plate a second meal with the same components on a dinner plate.
3. Use garnishes and/or sauces, flavored oils or vinegars in the manner that you have learned about in this chapter.

Evaluation

○ Support the ingredients that you chose and why you placed them in the positions that you did.
○ Have the group or class members evaluate these lunch and dinner plates according to their appearance, color, flow, garnish, height and shape.
○ Use a Data Sheet like the one that follows.

Culinary applications

How does plate size affect food perception? How would you use this information about plate size, appearance, color, flow, garnish, height and shape if preparing meals at a spa? Cafeteria? White tablecloth restaurant?

Data Sheet

Lunch plate	Dinner plate
Appearance	
Color	
Flow	
Garnish	
Height	
Shape	

6. Proportionality

Objective

○ To recognize the importance of proportion in healthy food presentation

Materials: A food magazine that features an entire meal that includes an appetizer, salad or soup, entree, dessert and beverage

Procedure

1. Locate a meal in a food magazine that includes an appetizer, salad or soup, entree, dessert and beverage with their yields, serving sizes and nutrition information. (If an entire meal cannot be found, then create a meal by using different courses from the magazine.)

2. Record each recipe's yield and serving size on a **Data Sheet** like the one that follows.
3. Revise the yields and serving sizes to create a healthier meal by using the information in this chapter. Be specific; support all of your answers.

Evaluation
- Based on the information in this chapter, are the serving sizes that are portrayed in the food magazine too large, too small or just right?
- If they are too large, then how should they be adjusted?
- Be specific; support all of your answers.

Culinary applications
Prepare a meal that consists of an appetizer, salad or soup, entree, dessert and beverage in healthy proportions as described in this chapter and in Chapter 1. How can this exercise be applied to other healthy meal preparations?

Data Sheet

Course	Serving size	Revised yield	Revised serving size	Adjustments
Appetizer				
Salad				
Soup				
Entree				
Dessert				
Beverage				

OVER EASY

This chapter focuses on culinary and baking basics: the fundamentals of what food science, nutrition and culinary professionals need to know for healthy product development, cooking and baking, and recipe and menu formulations. It serves as a foundation for additional information throughout this text on carbohydrates, lipids, minerals, proteins, vitamins and water and the foods and beverages that contain them.

For example, the information about dairy- and gluten-free cooking and baking in this chapter is intricately related to information on carbohydrate digestion in Chapter 4 and allergies in Chapters 5 and 9. Likewise, the information on sugar, fat, sodium and reduction in this chapter is echoed in Chapter 4 on carbohydrates, Chapter 6 on lipids, Chapter 7 on sodium, and Chapter 9 on diet and disease. Plus, you'll find recipes in Chapters 4 through 12 that incorporate the healthy techniques and procedures that were described in this chapter.

Cooking and baking healthy foods and beverages requires an array of healthy pantry, refrigerated and frozen foods and beverages, coupled with basic and specialized culinary and baking tools and equipment that are all featured in this chapter.

Healthy choices of meat, poultry and fish; methods for building flavor; general guidelines for cooking with culinary herbs and spices; components of a healthy plate, meal and menu; instructions for reducing, substituting and eliminating ingredients; and ideas for modifying cooking and baking techniques (including healthy heat applications) for creating and redoing recipes are all addressed in this chapter.

The cost of healthy eating, the Slow Food Movement and Chefs Collaborative and basic food safety are also highlighted to show that healthy food is affordable, accessible, an alternative to fast food, and a commodity that should be handled with care.

CHECK PLEASE

1. The process of heat transfer that transfers heat from a heat source to a pan or pot is called:
   a. convection
   b. conduction
   c. combination

   d. caramelizing

   e. radiation

2. The process of heat transfer that transfers heat through fluid is called:

   a. convection

   b. conduction

   c. combination

   d. caramelization

   e. radiation

3. The process of heat transfer without direct contact is called:

   a. convection

   b. conduction

   c. combination

   d. caramelization

   e. radiation

Essay Question

1. You have been asked to lower the fat in this list of ingredients. Describe three techniques that you can use. How would you rebuild the flavor? Support all of your comments.

EGGPLANT PARMESAN (SERVES 8)

Ingredients

Olive oil

2 pounds (about 2 large) eggplant, cut into ¼-inch slices

Salt

1 28-ounce can whole tomatoes, peeled 1 clove garlic, peeled and minced

⅓ cup *plus* more to equal ½-inch olive oil

Salt

Freshly ground black pepper

½ cup all-purpose flour

½ cup fine dry seasoned breadcrumbs

4 large eggs, beaten

1½ pounds whole-milk mozzarella cheese, sliced into ¼-inch rounds

1 cup Parmesan cheese, grated

1 packed cup fresh basil leaves

Directions

1. Preheat oven to 350°F.

2. Prepare 13 X 9 X 2-inch baking dish with olive oil.

3. Put eggplant slices in colander; sprinkle well with salt. Weigh down; drain for 1 to 2 hours.

4. Combine tomatoes, garlic, ⅓ cup olive oil, salt and pepper in food processor.

5. Combine flour and breadcrumbs in shallow bowl.

6. Pour beaten eggs in another shallow bowl.

7. Pour remaining olive oil to ½ inch in frying pan and heat.

8. Place eggplant in flour mixture and then in beaten eggs.

9. Fry eggplant in olive oil until golden brown on both sides; turn once and drain on paper towels.

10. Spread ⅓ of the tomato sauce in bottom of baking dish.

11. Top with ⅓ of eggplant slices, ⅓ of the mozzarella cheese, ⅓ of the Parmesan cheese and ⅓ of the basil leaves.

12. Stack two more layers in this manner; top with any remaining tomato sauce and Parmesan cheese.

13. Bake until cheese melts and top is slightly brown, about 30 minutes; let rest about 10 minutes before serving.

For additional questions, please see the *Culinary Nutrition* website at www.culinarynutrition.elsevier.com.

HUNGRY FOR MORE?

Chefs Collaborative   http://chefscollaborative.org
The Culinary Institute of America   http://www.ciachef.edu/
Johnson and Wales University   www.jwu.edu/
Slow Food USA   http://www.slowfood.com/
Hazard Analysis Critical Control Points (HACCP)
http://www.fda.gov/food/foodsafety/hazardanalysiscriticalcontrolpointshaccp/default.htm
US Department of Health and Human Safety   http://www.foodsafety.gov/
Dorenburg A, Page K. *Culinary Artistry.* New York: John Wiley, 1996.
Hass E. *FITFood: Eating Well for Life.* New York: Healthy Living Books, 2005.
Labensky SR, Van Damme E, Martel P, et al. *On Baking: A Textbook of Baking and Pastry Fundamentals.* New Jersey: Pearson/Prentice Hall, 2005.
Labensky SR, Hause AM. *On Cooking: A Textbook of Culinary Fundamentals,* 2nd ed. New Jersey: Prentice Hall, 1995.
The Culinary Institute of America. *Techniques of Healthy Cooking.* New Jersey: John Wiley, 2008.
Weil A, Daley R. *The Healthy Kitchen: Recipes for a Better Body, Life, and Spirit.* New York: Knopf, 2002.

TAKE AWAY
Slow Food and the Slow Food Movement

The concept of *slow food* is puzzling, since everyone should eat slowly for maximum enjoyment, normal digestion and absorption, and optimal nutrition. As the pace of life rapidly accelerates, the notion that we need a movement to restore the experience of eating slowly is suddenly not so puzzling. Fast and convenience foods and beverages are rapidly replacing sitdown meals because we live at such a high-speed pace.

> **Morsel** "When we no longer have good cooking in the world, we will have no literature, nor high and sharp intelligence, nor friendly gatherings, no social harmony." —Marie-Antoine Carême (French King of Chefs and the Chef of Kings, 1784–1833)

145

Historically, eating is a time to take a number of breaks in our days. Breakfast is a meal that is designed to break the fast between last night's dinner and the dawn of a new day. Lunch was originally designed as an ample meal called "dinner," and dinner was designed as a lighter meal called "supper" that was sometimes consumed late at night.

The midday meal is still traditional in some communities on weekends and festival days, and it is often based around the extended family. But due to such factors as more women in the workforce, school breakfast and lunch programs and meals on-the-run in airports and train stations, fast-food drive-ins and shopping malls, family meals are absent or they have taken on different characteristics. If people get together at all to eat, then chances are that it is fast. The Slow Food Movement addresses these issues.

The Slow Food Movement was founded by Carlo Petrini to resist and combat fast food. Its founding purpose was to preserve the culture of cuisine in ecological regions and the domestic animals, farming methods, foods, plants and seeds that are representative of these regions. Slow Food is a nonprofit, member-supported association that was officially founded in 1989. Since its inception, Slow Food has served to slow down the pace of food in modern life. Its ecological and gastronomic origins uphold local food traditions and localities.

Slow Food is concerned with where foods originate, how they are produced, and how they taste. Slow Food is also concerned with how consumers are affected by their food choices and how consumer food choices affect the rest of the world. Members of Slow Food are represented all over the globe.

Among the objectives of Slow Food are the celebration of local cuisines; education in gardening and ethical buying; formation and sustenance of seed banks with heirloom plant varieties; preservation and promotion of local and traditional food products; and the promotion of taste education. Slow Food also lobbies against agribusiness and the use of pesticides and genetic engineering and for organic farming.

Since Slow Food is a relatively young organization, it is hard to definitely determine its global impact. As a grassroots organization, it is really in its infancy. Statistics show that some European countries consume more organic foods and beverages than the rest of the world and that Slow Food may have been a part of this movement. Slow Food has been targeting youth to reintroduce the concepts of gardening and farming. This is so students can appreciate the journey and measures that help to put food on their plates.

Some critics of the Slow Food Movement feel that its efforts are elitist. This may be because it encourages the consumption of fresh foods and discourages cheaper methods of growing or preparing food (see "The cost of healthy eating" in this chapter). It is true that Slow Food emphasizes the production and consumption of local foods before the reliance on foods that must be transported or those that depend on energy, chemical and technological-intensive methods. This philosophy parallels Greenpeace and green parties and other antiglobalization movements, but it may not be feasible, at least at the present time, for feeding the masses.

Whether or not you choose to support the Slow Food Movement, the issues that it raises about preserving local foods and cultures and slowing down food experiences reveal provoking questions. As future nutrition, food science and culinary professionals, it is necessary to understand the factors that interfere with healthy eating as well as the factors that support it. Fast foods and healthy foods could be synonymous. The challenge is up to food and nutrition professionals, government agencies and associations like Slow Food to collaborate in their missions and visions [9,10].

The Chefs Collaborative

Morsel "Cuisine is when things taste like themselves." —Maurice Edmond Saillant [Curnonsky] (French writer and Prince of French Gastronomes, 1872–1956)

146

Like the Slow Food Movement, the *Chefs Collaborative* is relatively young. It was founded in 1993 by food professionals with common concerns about the sources of food. The Chefs Collaborative serves to provide its members with the means for running economical and sustainable food service businesses and to promote environmentally sound, flavorful and high-quality local ingredients for the nation's tables.

Not all of the members in the Chefs Collaborative are chefs. The US network represents a broad and independent range of food-related professionals, including culinary school instructors, distributors, farmers, fishermen, managers of large food service operations, ranchers, specialty store owners and others.

In its efforts, the Chefs Collaborative works with chefs and the greater food communities to foster a more sustainable food supply and to promote local foods. To these ends, the Chefs Collaborative supports diversity, local economies, seasonality and traditional practices.

Much like the Slow Food Movement, the Chefs Collaborative stands for foods that are fundamental to life, foods that nourish both the body and soul, and connect each of us to nature and to our communities. The Chefs Collaborative promotes foods that are delicious, local and seasonal, whole or with minimal processing, containing ingredients that are good for us and for the planet—the hallmarks of healthy cooking and eating.

The Chefs Collaborative also promotes biological and cultural diversity for our food supply, environment and health. By growing and harvesting foods that are close to their natural sources, it is implicit that we promote food sustainability and support both traditional and diverse agriculture.

The Chefs Collaborative has a farmer-chef program that includes chefs, consumers and farmers. This program serves to support small-scale artisan food makers, farmers and ranchers and informs its broad membership how to make sustainable purchasing decisions about the foods that they procure and consume.

As a result of its relationships between chefs and farmers and the strong belief in biodiversity and taste, the Chefs Collaborative is a partner with Slow Food and the American Livestock Breeds Conservancy in the alliance known as RAFT (Renewing America's Food Traditions). The RAFT Alliance brings together agricultural historians, local chefs, conservation activists, farmers, fishermen, nurserymen and ranchers. Like Slow Food, the program is young and the tasks are mighty.

As future nutrition, food science or culinary professionals, it is imperative that you see how associations such as the Chefs Collaborative can be impactful in promoting diversity, local economies, seasonality and traditional food practices. The future of our food supply and its equitable, safe and healthy dispersion is at stake, and we are all stakeholders [11,12,13].

References

[1] US Food and Drug Administration. Appendix B: additional requirements for nutrient content claims. <http://www.fda.gov/Food/GuidanceComplianceRegulatoryInformation/GuidanceDocuments/FoodLabelingNutrition/FoodLabelingGuide/ucm064916.htm/>; [accessed 02.02.08].

[2] foodprocessing.com food industry outlook: a taste of things to come. <http://www.foodprocessing.com/articles/2012/food-industry-outlook.html/>; 2012 [accessed 02.02.08].

[3] WebMD. Healthy eating and diet: portion size plate. <http://www.webmd.com/diet/healthtool-portion-size-plate/>.

[4] Ortiz EL. The encyclopedia of herbs, spices & flavorings. New York, NY DK Publishing; Reprint edition; 1994.

[5] US Food and Drug Administration. Safe eats—meat, poultry & seafood. <http://www.fda.gov/Food/ResourcesForYou/HealthEducators/ucm082294.htm/>; [accessed 02.02.08].

[6] US Department of Agriculture. <http://www.cnpp.usda.gov/>; [accessed 02.02.08].

[7] US Department of Agriculture. Diet quality of Americans in 1994–96 and 2001–02, as measured by the Healthy Eating Index—2005. <http://www.cnpp.usda.gov/Publications/NutritionInsights/Insight37.pdf/>; [accessed 02.02.08].

[8] The Nation. Walmart's fresh food makeover. <http://www.thenation.com/article/163396/walmarts-fresh-food-makeover/>; [accessed 02.02.08].

[9] Slow Food. <http://www.slowfood.com/>; [accessed 02.02.08].

[10] Petrini C. In: Slow food: collected thoughts on taste, tradition, and the honest pleasures of food. White River Junction: Vermont Chelsea Green Publishing; 2001.

[11] RAFT Alliance. <http://www.raftalliance.org/>; [accessed 02.02.08].

[12] Chefs Collaborative. <http://chefscollaborative.org/>; [accessed 02.02.08].

[13] Chefs Collaborative. <http://www.oldwayspt.org/sites/all/files/CC_1993_Charter.pdf%20.pdf/>; [accessed 02.02.08].

[14] US Census Bureau http://2010.census.gov/2010census/>; [accessed 02.02.10].

[15] US Census Bureau<http://www.census.gov/newsroom/releases/pdf/cb09-ff07.pdf> [accessed 02.02.10].

CHAPTER 4

Carbohydrate Basics: Sugars, Starches and Fibers in Foods and Health

Healthy Carbohydrate Choices, Roles and Applications in Nutrition, Food Science and the Culinary Arts

Culinary Nutrition. DOI: http://dx.doi.org/10.1016/B978-0-12-391882-6.00004-2

OBJECTIVES

1. Discuss the types of carbohydrates, their food sources and importance in the diet
2. Explain how carbohydrates are digested and metabolized by the body
3. Identify the dietary recommendations for total carbohydrates, sugar, whole grains and dietary fibers
4. Describe the roles of carbohydrates in lactose intolerance, gluten intolerance, diabetes, coronary heart disease and oral health, among other conditions
5. Apply the properties of starches, sugars, whole grains and dietary fibers to cooking and baking
6. Compare and contrast the functions of refined, enriched, fortified and whole grains in cooking and baking
7. Examine the properties of carbohydrate substitutes in cooking and baking and their effects in health and disease
8. Evaluate carbohydrate controversies
9. Assess the roles of carbohydrates in diseases
10. Judge the roles of carbohydrates in new product and recipe development, especially for specialized diets (i.e., gluten and lactose intolerance)

INTRODUCTION: CARBOHYDRATES
Sweet, Starchy and Fibrous

Rice, noodles and pasta, bread and breadstuffs, potatoes, corn and legumes . . . all of these basic foodstuffs have provided nourishment to people around the world for centuries. Rice, a staple cereal grain for much of the world, dates back thousands of years to India. The Chinese have consumed noodles for ages, long before the Italians created pasta. Bread and breadstuffs can be traced to prehistoric times. Potatoes were first cultivated in Central America, and then mariners brought potatoes to Europe, where they became widespread in northern diets. Corn dates back to pre-Columbian times in the Americas. Legumes have interwoven throughout early civilizations in Asia, Europe and the Americas.

> **Morsel** "Bread deals with living things, with giving life, with growth, with the seed, the grain that nurtures. It is not coincidence that we say bread is the staff of life."
> —Lionel Poilâne (French boulanger, 1945–2002)[1]

Some carbohydrates were initially not well received, such as potatoes. Potatoes are a member of the nightshade family, known for plants with druglike effects, including belladonna, mandrake and tobacco. When potatoes were first introduced into Europe around the 1500s their potentially poisonous effects were cause for concern—much like the introduction of some foods and beverages today.

As in the past, controversies still exist about these and other carbohydrates and their roles in the diet. Some versions of rice, noodles and pasta, breads and breadstuffs, potatoes, corn and legumes hardly resemble their predecessors. To help to sort out facts from fiction, nutrition, food science and culinary professionals must first understand the basics of carbohydrates and how they apply to today's diets.

What Are Carbohydrates?

Besides rice, noodles and pasta, breads and breadstuffs, potatoes, corn and legumes, carbohydrates are found in many other foods, including fruits, vegetables and dairy products. The origin of these foods and the carbohydrates that are contained in them is plants.

Plants use their green pigment, or *chlorophyll*, to trap energy from the sun. This energy is combined with carbon dioxide (a gas that is in the environment) and water to produce *glucose*, or sugar. The process is called *photosynthesis* (*photo* means "light" and *synthesize* means "to make"). Glucose supplies the body with energy. Glucose is found in the blood as **blood glucose** and is stored in the muscles and liver as **glycogen**. The storage form of glucose in plants is **starch.** When we eat foods with carbohydrates, they provide sugars (simple carbohydrates), starches (complex carbohydrates), and another type of carbohydrate, called *fiber*, which is the parts of plants that provide strength and support.

Once carbohydrates are digested and metabolized by the body, they release energy, which is essential for life. Certain body systems, such as the brain and the central nervous system, prefer the energy from carbohydrates before the energy that is derived from fats or proteins. While it is true that consuming fat and protein supplies energy, the processes are not as efficient as carbohydrate breakdown.

Carbohydrates provide the backbone of a plate or meal in many global cuisines. The USDA MyPlate guidelines that are featured in Chapter 1 recommend that fruits and vegetables make up about one-half of a plate.

In some countries protein has replaced carbohydrates as the star of the plate or meal. Too much of any nutrient is not considered healthy. In comparison to lean protein, most carbohydrate-containing foods contain less fat and no cholesterol—both which are associated with diseases such as coronary heart disease, diabetes and certain cancers. But current controversies suggest that too many carbohydrates can also lead to disease, from diabetes to obesity.

This chapter provides information about the different types of carbohydrates and their roles in the diet; the pros and cons of carbohydrate substitutes; how carbohydrates are digested, metabolized for energy and stored; the requirements for carbohydrates in normal nutrition; the problems with carbohydrates in relation to certain diseases; the importance of whole grains in the diet; the astounding variety of sugars, starches and fibers that chefs have at their disposal; and how food science and nutrition knowledge about carbohydrates can be applied to cooking and baking.

151

MAIN COURSES
Types of Carbohydrates: Sugars, Starches and Fibers

> **FOOD BYTE**
>
> Sugar has a long history. Cane sugar was first used in Polynesia and then in India as far back as 500 BC, where it was considered "a reed which gives honey without bees." Persian and Arabian conquerors then established sugar production in other lands, including North Africa and Spain. Sugar was later discovered by western Europeans during the Crusades in the eleventh century. The Portuguese and Dutch brought sugarcane to the Caribbean and South America during the 1500s and 1600s.
>
> "Sugar is sugar is sugar" is a common saying. The fact is that sugar exists in many forms with different properties in cooking and health. Sugar is considered a **simple carbohydrate**. The word *simple* refers to its chemical structure. Another name for a simple carbohydrate is a **monosaccharide** (mono means "one" and saccharide means an "organic compound"). Saccharides contain both sugars and starches. Three common monosaccharides include *glucose*, *fructose* and *galactose*. Glucose is the main form of sugar that circulates in the bloodstream and is the basic form of energy for the body. Fructose is a very sweet, naturally occurring sugar that is found in many fruits, vegetables and honey. It is also called fruit sugar. Galactose is found in dairy products, sugar beets, gums and mucilages (which are used as thickeners, gels and stabilizing agents). It is less sweet than glucose.
>
> Simple sugars can combine with other simple sugars and form *disaccharides*, or double sugars. Some common double sugars include *sucrose*, *maltose* and *lactose*. Sucrose, also known as table sugar, is a combination of glucose and fructose. It is naturally found in sugarcane and sugar beets. Maltose, or malt sugar, is the combination of two glucose molecules. Milk sugar, commonly known as

lactose, is a combination of galactose and glucose. Lactose is found in dairy products and is a by-product of cheese production. A summary of single and double sugars is found in Table 4-1.

TABLE 4-1 A Summary of Single and Double Sugars

Single Sugars	Double Sugars/Common Names
Glucose *plus* Fructose =	Sucrose (table sugar)
Glucose *plus* Glucose =	Maltose (malt sugar)
Galactose *plus* Glucose =	Lactose (milk sugar)
Glucose *plus* Fructose =	Sucrose (table sugar)

Simple and double sugars exist alone and in combination in foods and beverages. Some common foods and beverages with the average number of teaspoons of sugar per serving are shown in Table 4-2.

TABLE 4-2 Average Number of Teaspoons of Sugar Per Serving in Common Foods and Beverages

Foods and Beverages	Teaspoons Sugar per Serving
8 ounces 2% reduced-fat dairy milk	3 tsp
8 ounces 2% chocolate dairy milk	7
12 ounces cola	8
12 ounces fruit drink	12
1 plain doughnut	2
1 fig bar	5
6 Oreo-type cookies	6
10 jelly beans	7
½ cup ice cream	3
½ cup canned fruit in heavy syrup	4
1 serving (1/12) angel food cake	5
1 serving (1/16) frosted cake	6
1 serving (1/6) fruit pie	6

Source: [2].

Morsel "Just a spoonful of sugar helps the medicine go down." —Richard Sherman (songwriter), Robert Sherman (songwriter) and Clarence Brown [3]

TYPES OF SUGARS IN COOKING AND BAKING

There are many types of sugars available for cooking and baking. Their use depends on factors such as taste, texture and function. Some sugars are used in combination; others are used interchangeably; and still others can be replaced by sugar substitutes with similar characteristics. Some of these sugars and their applications in cooking and baking are shown in Table 4-3.

- *Beet sugar* is extracted from beets with hot water and an alkaline solution to remove any impurities. The mixture then undergoes evaporation, which concentrates the sugar into crystals. Different grades of white sugar and molasses, a thick, dark syrup, are produced. There is little nutritional difference between beet sugar and cane sugar, but the molasses in cane sugar processing does have some nutritional benefits.
- *Brown sugar* is produced during sugar refining when sugar crystals are mixed with molasses. **Refining** is the process by which the coarse parts of a food are removed. The more molasses that is in brown sugar, the deeper the color and the stronger the flavor.
- *Cane sugar* is produced from sugarcane that has been filtered and treated to remove the impurities, much like beet sugar. Molasses is also a by-product of cane sugar production. The sugar can then be processed into lighter grades. The size of the granules affects how quickly it dissolves and other functions.
- *Corn syrup* is a thick syrup that is made by processing cornstarch with acids or enzymes. Light corn syrup has been clarified, or made clearer, to remove color and cloudiness. Dark corn syrup generally has caramel coloring and flavoring added.

TABLE 4-3 Types of Sugars in Cooking and Baking	
Types of Sugar	**Uses in Cooking and Baking**
Baker's sugar	Sugaring doughnuts and cookies, fine crumb texture in commercial cakes
Bar, baker's, caster, superfine sugar	Delicately textured cakes, meringues, flavoring beverages, sweetening fruits
Beet sugar	Indistinguishable from white cane sugar, except in jams, marmalades
Brown sugar	Light: baking, butterscotch, condiments, glazes Dark: baked beans, gingerbread, mincemeat
Cane sugar	Wide cooking and baking applications
Corn syrup	Thickener, retains moisture and freshness; confectionery, ice cream
Date sugar	Does not dissolve when added to liquids
Decorating or coarse sugar	Adds sparkling appearance; confections, fondants, liquors
Fruit sugar	Dry mixes (gelatins, puddings, powdered drinks)
Granulated white sugar	Many cooking and baking applications depending on grain
High-fructose corn syrup	Processed foods, soft drinks
Invert sugar, invert syrup, trimoline	Retards sugar crystallization; retains moisture in packaged foods
Liquid sugar	Recipes that require sugar to be dissolved; adds brown color
Maple syrup	Baking, candy making, flavoring agent in some beers
Molasses, treacle, sorghum syrup	Adds color, flavor; gingerbread, baked beans
Powdered sugar, confectioner's sugar, icing sugar	Confections, icings, industrial baking, whipped cream
Raw sugar (barbados, demerara, muscovado, turbinado)	Light molasses flavor, color; tea, other beverages
Sugar cubes	Hot drinks, some alcoholic drinks

153

- *Fructose* is found naturally in berries, fruits, honey, melons and some root vegetables, such as beets, onions and sweet potatoes. It is available in crystallized and liquid forms.
- *Granulated sugar* is white refined sugar. It is made by dissolving raw sugar and purifying it with chemicals or by filtration. It is then dried to prevent clumping.
  - *Coarse-grained granulated sugar,* also called *sanding sugar, decorating sugar,* or *sugar nibs,* can add a "sparkle" to baked goods, candies and cookies. This is because it has large, irregular crystals that reflect light. Some types will not dissolve when exposed to heat.
  - *Normal-grained granulated sugar* is for common cooking and baking uses.
  - *Finer-grade granulated sugar,* such as *caste* or *superfine* (also called *baker's sugar* or *bar sugar*) dissolves quickly because it is so fine. It is useful in meringues and for flavoring beverages.
  - *Granulated cane juice,* a liquid by-product of the sugar production process, is consumed in some parts of the world. It is also dehydrated.
- *High-fructose corn syrup (HFCS)* is a type of corn syrup that has been processed by enzymes to increase the amount of fructose; then it is mixed with pure corn syrup. The balance of sugar comes from glucose. It is widely used in processed foods and soft drinks.
- *Invert sugar, invert syrup* or *trimoline* are sucrose-based sugars and syrups. They have been treated with enzymes or acids to split sucrose into glucose and fructose. Invert sugars and syrups are sweeter than sucrose, are less likely to form crystals, and are more **hygroscopic** (which means that they attract fluid and help products stay moist). For these reasons, invert sugar is valued by bakers.
- *Maple syrup* is made from the sap of maple trees. It is used in baking and candy making and as a flavoring agent in beer. Sucrose is the most common single sugar in maple syrup.

- *Molasses*, treacle or sorghum syrup is thick syrup that is produced from processing sugarcane or sugar beets into sugar. The quality of molasses depends on the age of the sugarcane or sugar beet, the amount of sugar that is extracted and the type of extraction.
- *Natural sugar* is unrefined sugar. Natural sugars are present in fruits, dairy products, grains, legumes, vegetables and animal muscles.
- *Powdered sugar*, confectioner's sugar or icing sugar is made by grinding white sugar into a fine powder. Sometimes an anticaking agent, such as cornstarch, is added.
- *Raw sugar* is made by clarifying or purifying sugar syrup with some chemical processing. Types of raw sugar include *demerara, muscovado* and *turbinado. Mill white sugar, plantation white sugar, crystal sugar* and *superior sugar* are types of raw sugar without colored impurities. They are bleached white by chemicals.
- *Sugar cubes* are made by mixing sugar crystals with sugar syrup.

SUGAR ON THE FOOD LABEL

The ending "-ose" on a food label usually indicates that a food product contains a sugar of some kind, such as glucose, dextrose, fructose, lactose, levulose, maltose, polydextrose or sucrose. Other names for sugar to look for on a food label include brown sugar, concentrated fruit juice sweetener, confectioner's sugar, corn syrup, corn sweeteners, date sugar, fruit juice concentrate, granulated cane juice, high-fructose corn syrup or sweeteners, honey, invert sugar, maltodextrin, maple syrup, molasses, powdered sugar, raw sugar and/or turbinado sugar.

Other terms for sweeteners that may appear on food labels include *added sugars, alternative sweeteners, nutritive sweeteners* and *nonnutritive sweeteners.* Added sugars are sugars and caloric sweeteners that are added to foods during processing or preparation. Alternative sweeteners are substances that are added to foods that contain little to no calories. They include nonnutritive sweeteners and sugar alcohols, such as mannitol, sorbitol and xylitol. Nutritive sweeteners contribute energy in the form of calories. Nonnutritive sweeteners are synthetic compounds that contribute an intensely sweet taste and few to no calories in comparison to white sugar. The FDA has approved the use of the nonnutritive sweeteners aspartame, acesulfame-K, neotame, saccharine and sucralose to sweeten foods and in substances that may come into contact with the mouth, such as toothpaste or mouthwash [4].

FOOD BYTE

The term *complex carbohydrates* was first used in the 1977 version of the *Dietary Goals for the United States*, prepared by the staff of the Select Committee on Nutrition and Human Needs. In this document, fruits, vegetables and whole grains were classified as complex carbohydrates, as compared to simple, refined carbohydrates, such as those found in sugars. The 2010 version of the USDA's *Dietary Guidelines for Americans* now focuses on whole grains and other fiber-rich foods.

STARCHES (COMPLEX CARBOHYDRATES)

Imagine as few as 10 or as many as 3,000 simple sugars linked into straight or branched chains or networks. These **complex sugar chains** and networks are called **complex carbohydrates** or **polysaccharides**. They are more commonly referred to as **starches**. Starches are where the bulk of energy is stored in plants. The richest starches are located in the seeds, such as grains; legumes, such as soybeans; root vegetables, such as cassava; and tubers, such as potatoes. These foods, which are often called "starchy," are summarized in Table 4-4.

Types of Starches in Cooking and Baking

Starches used in cooking and baking tend to fall into these categories: grains (cornstarch, rice and wheat flours); legumes (garfava and soy); and roots and tubers (arrowroot, potato starch and tapioca).

- *Arrowroot* is a finely textured, flourlike, gluten-free powder that comes from a tropical plant, native to the Americas. It is used as a thickener, much like cornstarch. Arrowroot has about 50 percent more thickening power than wheat flour. It is relatively tasteless and colorless. If overcooked, arrowroot will thin down and be less effective as a thickener.

TABLE 4-4 Types and Sources of Food Starches

Types of Food Starch	Source
Seeds	Grains such as corn, rice, wheat
Legumes	Soy, garfava
Modified food starches	Corn, potato, rice, tapioca, wheat
Root vegetables	Arrowroot, cassava, tapioca
Tuber vegetables	Potatoes, yams

- *Garfava* is a high-protein, gluten-free mixture of chickpea (garbanzo bean) flour and fava bean flour. It can be used as a thickener.
- *Potato starch* is a finely textured, flourlike, gluten-free powder that comes from the starchy portion of potatoes. It is used as a thickener, similar to arrowroot or cornstarch. It is best to mix potato starch with fluid before it is added to recipes, much like cornstarch.
- *Rice starch* is a finely textured, flourlike, gluten-free powder that comes from the endosperm (seed) of rice. It is not often used in Western countries.
- *Soy flour* is a high-protein, gluten-free flour that is made from roasted soybeans. It can be used as a thickener.
- *Tapioca* is a finely textured, flourlike, gluten-free powder that comes from the cassava tuber, or yucca root. It is also found in flake, granule, pearl and syrup forms. Tapioca is used as a thickener. When cooked, tapioca is translucent. If overcooked, tapioca may become sticky.
- *Wheat flour* is about 70 percent starch, and the rest is from gluten protein. For this reason, wheat flour does not thicken well. Wheat flour has a wheaty flavor and cloudy color due to the wheat gluten. If 1 tablespoon of cornstarch or potato starch is called for in a recipe, 1½ tablespoons of wheat flour may be needed for thickening.

155

FOOD BYTE

The word **starch** is derived from the Middle English word **sterchen**, which means "to stiffen." This is fitting, since starch can be used as a thickening agent to "stiffen" sauces when it is dissolved in fluid and heated. Some starches, when mixed with water and kneaded, stiffen into gluten, the protein that is responsible for giving bread and other baked goods their rigid structures. Gluten is also responsible for sensitivity and/or intolerance to barley, rye and wheat.

Starches on the Food Label

Starches are not listed on the Nutrition Facts Label of a food label. Instead, total carbohydrates, sugars and dietary fiber appear. Starches are listed in the ingredients on a food label. These may include amylose, amylopectin, arracacha, arrowroot, banana, barley, buckwheat, cassava, corn, fava, kudzu, lentil, maltodextrin, modified food starch, oca, polysaccharide, sago, sorghum, sweet potato, tapioca, taro, pea, potatoes, rice, wheat, yams and others. Global products have introduced a number of these starches into US and other diets.

DIETARY FIBER

FOOD BYTE

Fiber became a popularized nutritive substance in the 1970s when Dr. Denis Burkitt coined the phrase "the fiber hypothesis," in which he suggested that fiber can prevent certain diseases. Through Dr. Burkitt's research in Africa, he discovered that diseases that were common in Western cultures, such as colon cancer, coronary heart disease and diabetes, were uncommon in Africa. The differences were attributed to the high intake of fiber and the low intake of refined carbohydrates in Africa.

Dietary fiber is found in the leaves, seeds and stems from plants. There is not any dietary fiber in food from animals. Dietary fiber does not contain any calories, so it does not supply energy.

Dietary fiber is a polysaccharide like starch. Unlike starch, dietary fiber does not break down into single sugars. Instead, it passes through the gastrointestinal tract undigested, which supports healthy digestion. Other possible health benefits of dietary fiber include the prevention and management of adult-onset diabetes, certain cancers, coronary heart disease and digestive tract disorders.

The two main types of dietary fiber are *soluble* and *insoluble*. **Soluble fibers** dissolve or swell in fluid. **Insoluble fibers** do not dissolve or swell in fluids. Both types of fiber can be found in plant foods in a wide range of quantities.

A third type of dietary fiber is **resistant starch (RS).** Resistant starch is a form of starch that resists digestion in the small intestine due to its fibrous outer coat. It can produce some of the benefits of both soluble fiber and insoluble fiber. While sugars and starches are absorbed as glucose through the small intestine and used for short-term energy or stored, resistant starch passes into the large intestine, where it acts like dietary fiber. Resistant starch may contain some calories, but it does not raise blood sugar. Legumes, whole grains, unripe bananas, plantains and raw potatoes contain resistant starch. Resistant starch is also manufactured by chemical processes.

Soluble fibers are found in apples, barley, legumes, oats, prunes, rye and some root vegetables, such as onions and potatoes. They include algae (as carrageenan), beta-glucans, gums, mucilages and pectin. These soluble fibers appear in the ingredient list on food labels. They help provide texture and consistency to foods such as jellies (citrus pectin), salad dressings (guar gum) and ice cream (carrageenan).

> ### FOOD BYTE
> Another name for prune butter is lekvar. *Lekvar* is a very thick, jamlike puree of prunes (also known as dried plums) that is used to fill pastries, cookies and pierogies (Slavic dumplings). Lekvar is of East European origin and dates back before 1350. Prune puree is a useful ingredient in baking because it is filled with soluble fiber and is hygroscopic, or absorbs fluids.

Carrageenan comes from algae or seaweed. It is used for thickening instead of gelatin, so it is helpful in vegan diets. Carrageenan is a common ingredient in chocolate dairy milk, ice cream and yogurt. Beta-glucans are found in whole grains, including barley, oats and wheat and in baker's yeast and mushrooms. Food gums come from plants on land and sea, including barley, guar beans, other legumes and oats. Gums are also derived from microbial fermentation (xanthan) and synthesis (cellulose gum). Mucilages help conserve water and thicken. Among the richest sources of mucilages are cacti and flaxseeds.

Pectin is rich in underripe fruit. It helps to absorb water and gel. Pectin is used as a stabilizer and thickening agent in candies, frozen desserts, jams, jellies and preserves. Apples, berries, carrots, citrus fruits, pears and plums are good sources of pectin.

Soluble fibers may help delay the absorption of glucose from the bloodstream and lead to improved sugar tolerance in diabetics; slow the absorption of cholesterol and help to lower blood cholesterol in coronary heart disease; and provide fullness and satisfaction when they take up fluid and swell during digestion, which may benefit weight management.

Insoluble fibers include bran, flax, hemicellulose, lignans, nuts, seeds, the skin of fruits and vegetables and whole grains. The seeds and skin of fruits and vegetables are particularly good sources.

Hemicellulose can be found in bran and whole grains. Lignin is a woody fiber found in wheat bran and the seeds of fruits and vegetables.

Insoluble fibers help to increase bulk and soften the stool so it passes quickly through the large intestine. This feature makes it potentially beneficial in the prevention of digestive diseases, including colon cancer, diverticulosis and hemorrhoids. Insoluble fibers may also assist in weight management in that they speed the transit time of food in the intestines. For this reason, they may also be protective against gastrointestinal diseases. The research is ongoing.

Recipe: Berry Crumble

A crumble is a savory or sweet dish of British or Irish origin. It is composed of either meats and vegetables in a savory sauce or fruit that stews in its own juice; then it is topped with a crumbly mixture of fat (usually butter) and flour—plus sugar in the sweet version. The recipe for **Berry Crumble** *in the* **Recipe file** *which located within the* Culinary Nutrition *website at www.culinarynutrition.elsevier.com, is filled with soluble fiber from the oats and insoluble fiber from the sweetened berries. It is a heart-healthy dessert that boasts the cholesterol-lowering benefits of oats and the antioxidant value of berries. The finished dish is shown within the centerfold* **Photo file** *in Plate 4.1.*

Dietary Fiber Recommendations

It makes good sense to consume both soluble and insoluble fibers on a daily basis to achieve their combined health benefits. If a person consumes the recommended number of servings of fruits, vegetables and whole grains based on their daily caloric needs as detailed in Chapter 1, they should be consuming close to the amount of fiber that is needed daily.

According to the US Dietary Reference Intakes (DRIs) discussed in Chapter 1, the average female under the age of 50 needs 25 grams of fiber daily and the average male under 50 needs 38 grams of fiber daily. The daily fiber requirements decrease for people over 50 years of age: males require 30 grams of fiber daily and females require 21 grams of fiber daily. This is because total calorie needs decrease as people get older.

The recommendation for dietary fiber for children is that fiber intake should equal age in years plus 5 grams per day. For example, a 4-year-old child should consume 4 (years) plus 5 (grams of fiber) or 9 grams of fiber daily. Vegetable gum fiber supplements, which dissolve in fluids, are available as fiber supplements to the diet if warranted [5].

The sources and amounts of dietary fiber are shown in Table 4-5. A fiber-rich diet is shown in Table 4-6, with the amounts of foods and beverages that are needed to achieve the DRI recommendations for fiber.

Fiber Claims

The FDA regulates food products that carry the following health claim for fiber: *"Low-fat diets rich in fiber-containing grain products, fruits, and vegetables may reduce the risk of some types of cancer, a disease associated with many factors."* This claim is restricted to foods that are grain products, fruits or vegetables that contain dietary fiber; are low-fat; and are a good source of dietary fiber, without fortification [7].

Foods are consider a good dietary source of fiber if they contain at least 2.5 grams of fiber per serving and an excellent dietary source of fiber if they contain at least 5 grams of fiber per serving. In order for the terms "more" or "added fiber" to be used on a food label, a food needs to have at least 2.5 grams more or added fiber compared to the reference or regular food [8,9].

Too Much Fiber?

Can a person consume too much fiber? Anything in excess is not advisable. Soluble fibers are like sponges; they take up fluid and swell. If overconsumed excess soluble fiber could cause abdominal discomfort and dehydration. Too much insoluble fiber may cause foods to move through the intestinal tract quickly. There is a risk that calories and nutrients may be limited in absorption. Fiber supplements can be abused and lead to these conditions. Although some primitive cultures may consume as much as 60 grams of fiber daily, this amount from foodstuffs is uncommon.

Sources of Carbohydrates: Dairy Products, Fruits, Legumes, Vegetables and Whole Grains

CARBOHYDRATES IN FRUITS

The concept of food exchanges was discussed in Chapter 1. Food exchanges are particularly helpful in diabetic diets (which are discussed later in this chapter) and weight management. To review, a food can be

TABLE 4-5 Common Sources of Dietary Fiber	
Foods	Dietary Fiber (grams)
Fruits	
1 medium banana	3.9 g
1 medium apple with skin	3.3
1 medium orange	3.1
Vegetables	
1 cup raw carrots	3.1
1 cup cooked peas	8.8
1 cup green beans	4
Legumes	
1 cup cooked split peas	16.3
1 cup cooked garbanzo beans	12.5
1 cup baked Northern beans	10.4
Grains	
½ cup bran-type cereal	8.8
1 cup cooked oat bran cereal	5.7
1 slice whole grain bread	1.7

Source: [6].

TABLE 4-6 Fiber-Rich Diet	
Foods and Beverages	Dietary Fiber (grams)
Breakfast	
1 medium bran muffin	4.0 g
¾ cup cooked oatmeal	1.6
1 medium banana	1.8
1 cup soy milk	0
Lunch	
2 slices rye bread	4
2 ounces turkey breast	0
½ sliced medium tomato	0.8
Lettuce	0.4
1 medium apple	3
1 cup yogurt with fruit	1
1 fig bar	2
1 cup 2% reduced fat dairy milk	0
Dinner	
1 cup shredded carrot salad	3.1
1 skinless chicken breast	0
1 cup cooked brown rice	1.6
½ cup cooked broccoli	3
1 whole wheat roll	1.6
Snacks	
3 cups popped popcorn	4.5
8 graham crackers	3
12 ounces iced tea	0
1 cup hot chocolate	1
1 cup grapes	1.6
TOTAL	49.6 grams of fiber

"exchanged" for another food in a recipe or meal that has approximately the same number of calories and grams of carbohydrates, protein and fat. For example, a medium apple can be "exchanged" for a medium orange for about the same number of calories, carbohydrates, protein and fat.

The serving size for one fruit exchange is about 1 small piece of fresh fruit (about 4 ounces); ½ cup of canned unsweetened fruit or fruit juice; or ¼ cup of dried fruit. Each serving contains about 15 grams of carbohydrates, no significant protein, 60 calories, and no protein or fat. On average, fresh and frozen fruits have about 2 grams of fiber per serving or exchange. Dried fruits, such as raisins, apricots and prunes vary and have slightly more fiber per serving.

CARBOHYDRATES IN VEGETABLES

The serving size for one vegetable exchange is about ½ cup cooked nonstarchy vegetables or vegetable juice, or 1 cup of raw vegetables. Each serving of vegetables contains about 5 grams of carbohydrates, 2 grams of protein and about 25 calories. Vegetables contain 2 to 3 grams of dietary fiber per serving or exchange, on the average.

CARBOHYDRATES IN STARCHY VEGETABLES (POTATOES, BEETS, SQUASH, CORN, PEAS)

The serving size for one starchy vegetable exchange varies. It is about ½ cup cooked starchy vegetable if it is plain tasting. If it is naturally sweet, such as acorn squash, then it is less—about ¼ cup cooked. Each serving of starchy vegetables contains about 15 grams of carbohydrates, 0 to 3 grams of protein, 0 to 1 gram of fat and about 80 calories. On average, starchy vegetables contain 2 to 3 grams of dietary fiber per serving or exchange.

CARBOHYDRATES IN LEGUMES (COOKED BEANS, DRIED PEAS AND LENTILS)

The serving size for a legume exchange is about ½ cup cooked legumes. Each serving contains about 15 grams of carbohydrates, 0 to 3 grams of protein, 0 to 1 gram of fat and about 80 calories. Legumes average about 3 grams of fiber per serving or exchange, on the average.

> ### Recipe: Turkey Sausage, Beans and Greens
>
> *Legumes are versatile powerhouses of nutrients. They are typically high in folate, iron, magnesium and potassium; low in fat with no cholesterol; and a good source of protein, so they can be used as a meat substitute. The recipe for **Turkey Sausage, Beans and Greens** in the **Recipe file** which is located within the Culinary Nutrition website at www.culinarynutrition.elsevier.com, combines garbanzo or cannelloni beans, fresh kale or collard greens, and reduced-fat turkey sausage into a substantial and flavorsome entree. A vegetarian version can be made without the turkey sausage, since the soluble and insoluble fiber-rich ingredients in this hearty dish are quite satisfying.*

CARBOHYDRATES IN DAIRY PRODUCTS

The serving size for one dairy milk or milk product exchange (such as yogurt) is about 1 cup. Each serving contains about 12 grams of carbohydrate. The calories vary depending on the percent of fat in the milk or milk product. Milk and milk products do not contain dietary fiber, unless they are fortified.

The carbohydrates in 1 ounce of cheese also vary according to the fat content. One ounce of Parmesan cheese (1 tablespoon) contains about 0.2 gram of carbohydrates, while 1 ounce of cottage cheese contains about 6 grams of carbohydrates per serving.

CARBOHYDRATES IN GRAINS AND GRAIN PRODUCTS

159

The serving size for one grain exchange is about ½ cup cooked grain or 1 slice of bread. Each serving contains about 15 grams of carbohydrates, up to 3 grams of protein, and 1 gram of fat, and about 80 calories, unless fortified. Whole-grain products average about 2 grams of fiber per serving or exchange, unless fortified.

Refined, Enriched, Fortified Grains and Whole Grains

A number of food labeling designations for grains serve to distinguish their degree of wholeness and fortification. These include refined, enriched, fortified and whole.

A *refined grain* has undergone processing that removes the husk, bran and germ of the grain and leaves the endosperm, or starchy interior. An *enriched grain* is a refined grain that has been enriched with B vitamins (thiamin, riboflavin, niacin and folic acid) and iron as specified by the FDA. A *fortified grain* is a grain that has 10 percent or more of the Daily Value (DV) for specific nutrients. It can be a grain product or other food that is fortified to help prevent a nutrient deficiency (such as folic acid) or chronic disease (such as the reduction of spinal bifida through folic acid fortification). A *whole grain* is the entire cereal grain, with the husk, or outer inedible covering; bran, or fibrous protective covering; endosperm, or starchy interior; and germ, or fatty core, all intact.

> **Morsel** "The breakfast food idea made its appearance in a little third-story room on the corner of 28th Street and Third Avenue, New York City. . . . My cooking facilities were very limited, [making it] very difficult to prepare cereals. It often occurred to me that it should be possible to purchase cereals at groceries already cooked and ready to eat, and I considered different ways in which this might be done."
> — John Harvey Kellogg (Kellogg's cereal industrialist,1852–1943)

Because the fat in the germ can become rancid, refined grains may have a longer shelf life than whole grains. Whole grains may need refrigeration or freezing to help prevent deterioration and rancidity. Preservatives, such as calcium or sodium propionate, are sometimes used to add shelf life and prevent mold and staleness.

TABLE 4-7 Comparison of Ingredients Lists in Grain Products

Grain product #1	Grain product #2
Ingredients: 100% whole wheat flour, water, yeast, wheat gluten, canola oil, salt	Ingredients: Wheat flour, water, molasses, yeast, wheat gluten, canola oil, salt, vitamins (thiamin hydrochloride, folic acid), minerals (iron, zinc oxide)

WHOLE GRAINS

Enriched and fortified grains contain nutrients that are added back during processing, such as niacin, vitamin B6, magnesium, manganese, phosphorus and selenium. In contrast, whole grains are "nutrient packages" with their four nutrient-rich parts still intact.

The bran in whole grains contains insoluble dietary fibers, B vitamins, 50 to 80 percent of the grain's minerals (including iron, copper, zinc and magnesium), and phytochemicals, or protective plant substances. The germ contains B vitamins, trace minerals, unsaturated fats, phytochemicals and antioxidants, such as vitamin E. The endosperm is full of complex carbohydrates, protein and smaller amounts of B vitamins.

Common whole grains include brown rice, oatmeal, popcorn and 100 percent whole wheat flour. Common refined grains and grain products that may be enriched or fortified include white rice, white bread and many types of pastas. Color is not an indicator of whole grains. For example, cereals and breads can be sprayed with molasses to look brown. White bread may contain a type of white fiber and have higher fiber content than some brown breads.

Read the ingredient list to make sure that the first ingredients are whole grains. Look for the terms "100% whole grain, whole wheat or whole meal" in the topmost positions. If the first ingredients are listed as "contains whole grain, enriched wheat or grain flour, made with whole grain, multigrain, or stone-ground" the food product may not be 100 percent whole grain.

In Table 4-7, the first ingredient list indicates 100 percent whole-grain flour as the first ingredient. The second ingredient list indicates wheat flour and molasses for coloring, and it is enriched with thiamin, folic acid, iron and zinc. The first food product is 100 percent whole grain.

Whole-Grain Recommendations and Claims

Healthy People is a consortium of agencies and organizations that produce 10-year, science-based, national objectives for improving the health of all Americans [10]. One of the objectives of *Healthy People 2010* is to increase the proportion of whole grains in the diets of people aged 2 years and older.

The *US Dietary Guidelines for Americans* are the cornerstone of US nutrition policy and nutrition education activities. According to the *2010 US Dietary Guidelines*, adults should consume at least half of all grains as whole grains and increase their whole-grain consumption by replacing refined grains with whole grains.

While Americans eat plenty of grains and grain products, most of those that are consumed are refined rather than whole. Adults are encouraged to consume at least three 1-ounce servings of whole grains daily. Serving sizes of common whole grains and whole-grain products that equal 1-ounce servings are shown in Table 4-8 [11].

Food products that contain 51 percent or more whole-grain ingredients by weight and with limited amounts of fat, cholesterol and sodium may carry this FDA-approved health claim:

> Diets rich in whole-grain foods and other plant foods, and low in total fat, saturated fat and cholesterol, may reduce the risk of heart disease and certain cancers.

Whole-grain oat or foods with psyllium fiber (soluble fiber) may also claim:

> Soluble fiber, as part of a diet low in saturated fat and cholesterol, may reduce the risk of heart disease.

Foods that bear a psyllium fiber health claim must also display a statement on the label that explains the need to consume them with adequate amounts of fluids [7,12,13].

TABLE 4-8 Serving Sizes of Common Whole-Grain Foods and Food Products

Whole Grains	Serving Sizes That Equal 1 Ounce of Whole Grains
Brown rice	½ cup cooked
Whole-grain bagel	½ or 1 ounce
Whole-grain bread	1 slice or 1 ounce
Whole-grain cereal	½ cup cooked or 1 ounce ready-to-eat
Whole-grain cracker	5 to 7 small crackers or 1 ounce
Whole-grain muffin	1 small or 1 ounce
Whole-grain pancake or waffle	1 small or 1 ounce
Whole-grain pasta	½ cup cooked
Whole-grain pita bread	½ or 1-ounce
Whole-grain tortilla	1 small or 1 ounce
Popcorn	3 cups

Source: [11]

How to Increase Whole Grains in Cooking and Baking

Substituting whole grains for refined grains in cooking and baking requires trial and error. It is not measure for measure. That is because whole grains tend to be heavier, with different properties and flavor than refined grains. These recommendations call for experimentation for best results.

- Substitute whole wheat flour for up to ⅓ to ½ of the refined wheat flour in some cookie, muffin, quick bread and pancake recipes. The recipe can be repeated with more whole wheat flour if the color, texture and taste are not compromised.
- Add an extra 1 teaspoon of liquid per 1 cup of whole wheat flour to a recipe because the bran absorbs liquid.
- Mix whole wheat yeast bread dough and let it rest about 15 minutes to absorb any liquid; add more liquid if needed before kneading.
- Instead of whole wheat flour, add up to 20 percent of another whole-grain flour, such as sorghum, to some recipes. This amount equals about ¼ of the refined wheat flour that is called for in the recipe.
- Use white whole wheat flour or whole wheat pastry flour for the total amount of all-purpose flour in some cookie, muffin, quick breads and pancake recipes. White whole wheat flour is a whole grain and is nutritionally similar to red whole wheat flour but lacks the pigmentation.
- Replace about ⅓ of the refined wheat flour in some recipes with quick oats or old-fashioned oats. Add about ½ to ¾ cup of uncooked oats to each pound of ground beef or ground turkey in burger or meatloaf recipes.
- Use whole cornmeal in cornbread, corncakes or corn muffins.

161

Recipe: Polenta Bites

Fresh corn is usually considered a vegetable, and dried corn (including popcorn) is considered a gluten-free grain. Make sure that corn flour, corn grits, cornmeal, or polenta is labeled "whole corn" or "whole-grain corn" for the most nutrients, including antioxidants and carotenoids. The recipe for **Polenta Bites** *in the* **Recipe file** *which is located within the Culinary Nutrition website at www.culinarynutrition.elsevier.com, uses coarse ground yellow cornmeal along with assertive Asiago or Parmesan cheese, garlic, onions and mushrooms for flavorful "bites" that tantalize the appetite without overpowering it. The finished dish is shown within the centerfold* **Photo file** *in Plate 4.2.*

- Add barley, corn, millet, oat or rice bran to some batters in small quantities. Add about 1 teaspoon of liquid per 1 cup, since the bran absorbs liquid.
- Substitute whole grains for part of the refined grains in savory recipes, such as pilafs or risottos. Grains from which to choose include barley, brown rice, bulgur, millet, quinoa, sorghum or whole wheat couscous.
- Add about ½ cup of cooked whole grains, such as barley, brown rice, bulgur, rye or wheat berries, or wild rice to soup or stuffing.

- Add cooked whole grains to salads, such as *tabbouleh*, a Middle Eastern salad that is made with bulgur (cracked wheat). Couscous, quinoa or wheat berries can be combined with cooked or raw vegetables.
- Use breakfast-type hot and cold cereals that are made with whole grains, such as amaranth, kamut, quinoa or spelt. *Muesli* is a Swiss breakfast cereal made from uncooked oats, fruits and nuts.
- Use whole-grain pasta or pastas that are blends of whole grains and enriched or fortified wheat flour.
- Use a combination of whole-grain and fortified or enriched white breads. Refrigerate or freeze what is not immediately used.
- Make snack mixes with mixed whole-grain cereals and/or popcorn.

FOOD BYTE

Some sugar substitutes were discovered quite by accident. *Saccharine* was discovered about 130 years ago by scientists who were experimenting with some substitutes for coal tar. *Aspartame* was discovered in the 1960s by a chemist who was working on an ulcer drug. *Sucralose* (marketed as Splenda®) was discovered in 1976 by a graduate student who was testing some other compounds [14].

Carbohydrate Substitutes

A *substitute* is a "stand-in" that takes the place for the function of something else. If the carbohydrates from fruits, vegetables, legumes and whole grains are so important in our diet, then why should we consume carbohydrate substitutes? This is because carbohydrate substitutes allow us to consume some sweet and starchy foods without all of the calories they would normally provide. Also, carbohydrate substitutes provide options for diabetics who need to watch the total amount of carbohydrates in their diet.

SUGAR SUBSTITUTES

Sugar substitutes are not a modern phenomenon. They date back to the late 1800s when a chemist accidentally discovered the sweetness of a coal tar derivative and called it "saccharine." The use of saccharine increased during the sugar shortage of World War I and again during the 1960s, when dieting became popular in the United States [15].

High-Intensity Sweeteners

High-intensity sweeteners, are generally nonnutritive, noncaloric and nonmetabolized. They pass through the body unchanged. High-intensity sweeteners approved by FDA include acesulfame-K, aspartame, neotame, saccharin, sucralose and tagatose.

- *Acesulfame potassium (acesulfame-K)* is a potassium salt that is about 200 times sweeter than sucrose. Acesulfame-K is stable at high temperatures and soluble in water. It is an all-purpose sweetener that is used in baked goods, candies, chewing gum, desserts, diet drinks, gelatins, puddings and as a tabletop sweetener in *Sweet One* and *Swiss Sweet*. Since it may leave a slight aftertaste, acesulfame-K is often combined with other sweeteners.
- *Aspartame* is a blend of the amino acid aspartic acid and a form of phenylalanine that is about 200 times sweeter than table sugar. Aspartame is not heat stable. It is an all-purpose sweetener that is used in beverages, breath mints, chewing gum, cocoa mixes, frozen desserts, gelatins, puddings, powdered soft drinks and as a tabletop sweetener in Equal. The FDA has confirmed it is safe to consume, except by anyone with *phenylketonuria*, a genetic disorder of the metabolism [16].
- *Neotame* is a blend of the amino acids aspartic acid and phenylalanine. It is 7,000 to 13,000 times sweeter than sucrose. Neotame is stable at high temperatures. It is a general all-purpose sweetener that has both cooking and baking applications. Neotame is used in baked goods, beverages, candies, chewing gum, dairy products, frozen desserts, puddings, yogurt-type products and as a tabletop sweetener.
- *Saccharine* is produced from a naturally occurring substance in grapes. It is about 300 to 500 times sweeter than sucrose. It is often blended with other sweeteners to mask its aftertaste. Saccharine is heat stable. It is used in baked goods, beverages, candies, chewing gum, jams, medicines, soft drinks, toothpaste and as a tabletop sweetener in Sweet'N Low® and Sweet 10®.

- *Sucralose* begins as sucrose and then is chemically altered, producing about 600 times the sweetness of sucrose. It is stable at most temperatures. Sucralose is a general, all-purpose sweetener that is used in baked goods, beverages, candies, canned fruits, cereals and cereal bars, chewing gum, condiments, dairy products, desserts (as light ice cream, popsicles and puddings), jams, nutritional products and dietary supplements, salad dressings, snack foods, syrups and condiments (as light maple syrup and low-calorie jams and jellies) and as a tabletop sweetener in Splenda®. Sucralose-sweetened tabletop sweeteners may contain other carbohydrates for texture and volume.

  Sucralose may be used in place of or in combination with sucrose in baked goods. Caramelization, cooking time, flavor, moisture retention, texture and volume may vary. Complete substitution of sucralose for sugar is possible in some beverages, cheesecakes, fruit pie fillings, glazes and sweet sauces.

- *Tagatose* is similar in sweetness and physical bulk to sucrose, but it is metabolized like other high-intensity sweeteners. Tagatose is used in chewing gum, dairy products, diet soft drinks, frostings, frozen yogurt, hard and soft confectioneries, health bars, nonfat ice cream and ready-to-eat cereals. Due to its bulk, tagatose can be used in small amounts in baking and products that are subjected to high temperatures.

Sugar substitutes are also discussed in Chapter 9 in regards to disease prevention and diet maintenance.

Natural Sweeteners

Natural sweeteners, in comparison to nonnutritive sweeteners, contain calories and nutrients, are metabolized, and change as they pass through the body. They include *agave nectar, brown rice syrup, date sugar, honey, maple syrup, molasses and blackstrap molasses, sorghum syrup* and *stevia*.

- *Agave nectar or syrup* is from the agave plant, which is also the source of tequila. It is about 1½ times as sweet as white sugar. Agave comes in many flavors and colors, from light and mild to dark and strong. Blue agave is the most common.

  Agave dissolves quickly, so it can be used to sweeten cold beverages. Some adjustments may be needed when using agave nectar in baking. These include increasing flour or cornstarch by about ¼ cup; reducing other liquids in the recipe by about 1 ounce; thoroughly oiling baking or muffin pans; reducing oven temperature by about 25 F; and increasing baking time by about 5 to 10 minutes. Cookies will not come out crispy but rather will have a cakelike texture, since agave retains moisture. About ¾ cup of agave syrup equals about 1 cup of white sugar in sweetening.

  Agave is a vegan alternative for honey. Since agave has only a mild effect on blood sugar, it is favored in carbohydrate-restricted diets.

- *Brown rice syrup* is made by heating brown rice with enzymes. In the process, about 50 percent of the rice starches are converted into sugars; the liquid is strained and the syrup remains. Brown rice syrup is about half as sweet as white sugar. It has a mild, butterscotch flavor. Brown rice syrup can be used in cookies, muffins and puddings; as a syrup for pancakes and waffles; and as a sweetener for iced tea and rice milk.

  In general, substitute 1¼ cups of brown rice syrup for 1 cup of white sugar and reduce the liquid in a recipe by about ¼ cup. Brown rice syrup is gluten-free and suitable for vegans.

- *Date sugar* is made from pulverized dates. It contains some fiber and minerals. The date pieces do not dissolve in liquids or melt like other sugars, so the use of date sugar is limited.

  One cup of date sugar equals about 1 cup of white or brown sugar, but the flavor of date sugar is strong and it is expensive.

- *Honey* is made by honeybees from the nectar of flowers. It is sweeter and has more calories than white sugar. Honey contains some enzymes and minerals. If honey if used in baked goods, it may slightly add to the rising time of the dough.

  Use about ¾ cup of honey for 1 cup of white sugar in recipes and reduce the amount of liquid by about 3 to 4 tablespoons. When baking, if baking soda is called for in a recipe, it may need to be reduced by about ½ of a teaspoon. Like agave nectar, cookies made with honey will have a soft texture.

- *Maple syrup* is made by boiling down sap from maple trees until the sugars condense into thickened syrup. Natural maple syrup contains minerals, such as calcium and potassium. Maple syrup is also manufactured by combining corn syrup, maple flavoring and coloring. Manufactured maple syrup may not contain the same level of minerals as natural maple syrup.

  Use about ¾ cup of maple syrup for each 1 cup of white sugar in recipes and reduce the amount of liquid by about 3 to 4 tablespoons.

- *Molasses* is the thick syrup that remains after sugar beets or sugarcane is processed to make white sugar. The type of molasses depends on the maturity of the sugar beet or cane, the amount of sugar that is removed, and the extraction process.

   About 1 1/3 cups of molasses can be substituted for 1 cup of white sugar in some recipes. Reduce the amount of liquid by about 5 tablespoons. Since molasses is more acidic than white sugar, add 1/2 teaspoon of baking soda per 1 cup of molasses in baking. In general, replace no more than half of the white sugar in recipes with molasses since it imparts a dark color and strong flavor.

- *Blackstrap molasses* contains the least amount of sugar in the molasses group of sweeteners, with some vitamins and minerals. Blackstrap molasses is mild in sweetness and bitter-tart. It is used both to sweeten and color foods, particularly baked goods.

- *Sorghum syrup*, sometimes mistaken for blackstrap molasses, is also a by-product of the sugar-making process. Sorghum syrup comes from sorghum cane. It contains calcium, iron and potassium.

   Sorghum syrup can be substituted in equal quantities in recipes that call for honey, corn syrup, maple syrup or molasses, such as in baked beans, barbecue sauce or gingerbread. Sorghum syrup has a distinct taste that may not be a suitable substitute in some recipes.

- *Stevioside (stevia)*, a plant in the sunflower family (also known as sugarleaf and sweetleaf), is as much as 300 times sweeter than white sugar. Initially, stevia had a bitter, licorice-like aftertaste, but the sweetest parts of the plant are now used.

   Stevia does not caramelize or crystallize. It is used to sweeten beverages, cereal, coffee and tea, fruit and yogurt and as a tabletop sweetener in PureVia® and Truvia®. Stevia has only a minor effect on blood sugar, so it is favored in carbohydrate-controlled diets. In general, ¼ teaspoon of powdered stevia extract, or 2 tablespoons whole-leaf stevia, equals about 1 cup of white sugar in sweetening.

Sugar Alcohols

A **sugar alcohol** is a sugar with an alcohol group attached to it. They include erythritol, lactitol, maltitol, mannitol, sorbitol and xylitol—identified by their "ol" suffix.

Sugar alcohols are reduced-calorie sweeteners. They are not as sweet as white sugar and they have fewer calories. On the average, sugar alcohols provide about one-half of the calories of white sugar. Sugar alcohols are poorly absorbed into the bloodstream from the small intestine, so they only cause a small change in blood sugar. This is meaningful to diabetics. Foods and beverages with sugar alcohols should be taken into account when estimating the total amount of carbohydrates in a diabetic diet. The American Diabetes Association offers guidelines [17].

Due to their poor absorption, if too many sugar alcohols are ingested, they can lead to gas or diarrhea. This may be the case if sugar alcohols are overconsumed in beverages and sweets.

Sugar alcohols are not broken down by the bacteria in the mouth, so they do not lead to dental cavities. That is why chewing sugarless gum actually prevents teeth from decay, and due to the chemical structure of sugar alcohols, they actually leave the mouth feeling cool! Besides chewing gum, sugar alcohols are found in some candies, cookies, ice cream and puddings. Sugar alcohols do not brown, nor do they caramelize when heated, so they have limited value to cooks. In food product development, sugar alcohols are sometimes used to mask the bitter aftertaste of other sweeteners.

STARCH SUBSTITUTES
Modified Food Starches

Grain starches, such as cornstarch, rice starch and wheat flour, and root starches, such as arrowroot, potato and tapioca, have versatile properties in cooking. When heated, these grain and root starches become soluble in water. They swell, thicken and stabilize foods such as custards, gravies, pie fillings, puddings, salad dressings, sauces and soups.

Grain and root starches are not always consistent or stable; plus, they may not bind in certain preparations, such as in gels. Partially to overcome these disadvantages, food manufacturers have created **modified food starches** that can withstand excessive heat, acid or freezing temperatures. Modified food starches should not be confused with **genetically modified** starch from genetically engineered plants.

Food starches can be modified by chemical or physical means. Some food starches can be modified to dissolve and disperse immediately in fluids; others can be modified to dissolve and disperse without cooking or to hold emulsions more effectively. Modified food starches are also used as anticaking agents, fat substitutes and humectants to keep foods moist. Modified food starches should be avoided by people who have celiac disease, unless the food is labeled gluten-free.

FIBER SUBSTITUTES

Soluble fiber substitutes include *inulin, psyllium seed husk (psyllium)* and *vegetable gums*. They are used to help lose weight, lower blood cholesterol, reduce the risk of colon cancer and treat gastrointestinal disorders.

Inulin is a fiber that is found in the roots and rhizomes (underground stems) of plants. It promotes the health of intestinal bacteria, so it is used as a prebiotic. Inulin ranges from bland to mildly sweet. It contains about ¼ of the calories of white sugar per gram, with minimal effect on blood sugar, so it may be suitable for diabetics. Inulin can be used to replace sugar, fat and flour in some food preparations. Large quantities can lead to bloating or gas.

Psyllium seed husk (psyllium) is the fibrous seed coating of a plant native to India. Psyllium is soluble in water; it expands and become sticky and glutinous. It is indigestible in humans. Psyllium is used to relieve gastrointestinal disorders and shows promise in lowering cholesterol and in diabetes management.

The FDA permits that a food product with 1.7 grams of psyllium seed husk soluble fiber (or 0.75 grams of oat or barley fiber) can carry an approved health claim that states that regular consumption of that product, in conjunction with a diet low in saturated fat and cholesterol, may reduce the risk of heart disease. Specifically, the claim must read as follows:

> Soluble fiber from foods such as [the name of the soluble fiber source; and, if desired, the name of the food product], as part of a diet low in saturated fat and cholesterol, may reduce the risk of heart disease. A serving of [name of the food product] supplies _____ grams of the [necessary daily dietary intake for the benefit soluble fiber from [name of the soluble fiber source] necessary per day to have this effect. [13]

Vegetable gum fibers are found in the woody parts and seed coatings of plants. They include agar, carrageenan, gum arabic, guar gum and acacia gum, among others. Vegetable gums are used in the food industry as emulsifiers, gelling agents, stabilizers and thickening agents. Some vegetable gums are available in powdered forms that dissolve easily in fluids with little to no aftertaste. Due to their thickening potential, vegetable gums can be useful in gluten-free foods and diets.

165

CARBOHYDRATES IN COOKING AND BAKING

Sugars, starches and fibers from the plant kingdom offer a world of cooking and baking possibilities. To begin, many are *hygroscopic*, which means that they easily mix with water and other fluids, both making and keeping foods moist.

Sugars lend flavor and color to foods and beverages. In fact, sugars provide such an essential taste that they have their own sweet sense of taste, as described in Chapter 1. And starches help to provide texture and bulk. If either of these carbohydrates is reduced or eliminated from cooking, and especially from baking, the final products may suffer.

Starches readily absorb cooking water and swell, such as cooked rice or barley. When they cool, the starch molecules rebound, or stick together and form a moist gel. These cooked and cooled features of starches provide endless culinary applications.

Stored animal starch, called glycogen, and its role in energy metabolism—specifically sports nutrition—is discussed more fully in Chapter 10. Glycogen is where animals store carbohydrates for energy. It is a small component of animal tissue, but it might affect the texture of the animal protein.

While cooking helps to soften starch, cellulose is left pretty much intact, so cooking with fibrous grains, legumes, vegetables and fruits can literally be tough. Some vegetables and fruits can be peeled. Grains and legumes may require longer cooking time to soften, but not dissolve.

Pectin is partly water-soluble, so cooking vegetables and fruits with pectin will help to soften them. When pectin is extracted from apples and citrus fruits, it can be used for thickening sauces, jams and jellies.

The use of gums in cooking and baking, such as guar gum, locust bean gum, or xanthan gum, is helpful in thickening, gelling, stabilizing emulsions and forming smooth consistencies in candies and frozen confections. Some can be used in vegan diets in place of gelatin that is an animal by-product.

How Carbohydrates Work in the Body: Carbohydrate Digestion and Metabolism

Carbohydrate digestion and metabolism are described in Chapter 1. A review of the process follows. Starting in the mouth, by way of the esophagus, stomach and small intestine, sugars and starches are cleaved, or broken down through chemical and physical digestion, and converted into single sugars for absorption into the bloodstream.

Morsel *"It is more important to eat some carbohydrates at breakfast, because the brain needs fuel right away, and carbohydrate is the best source."* —Andrew Weil, MD (holistic physician, 1942–)

In the mouth, *salivary amylase*, an enzyme found in saliva, serves to moisten food and begin the digestion process. Partially digested sugars and starches then pass into the stomach, where some additional breakdown occurs. In the small intestine, *pancreatic amylase* is secreted by the pancreas into the first section of the small intestine, which helps to break down starches into double sugars: lactose, maltose and sucrose. Then other intestinal enzymes break down these double sugars into single sugars: glucose, fructose and galactose. These single sugars are all finally converted into glucose, which is then absorbed through the small intestine into the bloodstream.

The glucose is then delivered to the liver by the bloodstream, where it is stored or sent to the body cells for energy. Think of the liver as a blood sugar regulator: it dispenses blood sugar as the cells require it. When there is too much sugar in the bloodstream (hyperglycemia), as in diabetes, the hormone insulin helps to remove sugar from the bloodstream and move it into the cells for storage. In Type I diabetes, the body cannot produce insulin, and this is why people who have Type I diabetes must inject insulin to assist this process. If blood sugar is too low (hypoglycemia), another hormone called glucagon helps to break down glycogen (stored glucose) and send glucose into the bloodstream. Some glucose can be made from protein and fats, but the body prefers the glucose that is made from carbohydrates. In Type II diabetes, the body may make some insulin, but it may be ineffective.

Some carbohydrates are digested and metabolized slowly, and others relatively fast. This is determined to some degree by the composition of the carbohydrates and how "resistant" they are to enzymes. A simple sugar is much less resistant than a complex carbohydrate, or starch, so it is digested and metabolized faster. The presence of food, stomach acid and soluble fiber also slows down the digestion and absorption of carbohydrates. If a person consumes foods that are high in fiber, such as whole grains and legumes, they may take longer to digest and metabolize than simple sugars. While they will probably not provide quick energy, they may provide sustained energy.

Carbohydrates in Health: Dietary Carbohydrate Recommendations

Now that the importance of carbohydrates in the diet has been established, how many carbohydrates should be consumed on a daily basis for overall health and disease prevention? If a person consumes too many carbohydrates, will the excess lead to obesity and diseases such as cardiovascular disease, diabetes and certain cancers?

TOTAL CARBOHYDRATES

The 2010 US Dietary Reference Intake values recommend that daily carbohydrate intake range from 45 to 65 percent of total calories. An inactive, smaller-framed person may only need 45 percent of his or her total calories from carbohydrates, while a larger-framed, more active person may need a greater percentage. A method for determining carbohydrate needs for a theoretical woman and man is shown in Table 4-9 [11].

If a person consumes an average of 2,000 calories a day, about 6 ounces of grains or grain products are recommended, with one-half of this amount, or 3 ounces, from whole grains. One ounce of grains or grain products is approximately equal to:

- ½ bagel
- 1 slice bread
- ½ cup cooked cereal
- 1 cup dry cereal
- ½ English muffin

TABLE 4-9 How to Determine Carbohydrate Needs		
Age and Gender	19- to 30-Year-Old Women	19- To 30-Year-Old Men
Activity level	Sedentary	Active
Estimated daily calorie need	2,200 calories	3,000 calories
Multiplied by	0.45 (lower end of nutritional recommendation for carbohydrates in a daily diet, expressed as a decimal)	0.65 (higher end of nutritional recommendation for carbohydrates in a daily diet, expressed as a decimal)
Total	990 calories of carbohydrates daily	1,950 calories of carbohydrates daily

Source: [11].

- ½ cup cooked pasta or rice
- 3 cups popped popcorn
- 6-inch tortilla

Carbohydrate needs are based on age, gender, activity level and caloric needs [18].

According to the *2010 US Dietary Guidelines for Americans*, sedentary women aged 19 to 30 years require about 1,800 to 2,000 calories daily; 2,000 to 2,200 calories daily if they are moderately active; and 2,400 calories daily if they are active. Sedentary women aged 31 to 50 years require about 1,800 calories daily; 2,000 calories daily if they are moderately active; and 2,200 calories daily if they are active. Sedentary women aged 51 and older require about 1,600 calories daily; 1,800 calories daily if they are moderately active; and 2,000 to 2,200 calories daily if they are active.

Sedentary men aged 19 to 30 years require up to 2,600 calories daily; 2,800 calories daily if they are moderately active; and 3,000 calories daily if they are active. Sedentary 31- to 50-year-old men require up to 2,400 calories daily; 2,600 calories daily if they are moderately active; and 2,800 to 3,000 calories daily if they are active. Sedentary men aged 51 and older require up to 2,200 calories daily; 2,400 calories daily if they are moderately active; and 2,800 calories daily if they are active.

The following formula is for applying the recommendation of 45 to 65 percent of total calories from carbohydrates to two of these calorie levels. This formula can also be used for other calorie levels. To determine the *grams* of carbohydrates needed daily, divide the total number of calories by 4 (1 gram of carbohydrate equals 4 calories):

990 calories of carbohydrates daily/4 calories per gram = 247.5 grams of carbohydrates daily
1,950 calories of carbohydrate daily/4 calories per gram = 487.5 grams of carbohydrates daily

Some foods and beverages that meet these two daily carbohydrate requirements are shown in Table 4-10. In general, an active man requires almost twice the amount of carbohydrates as a sedentary woman to meet his daily needs. If daily activity is reduced, then carbohydrate intake will need to decrease. Excess carbohydrate calories beyond daily needs may increase body weight, just like excess fat or protein in the diet.

A diet planning tool that outlines carbohydrate consumption is the USDA Food Patterns, which identifies the daily amounts of nutrient-dense foods to consume from five major food groups and their subgroups, including carbohydrates (dairy products, fruits, grains and vegetables). These food patterns were developed to help people execute the *2010 Dietary Guidelines* recommendations.

The recommended amounts and limits of carbohydrates at 12 calorie levels, ranging from 1,000 calories to 3,200 calories, can be found at http://www.cnpp.usda.gov/USDAFoodPatterns.htm.

ADDED SUGARS

The *2010 US Dietary Guidelines for Americans* recommends that added sugar intake ranges from 10 to 25 percent of total calories. This amounts to about 3 to 12 teaspoons of added sugar daily, depending on the

TABLE 4-10 Foods and Beverages That Meet Daily Carbohydrate Needs

Foods and Beverages	Amounts of Carbohydrates (grams)
1 cup cooked oatmeal	25 g
1 cup frozen low-fat yogurt	37
1 medium banana	27
1 medium apple	32
½ cup cooked garbanzo beans	22
½ cup cooked brown rice	22
2 cups skim milk	24
2 slices whole wheat bread	26
2 cups popped popcorn	38
Total	253
2 cups cooked oatmeal	50
2 cups frozen low-fat yogurt	74
2 medium bananas	54
2 medium apples	64
1 cup cooked garbanzo beans	44
1 cup cooked brown rice	44
3 cups skim milk	36
4 slices whole wheat bread	52
4 cups popped popcorn	76
Total	494

TABLE 4-11 Calorie Levels, Added Sugar and Food Equivalents

Calories	Added Sugar (teaspoons)	Food Equivalents
1,600 cal	3 tsp	½ cup ice cream; ½ cup 2% chocolate dairy milk
1,800	5	½ cup sherbet; 1 ounce fudge
2,000	8	2-ounce chocolate bar; 12-ounce cola drink
2,200	9	10-ounce fruit punch drink
2,400	11	16-ounce chocolate milkshake

daily calorie level. Based on an average daily calorie intake of 2,000 calories, this equals about 8 teaspoons of added sugar. There are about 8 teaspoons of sugar in a 2-ounce chocolate bar and a 12-ounce cola drink. Other calorie levels, added sugars and food equivalents are shown in Table 4-11. This shows that foods with added sugars can be consumed in a calorie-controlled diet. The remaining calories should come from nutrient-dense foods.

How can this information be applied to cooking and baking? If you oversee the foods and beverages for sedentary people at a weight loss spa, then you may have to adjust the recipes or meals to provide just 45 percent of the total calories from carbohydrates. If you manage the foods and beverages at a training clinic for athletes, then you may have to adjust the recipes or meals to provide as much as 65 percent of the total calories from carbohydrates. You can use the USDA National Nutrient Database for Standard Reference at http://ndb.nal.usda.gov/ to determine the number of grams of carbohydrates in foods and beverages for recipe and menu development.

Carbohydrates in Disease: Lactose Intolerance, Gluten Intolerance, Coronary Heart Disease, Diabetes, Hypoglycemia and Obesity

LACTOSE INTOLERANCE

The use of dairy products in cooking and baking and how to adjust recipes if dairy products are eliminated due to allergies, religious constraints or other reasons are discussed in Chapter 5. By understanding the symptoms that are associated with *lactose intolerance,* one can see why cooking and baking without dairy products is critical for certain segments of the population.

TABLE 4-12 Lactose in Common Dairy Products

Dairy Products	Servings	Lactose (grams)
Low-fat cottage cheese	1 cup	7–8 g
Ice cream	1 cup	9–10
Low-fat yogurt	1 cup	11–15
2% reduced-fat dairy milk	1 cup	9–13
2% reduced-fat, lactose-reduced dairy milk	1 cup	3.3
Parmesan cheese	1 ounce	0.7–0.8
Swiss cheese	1 ounce	1

The milk sugar *lactose* is fundamental to dairy milk and milk products. It is the milk sugar and not the dairy product itself that causes lactose intolerance. Lactose intolerance is the inability to digest, metabolize and absorb lactose that produces gastrointestinal symptoms such as pain and gas.

There is a higher incidence of lactose intolerance in countries where dairy products are not commonly consumed. These include Africa, Asia, Central America and the Middle East. Lactose intolerance may increase with age if there is a reduction or absence of the enzyme *lactase*, which is responsible in the breakdown of lactose.

Why Are Some People Lactose Intolerant?

Lactose is a double sugar, made up of two single sugars, glucose and galactose, that are linked together. Lactose must be broken down into these single sugars to be metabolized for energy. The enzyme lactase, which is located in the lining of the small intestine, is responsible for this division. If a person does not produce enough lactase, then lactose cannot be broken down and glucose and galactose cannot be absorbed through the small intestine into the bloodstream for energy. Instead, lactose collects in the small intestine. Intestinal bacteria metabolize lactose, which causes it to ferment and produce a range of symptoms, including cramping, bloating, diarrhea and/or gas. Most people with lactose intolerance need to avoid or eliminate lactose and therefore most dairy products. Individual responses may vary.

A lactase deficiency can also be caused by diseases that destroy the lining of the small intestine and lactase. Such is the case in *celiac sprue disease. Celiac disease* is an autoimmune disorder in the small intestine. It is caused by a reaction to the protein in wheat and other common grains, such as barley and rye. This reaction causes an inflammatory response in the small intestine, which interferes with nutrient absorption. The most effective treatment is a gluten-free diet.

Celiac disease damages the *villi,* or hairlike structures that line the small intestine. Once a gluten-free diet is followed and celiac disease is under control, the villi may be able to recover. It is also important to distinguish lactose intolerance from a *milk allergy,* which is an abnormal immune response, usually to the protein in dairy milk and milk products.

Where Is Lactose?

Human milk is high in lactose. Cow, goat, buffalo, sheep and yak milk all contain about the same amount of lactose—around half that of human milk. Fat-reduced and fat-free dairy products tend to have slightly higher lactose content, since they may have added milk solids, as do some butter products.

Hard cheese, such as Parmesan or Swiss; fermented cheese (partially broken down by bacteria); soft cheese; and ice cream may contain less lactose and be better tolerated. Some buttermilk, sour cream and yogurt products contain lactase, produced by bacteria in their manufacture, and also may be tolerated by some people. Certain brands contain additional milk solids and may not be tolerated. Table 4-12 lists the amount of lactose in some common dairy products.

As a food additive, lactose is found in both dairy and nondairy food products. It contributes to coagulation, flavor and texture. Food additives with lactose include lactoserum, margarine, milk solids, modified milk ingredients and whey. They may be found in nondairy foods, including processed breads, meal-replacement products, and meats, so it is important for people who are lactose intolerant to carefully read food labels. Kosher products that are labeled *pareve* are free of milk. But if a "D" (dairy) is present next to the circled "K" (Ⓚ for kosher), then the food likely contains some milk solids.

Bean, grain and nut milks, such as soy, oat, rice and almond, are marketed as dairy milk replacement beverages. Unless they are fortified with the nutrients found in dairy milk, especially calcium and vitamin D, they may fall short nutritionally.

For example, some brands of rice milk have only 1 gram of protein and 20 milligrams of calcium per cup, versus 8 grams of protein and 291 milligrams of calcium per cup of dairy milk, unless they are fortified. Plus, some brands of rice milk have as much as three times the carbohydrates as dairy milk—usually for sweetening. Some brands of almond milk are lower in total carbohydrates and sugars, depending on their formulations.

Lactase drops and tablets can be taken before dairy products are consumed to aid digestion. Lactose-intolerant individuals should experiment taking these products at different times and in different dosages for maximum effectiveness. The advantage of using lactase drops and tablets is that a person may still be able to digest some dairy products and benefit by their nutrients. A person can live without lactose in their diet, but he or she cannot live healthfully without the nutrients that dairy products supply.

Morsel "If thou tastest a crust of bread, thou tastest all the stars and all the heavens." —Robert Browning (English poet and playwright, 1812–1889)

From a culinary perspective, dairy products, including milk, cheese, cream, ice cream and yogurt, provide a wide range of culinary possibilities. Doing without dairy products in cooking and baking is achievable, but challenging. Refer to Chapter 5 to help with solutions to the challenges that lactose-free cooking present.

GLUTEN INTOLERANCE

170

Gluten intolerance is an inability of the body to tolerate gluten, the protein in certain grains, including wheat, barley or rye. It is different from a *wheat allergy*, which is a sudden and severe onset of allergic reactions, including such symptoms as asthma and other breathing difficulties, coughing and/or projectile vomiting. A wheat allergy can be life-threatening to people who are allergic to wheat.

As previously discussed, gluten intolerance is a symptom of celiac disease, an autoimmune disorder in genetically predisposed people that affects the small intestine. An autoimmune disorder or disease is due to an aggressive immune response to substances that are normally present in the body and the environment. In the case of celiac disease, these substances are wheat and other grains.

Symptoms of celiac disease may include anemia, diarrhea, fatigue and weight loss. If it is present in children, celiac disease may cause failure to thrive due to nutrient malabsorption and subsequent nutrient deficiencies. As the small intestine becomes increasingly damaged, lactose intolerance may also occur.

Gluten intolerance is due to *gliaden*, a gluten-type protein that is found in wheat, barley, rye and other related grains. When gliaden is ingested, the autoimmune system reacts with the tissues in the small intestine and produces an inflammatory response. The *villi*, small hairlike projectiles that normally protrude from the intestinal wall, become too flattened to assist nutrient absorption into the bloodstream. A screening exam confirms this condition.

There is no known cure for celiac disease. People who have celiac disease run the risk of nutrient deficiencies, including vitamins A, D, E and K; folic acid and vitamin B12; and the minerals calcium and iron. Additionally they may suffer from abdominal bleeding, anemia and/or osteoporosis.

Common and "ancient" grains implicated with gluten intolerance include barley, bulgur, couscous, einkorn, emmer, farro, kamut, kasha, matzo meal, rye, spelt, triticale and any type of wheat (including durum, farina, graham flour and semolina). Some people also respond negatively to oats, since they may be contaminated with wheat. Individualized diets are recommended.

Tolerated grains may include corn, millet, quinoa, rice, sorghum and teff. Pure buckwheat and amaranth may also be tolerated because they are not botanically considered grains. Potato and legume starches, such as soy, are often used in combination with tolerated grains to duplicate the characteristics of wheat products.

If a person follows a strict, gluten-free diet, the small intestine may have time to heal and symptoms may subside. This is why it is so important to read food labels and to learn about the "hidden" ingredients in foods that may contain gluten, such as artificial and natural flavorings, hydrolyzed plant or vegetable proteins, or modified food starches. Some of these ingredients may be found in beer, cold cuts, egg substitutes, frozen yogurt and yogurt drinks, salad dressings and other foods. Trial and error, elimination of suspected foods, and replacement by tolerated foods are recommended.

A wide range of gluten-free products are currently available. As more people are diagnosed with gluten sensitivity or intolerance, this will necessitate more gluten-free options and cooking and baking adaptations [19,20].

DIABETES

Diabetes is the common name for *diabetes mellitus,* one of the oldest known diseases. Since antiquity, the condition has been described as the need to "siphon" or discharge large amounts of honey-scented urine. Early symptoms of diabetes may include excessive thirst and urination and sugar in the urine. Other symptoms may include blurry vision, increased fatigue, irritability and/or unusual weight loss.

There are three types of diabetes: Type I diabetes, also called juvenile diabetes; Type II diabetes, also called adult onset diabetes; and gestational diabetes, also called the diabetes of pregnancy. Type I diabetes is due to inadequate insulin production by the beta cells of the pancreas. It usually occurs when people are young, which is why it is called juvenile diabetes. It is an autoimmune disease, much like celiac disease. There is no known cure for Type I diabetes at this time. Treatments for Type I diabetes include programmed insulin injections and blood sugar management through diet and exercise.

Type II diabetes is due, in part, to insulin resistance, which means that the pancreas may produce enough insulin but that something may interfere with insulin from reaching the targeted tissues. Also, the pancreas may tire from working so hard to sustain a high level of insulin to remove sugar from the bloodstream, so it may eventually function abnormally. Treatments for Type II diabetes include diet prescription, weight management, increased activity, oral medications to assist with glucose control and insulin injections, if required.

Gestational diabetes also involves insulin resistance, which is probably driven by predisposition to the disease and hormonal fluctuations during pregnancy. Gestational diabetes often disappears when the pregnancy is over.

Long-term effects of diabetes with poor blood sugar management may include disorders of the cardiovascular and digestion systems, eyes, feet, kidneys, nerves, sexual functions, skin, teeth and gums and produce increased risks for heart disease and bone and joint disorders, among other conditions.

Children, Teens and Type II Diabetes

Type II diabetes is a condition that is normally associated with age, obesity and poor nutrient intake. It has become more prevalent in children and teens. There appears to be a host of behavioral, environmental and social factors that may predispose children and teens to Type II diabetes.

Puberty is an important factor. This may be due to fluctuations in hormone levels, which may cause insulin resistance and decreased insulin action. Obesity is another speculated factor. The condition of extra body fat in children and teens, like obese adults, can lead to insulin resistance. Both obese children and obese adults may produce too much insulin, and when the need arises, they may be unable to produce even more insulin. Other factors that may contribute to Type II diabetes in children and teens include a family history of Type II diabetes and an ethnic background of African-American, American Indian, Asian, Hispanic or Pacific Islander origin.

Recipes, meals and menus should be developed that highlight the importance of healthy eating for the entire family, not just the diabetic. Other considerations should incorporate culture, family resources and lifestyle. Increased activity is essential to weight loss and control of Type II diabetes in children and teens. This is because exercise speeds up calorie expenditure and promotes weight loss and body fat—thus, increased insulin sensitivity.

If diabetes is not managed, uncontrolled blood sugar can cause *hypoglycemia,* or low blood sugar, which can cause blood vessel and nerve damage. In turn, this damage can lead to cardiovascular disease; retinal damage,

171

which can lead to blindness; chronic renal disease, which can lead to kidney failure; and poor wound healing, which can lead to *gangrene*, which is decay of body tissues due to insufficient blood supply, with possible amputation.

Medical nutrition therapy (MNT) helps to prevent diabetes, manage existing diabetes and slow the development of diabetes complications through healthy food choices, physical activity and weight loss when warranted. It is usually done through the guidance of registered dietitians (RDs) as licensed by their state of practice.

The goals of MNT are to maintain a person's normal blood glucose levels, blood fats and blood pressure; modify their nutrient intake and lifestyle; account for any personal and cultural preferences; and maintain his or her pleasure of eating. For Type I and gestational diabetes, MNT also serves to meet the nutritional requirements of children and pregnancy. For Type II diabetes, MNT also serves to help normalize blood sugar control and to promote self-management.

Food and Nutrition Recommendations for People with Diabetes

In the past, diabetes management consisted of prescribed amounts of food and beverages at set times to match prescribed amounts of insulin. Today's recommendations consist of attention to total daily carbohydrates, with prudent food and nutrition guidelines that both patients and families can follow. More information on creating recipes and meals for diabetics can be found in Chapter 9.

- Eat vegetables for fiber and nutrients.
- Focus on nonstarchy vegetables, such as deep leafy greens and those in the cruciferous family, such as broccoli and cabbage.
- Eat whole fruit for fiber and nutrients.
- Do not drink too much fruit juice or eat too much dried fruit. Both fruit juice and dried fruit contain concentrated sugars.
- Eat whole grains before processed grain products for fiber and nutrients.
- Include cooked beans, lentils and peas for fiber, protein and nutrients.

Recipe: Vegetarian Chili

*Vegetarian chili is usually a fusion of vegetables, legumes and spices, often in a tomato-based stew. Chili does not require meat to be flavorful or nutritious. In the **Vegetarian Chili** recipe in the **Recipe file**, which is located within the Culinary Nutrition website at www.culinarynutrition.elsevier.com, carrots, garlic, mushrooms, onions and bell and chipotle peppers intermingle with basil, chili powder, cumin and oregano for a substantial and mouthwatering experience. Other than flavor, capsaicin, the active component in chili peppers, may stimulate fat metabolism and reduce cholesterol and triglyceride levels. Generally, the hotter the chili pepper, the more capsaicin that it contains. The finished dish is shown within the centerfold **Photo file** in Plate 4.3.*

- Include fish two to three times a week for lean protein and healthy fats.
- Choose low- and nonfat dairy products for protein and nutrients.
- Choose lean meats for lean protein and nutrients. Trim the fat and remove the skin wherever possible.
- Choose water, reduced-sugar and/or sugar-free beverages.
- Choose liquid oils before solid fats for cooking.
- Reduce high-calorie snack foods and desserts.
- If alcohol is consumed, do so in moderation and preferably with meals.
- Watch portion sizes.

The Role of Nutrition, Food Science and Culinary Professionals in Diabetes Management

While there is no longer a "diabetic diet," it is still important for nutrition and culinary professionals to understand the significance of meal planning for diabetics. Meal plans should account for such factors as age, activity level, ethnicity, medical history, medications, nutrition comprehension and weight management. A team approach by registered dietitians and chefs who develop recipe, meal and menu plans offers promising strategies. The development of new food products for diabetics continues to be in demand.

There may be some misconceptions about planning meals and cooking for people with diabetes. Diabetics can eat foods and drink beverages with sugar. However, they should be consumed in moderation with other foods that take longer to digest, such as lean protein and healthy fats, to help slow their effects on blood sugar. The total amount of carbohydrate spread across the day must also be taken into consideration.

Diabetics can also consume refined starches, such as enriched white bread or potatoes, in moderation. All carbohydrates raise blood sugar, including whole grains, which take longer to digest. That is the reason why half of total grains and grain products each day should be from whole grains.

Specialty diabetic food products may not be necessary if a diabetic diet is well planned and closely put into practice. They do offer some sweet options with little to no effect on blood sugar.

HYPOGLYCEMIA

Hypoglycemia, or low blood sugar, has many suspected causes, including poor blood sugar management that is associated with diabetes. Symptoms of hypoglycemia may include feeling cold, shaky, tired or weak. While these symptoms may be associated with other conditions, true hypoglycemia can be diagnosed by a medical test.

If chronic and undiagnosed, an inadequate supply of glucose to fuel the brain can lead to neurological problems, unconsciousness and even death. This is another convincing reason why it is critical for diabetics to regulate their diet and manage their blood sugar. To guard against hypoglycemia, people with diabetes can carry quick sources of sugar such as hard candies or sugar packets that can be dissolved in fluid for rapid digestion and absorption.

CORONARY HEART DISEASE, OBESITY AND METABOLIC DISEASE

The relationship of refined carbohydrates and coronary heart disease is controversial. Re-examination of carbohydrate digestion and metabolism is helpful. During digestion, carbohydrates are broken down into sugars that can be metabolized for energy and other functions or stored. Too many carbohydrates in the diet can cause more carbohydrate to be stored by the body than metabolized for energy. This condition may contribute to obesity, which is one of the risk factors that are associated with coronary heart disease.

173

Morsel "It's so logical and so simple. Fat is the backup fuel system. The role it plays in the body is that when there's no carbohydrate around, fat will become the primary energy fuel. That's pretty well known." —Robert Atkins (physician and creator of the Atkins Diet, 1930–2003)

Obesity is also one of the risk factors that is associated with Type II adult-onset diabetes. In this state, the pancreas produces insulin, but something interferes with the ability of insulin to transport sugar into the cells, so blood sugar is elevated. The condition of obesity or body fatness may be one of the contributing factors to this interference.

Obesity and diabetes are also two risk factors of the condition *metabolic syndrome.* High blood pressure, high blood fats (particularly triglycerides), and low levels of protective HDL cholesterol are other risk factors. People who exhibit many of these symptoms and are diagnosed with metabolic syndrome may have a higher risk of coronary heart disease than those with risk factors.

In the "Take away" section in this chapter, information is provided about the controversies that surround low-carbohydrate, high-protein diets in relation to coronary heart disease and weight management. When total carbohydrate consumption is reduced, in their absence fats are metabolized for energy. This reduces fats in the bloodstream and, in turn, the risks of metabolic syndrome and coronary heart disease.

The reason why low-carbohydrate diets are controversial is that higher protein and fat consumption have historically been correlated with elevated blood fats, especially cholesterol, and coronary heart disease. Moreover, *homocysteine,* a substance associated with higher-protein diets, has been linked with coronary heart disease. Homocysteine is produced during protein digestion.

B vitamins help to convert homocysteine into amino acids, the building blocks of protein. B vitamins are found in breads, cereals, grains, green leafy vegetables and legumes—many of the foods that are either reduced or eliminated on low-carbohydrate diets. If homocysteine is not converted into amino acids, it can build up and damage the lining of the arteries, including the coronary arteries, and accelerate the development of blood clots.

In summary, having too few or too many carbohydrates in the diet may affect blood fats and contribute to coronary heart disease. Refined carbohydrates may be underlying factors in the development and progression of coronary heart disease. Whole-grain carbohydrates and fruits and vegetables with fiber, vitamins and minerals may help lower blood fats and protect the initiation and advancement of coronary heart disease, obesity and other degenerative conditions. Like other aspects of a healthy diet, moderation rules [21].

Bite on This: whole-grain cooking

Whole grains should be rinsed thoroughly to remove dirt and grit, whether purchased in bulk or individually packaged. Most brown long-grain rice, converted rice and white long-grain rice do not require rinsing, since they are generally clean. Soaking whole grains a few hours or overnight is optional; it can soften the grains, remove some of the starchiness, and speed up the cooking time. Generally, cracked, rolled and other processed grains do not require soaking.

The soaking water can be discarded, or the whole grains can be cooked right in it. Bring the water and the whole grains to a boil, reduce the heat to a simmer, and cover the pot. Do not lift the cover until the cooking time is completed, as shown in Table 4-13. This can take from 20 minutes to one hour, depending on the toughness of the seed coat. The whole grains should be slightly chewy when fully cooked. Once cooked, gently fluff and separate the whole grains with a fork. Then replace the cover, and let the whole grains continue to steam for about 5 to 10 minutes before serving.

For a nutty flavor, the whole grains can be lightly toasted in a dry pan until browned. Then they can be added to water or other cooking liquids, such as juice, stock or wine and cooked until the grains are softened but not mushy in texture.

174

Whole grains	Calories (cal)	Carbohydrates (grams)	Protein (grams)	Fat (grams)	Fiber (grams)	Gluten
Amaranth	170 cal	29 g	7 g	2 g	3 g	No
Barley	176	38	5	0.5	7.8	
Buckwheat	146	31	6	1.5	4.25	No
Kamut	94	20	4	1	3	
Millet	150	34	5	1.5	3	No
Rolled Oats	77	13	3	1	2	
Popcorn	120	21	4	3	4	No
Quinoa	140	25	5	2	4	No
Rice	191	39	4	2	0.2	
Brown Rice	171	36	4	1	1.5	No
Wild Rice	143	30	6	0.5	2.5	No
Rye	141	29	6	1	6	
Spelt	140	31	6	1	3	
Teff	182	37	6	1.4	3.7	No
Wheat	157	34	6	0.7	5.8	
Bulgur Wheat	150	33	5	0.5	4	
Couscous	162	33	5.5	0.2	2	
Cracked Wheat	140	29	5	0	6	

TABLE 4-13 Nutrients in Whole Grains (Based on ¼ Cup Dry)

Source: [22].

Bite on This: ancient grains

Many whole grains are ancient grains, which means they have been used since antiquity. Some ancient grains are favored in today's cooking because of their interesting colors, flavors and textures. Several ancient grains, like whole grains, are intact with their germ, endosperm, bran and husk. Ancient grains have a wealth of nutrients, fibers and protective phytochemicals, and numerous culinary applications.

> **Morsel** "Look at the amaranth: on tall mountains it grows, on the very stones and rocks and places inaccessible." —Amarantos (Greek folk song)

- **Amaranth** is an 8,000-year-old crop that was called a "super food" by the ancient Aztecs. It was fed to runners and warriors for energy and athletic performance. Ancient amaranth is still reportedly grown in Mexico; other strains are grown in Guatemala, India and Peru. Amaranth is a pseudo-grain, like quinoa, which means that it is not a true grain. Instead, amaranth is a group of herbs.
- **Nutritional value:** Amaranth contains notable amounts of calcium, fiber and iron, and a full range of amino acids, which makes it a source of high-quality protein. It has more complete protein than some other cereal grains, such as oats, rye or wheat.
- **Culinary uses:** Amaranth is a popular snack food in Mexico; it is sometimes mixed with chocolate or puffed rice. Amaranth seeds can be ground into flour, made into bread, and flaked for use in cereals. Because it is a complete protein, amaranth can be used as a vegetarian entree, paired with vegetables and legumes, if desired.
- **Barley** was cultivated around the Dead Sea as much as 9,500 years ago. It was a staple cereal grain along with einkorn and emmer wheat and was used to make bread and beer.
- **Nutritional value:** Barley is rich in nutrients. It contains amino acids; vitamins B1, B2, B6, C and folic acid; the minerals calcium, copper, iron, magnesium, manganese, potassium, sodium and zinc; and the antioxidant beta carotene.
- **Culinary uses:** Barley can be used in chili, salads, side dishes, soups and stews; as a stuffing for peppers, poultry and tomatoes; and mixed with cooked legumes in vegetarian "meatloaf." Barley is an ingredient in beer and whisky production, and a small amount of barley is used as a coffee substitute. Barley has a rich, nutlike flavor and an appealing chewy, pasta-like consistency. It contains gluten, like rye and wheat.

> **Morsel** "Eat only barley [diet of bread and water]." —Aristophanes (Greek playwright, 448–380 BC)

- **Buckwheat** is technically a herb, like amaranth. Buckwheat originated in Asia, where it is commonly used today in buckwheat noodles. Buckwheat groats are smashed hulled buckwheat seeds, which have widespread use in Eastern Europe.
- **Nutritional value:** Buckwheat is rich in iron, selenium and zinc and some antioxidants. It does not contain gluten, so buckwheat is useful in gluten-free cooking and baking and gluten-free products, including gluten-free buckwheat honey and beer.
- **Culinary uses:** Buckwheat can be made into buckwheat flour, which can be used in a variety of baked goods, including breads, cookies, crackers and muffins, and in pancakes and waffles. Buckwheat can be mixed with other grains in breadstuffs, pilafs and other preparations. **Kasha** is a pilaf made with toasted buckwheat groats.
- **Kamut** is a large grain, similar to durum wheat and spelt. Kamut may have been used throughout Egyptian history, but there is no proof of its age. Plus, ancient Egyptians grew only emmer wheat.
- **Nutritional value:** Kamut has a higher nutrient profile, including 30 percent more protein, than wheat. Kamut may be tolerated by people who have wheat allergies but not by those who are gluten intolerant. While kamut contains gluten, it is highly water soluble, which may make it easier to digest than durum or hard wheat.
- **Culinary uses:** Because kamut is such sturdy wheat, it requires a long simmering time to soften, and it holds up in slow cookers. Kamut can be found in breads, breakfast cereals, pastas and even kamut-based beverages. It has a full flavor.
- **Millet** is actually a group of grains that are the principal food sources in desert regions of the world. Millet was reportedly harvested on the upper Nile River near Sudan and in China around 6000 BC. Today, millet flour is used in western India to make **chapatti**, a dense whole-grain bread, and **roti**, a flat, thin cake. Millet is used to make beer in east Africa, a fermented drink similar to beer in the Balkan Peninsula, and also porridge.

- **Nutritional value:** Millet contains protein, fiber, the B-complex vitamins and vitamin E, and the minerals iron, magnesium, phosphorous and potassium. Millet is higher in fat than wheat, but about half of its fat is polyunsaturated. Millet does not contain gluten, so millet is an acceptable grain for gluten-free diets.
- **Culinary uses:** Millet can be used in casseroles, pilafs, risottos, soups, stews and stuffings. It is fairly interchangeable with buckwheat, quinoa or rice. Millet is mildly sweet with a nutlike flavor.
- *Modern wheat* is derived from three wheat varieties that been harvested in Europe and the Near East for over 9,000 years. These are *einkorn, emmer* and *spelt.*
  - *Einkorn*, a tough grain, is a precursor of durum wheat. It was grown in Europe about 11000 BC. Other evidence of einkorn farming was found in southeast Turkey and Jericho. Einkorn is rarely grown today.
  - *Emmer*, also known as *farro*, is another precursor of durum wheat. It was a farming staple in ancient Egypt and Turkey. Emmer is still farmed today for both human food and animal feed.
- **Culinary uses:** Emmer bread is consumed in Switzerland. In Italy, farro is used as a side dish and in soup. Farro flour is used in making pasta and in soup. It has an earthly taste and gritty texture.
  - *Spelt*, another precursor of durum wheat, is thought to have originated in Mesopotamia about 9000 BC. It is believed that only emmer and einkorn preceded spelt in domestication. Spelt's grains are longer and pointier than durum wheat, with stronger husks. Because spelt is closely related to wheat, it is not a substitute for people who are gluten intolerant.
- **Culinary uses:** Spelt is accessible as flour or grain. It can be used in casseroles, cookies, crackers, hot breakfast cereals, pasta, pilafs and stuffings. Spelt is available in a coarse, pale bread, similar in color and texture to light rye bread but slightly sweeter and nuttier in flavor. The Dutch distill gin that is made with a spelt base, and Bavarians brew beer that is made from spelt. In Germany, unripe spelt grains are dried and consumed as *Grünkern*, or "green grain." Spelt has a distinctive nutty flavor.
  - *Oats* date back to around 2000 BC in the Middle East. Oats are better able to withstand harsh growing conditions than wheat and barley. This made oats a valuable grain for feeding the poor who lived in disadvantaged regions. Contrary to oatmeal, oats have a hard hull. Hulled oats, or oat groats, look like rye or triticale wheat.
- **Nutrition value:** Oats may be consumed in moderation by people who are allergic to wheat. But some commercial oats may be contaminated with wheat or barley. Oats have both soluble and insoluble fibers and may be useful in lowering cholesterol and reducing the risk of coronary heart disease (see Chapter 9). They are higher in polyunsaturated fatty acids than wheat and are also rich in B vitamins and the antioxidant vitamin E.
- **Culinary uses:** Cooked whole oats or oat groats can be used as a hearty side dish. Rolled oats can be transformed into breakfast cereals such as muesli or granola. Cooked oats can be prepared as porridge or hot cereal. Pulverized oats can be used as flour for oatcakes, oatmeal cookies or oat bread. Fast-cooking oats can function as a thickener in soups. Oats are used in Britain for brewing beer, such as oatmeal stout.
- *Quinoa* is not a true grain, much like amaranth and buckwheat. It is technically a fruit because it contains a seed. The Incas referred to quinoa as the "Mother Grain" because it was thought to be very healthy and promote longevity. Quinoa has been grown in the Andes mountain regions of South America, especially around Bolivia, for more than 5,000 years. It is often referred to as a "super food",
- **Nutritional value:** Like amaranth, quinoa is one of the few plant foods that provide complete protein with a balanced mixture of all of the essential amino acids. Quinoa is also a very good source of manganese and a good source of copper, iron, magnesium and phosphorus. It is gluten-free.
- **Culinary uses:** Quinoa can be used like rice as a side dish, such as pilaf; in grain salads; and in stuffings. Since quinoa is a complete protein food, it can be used as a base for vegetarian entrees. Quinoa flour can be combined with potato starch, sorghum flour or tapioca to create a gluten-free baking mix. Quinoa is also processed into flaked cold cereals like amaranth.
- *Teff* is a tiny grain that comes in brown, red and white varieties. Because it is so tiny, the entire grain must be milled because there is no way to remove the germ or the husk. Teff has

been a staple of Ethiopian cooking for thousands of years. It is the main ingredient in *Injera,* a traditional flat bread. In the United States, Teff is primarily grown in Idaho.

- **Nutritional value:** Teff has more calcium and iron than millet, oats, rice or wheat, and it is a rich source of other minerals such as boron, copper, magnesium, phosphorous and zinc. Teff is higher in protein than wheat or barley. Because teff is gluten-free, it is a good choice for people who need to avoid gluten and wheat.
- **Culinary uses:** Teff is a versatile grain that can be boiled and prepared as a simple hot breakfast cereal; ground and used as flour in cereals and baked goods, such as breads, cookies and crackers; added as a thickener for sauces or stews; and sprouted and integrated into salads and sandwiches. It has a distinctive sweet and malty flavor.
- *Triticale* is a hybrid of wheat and rye. It combines the high-yield characteristics of wheat, with the environmental tolerance and disease resistance of rye. Triticale was first bred in Scotland and Sweden during the late nineteenth century. Today, triticale is grown mostly as animal feed, although some is used in flour and breakfast cereals.
- **Nutritional value:** The protein content of triticale is higher than wheat, while the gluten content of triticale is less than wheat. It cannot be used by those who are gluten sensitive.
- **Culinary uses:** Triticale is available in whole-grain, flake and flour forms. It is found in baked goods such as breads, cookies and crackers, and in cereals, pancakes and waffles. Triticale berries (the entire grain) can be sprouted and added to salads. It has an earthy flavor and aroma.

Bite on This: carbohydrates and oral health

Dental caries, or tooth decay, is an infectious disease that damages the structure of teeth. In this condition, oral bacteria change carbohydrates in the mouth into acids that demineralize the teeth. *Cavities,* or holes in the teeth, may result. If untreated, dental caries may cause infection, pain or tooth loss.

Periodontal disease (periodontitis), or gum disease, is an infectious disease that damages the gums. In this condition, oral bacteria attack the ligaments and bone that anchor the teeth. Bone loss can occur, which may cause pockets of space between the gums and teeth and increase the risks of infection. Periodontitis can increase the need for bone and gum grafts and lead to tooth loss.

When carbohydrate-containing foods and beverages adhere to the teeth, they damage tooth surfaces, settle in spaces between teeth, and initiate the decay process. Sticky carbohydrates, such as candy or cola, are more likely to cause damage and decay.

Specifically, oral bacteria break down saliva, the fluid that keeps the mouth moistened and helps in the digestive process. Saliva is the "glue" that helps oral bacteria adhere to the teeth and form *dental plaque,* a sticky, colorless biofilm. Once plaque accumulates, it may harden into calculus or tartar. If plaque accumulates beneath the gum line, it may lead to or aggravate periodontitis. Regular dental visits will ensure that this dental plaque is removed from the teeth before it damages them.

Dental plaque may not be obvious. It is clear and gelatinous, thanks to saliva. When a person eats carbohydrates *of any kind,* the bacteria ferment, or break down, these carbohydrates to provide their own food sources. A by-product of this fermentation is lactic acid, which may etch away at the teeth and strip them of the minerals that protect them. Once the teeth have lost their natural defense, the bacteria are then free to advance into the teeth and cause decay and cavities. If dental plaque is removed or cavities are filled, this can result in tooth loss and/or gum disorders.

To try to prevent or curtail dental problems, cut back on total carbohydrates consumption, not just sugars. As discussed, starches are made of many sugars, and their chemical and physical breakdown begins in the mouth. Bacteria prefer carbohydrates for their food, particularly sucrose, or table sugar. That is why cutting down on refined sugars may decrease dental caries.

Remember to look for the ending "-ose" on a food label when determining if a food product contains sugar. Potentially cavity-causing sugars can also be found in corn syrup, honey, maple syrup and molasses. Because these substances are sticky, they have the potential of adhering to the teeth even more than granular sugars. Consumption of regular soda, powdered beverages with sugar, and 100 percent fruit juices may also increase the risk of dental caries. Drinking beverages such as these with a meal or snack and/or brushing your teeth after consuming high-sugar foods and beverages may help reduce the adherence of sugar [23].

The fermentation action of bacteria on starches takes longer than sugars. If starches are also sticky, such as cupcakes with frosting or glazed sweet rolls, then the food particles and sugars can become lodged between the teeth and gums. Unless you brush your teeth right away, these captured particles are perfectly situated for oral bacteria to ferment the carbohydrates.

A diet with lean meats and foods high in fiber, especially fresh fruits and vegetables, helps to cleanse the teeth of food particles and sugars and decrease the incidence of cavities. The fibers from fresh fruits and vegetables help to counteract the dental caries–causing effects of carbohydrates. Fiber helps to clean the teeth, much like windshield wipers clean the windshield of a car.

The more people eat over the course of a day, the more they are exposed to carbohydrates because they are so prevalent in most diets. Frequent snacking, especially with carbohydrate-containing foods and beverages such as candy and soda, provides an endless amount of carbohydrates for the oral bacteria. It is best to choose snacks with more protein, including lean meats, lower-fat cheeses, dry-roasted nuts, low-fat dairy milk or plain low-fat yogurt. Despite their carbohydrate content, dairy products may have a neutral effect on dental caries due to their protein content.

Consuming a nonsugar beverage with snacks helps to flush away food particles. So does swishing your mouth with water or brushing and flossing after eating, which are essential practices of good oral hygiene

SERVE IT FORTH

Adapting recipes to meet consumer preferences is part food science and part culinary artistry. Although some basic guidelines can be provided, testing and tasting are the best strategies. You will use the Basic Muffins recipe to make muffin variations that are whole grain, reduced in carbohydrates, lactose-free, gluten-free, high in fiber, and that have a low Glycemic Index (GI). Record your observations, and then answer the questions that follow each activity.

Some breadstuffs are both lactose-free and gluten-free, or high-fiber with a low GI. These activities are filled with tips and techniques to assist in their development.

BASIC MUFFINS

Ingredients

Nonstick cooking spray
1¾ cup all-purpose flour
3 teaspoons baking powder
2 tablespoons white sugar
1 cup 2% reduced-fat dairy milk
½ teaspoon salt
3 tablespoons melted sweet butter or vegetable oil (like canola)
1 large egg

Directions

1. Preheat oven to 425°F.
2. Spray a 12-cup muffin tin with the nonstick cooking spray.
3. Sift the flour, baking powder and white sugar together into a medium bowl; set aside.
4. Beat the egg in a small bowl until light and fluffy.
5. Slowly blend the milk and butter or oil into the beaten egg.
6. Add the egg mixture to the dry ingredients; stir only until combined and moistened.
7. Spoon the batter into the prepared muffin cups; fill each cup half full.
8. Bake about 20 to 25 minutes, or until lightly browned.

Yield: 12 (2-inch) muffins

Making Basic Muffins Whole Grain

The flour in this recipe is all-purpose white flour. To make these muffins whole grain, 100 percent whole wheat flour may be substituted. However, this substitution may lead to dense muffins. To compensate, try substituting 100 percent whole wheat flour for ⅓ to ½ of the all-purpose flour and note the results. Or try sifting the 100 percent whole wheat flour one or two additional times to help incorporate more air. Also, mix the ingredients as little as possible to avoid forming gluten which will toughen the muffins.

- What are the results of these adjustments?
- What other changes can be made to this recipe to make these muffins whole grain?
- How will the sensory characteristics of appearance, taste and texture be affected by these changes?

Making Basic Muffins Low Carbohydrate

The total amount of carbohydrates in this recipe reflects the amounts of flour, sugar and dairy milk. If any of these ingredients are reduced, the texture and color may suffer because each of these ingredients has specific functions. A sugar substitute, such as one that is featured in this chapter, can be used to reduce the amount of sugar in this recipe. However, the recipe will need to be adjusted.

Use the amount of sugar substitute that equals 2 tablespoons of white sugar. Keep in mind that sugar has specific functions in baking: it contributes to browning and texture (because it retains moisture). Baking with a sugar substitute may cause the muffins to be drier, puffier and sweeter than muffins that are made with table sugar. Some sugar substitutes are designed for baking. Specific information for their use can be found on the package or company website.

- What are the results of these adjustments?
- What other changes can be made to this recipe to reduce carbohydrates?
- How will the sensory characteristics of appearance, taste and texture be affected by these changes?

Making Basic Muffins Lactose-Free

A nondairy product, such as low-fat soy milk, can be substituted in an equal amount for the 2% reduced-fat dairy milk in this recipe. Full-fat soy milk may contribute too much fat. Nonfat legume or grain milks, such as rice milk, may be too thin, and the muffins may be too dry. Compare the Nutrition Facts Panel to make sure that the substitute is equal in fat. Most butter has milk solids. You will need to substitute vegetable oil or use a melted vegetable shortening that does not contain milk solids. It is important to read the ingredients list on the label to ensure that the products that are substituted are suitable for lactose-free baking.

- What are the results of these adjustments?
- What other changes can be made to this recipe to make it lactose-free?
- How will the sensory characteristics of appearance, taste and texture be affected by these changes?

Three additional activities can be found within the *Culinary Nutrition* website at www.culinarynutrition.elsevier.com.

WHAT'S COOKING?

1. **Sugars (within starches)**
   Objectives
   ○ To detect the sugars that are contained in some starches
   ○ To determine if the fibers in starchy foods inhibit the ability to detect sugars
   Materials
   Soda cracker, rice cake, rye-crisp type 100 percent whole-grain cracker, glass and water
   Procedure
   Chew the soda cracker and let the residue stay in your mouth for a few minutes without swallowing; then swallow. Take a mouthful of water to swish out your mouth. Repeat the exercise with the rice cake and then again with the whole-grain cracker.
   Evaluation
   Note if the taste of *each* of the crackers changes as you leave their residue in your mouth. Is there any difference in taste before, during and after chewing each cracker? If so, to what do you attribute these differences? Similarities? How do your conclusions compare and contrast to cooked starches, such as rice or barley?
   Culinary applications
   How can this information be applied to new product or recipe development?

2. Fibers (breads)

Objective

○ To compare and contrast the insoluble fibers in breads

Materials

One slice each of 100 percent whole-grain bread, wheat flour or light wheat bread and white bread

Procedure

Take a scoop out of the inside of one of the slices of bread. Try to form a ball with it, using the palms of your hands. Repeat this exercise with each of the other two slices of bread.

Evaluation

Insoluble fiber generally consists of short fibers, which are characteristic of wheat bran. Bread with insoluble fiber should crumble when rubbed into a ball. Soluble fiber generally consists of longer fibers, characteristic of gums and pectin. Bread with soluble fiber may form a semisolid ball when compacted. Which bread do you think has the most insoluble fiber? Soluble fiber? You can repeat this experiment with mixed-grain bread and/or high-fiber white bread. What conclusions can you apply to recipes with fiber?

Culinary applications

How can this information be applied to new product or recipe development?

3. Starches (root starches)

Objectives

○ To compare the properties of starches

○ To contrast the *solubility* (the amount of a substance that can be dissolved in a solvent) of starches in water

Materials

Arrowroot, cornstarch, potato starch, tapioca, white flour; water, 5 bowls, measuring cup and measuring spoons, pot, burner, stove or microwave

Procedure

Put 1 cup of cool water in each of the 5 bowls. Add 2 tablespoons of one of the starches to the first bowl. Do not mix. Repeat with each of the other starches and the flour. If you have access to a burner, oven or microwave, gently warm each of the solutions.

Evaluation

Note the rate that each of these starches dissolves in the cool water. If warmed, note the effect(s) that heat has on each of the starch solutions. What conclusions can you make about the solubility of each of the starches? How to they compare in solubility to flour? Can you make any conclusions about the properties of starches in cooking based on what you observed?

Culinary applications

How can this information be applied to new product or recipe development?

4. Gluten (flours)

Objective

○ To become familiar with different types of flour and gluten content

Materials

Any of the following flours: all-purpose flour, bread flour, gluten flour, instant flour, pastry flour and whole wheat flour; water (½ to ¾ cup for each type of flour); bowls (1 bowl for each type of flour); measuring cup; sieve or cheesecloth; oven; and nonstick baking sheet or nonstick baking spray.

Procedure

Put 1 cup of each of the flours into separate bowls. Slowly add about ½ to ¾ cup of water to each of the bowls. Knead each mixture until it forms a soft, rubbery ball of dough. Let the dough rest about 10 minutes. Run cold water over each of the dough balls. You may need a sieve or cheesecloth for the more delicate dough.

Evaluation

As you run the cold water over each of the dough balls, note if the water turns milky. If it does, rate the degree of milkiness of each dough ball. If the water no longer becomes milky, what does this indicate about each of the dough balls?

Are there differences in the sizes and the textures of each of the dough balls? Put the dough balls on a nonstick baking sheet or one that has been sprayed with nonstick cooking spray. Bake the dough balls in a 450°F oven about 15–30 minutes. What happens to each of the dough balls? Why? How can you apply this information to cooking? Baking? Gluten-free cooking and baking?

Culinary applications
How can this information be applied to new product or recipe development?

5. Carbohydrates on the food label (labels)

Objectives
- ○ To identify sugars, starches and fibers on food labels
- ○ To determine if foods are an excellent, an average or a poor source of fiber

Materials
Two food labels from breakfast cereal, including the Nutrition Facts Panel and the list of ingredients

Procedure
Make a copy of the following information for each of the breakfast cereals: serving size, calories per serving, total carbohydrate, dietary fiber, sugars and the %DV of total carbohydrate and fiber

Evaluation
a. Make sure that the serving sizes of both breakfast cereals are equal (i.e., if one cereal is a ½ cup serving and one is a ¼ cup serving, you will need to double the serving size of the second breakfast cereal so the servings are equal).
b. List all of the ingredients in the first breakfast cereal that contain carbohydrates. Circle those that contain sugar. Repeat this exercise for the second breakfast cereal.
c. What are the sugars in the first breakfast cereal? The second breakfast cereal? Which cereal has more sugars?
d. Which cereal contains the most total carbohydrate per serving? Dietary fiber?
e. Rate the carbohydrate and fiber according to their DVs.
f. If a food has 5 percent or less of the DV of a nutrient, it is considered to be low in that nutrient. It is considered a good source of a nutrient if it has between 10 and 19 percent of the DV of a nutrient. If a food has more than 20 percent of the DV of a nutrient, it is considered high in that nutrient. The DVs are based on a 2,000-calorie diet [24]. Compare the remaining DVs of both cereals. Which of their DVS are noteworthy?
g. Based on your conclusions, which of these breakfast cereals do you consider to be more nutritious and why?

Culinary applications
How can this information be applied to new product or recipe development?

6. Carbohydrate substitutes

Objectives
- ○ To determine the presence of sugar substitutes in beverages
- ○ To compare the taste and solubility of sugar substitutes to white sugar in beverages

Materials
Sugar substitutes such as acesulfame potassium (Sunett®, Sweet One®), aspartame (Equal®, NutraSweet®), saccharin (SugarTwin®, Sweet'N Low®) or sucralose (Splenda®) that dissolve in cold liquid; table sugar; unsweetened iced tea; glasses; teaspoon

Procedure
Fill each glass with 12 ounces of unsweetened iced tea. Add one packet of sugar substitute to each glass of iced tea. Add 2 teaspoons of white sugar to one of the glasses of iced tea. Stir each mixture well.

Evaluation
a. Compare how each sugar substitute dissolves in the iced tea. Contrast your observations with the rate that white sugar dissolves.
b. Compare the tastes of each glass of sugar substitute–sweetened iced tea.
c. Contrast each of these tastes with the white sugar–sweetened iced tea.

Culinary applications
How can this information be applied to new product and recipe development of sugar-sweetened and sugar-reduced beverages?

181

OVER EASY

In a time that finds people struggling with weight control, diet and disease, much focus has been directed to individual nutrients and their effects on weight and disease management. Carbohydrates have been in the limelight for their suspected and confirmed roles in obesity, cardiovascular disease, celiac disease and gluten intolerance, dental caries, diabetes, lactose intolerance and metabolic syndrome, among other conditions.

No single nutrient causes all of these conditions, nor is there just one nutrient that fixes them. Sugars and starches do not cause overweight, but eating too much of any of these carbohydrates may contribute to weight gain. If not counterbalanced with exercise, these extra pounds may lead to obesity. Likewise, eating too many carbohydrates does not cause cardiovascular disease or diabetes. Rather, they may lead to overweight, which may predispose certain individuals to these diseases. People who are lactose or gluten intolerant are best served by eliminating lactose and gluten, and people who are prone to dental caries should practice proper dental hygiene.

CHECK PLEASE

1. The single sugar that is the building block of carbohydrates is:
   a. sucrose
   b. fructose
   c. glucose
   d. lactose
   e. maltose

2. The double sugar that is present in dairy products is called:
   a. sucrose
   b. lactose
   c. galactose
   d. maltose
   e. fructose

3. The protein called gluten that is found in most wheat products is also found in:
   a. corn
   b. rice
   c. soy
   d. barley
   e. potatoes

182

ESSAY QUESTION

1. Which two ancient grains are considered "super foods" but are not really grains? If they are not grains, in which plant families are they found? Why are they considered super? How would you use them in recipes? In meals?

For additional questions, please see the *Culinary Nutrition* website at www.culinarynutrition.elsevier.com.

HUNGRY FOR MORE?

American Diabetes Association   http://www.diabetes.org www.diabetes.org
Calorie Control Council   www.caloriecontrol.org
Celiac Sprue Association   www.csaceliacs.org
Corn Refiners Association   www.corn.org
Gluten Intolerance Group of North America   www.gluten.net
Glycemic Index of Foods   www.glycemicindex.com
International Food Information Council (IFIC)   www.ific.org
National Dairy Council   www.nationaldairycouncil.org
National Institute of Diabetes and Digestive and Kidney Diseases   www.nlm.nih.gov
The Sugar Association, Inc.   www.sugar.org
Wheat Foods Council   www.wheatfoods.org
The Whole Grains Council   www.wholegrainscouncil.org

TAKE AWAY
The Carbohydrate and Diet Debate

Despite the fact that carbohydrates make up most of the food that is consumed around the world, some skeptics still question its role in healthy diets. Carbohydrates have been implicated in a number of diseases, which include coronary heart disease, diabetes and obesity. The concept of a low-carbohydrate diet to lose weight and prevent disease has been popularized for many years. Does it have merit, and if so, is it safe?

LOW-CARBOHYDRATE DIETS

Low-carbohydrate diets restrict carbohydrate consumption and replace carbohydrate calories with proteins and fats in a variety of combinations. The theories behind low-carbohydrate, high-protein diets are not new. In the late 1960s, quick weight loss was promised by Dr. Irwin Stillman, who created the Stillman Diet. This diet was popularized in his book *The Doctor's Quick Weight Loss Diet.*

Following the success of this diet, Dr. Robert Atkins created a low-carbohydrate diet plan that was promoted in his book *Dr. Atkins' Diet Revolution.* In the early 1970s, excess protein and dietary fat were considered to be dangerous, so initially the Atkins Diet was cautiously received. That was until the 1990s, when Dr. Atkins wrote the book *Dr. Atkins' New Diet Revolution*, which received popular acclaim, despite continued medical scrutiny [25,26].

While the pros and cons of the Atkins Diet were being debated, Dr. David Jenkins, a professor of nutrition from the University of Toronto, developed the Glycemic Index, which is a measure of how carbohydrates affect insulin in the body.

As discussed in this chapter, insulin is a hormone that is required for sugar to be transported into the cells for energy. Simple carbohydrates, such as sugar, are digested and absorbed relatively fast by the body. Their demand for insulin is higher than some starches, which are digested and absorbed slower than sugars. Based on the Glycemic Index, carbohydrates were considered "good" if they had a lower insulin demand and "bad" if they had a higher insulin demand. Additionally, the ratio of carbohydrates to proteins and fats in the diet was questioned [27].

THE GLYCEMIC INDEX

According to the Glycemic Index, foods are ranked according to how fast they are digested into glucose and how much each food causes blood glucose to rise. Glucose is used as the standard at GI = 100. Pure sugar creates the greatest rise (it is ranked at 121), and then cereals (about 60–75 GI), fruits (about 40–65 GI), dairy products (about 30–40 GI), and finally legumes with the least potential rise in blood glucose (about 15–35 GI). Some root vegetables, such as potatoes, can be as high as 70–90 GI.

The Glycemic Index values of sample foods are shown in Table 4-14. Also, the composition of a meal can affect the glycemic response, meaning that if a low-GI food is combined with a high-GI food, the blood glucose level response may be equalized. Other factors that can affect the GI include the location where the food was grown, the degree of ripeness of a food, and the extent of food processing.

TABLE 4-14: Glycemic Index Values of Sample Foods

Low Glycemic Index Foods (rank of 55 or less): Apples, baked beans, bran cereal, brown rice, carrots, legumes, lentils, milk, oats, oranges, peaches, sweet potatoes, tomatoes and yogurt

Intermediate Glycemic Index foods (rank of 56–69): Bananas, cream of wheat-type cereal, ice cream, orange juice, instant oatmeal, pineapple, popcorn, raisins, rye bread and shredded wheat-type cereal

High Glycemic Index foods (rank of 70 or more): Bagels, breakfast cereals (other than whole grain), honey, jelly beans, mashed potatoes, pancakes, pretzels, rice, soft drinks, waffles, watermelon and white bread

> **Recipe: Warm Whole-Grain Pasta Salad with Spinach, Berries and Balsamic Vinaigrette**
>
> *The recipe for **Warm Whole-Grain Pasta Salad with Spinach, Berries and Balsamic Vinaigrette** in the **Recipe file** which is located within the Culinary Nutrition website at www.culinarynutrition.elsevier.com, uses whole-grain pasta with a 45 GI, spinach with a 15 GI, and berries with a 32 GI. It is considered a low–Glycemic Index recipe, due in part to the fiber content of the whole-grain pasta, spinach and berries. Be sure to follow the package instructions because some whole-grain pasta requires a longer cooking time than pasta that is made with enriched wheat or all-purpose flour. There is an appealing interplay of warm pasta against room-temperature vegetables and fruits in this recipe that heightens interest and sensory satisfaction. The finished dish is shown within the centerfold **Photo file** in Plate 4.4.*

In the 1990s, the US dietary recommendations proposed as much as 55 to 60 percent of the US diet should come from carbohydrates. Today, some low-carbohydrate, high-protein diets recommend that as little as 30 percent of the diet come from carbohydrates. Other diets advise between 40 and 50 percent carbohydrate, such as the Zone Diet and the South Beach Diet. Questions still remain about the exact proportions of carbohydrates, protein and fat in a healthy diet [28]. To understand controversies that surround low-carbohydrate diets, one must look closely at how they work.

HOW LOW-CARBOHYDRATE DIETS WORK

A person's blood sugar level must be maintained within a certain range in order to have enough energy to think and for the body to function. Insulin, a hormone that is produced in the pancreas, helps to move digested and metabolized sugar from the bloodstream into the cells for energy or storage.

This process reduces the blood sugar level to normal. If the pancreas does not produce enough insulin (as in diabetes), the sugar in the bloodstream may remain elevated. Elevated sugar in the bloodstream may damage small blood vessels in the body and increase the risk of blindness, heart attack, infections, kidney disease, stroke and wound healing.

The argument for low-carbohydrate diets is that they are less stressful on the pancreas and insulin production than higher-carbohydrate diets. If the body runs out of stored carbohydrates, the liver produces a type of fat called *ketones* that can be converted into energy. This process of energy conversion is called *ketosis*. When a diet is higher in protein and fats and lower in carbohydrates, it encourages ketosis. A person can tell if he or she is in ketosis because breath, sweat and urine may smell of ketones.

Another argument for low-carbohydrate diets is that in Westernized countries, such as in the United States, the diet is high in refined carbohydrates, and the amount of carbohydrate that the body cannot use for energy may be converted into fat. By reversing the composition of the diet and having more protein and fats than carbohydrates, the body may be able to burn fat for energy and weight loss may result.

ARE LOW-CARBOHYDRATE DIETS SAFE?

Critics of low-carbohydrate diets contend that they may lead to weakness or fatigue and reduced athletic performance. Vitamin and mineral deficiencies may follow. A serious acidic condition in the blood may develop from ketosis, which may lead to coma or even death.

LONG-TERM EFFECTS

Another criticism of low-carbohydrate diets has to do with the effects of these diets over time. Questions have been raised about the increased risk of cancer, coronary heart disease, gout, high blood pressure, kidney stones and osteoporosis that are associated with these diets. While low-carbohydrate diets can be traced back to the 1800s, the long-term implications have not been established because diets such as these are so difficult to maintain.

Since little agreement exists regarding the long-term safety of low-carbohydrate diets, this is why the carbohydrate diet debate is ongoing. Until all the research is conclusive, a diet that includes most foods and beverages in moderation still appears the wisest dietary approach. Individualized lower-carbohydrate diets may be designed and implemented as warranted [29].

"Got Milk?"

The "Got milk?" advertising campaign has promoted the consumption of dairy milk since 1993. The fluid milk processors in California appropriated a small portion of the sale of each gallon to advertising, marketing, promotion and public relations. This led to the development of the California Milk Processor Board (CMPB) and the "Got milk?" campaign [30–32].

The advertisements, as seen in many media, depict famous and ordinary people who drink dairy milk, evidenced by their milk "moustaches." Milk consumption rose the highest it had been for 20 years partly as a result of this campaign.

The campaign was criticized by a nonprofit group who opposed the use of animal products as food. This public protest was partially responsible for the controversy about the importance of dairy milk in the human diet after an infant is no longer breast or formula feeding. This is because humans are the only species who consume the milk from another species as they grow to adulthood.

Normally, mammals reduce their production of the enzyme lactase when they wean their young. Globally, in non-dairy-dependent countries, the production of lactase drops significantly. In dairy-dependent countries, such as the United States, lactase production may continue throughout life, except among certain ethnicities [33].

Some people of African, Asian, Hispanic and Native American descent are more likely to develop lactose intolerance at a young age. Most of the world does not consume dairy products. Still, the *2010 US Dietary Guidelines* recommend 2 cups of low-fat or fat-free dairy milk or equivalent milk products, such as yogurt, daily for children 2 to 3 years old, 2½ cups for children 4 to 8 years of age, and 3 cups for people 9 years of age and older.

Dairy milk is a storehouse of nutrients. It contains nine essential nutrients, with 10 to 30 percent of the DV for these nutrients, which are shown in Table 4-15.

One cup (8 ounces) of nonfat white dairy milk contains about 83 calories, 8 grams of protein, 12 grams of carbohydrates (including 12 grams of sugar), 0.4 gram of total fat, 5 milligrams of cholesterol and 103 milligrams of sodium. The human body requires calcium, carbohydrates, fats, protein, vitamins and minerals, not dairy milk or dairy products per se. Other foods and beverages, such as fortified legume and grain beverages, provide an array of these nutrients in varying amounts. For example, 1 cup (8 ounces) of nonfat soy milk contains about 70 calories, 6 grams of protein, 8 grams of carbohydrates (including 6 grams of sugar), 2 grams of total fat, 0 milligrams of cholesterol and 119 milligrams of sodium.

In comparison, 1 cup (8 ounces) of rice milk contains about 120 calories, 1 gram of protein, 23 grams of carbohydrates (including 10 grams of sugar), 2.5 grams of total fat, 0 milligrams of cholesterol and 100 milligrams of sodium [34]. If you choose to substitute a nondairy beverage for dairy milk, make sure it is fortified with calcium and other nutrients that may include vitamins A, D and/or B12 and the mineral iron.

TABLE 4-15 Nutrients in 8 Ounces of Fat-Free White Dairy Milk

Nutrients	Daily Values
Calcium	30%
Riboflavin	26%
Vitamin D	25%
Phosphorus	25%
Vitamin B12	22%
Protein	16%
Potassium	11%
Vitamin A	10%
Niacin	10%

If nondairy beverages are used to replace dairy milk in the diet, they should be fortified with at least 30 percent of the DV for calcium per serving. This amount equals the calcium per serving that one 8-ounce glass of dairy milk supplies. The body needs a certain concentration of calcium in the bloodstream to function properly. When blood calcium is low, the body extracts calcium from its bones to keep blood calcium within the normal range. If calcium in the bones is not regularly replaced, people can develop osteoporosis, or brittle bones, that may fracture and cause other complications. The controversies that surround the "Got milk?" campaign have brought the critical issue of calcium to the forefront.

References

[1] Poilane. <http://www.poilane.com/index.php?passer=1&directshop=1/>; [accessed 03.09.08].

[2] Nutrient Data Laboratory. <http://www.ars.usda.gov/SP2UserFiles/Place/12354500/Data/Add_Sug/addsug01.pdf/>; [accessed 03.09.08].

[3] Sherman RB, Sherman RM. "A Spoonful of Sugar." From Mary Poppins; 1964.

[4] American Dietetic Association Use of nutritive and nonnutritive sweeteners. J Am Diet Assoc 2004;104(2):255–75.

[5] Institute of Medicine, Food and Nutrition Board . In: Dietary reference intakes for energy, carbohydrate, fiber, fat, fatty acids, cholesterol, protein, and amino acids. Washington, DC: National Academy Press; 2010.

[6] US Department of Agriculture (USDA). National nutrient database for standard reference. <http://www.nal.usda.gov/fnic/foodcomp/Data/SR17/wtrank/sr17a291.pdf/>; [accessed 03.09.08].

[7] US Food and Drug Administration (FDA). Guidance for industry: a food labeling guide. <http://www.fda.gov/Food/GuidanceComplianceRegulatoryInformation/GuidanceDocuments/FoodLabelingNutrition/FoodLabelingGuide/ucm064919.htm/>; [accessed 03.09.08].

[8] US Food and Drug Administration (FDA). Definitions of nutrient content claims. <http://www.fda.gov/Food/GuidanceComplianceRegulatoryInformation/GuidanceDocuments/FoodLabelingNutrition/FoodLabelingGuide/ucm064911.htm/>; [accessed 03.09.08].

[9] US Food and Drug Administration (FDA). Nutrition facts label programs and materials. <http://www.fda.gov/Food/ResourcesForYou/Consumers/NFLPM/default.htm/>; [accessed 03.09.08].

[10] US Department of Health and Human Services. Nutrition and weight status. <http://healthypeople.gov/2020/topicsobjectives2020/objectiveslist.aspx?topicId=29/>; [accessed 03.09.08].

[11] US Department of Agriculture (USDA). Dietary guidelines for Americans. <http://www.cnpp.usda.gov/DGAs2010-PolicyDocument.htm/>; 2010 [accessed 03.09.08].

[12] Whole Grains Council. <http://wholegrainscouncil.org/whole-grain-stamp/government-guidance/>; [accessed 03.09.08].

[13] http://www.cfsan.fda.gov/~dms/flg-6c.html

[14] Selim J. The chemistry of artificial sweeteners. Discover Magazine. <http://discovermagazine.com/2005/aug/chemistry-of-artificial-sweeteners/>; [accessed 03.09.08].

[15] Myers RL. In: The 100 most important chemical compounds: a reference guide. Westport, CT: Greenwood Press; 2007.

[16] US Department of Agriculture (USDA). USDA national nutrient database for standard reference. <http://www.accessdata.fda.gov/scripts/cdrh/cfdocs/cfcfr/CFRSearch.cfm?fr=201.21/>; [accessed 03.09.08].

[17] American Diabetes Association (ADA). Sugar alcohols: reduced calorie sweetners. <http://www.diabetes.org/food-and-fitness/food/what-can-i-eat/sugar-alcohols.html/>; [accessed 03.09.08].

[18] Office of Disease Prevention and Heath Promotion. Dietary guidelines for Americans. <http://www.health.gov/DietaryGuidelines/dga2005/document/default.htm/>; 2010 [accessed 03.09.08].

[19] National Institutes of Health. Celiac disease—sprue.<http://www.nlm.nih.gov/medlineplus/ency/article/000233.htm/>; [accessed 03.09.08].

[20] Celiac Sprue Association. <http://www.csaceliacs.info/>; [accessed 03.09.08].

[21] Berge AF. How the ideology of low fat conquered America. J Hist Med Allied Sci 2008;63(2):139–77.

[22] US Department of Agriculture. USDA national nutrient database for standard reference. <http://ndb.nal.usda.gov/>; [accessed 03.09.08].

[23] Marshall TA, Levy SM, Broffitt B, et al. Dental caries and beverage consumption in young children. Pediatrics 2003;112:e184–191.

[24] http://www.fda.gov/food/labelingnutrition/consumerinformation/ucm078889.htm

[25] The Stillman diet - History of diets, Part 12 - protein diet Men's Fitness; 1967. http://edinformatics.com/health_fitness/low_carb_diet.htm; http://www.highbeam.com/doc/1G1-102140891.html

[26] June 2003. The History of the Atkins Diet, A Revolutionary Lifestyle in Low carbohydrate diet <https://www.diabetesdaily.com/wiki/Low-carbohydrate_diet>.

[27] Jenkins DJ, Wolever TM, Taylor RH, et al. Glycemic index of foods: a physiological basis for carbohydrate exchange. Am J Clin Nutr 1981;34(3):362–6.

[28] Bio-Medicine. <http://www.bio-medicine.org/medicine-news-1/ADA-Issues-New-Clinical-Practice-Recommendations-8877-1/>; [accessed 03.09.08].

[29] Bradley U, Spence M, Courtney CH, et al. Low-fat versus low-carbohydrate weight reduction diets effects on weight loss, insulin resistance, and cardiovascular risk: a randomized control trial. Diabetes 2009;58:2741–8.

[30] California Milk Processor Board: Got Milk? <http://www.gotmilk.com/>; [accessed 03.09.08].

[31] Advertising Educational Foundation. <http://www.aef.com/on_campus/classroom/case_histories/3000/>; [accessed 23.11.10].

[32] Sunset B. Got milk? campaign. <http://marketing-case-studies.blogspot.com/2008/04/got-milk-campaign.html/>; [accessed 23.11.10].

[33] Morahan L. PETA anti-milk campaign has little impact on milk consumption. <http://cnsnews.com/node/4262/>; [accessed 03.09.08].

[34] US Department of Agriculture (USDA). USDA national nutrient database for standard reference. <http://www.nal.usda.gov/fnic/foodcomp/Data/SR21/nutrlist/sr21w303.pdf>; [accessed 03.09.08].

CHAPTER 5

Protein Basics: Animal and Vegetable Proteins in Food and Health

Healthy Protein Choices, Roles and Applications in Nutrition, Food Science and the Culinary Arts

Culinary Nutrition. DOI: http://dx.doi.org/10.1016/B978-0-12-391882-6.00005-4

OBJECTIVES

1. Discuss what protein is and why it is essential to the human body
2. Explain the sources and functions of protein in the human body
3. Describe how protein is digested and metabolized by the human body
4. Apply the US protein recommendations for normal and specialized needs
5. Describe the roles of protein in food allergies and sensitivities
6. Explain the use of protein in vegetarian and vegan diets
7. Relate complementary protein concepts to cooking and baking
8. Explain the different sources of soy protein, their roles in the diet and uses in cooking and baking
9. Evaluate protein controversies
10. Compare and contrast the advantages and disadvantages of higher protein diets

INTRODUCTION: ANIMAL AND VEGETABLE PROTEINS IN FOOD AND HEALTH
Proteins

Protein is more than meat, poultry, fish, eggs, dairy milk and dairy products, or vegetables. Protein is the building blocks inside these foods that are indispensable to life. It is not surprising that the Greek root for protein is *prota*, which means "of primary importance."

> **Morsel** "Poultry is for the cook what canvas is for the painter."
> —Anthelme Brillat-Savarin (French epicure, gastronome, lawyer and politician, 1755–1826)

Protein was first discovered and named by chemists in the 1800s. Protein was noted for its central role in living organisms in the early 1900s and identified by its structure in the 1950s. The first proteins that were studied were *urease*, an enzyme; *insulin*, a hormone; and *hemoglobin* and *myoglobin*, blood and muscle proteins that help to identify the many functions that protein has in the human body [1,2].

Amino acids, the structural building blocks that exist in these and other proteins, are responsible for bodily functions and ultimately for life. These microscopic amino acids are the fundamental units of the protein foods that you consume: beef, dairy products, fish, lamb, legumes, nuts and seeds, pork, poultry, seafood, vegetables and even some fruits!

This chapter examines the sources and functions of protein in the human diet. It compares and contrasts animal versus vegetable proteins and their roles in health and disease, especially food allergies. You will learn about some proteins that might be new to you, such as meat analogs, sea proteins and soy foods. You will see how to select, prepare, cook and bake with these unusual and more familiar types of protein. You will determine how much protein is needed daily, and how this translates into food selection. You will realize how a little bit of great-tasting protein can be extended in recipes and that too much protein may actually be risky to one's health. Finally, you will experience how the magic of food science and the artistry of cooking help to transform protein foods into delicious recipes.

The Protein Predicament

What is considered enough protein in the human diet? What is too little or too much protein? How much protein should be consumed in relation to carbohydrates or fats? These have been ongoing questions since the discovery of protein, and they continue to be controversial today.

Protein needs are based on many factors, and what is safe and adequate for one person may not be for another. Like other nutrients in a normal diet, moderation is key. There are situations that require more protein and conditions that cause protein "wasting" or loss and protein overload.

A solid foundation that is grounded in the science of protein is essential for understanding the role of protein in health and disease and for translating this information into nutrition recommendations and culinary applications. The "Protein Predicament" will be revisited at the end of this chapter so educated conclusions and actions can be made.

MAIN COURSES
A Protein Primer: Protein Types, Sources and Functions

Proteins are complex, organic molecules. When acid, air, heat or salt are applied to proteins, they become functional and are able to perform their many roles in the human body. There are literally hundreds of proteins in food and in the human body. Protein can be found in animals, plants, microorganisms and laboratories—both scientific and kitchen labs where food scientists and chefs are "cooking up" new proteins.

Like carbohydrates and lipids, protein provides energy, which means that protein contains calories. Unlike carbohydrates and lipids, protein contains *nitrogen*, an element that is essential to many biological processes and functions, especially growth and development.

Nitrogen is also essential to plants' growth and development. Plant fertilizer often contains nitrogen, since this element is often the most important determinant of plant development and crop yield.

PROTEIN FUNCTIONS

Protein serves a number of bodily functions, including growth, maintenance, repair and structure; regulation of body processes; and energy.

Growth, Maintenance, Repair and Structure

Protein provides the building materials to help the body grow, maintain health and repair itself. Protein also supplies the body's structures found in bones, hair, ligaments, membranes, muscles, organs, skin, teeth and tendons. When you lose a few strands of hair and see new hair grow in or when you cut yourself and see the cut heal, these are signs of proteins at work.

Regulation of Body Processes

Protein helps make *enzymes*, *hormones* and *antibodies*, substances that assist the body's many processes.

- *Enzymes* are compounds that help to speed up chemical reactions. For example, *salivary amylase*, an enzyme in saliva, helps to digest protein in the mouth, and *lactase*, an enzyme in the small intestine, helps to break down the milk sugar lactose in the small intestine.
- *Hormones* are chemical messengers that help to regulate the body's activities, such as growth, hunger and metabolism. Hormones are specific to certain tissues or organs, and they prefer to keep conditions normal. For example, *insulin* and *glucagon* are hormones that help to regulate (or stabilize) blood sugar, and the *thyroid* hormone helps to regulate (or normalize) metabolism.
- *Antibodies* are specialized proteins that help to fight infections. They are intricately involved in the body's immune response. If the body does not have enough protein, it may not be able to produce enough antibodies to combat disease. For example, *immunoglobulin E (IgE)* is an antibody that recognizes and neutralizes allergens like those found in food or the environment.

Protein helps to control the *balance of fluids* throughout the body. It keeps the optimal concentration of fluids inside and outside of the cells and body tissues. Too much fluid and cells will rupture; too little and they will shrink, which affects their ability to function.

Protein helps monitor the body's *acid-base balance*. Both acids and bases must be regulated carefully in the bloodstream so they are stable. This is because body cells and organs function best when internal conditions are constant. The blood is neutral, which means it is neither too acidic nor too basic, because protein acts as a buffer to maintain this balance. Protein also protects the body from *acidosis*, a potentially fatal acidic condition in the bloodstream.

191

Protein helps to *transport substances* throughout the body and inside and outside the cells. There is an intricate pumping system in the cells that is dependent on protein. This system moves sodium and potassium between and among the cells. If this balance is disturbed, it can be fatal.

Energy

In the absence of carbohydrates, protein can be metabolized into energy. In Chapter 1, it was noted that one gram of protein supplies four calories, just like carbohydrates. If the body needs energy, then the protein that is stored in the blood, liver, muscles and skin can be converted into energy. But the body prefers carbohydrates to proteins.

> **Morsel** "The rich eat the meat; the poor eat the bones." —Yiddish proverb

TYPES OF PROTEIN

The two main types of protein are protein from animals and protein from plants. Animal protein is found in beef, dairy products, eggs, fish, lamb, pork, poultry, seafood and products that are made from these foods. Animal proteins are considered to be *complete*, or *high-quality*, *protein*, because they have all of the essential amino acids that are needed by humans.

Plant proteins are found in legumes, nuts, vegetables, seeds, some fruits and the products that are made from these foods. Plant proteins are considered *incomplete*, or *lower-quality protein*, because they are missing some of the essential amino acids that are needed by humans. There are some exceptional vegetable proteins that contain all of the essential amino acids. These include soybeans and two grains: amaranth and quinoa.

Amino Acids: The Building Blocks of Protein

Proteins are large chemical structures that are made of smaller building blocks called *amino acids*. Amino acids contain a basic structure that can be used by the body for energy and two side groups: one that contains nitrogen and one that contains an acid. When protein is digested, it is broken down into each of these components that the body uses for its many functions. In healthy people, most of the protein is used, stored or recycled.

There are 20 amino acids that make up most of the protein in the body. Healthy humans can make 11 of these amino acids from substances that already exist in the body. These are called *nonessential amino acids*. The human body cannot make 9 amino acids, which must be supplied from the diet. These are called *essential amino acids*. If a person does not consume these essential amino acids, then the body may not be able to meet all of its physiological needs.

Complementary Proteins

Incomplete plant proteins can be matched with other incomplete or complete plant protein to complete their amino acids. This process is called *protein complementation.* Chefs and home cooks may unknowingly complement plant proteins in their recipes. For example, simply spreading peanut butter on whole-grain bread combines the incomplete proteins of both of these foods to produce a full spectrum of amino acids.

Food scientists may intentionally complement plant proteins through protein technology in the development of new products. For example, some wheat pastas contain soy or other legume flours that create products with all of the essential amino acids.

It was once thought that incomplete proteins had to be complemented at each meal. In general, if a person consumes a well-balanced diet with enough calories—one that does not depend heavily on fruits, some tubers (such as sweet potatoes or cassava), or refined fat, flour and sugar—there is little danger of protein deficiency [3]. Table 5-1 shows some examples of protein complements in food preparation and cooking.

192

TABLE 5-1 Protein Complementation in Food Preparation and Cooking

Foods with Incomplete Amino Acids	Protein Complements	Examples
Whole-grain hot or cold breakfast cereal	Dairy milk or fortified soy milk	Cooked oatmeal with dairy milk or fortified soy milk
Whole-grain pancakes or waffles	Dairy yogurt or fortified soy yogurt	Buckwheat pancakes or waffles with dairy yogurt or fortified soy yogurt
Other whole grains	Dairy cheese or fortified soy cheese	Lasagna or macaroni and cheese made with dairy cheese or fortified soy cheese
Whole-grain bread or rolls	Almond, cashew, peanut or soy "butter"	Peanut butter sandwich on whole-grain bread or rolls
Whole-grain bread or rolls	Dairy cheese or fortified soy cheese	Cheese sandwich on whole-grain bread or rolls
Legume soup	Whole-grain crackers	Split pea or lentil soup with whole-grain crackers or croutons
Whole-grain pasta or brown rice	Dairy cheese or fortified soy cheese, cooked legumes, nuts and seeds	Minestrone soup with pasta, chick peas and Parmesan cheese or Arroz con Queso (rice with cheese)
Brown rice	Legumes	Hopping John (Caribbean black-eyed peas and rice) or red beans and rice
Corn tortillas	Dairy cheese or fortified soy cheese, cooked legumes	Corn tortillas with vegetarian refried beans and dairy cheese or fortified soy cheese
Potatoes	Dairy cheese or fortified soy cheese green leafy vegetables	Stuffed potatoes with dairy cheese or fortified soy cheese sauce and broccoli or spinach
Nuts and seeds	Cooked legumes, grains, dairy cheese or fortified soy cheese, green vegetables	Falafel with tahini (chick pea patties with sesame seed sauce), or broccoli with pesto sauce

Protein in Cooking and Baking

The amino acids in protein have important functions in cooking and baking. They are involved in the browning of protein foods at high temperatures, such as meat.

The Maillard reaction between protein and carbohydrates helps to create complex and meaty flavors, thanks to the nitrogen and sulfur in amino acids. Some of the shorter-chain amino acids, called *peptides*, have their own tastes. Fermented foods such as cured pork products, cheese and soy contain partially broken-down proteins with a distinctive savory taste due to the amino acid *glutamic acid.* Glutamic acid is also found in tomatoes, seaweeds, mushrooms and monosodium glutamate (MSG), the salt of glutamic acid. Amino acids that contain sulfur, such as *cysteine* and *methionine*, found in dairy products, eggs, fish, legumes, poultry, pork and sausage, create a meaty and sometimes egglike taste when heated.

Amino acids can absorb and hold water. This feature is important in both cooking and baking. Wheat protein can absorb water and form gluten, a tough protein that does not dissolve in water. Gluten is an important structural protein in baked goods such as breads. The protein in meat fibers is also tough, but it can be broken down by acids, agitation, heat or salt. The protein in eggs and milk is weaker and more soluble, which means that their bonds easily break down in liquid.

Protein is added to food products to boost the protein content and sometimes to control the carbohydrate and fat content. Soy, wheat and whey proteins are commonly added to baked items in food product development for flavor, functionality and nutritional value. In home kitchens, nonfat dry milk powder, powdered egg or egg white, soy protein powder and whey can be added to recipes to boost protein. Adjustments may have to be made in both commercial labs and home kitchens for taste and texture.

FOOD BYTE

There are more than 180 species of pigs that are found on every continent, except Antarctica. It is no wonder that pork is the world's most widely eaten meat and that hogs are a source of nearly 40 drugs and pharmaceuticals. While pigs are thought to be dirty, they actually keep themselves pretty clean. Their skin even replicates human skin [4,5].

SOURCES OF PROTEIN

Protein is abundant in foods and beverages from animals, including meat, poultry, fish and seafood, eggs and dairy products, and foods and beverages from plants, including legumes, vegetables and grains and nuts and seeds.

Meat, Poultry, Fish and Seafood

Morsel *"Beef is the soul of cooking."* —Marie Antoine Careme (French King of Chefs and the Chef of Kings, 1784–1833)

Animal proteins, found in meat, poultry, fish and seafood, provide excellent, high-quality protein, vitamin B12, and the minerals iron and zinc. One 4-ounce serving of animal protein, such as a 4-ounce beefsteak, chicken breast or pork chop, contains about 30 grams of protein. Other nutrients, including calories and fat vary.

Eggs

Eggs are nutrient-dense, with about 7 grams of protein per large egg at only 75 calories. Eggs contain 13 essential nutrients. These include the vitamins folate, riboflavin and vitamin D; the minerals calcium, phosphorus, iron, iodine, selenium and zinc; the phytonutrients lutein and zeaxanthin; and choline, a vitamin-like substance.

Recipe: Mushroom and Potato Frittata

*Eggs have been dubbed "Nature's Perfect Food" because they are naturally housed inside shells, provide a powerhouse of nutrients, offer a wide array of functionality and versatility in cooking and baking, meet formulation requirements in product development, and are relatively inexpensive. The recipe for **Mushroom and Potato Frittata** is in the **Recipe file** which is located within the Culinary Nutrition website at www.culinarynutrition.elsevier.com, pairs eggs with flavorsome mushrooms, simple potatoes and fresh herbs in an open-faced omelet that is adaptable for many meals, day or night. The finished dish is shown within the centerfold **Photo file** in Plate 5.1.*

Dairy Products

Dairy products are excellent sources of high-quality protein; vitamins, including niacin, phosphorus, potassium, riboflavin, vitamins B12 and D; and minerals, including calcium, magnesium, phosphorus, and potassium.

One 4-ounce serving of low-fat (2%) cottage cheese has about 15 grams of protein; 1 cup of plain nonfat yogurt has about 12 grams of protein; 1 cup of fat-free dairy milk has about 8 grams of protein; and 1 cup of vanilla ice cream has about 4 grams of protein. Calories and other nutrients vary.

Legumes

Garbanzo beans (chick peas), kidney beans, lima beans and other legumes, and peanut butter provide lower-quality, incomplete protein, while soybeans provide complete protein. Legumes are also a good source of fiber; the B vitamins, especially folate; and the minerals calcium, iron, selenium and zinc. One-half cup of cooked legumes contains about 8 grams of protein, as does ½ cup of tofu (soybean curd) and 2 tablespoons of peanut butter. There are about 125 calories in ½ cup of cooked legumes and about 200 calories in 2 tablespoons of peanut butter.

Vegetables and Grains

Vegetables, such as broccoli and spinach, and grains and grain products, such as rice and bread, provide lower-quality, incomplete protein. One-half cup of cooked vegetables, 1 slice of bread and ½ cup of cooked grains range in protein from 2 to 6 grams. If they are fortified, the protein may be higher. Calories and other nutrients vary.

Nuts and Seeds

Two tablespoons of nuts or seeds contain about 2 to 3 grams of protein; vitamins, including vitamins A and E; minerals, including phosphorous and potassium; and fiber. Nuts and seeds are high in fat in proportion to their protein content. There are about 100 calories in 2 tablespoons of nuts. The protein content of common foods is shown in Table 5-2.

PROTEIN DIGESTION AND ABSORPTION

Protein digestion begins in the mouth. The teeth cut and tear complex protein molecules, found in such foods as beef or poultry, and grind them to a pulp. This is called *physical digestion.* Then saliva mixes with the pulverized protein to soften it.

Once this softened protein is swallowed, it heads through the esophagus and into the stomach, where *hydrochloric acid*, a strong acid, and *pepsin*, an enzyme, help to unravel the protein complex into smaller segments. The stomach has a protective coating that prevents hydrochloric acid from burning through it. This process is called *denaturation.* Denaturation also happens to proteins in cooking when acid, agitation, air bubbles, heat or salt are applied.

Then the protein segments move into the small intestine, where other enzymes split them into amino acids. The amino acids now move through the intestinal wall with the help of villi, little hairlike projections, to be absorbed into the bloodstream. The blood carries amino acids to the liver, where some are stored, and to

195

TABLE 5-2 Protein Content of Common Foods		
Foods	**Serving Sizes**	**Protein (grams)**
Beef round roast, cooked	3 ounces	25
Bread, white	1 slice	3
Broccoli, cooked	½ cup	3
Cheddar cheese	2 ounces	14
Chicken, white meat, cooked	3 ounces	30
Cottage cheese	½ cup	14
Egg, whole	1 egg	6
Fish (as flounder, halibut), cooked	3 ounces	12
Hot dog, cooked	2 ounces	7
Legumes (as kidney, lima, garbanzo)	½ cup	8
Milk, 2%	1 cup	8
Mozarella cheese	2 ounces	12
Lamb, cooked	3 ounces	21
Pasta, cooked	½ cup	3
Peanut butter	2 tablespoons	8
Pork roast, cooked	3 ounces	21
Rice, brown, cooked	½ cup	5
Sausage, cooked	1 patty	5
Shrimp, cooked	12 large	17
Soymilk	1 cup	6
Tofu	3 ounces	8
Tortilla, corn	1 tortilla	2
Tuna, canned	3 ounces	24
Turkey, white meat, cooked	3 ounces	28
Yogurt, low-fat	8 ounces	12

other body sites, where they are reformulated for many bodily functions, repair and maintenance. The residue then passes into the large intestine for excretion, but usually very little remains.

Determining Protein Needs

The amount of protein needed on a daily basis is determined by a person's body weight. The Recommended Dietary Allowance (RDA) for protein for healthy adults is 0.4 gram of protein per pound of body weight per day (0.4 gram/pound of body weight/day). The RDA is actually based on 0.8 gram of protein per kilogram of body weight per day (0.8 gram/kilogram of body weight/day). To determine body weight in kilograms, divide body weight in pounds by 2.2 (2.2 pounds = 1 kilogram).

The following examples show how to calculate the daily protein requirements for a vegetarian woman and a man who eats meat, and how these requirements can be met through protein-rich food choices.

Example 1

Daily protein requirement for 135-pound vegetarian woman:

135 pounds of body weight × .4 gram of protein per pound = 54 grams of protein daily

Therefore, a vegetarian woman who weighs 135 pounds will need about 54 grams of protein daily. The following shows how to convert 54 grams of protein into servings of food and beverages to fulfill her daily protein need:

Food or Beverage	Amount of Protein (in grams)
2 cups 2% milk	16
1 cup low-fat yogurt	12
2 tablespoons peanut butter	8
2 slices whole-grain bread	6
½ cup tofu	9
1 cup cooked brown rice	5
½ cup fresh broccoli	3

Total = 59 grams of protein × 4 calories of protein/gram = 236 calories from protein daily

Example 2

Daily protein requirement for 180-pound man who eats meat:

180 pounds of body weight × .4 gram of protein per pound = 72 grams of protein daily

Therefore, a man who eats meat who weighs 180 pounds will need about 72 grams of protein daily. The following shows how to convert 72 grams of protein into servings of food and beverages to fulfill his daily protein need:

Food or Beverage	Amount of Protein (in grams)
1 cup 2% milk	8
2 large eggs	12
2 sausage patties	10
2 slices whole-grain bread	6
2 cups cooked pasta	10
3 ounces lean ground beef	24
1 ounce mozzarella cheese	6

Total = 76 grams of protein × 4 calories of protein/gram = 304 calories from protein daily

Both the woman who follows a vegetarian diet and the man who eats meat can meet their daily protein needs by consuming a variety of plant or animal foods. Protein needs may increase if someone is ill and cannot eat; has sustained blood loss or burns; is dieting and eliminates certain foods and beverages; is pregnant, lactating or rapidly growing, such as during infancy or adolescence; or is building muscle, such as in weight lifting. An additional serving or two of a protein-rich food or beverage, such as meat, poultry and dairy or fortified soy milk, may be sufficient. Unusual needs for protein should be addressed and individualized.

PROTEIN IN THE DIET

According to the Institutes of Medicine, the health division of the National Academy of Sciences, the Acceptable Macronutrient Distribution Range (AMDR) for protein is 10 to 35 percent of daily calories. The lower percentage is for people with reduced protein needs, such as the elderly. The higher percentage is for people with increased protein needs, such as triathletes [6,7].

Based on 2,000 calories daily (the standard reference caloric intake that the FDA uses on the nutrition label), this range equates to about 200 to 700 total calories from protein daily:

$$2,000 \text{ calories} \times .10 \, (10\% \text{ expressed as a decimal}) = 200 \text{ calories from protein daily}$$
$$2,000 \text{ calories} \times .35 \, (35\% \text{ expressed as a decimal}) = 700 \text{ calories from protein daily}$$

By using the examples of the vegetarian woman and the man who consumes meat, both the woman and the man meet the AMDR for protein. The AMDR for protein (10 to 35 percent of total calories daily, or 200 to 700 calories daily, based on 2,000 total daily calories):

Vegetarian woman: 59 grams of protein × 4 calories of protein / gram = 236 calories from protein daily
Man who eats meat: 76 grams of protein × 4 calories of protein / gram = 304 calories from protein daily

If their protein needs increase—for example, if the woman becomes pregnant or the man engages in strenuous sports training—they will need more protein. This amount should be based upon their increased body weight and protein demands.

> **Morsel** "The way you cut your meat reflects the way you live." —Confucius (Chinese social philosopher and thinker, 551–479 BC)

197

PROTEIN CONSUMPTION PATTERNS

Protein consumption has increased steadily in the United States since the 1950s. Most of the protein consumed today is from animal protein. A serving of animal protein is considered to be just 2 to 3 ounces. The average restaurant serving may be two to four times larger, and meat is central to the plate [8–10].

By reducing animal protein and incorporating plant proteins from baked goods, cereals and other grain products, legumes, nuts, pasta and potatoes, Americans will diversity their protein intake and consume less cholesterol, saturated fat and probably calories. This is because there is no cholesterol in plants, animal protein has more saturated fat than most vegetable protein, and fat is calorie-dense, with twice the calories of protein and carbohydrates. Too much vegetable protein above the daily protein need can also contribute to excess calories.

PROTEIN ON THE FOOD LABEL

The protein content of a food or beverage is listed on the Nutrition Facts Panel. It is shown as both grams per serving and the percent Daily Value (DV) for protein. Based on a 2,000-calorie diet, the DV for protein is 50 grams per day, or 200 calories. Table 5-3 shows where protein is listed on the Nutrition Facts Panel.

According to the Nutrition Facts Panel, one slice of whole-grain bread contains 3 grams of protein, or 8 percent of the DV for protein.

To determine the percentage of total calories from protein in one slice of whole-grain bread, use the following information:

- 1 gram of protein contains 4 calories.
- 3 grams of protein (in 1 slice of whole-grain bread) × 4 calories of protein/gram = 12 calories of protein in one slice of whole-grain bread
- 12 calories of protein in one slice of whole-grain bread/69 total calories per slice = .17 × 100 (multiply by 100 to change the decimal to percent) or 17% protein

TABLE 5-3 Nutrition Facts for One Slice of Whole-Grain Bread		
Calories and Nutrients	**Amounts Per Serving**	**% Daily Values**[a]
Calories	69	
Calories from fat	10	
Total fat (grams)	1	2%
Saturated fat (grams)	0	1%
Trans fat (grams)	0	
Cholesterol (grams)	0	0%
Sodium (milligrams)	109	5%
Total carbohydrate (grams)	11	4%
Dietary fiber (grams)	2	8%
Sugars (grams)	2	
Protein (grams)	3	8%
Vitamin A		0%
Vitamin C		0%
Calcium		3%
Iron		4%

Source: *[11].*
[a]Percent Daily Values are based on a 2,000-calorie diet. DVs may be higher or lower depending on your calorie needs. If void, no Daily Values are established.

Therefore, one slice of whole-grain bread contains 17 percent protein. This percentage tells you that less than 20 percent (one-fifth) of a slice of whole-grain bread is made from protein. Carbohydrates and lipids contribute the remaining calories, since vitamins and minerals do not contain calories. If you want a slice of bread with more protein, then you need to choose one with more than 3 grams of protein per slice.

According to the FDA, based on a 2,000-calorie daily diet and the DV for protein at 50 grams/day, a food product can bear the following claims:

"**High**" "**Rich In**," or "**Excellent Source Of**" if the product contains 20% or more of the DV, or 10 grams of protein per standard serving
"**Good Source**" "**Contains**," or "**Provides**" if the product contains 10% to 19% of the DV, or 5 grams of protein per standard serving
"**More**," "**Fortified**," "**Enriched**," "**Added**," "**Extra**," or "**Plus**" if the product contains 10% or more of the DV per standard serving [12].

The ability to read food labels and convert this information into food and dietary advice is important in recipe, meal and diet planning, both for healthy and restrictive diets. You can use this information to compare the grams of protein and the percent DV on the Nutrition Facts Panel to find products with the highest protein and the least total fat, saturated fat, cholesterol and calories.

Protein in Health and Disease

The RDA for protein should be adequate to supply a healthy body with the protein it needs for its many functions. If protein is not supplied by the diet, then the body will draw protein from its stores—muscles, organ systems and cells, with major concentrations of protein in the muscle cells. The heart is a muscle, and too little protein in the diet can stress the heart.

If enough protein is consumed to meet bodily needs, this keeps the body in *nitrogen equilibrium.* Nitrogen, an important element in the protein molecule, is a measure of healthy protein status. During starvation, severe illness or injury, *negative nitrogen balance* may occur. Protein can restore equilibrium. During periods of growth, such as pregnancy, infancy and puberty, hormones may stimulate *positive nitrogen balance* to meet increased protein needs. Once growth slows or stops, protein needs normalize.

PROTEIN MALNUTRITION

Malnutrition is a condition that occurs when insufficient nutrients are consumed. *Protein malnutrition* is an insufficient intake of protein to maintain protein equilibrium in the body. It is more prevalent in third-world countries where protein and energy (calories) are limited. This is another form of malnutrition called *protein-energy malnutrition (PEM)*. The characteristic appearance of people with PEM is extreme thinness because the muscles have shrunk in size. *Edema*, swelling in the stomach and legs from fluid that has leaked out of the blood vessels, may also be present. PEM may also be found in poverty-stricken areas of the United States, in undernourished hospital patients, and in people with AIDS, anorexia, cancer and end-stage renal disease (ESRD) [10].

Too much protein in the diet may also cause malnutrition, because it may displace other nutrients, such as carbohydrates, and add too many calories, fats and cholesterol. The liver and kidneys may become burdened and enlarge, which compromises their functions. More calcium is excreted in the urine, which increases the need for dietary calcium. If calcium-rich foods and beverages are not consumed, then calcium may be drawn from the blood and bones. Excess protein in the diet may also contribute more dietary sodium, since this mineral is naturally present in protein foods. Too much sodium can upset the normal balance of sodium and potassium in the blood and cells, with potentially serious effects.

> **Morsel** "How foolish is man to believe that abstaining from flesh and eating fish, which is so much more delicate and delicious, constitutes fasting."
> —Napoleon Bonaparte (French military and political leader, 1769–1821)

Vegetarian and Vegan Diets

Vegetarian diets are based on plant proteins from legumes, grains, nuts and seeds, vegetables and fruits. Most vegetarian diets exclude some type of animal protein. *Lacto-ovo vegetarians* include dairy products and eggs (*lacto* is Latin for "milk," and *ovo* is Latin for "eggs") but exclude meats; *lacto vegetarians* eliminate eggs; *ovo vegetarians* eliminate dairy products; *vegans* eliminate all animal products, including dairy products and eggs; and *pesco-vegetarians* consume fish. Some people may call themselves vegetarians but will still consume some animal protein, such as poultry.

People select vegetarian diets for a variety of reasons that may include aesthetic, cultural, economical, environmental, ethical, moral, religious, societal, political, tasteful and/or healthful. The healthful benefits of vegetarian diets are featured next.

HEALTHFUL BENEFITS OF VEGETARIAN DIETS

If a vegetarian diet is well planned, it can meet a person's nutritional needs and may provide additional healthful benefits. Vegetarian diets may be higher in fiber, some vitamins, and minerals and phytonutrients than nonvegetarian diets. These features may offer them some protective factors against certain diseases, such as cardiovascular disease, cancer, diabetes and hypertension. Religious and cultural groups who follow vegetarian diets, such as the Seventh-Day Adventists, have demonstrated lower rates of these diseases [13].

A well-planned vegetarian diet with plenty of fiber may also have weight management benefits. This is because vegetables are more nutrient-dense and lower in calories than some meats, and vegetable fibers are filling. However, a poorly chosen vegetarian diet that is filled with refined carbohydrates and fats may contribute excess calories and create nutrient deficiencies.

CONCERNS ABOUT VEGETARIAN DIETS

Several stages of the life cycle require especially careful vegetarian diet planning. These include pregnancy, lactation, infancy, childhood, adolescence and aging. A pregnant vegetarian woman requires more calories, protein, vitamins, and minerals, especially vitamins D and B12, and the minerals calcium, iron and zinc. A lactating vegetarian woman requires about the same amount of protein as pregnancy; her vitamin B12 requirement is higher, while her need for iron and calories is lower.

Vegetarian infants and children may not thrive or reach their growth potential. Care must be taken to provide enough high-quality protein and calories for growth and development, and vitamins D and B12 for bone development and normal functioning of the brain and nervous system. Vegetarian teens may not have high enough nutrient levels to meet their increased growth and athletic demands. Protein and calories are especially significant. Vegetarian seniors may be short on vital nutrients to maintain their health and prevent disease. While their calorie and protein needs may decrease, their requirements for certain vitamins and minerals, such as vitamin D and calcium, may rise.

Vegetarian Diet Guidelines

No matter what age, vegetarians should consume enough calories to maintain their ideal body weight, as described in Chapter 1. Vegetarians must also consume enough protein based upon their body weight and adequate amounts of vitamins B12 and D, and the minerals calcium, iron and zinc. A number of meal-planning tools to meet these nutrient requirements have been developed specifically for vegetarians. Figure 5-1 shows the vegetarian food guide pyramid [14].

VEGETARIAN FOOD GROUPS AND RECOMMENDED SERVINGS

The recommended numbers of daily servings for vegetarians and sample serving sizes follow. Numbers of servings may vary according to caloric needs.

- Six servings of grain foods, including breads, cereals and cooked grains. Grains should be whole grain and fortified.
  One serving = 1 slice bread, ½ cup cooked cereal, 1 ounce ready-to-eat cereal

- Five servings of protein-rich foods, including legumes, nuts, higher-protein grains and vegetables.
  One serving = ½ cup cooked legumes, ½ cup tofu or tempeh, 2 tablespoons nut butter, ¼ cup nuts, 1 ounce meat substitute

- Four servings of vegetables, including cooked and raw vegetables and vegetable juice.
  One serving = ½ cup cooked vegetables, 1 cup raw vegetables, ½ cup vegetable juice

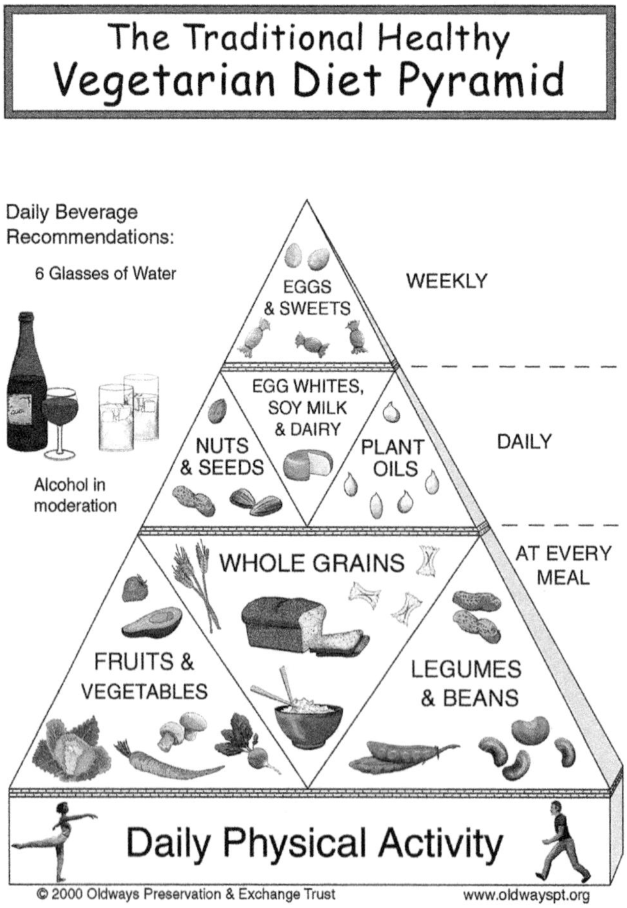

The Traditional Healthy
Vegetarian Diet Pyramid

Daily Beverage Recommendations:

6 Glasses of Water

EGGS & SWEETS — WEEKLY

EGG WHITES, SOY MILK & DAIRY

NUTS & SEEDS

PLANT OILS — DAILY

Alcohol in moderation

WHOLE GRAINS — AT EVERY MEAL

FRUITS & VEGETABLES

LEGUMES & BEANS

Daily Physical Activity

© 2000 Oldways Preservation & Exchange Trust   www.oldwayspt.org

FIGURE 5-1
Vegetarian food guide pyramid.

- Two servings of fruits, including cooked, raw, dried and fruit juice.
  One serving = 1 medium piece fruit, ½ cup chopped fruit, ½ cup fruit juice, ¼ cup dried fruit

- Two servings of fats, including omega-3 fats, and emphasizing liquid fats.
  One serving = 1 teaspoon oil, soft margarine or mayonnaise, about 5 nuts, 1 tablespoon seeds

CALCIUM, IRON, ZINC, VITAMIN D AND VITAMIN B12

Certain vitamins and minerals are difficult to obtain in vegetarian diets and are even harder to attain in vegan diets. This is because they are mainly available from animal foods and beverages. They include calcium, iron, zinc, vitamin D and vitamin B12. Calcium and vitamin D are plentiful in dairy products, and iron, zinc and vitamin B12 are abundant in meats. When dairy products and meats are omitted from the diet, it is challenging to consume the right foods in correct quantities to meet these nutrient requirements. The RDA for calcium for healthy adults is 1,000 milligrams. Vegetarian sources of calcium include the following:

Foods	Calcium in Milligrams (mg)/Serving
Calcium-fortified orange juice	350 mg/cup
Calcium-fortified rice drink	300 mg/cup
Calcium-fortified soy milk	200–300 mg/cup
Calcium-fortified cereal and snack bars	200 mg/bar
Bok choy, collards, kale, turnip greens	160–200 mg/1 cup cooked
Instant oatmeal	165 mg/1 packet
Tofu	130 mg/½ cup
Almonds	126 mg/½ cup
Calcium-fortified waffle	122 mg/1 waffle
Broccoli	94 mg/½ cup
Corn tortilla	52 mg/1 medium
Legumes	50 mg/½ cup cooked

The RDA for iron for healthy adults is 8 milligrams for men and 18 milligrams for women. Vegetarian sources of iron include the following:

Foods	Iron in Milligrams (mg)/Serving
Instant cream-of-wheat	8.2 mg/¾ cup cooked
Spinach	3.2 mg/½ cup cooked
Lima or navy beans	2.3–2.5 mg/½ cup cooked
Prune juice	2.3 mg/¾ cup
Swiss chard	2.0 mg/½ cup cooked
Oatmeal	1.6 mg/1 cup cooked
Dried figs	1.3 mg/¼ cup
Green peas	1.3 mg/½ cup cooked
Wheat bread	.94 mg/1 slice
Apricots	.82 mg/5 dried halves
Raisins	.76 mg/¼ cup
Broccoli	.65/½ cup cooked

The RDA for zinc for healthy adults is 11 milligrams for men and 8 milligrams for women. Vegetarian sources of zinc include the following:

Foods	Zinc in Milligrams (mg)/Serving
Dry-roasted soybeans	4.0 mg/½ cup
Enriched cereal	3.1 mg/¾ cup
Peanuts	1.7 mg/¾ cup
Black beans and black-eyed peas	1.0–1.1 mg/½ cup cooked

Foods	Zinc in Milligrams (mg)/Serving
Tofu	1.0 mg/½ cup
Green peas	.75 mg/½ cup cooked
Spinach	.68 mg/½ cup cooked
Whole-wheat bread	.55 mg/1 slice

The RDA for vitamin D for healthy adults is 600 IU (15 mcg) for men and women. Vegetarian sources of vitamin D include the following:

Foods and Beverages	Vitamin D in Micrograms (mcg)/Serving
Fat-free milk	2.5 mcg/1 cup
Fortified margarine	.5 mcg/1 tsp
Fortified cereals	.6-3 mcg/serving
Fortified soy foods	1–2.5 mcg/serving

There are no dependable unfortified sources of vitamin D from plants. Vitamin D is made when the skin is exposed to sunlight and a chemical transformation takes place. Some fortified vegan products contain D2, which has a different form and function in the body than naturally occurring vitamin D with D3 (cholecalciferol), synthesized by humans when skin is exposed to sunlight.

The RDA for vitamin B12 for healthy adults is 2.4 micrograms for men and women. Lacto-ovo sources of vitamin B12 include the following:

Foods and Beverages	Vitamin B12 in Micrograms (mcg)/Serving
Cottage cheese	2 mcg/1 cup
Fat-free milk	.9 mcg/1 cup
Egg	.5 mcg/1 whole

The only dependable unfortified sources of vitamin B12 are meats, dairy products and eggs. Fermented soy foods, such as tempeh, algae and seaweeds, claim to be sources of vitamin B12, but their content may vary. Some fortified foods, such as breakfast cereals, may vary in vitamin B12 formulation and nutritional yeast products may vary in vitamin B12 bioavailability. Bacteria that live in the large intestine can synthesize vitamin B12, but it is not available for absorption through the small intestine like other nutrients [15].

VEGETARIAN RECIPE AND MEAL PLANNING

Legumes, vegetables, grains and starchy vegetables such as potatoes can be afterthoughts when meat is the star of the plate. In some countries, meat is used in smaller proportions compared to grains and vegetables, and it occupies a less important place in a meal. In other cuisines, meat may be totally absent. The nutritional balance and satisfaction of the entire meal is key.

When planning vegetarian meals, grains, legumes, and starchy vegetables provide the foundation. Start with a grain with complete protein, such as amaranth or quinoa, and then build the side dishes, such as cooked lentils or spinach, around or over it. Or use a single item, such as a slice of cooked eggplant, portobello mushroom or tomato half as the focal point, and add some small timbales of cooked grains. If dairy products, eggs or soy are in a recipe, there is less need to complement the vegetable proteins. If the recipe is vegan, complementary grains, legumes, and vegetables boost nutrients and enhance taste. Suggested serving sizes for meal planning are provided in the "Vegetarian food groups and recommended servings" section. A sample daily lacto-ovo vegetarian menu is shown in Table 5-4, with adaptations for vegans.

VEGETARIAN COOKING

Vegetarian cooking is more than just omitting meat; it also means finding substitutes for different types of meat, dairy products, eggs, gelatin and other animal-based ingredients.

TABLE 5-4 Sample Daily Lacto-Ovo Vegetarian and Vegan Menus

Lacto-ovo Vegetarian Menu	Vegan Adaptations
Breakfast	
1 cup fortified whole-grain cereal	
1 cup nonfat dairy milk	Fortified soy milk
½ cup sliced banana slices	
1 slice whole-grain toast	
1 teaspoon margarine	Fortified soy margarine
Lunch	
1 cup mixed-vegetable soup	
1 whole-grain pita bread filled with	
½ cup hummus, lettuce, tomato	
Dinner	
½ cup cooked quinoa or amaranth	
1 cup cooked broccoli	
1 medium orange	
Snack	
1 cup nonfat plain yogurt	Fortified soy yogurt
½ cup berries	
½ cup roasted soy nuts	
Daily totals	
Calories:	2,407 calories	2,570 calories
Carbohydrates:	394.4 grams	417.4 grams
Fiber:	50.8 grams	54.5 grams
Protein:	104.8 grams	102.7 grams
Total fat	53.8 grams	63.5 grams
Saturated fat	8 grams	9.1 grams
Cholesterol	9.8 milligrams	0 milligrams
Polyunsaturated fat	20.7 grams	25.1 grams
Monounsaturated fat	18.5 grams	21.2 grams
Sodium	2,402 milligrams	2,344.2 milligrams
Calcium	1,333.8 milligrams	942.7 milligrams
Iron	35.8 milligrams	41.0 milligrams
Zinc	18.7 milligrams	17.2 milligrams
Vitamin B12	2.8 micrograms	3 micrograms
Vitamin D	100.5 IU	39.2 IU

203

To Replace Meat

Tofu (soy "cheese"), tempeh (cooked and fermented soybeans) and texturized soy protein (TSP) replicate the complete amino acids that are found in meats. Tofu, tempeh, and TSP can be used in savory dishes, and tofu can also be used in sweet desserts and beverages. Some varieties of tofu are shelf-stable. Seitan (wheat protein) is a meaty-tasting vegetarian alternative to meat, but its protein profile is incomplete. Since seitan is made from wheat, a good protein complement is legumes.

To Replace Dairy Products

Nut, rice or soy nondairy beverages (often called "milk") can be used in place of dairy milk in some recipes. Use unflavored plant beverages for savory recipes. Almond, coconut and oat "milks" can be used in dessert recipes because they often contain sweeteners, such as evaporated cane juice. Some vegetarian cheese alternatives can be found without casein (a milk derivative). Crumbled tofu can be used to replace cottage or ricotta cheese in some recipes, and nutritional yeast, which has a meaty flavor and taste, can be used like Parmesan cheese.

To Replace Eggs

Some commercial egg replacers are vegetarian, but their usefulness in recipes can vary. This is because eggs perform a variety of functions. In cakes, eggs serve as a leavening agent. In cookies and muffins, eggs act as a binder and add moisture. In mayonnaise and quiche, eggs are paramount; however, plain tofu may be a good substitute. Plain tofu can also be used in recipes that require several eggs.

Tofu lends creaminess, but it does not provide rise to a recipe. To avoid lumps in the final product, puree tofu before adding it to a recipe. If a recipe needs more binding, add 2 to 3 tablespoons of arrowroot, cornstarch, instant potato flakes, mashed sweet or white potatoes, potato starch, tomato paste, whole wheat flour or ¼ cup silken tofu pureed with 1 tablespoon of flour for each whole large egg.

To Replace Gelatin

Gelatin is an animal product, so it is not suitable as a thickener in vegetarian cooking and baking. Some kosher gelatins are vegetarian. *Agar-agar*, a flavorless gelling substance made from cooked and pressed seaweed, may be substituted for gelatin in equal amounts. Agar-agar does not need refrigeration to gel. For a firmer gel, add more agar-agar; for a softer gel, add more liquid. *Carrageen*, a seaweed-based gelling substance, can be used for soft gels and puddings. One ounce of carrageen will gel about 1 cup of liquid.

Other specialized ingredients such as the following can be used to replicate the flavors and textures that are common in meat-based diets:

- *Agar or agar-agar* is a vegetarian gelatin substitute that is used as a thickener for jellies, ice cream and soups. Use agar in recipes that call for egg whites. To mimic whipped egg whites, dissolve 1 tablespoon of agar powder in 1 tablespoon of water; whip, chill and whip the mixture again.
- *Agave syrup* is a sweetener from the agave plant that is native to Mexico. It can be used in place of honey in some recipes. Since honey is produced by bees, some vegetarians exclude it. Agave syrup is sweeter than honey but thinner.
- *Carob* is actually a legume that can be used in place of chocolate in some recipes. It is milder and less bitter than chocolate, and it pairs well with fruit in desserts.
- *Flaxseeds* have a nutty taste and chewy texture. They take on the properties of eggs and fat in some recipes. For each egg, mix 1 tablespoon of ground flaxseeds with 3 tablespoons of water; let the mixture blend together for a few minutes. Ground flaxseeds may cause a recipe to be chewy with less volume, and baked goods may brown more quickly.
- *Kudzu* is a starchy powder like arrowroot or cornstarch that is used to thicken gravies, sauces, and stews.
- *Liquid amino acids* are a nonfermented soy sauce alternative, with a meatlike, umami-rich flavor. They can be used to flavor hearty dishes such as braises, chili, soups and stews
- *Mushrooms*, such as shiitake or portobello, whether fresh or dried and reconstituted, provide meaty texture and the earthy taste of umami.
- *Nut "butters,"* such as almonds, cashews or other nuts, may be used in place of butter in equal amounts in some recipes. While peanut butter is a legume, it is sometimes used as nut butters.
- *Pectin* is a natural gelling agent that is found in citrus fruits, including lemons and limes; berries, such as blackberries, cranberries and red currants; and treetop fruit, especially apples and quinces.
- *Sea vegetables*, such as alaria, arame, dulse, hijiki, kelp, kombu and nori, provide a depth of flavor and saltiness to vegetarian recipe, whether fresh or dried. Sea vegetables add iodine, vitamin K, folate, magnesium, calcium and iron to vegetarian diets.
- *Vegetable broth or stock* can replace beef, poultry or fish stock in some recipes.

Soybeans

One of the most versatile vegetarian foods that can replicate the flavor and texture of meat is the soybean. Like meat, soybeans contain all of the essential amino acids, but unlike meat, soybeans do not contain any cholesterol, because it comes from plants.

The nutritional and health values of soy have been admired for hundreds of years. Soybeans were first cultivated in China over 3,000 years ago. Their use spread throughout Asia, where soybeans are still prominent in many forms of Asian cuisine today.

204

Soybeans were first introduced to the United States in the 1700s as a crop for livestock and only became recognized as a food crop in the 1920s. Today, soybeans serve as a feed crop and a food crop. Food technology has created a world of soy products for US consumption that barely resemble the soybean of antiquity.

Soybeans have unique properties. They are 40 percent protein, 35 percent carbohydrate and 25 percent lipid—which makes them almost half protein. Soybeans are relatively low in carbohydrates and high in fiber, and their lipids contain healthful omega-3 fatty acids.

One-half cup of cooked yellow soybeans contains about 150 calories, 14 grams of protein, 9 grams of carbohydrates, 8 grams of fat, with only 1 gram of saturated fat, 5 grams of dietary fiber, 90 milligrams of calcium, 46 milligrams of folate and 4 milligrams of iron [15–17].

SOY FOODS

Many types of soy foods are available in US food markets and ethnic grocers. Brands vary, and freshness matters. These include, but are not limited to, the following foods and beverages. This is because soy has so many applications. Versatile soybeans in one form or another can be found in cereal, potato chips, coffee, ice cream, nondairy creamer, protein and meal replacement bars, pasta and nondairy whipped topping. Check the labels for nutrition information and "sell by" dates to find the best soy product for nutrition and taste.

- *Cultured soy yogurt* is soy-based yogurt with a creamy texture that is similar to traditional dairy-based yogurt. One 6-ounce serving contains about 7 grams of protein and about 150 to 200 calories.
- *Edamame* (Chinese and Japanese) are green soybeans that have been harvested when they are about 80 percent mature. Edamame are bigger and sweeter than traditional soybeans. One-half cup of edamame provides about 8 grams of protein and about 100 calories.
- *Miso* (Japanese), *Chiang* (Chinese) or *Chao Doo* (Vietnamese) is thick, fermented soybean paste. Miso is made by fermenting rice, barley and soybeans with salt and a vitamin B12 bacteria starter in cedar vats for one to three years. Like wine and cheese, miso varies in aroma, color, flavor and texture, depending on the length of fermentation and additional ingredients. One tablespoon of miso contains about 2 grams of protein and about 25 calories. Miso also contains vitamin B12, copper, manganese and zinc.
- *Natto* is made of fermented, cooked whole soybeans. It has a nutrient profile that is similar to miso. Natto is strong smelling with a cheeselike texture and sticky, gelatinous coating. It is primarily used as a spread or in soups. One tablespoon of natto provides about 2 grams of protein and about 27 calories.
- *Processed soy foods look*, feel and taste like the foods they replicate: bacon, bologna, butter, cheese, chips, ground meat, hot dogs, ice cream, milk, sausages and yogurt. While they may resemble these foods, they are not chemically or nutritionally similar. Soy foods have no cholesterol. They may be higher in fiber, some vitamins and minerals, and phytonutrients than animal-based products. They may also be higher in fat and sodium, so check the labels. Protein and calories vary.
- *Seitan* is also known as wheat gluten. It is made by washing wheat flour dough until the starch dissolves. Seitan is an alternative to tofu in Asian, Buddhist, macrobiotic and vegetarian cuisines. One-third cup of seitan has about 23 grams of protein and 160 calories.
- *Soy butter* is a processed spread that is made from fresh roasted whole soybeans. It is similar to peanut butter in both taste and texture, but it has less total fat and saturated fat. Soy butter can be used as a substitute for peanut butter. Two tablespoons of soy butter contain about 7 grams of protein and 170 calories, and it is cholesterol-free.
- *Soy flour* is made from defatted soybeans. It is used in the production of soy protein isolate for other soy-based foods. Soy flour comes in full-fat, low-fat and defatted varieties. One tablespoon of defatted soy flour has about 6 grams of protein and 41 calories.
- *Soy-based infant formulas* are designed for babies who are allergic to cow's milk. The nutrients replicate those in breastmilk. Soy-based infant formulas were first introduced into the United States in the early 1900s. Protein and calories vary. Many are fortified with iron and other minerals and vitamins.
- *Soy lecithin* is extracted from soybean oil. Its primary component, choline, is vital for cell membranes, and it has many reported health benefits from cognition to cardiovascular. Soy lecithin is used as an emulsifier or stabilizer in cooking and baking. It helps to solidify margarine and provides texture and consistency to chocolates, coatings and salad dressings. One tablespoon of soy lecithin has 0 grams of protein and about 53 calories [18].

- *Soybean meal* remains after soy oil is extracted from whole soybeans. Per cup, soybean meal is about 30 to 50 percent protein. It is mostly used for feeding poultry, swine and fish.
- *Soy milk* is an emulsion of oil, water and soy protein. It is produced by soaking dry soybeans and then grinding them with water. Soy milk contains about the same amount of protein as cow's milk but is lactose-free, with little saturated fats and no cholesterol. Soymilk is often fortified with protein, vitamins and minerals—especially vitamin D and calcium. A comparison of soy milk and dairy milk is shown in Table 5-5.
- *Soybean oil* is made from soybeans that have been cracked, rolled into flakes, solvent-extracted and refined. It is found in both liquid and partially hydrogenated forms that are sold as ``vegetable oil," and it isused in a wide variety of processed foods. Soybean oil contains mostly unsaturated fatty acids that oxidize easily. For this reason, soybean oil is undesirable for restaurant use. One tablespoon of soybean oil contains about 120 calories and practically no protein.
- *Soy sauce* (Chinese), *Shoyu* or *Soya Sauce* (Japanese) is a fermented sauce that is made from soybeans, roasted grains, water and salt. Soy sauce is high in sodium, but a reduced-sodium variety is available. It contributes a savory, umami flavor to foods. One tablespoon of soy sauce contains about 9 calories and 1 gram of protein.
- *Tempeh* is made from cultured and fermented soybeans that are formed into chunky, tender soybean "cakes." The soybeans are sometimes mixed with rice or millet. Tempeh is high in protein and dietary fiber; it contains some vitamin B12 from fermentation in addition to calcium and iron. One-half cup of tempeh provides about 19 grams of protein and 200 calories.
- *Texturized soy or vegetable protein (TVP)* is a meat substitute that is made from defatted soybean flour. It can be used in many ways in recipes because TVP takes on the texture and flavor of the ingredients that it replaces, such as ground meat in chili, hamburger, Sloppy Joes, spaghetti and taco recipes. One-half cup of dry TVP supplies about 24 grams of protein and 160 calories.
- *Tofu* (Japanese), *doufu* (Chinese) or bean curd is made by curdling fresh, hot soy milk with a coagulant and then pressing the curds into cheeselike blocks. Tofu comes fresh and processed, in soft/silken, firm and extra-firm varieties, and it has a range of culinary applications, depending on its texture. Tofu is low in saturated fats, with no cholesterol. It contains calcium, copper, iron, manganese and magnesium. One-half cup of tofu supplies about 8 grams of protein and 80 calories.

COOKING AND BAKING WITH SOYBEANS AND SOY FOODS

Soybeans and soybean products have unique aromas, tastes and textures. While they can be substituted for dairy milk, cheese and meat products in some recipes, they may feel, smell, react and taste differently. Using the freshest soybean products will help to guard against any off-flavors. Ingredient adjustments may be necessary.

The protein in soybeans is heat stable, which allows it to withstand heat processing into soy milk, tofu, TVP, and most heat applications in cooking and baking. The following are some specific uses of soy foods in cooking and baking:

- *Edamame* pods are commonly boiled or steamed and then salted and served whole and as an appetizer or snack. The green soybeans are easily popped out of their pods, which are discarded. Edamame are also available without the pods and are a versatile ingredient, lending color, taste and texture to cold or hot savory dishes.

TABLE 5-5 Nutrients in 2% Fat Soy Milk Compared to 2% Fat Dairy Milk	
8 Ounces 2% Fat Soy Milk	**8 Ounces 2% Fat Dairy Milk**
100 calories	120 calories
3.5 grams total fat	5 grams total fat
0.5 grams saturated fat	3 grams saturated fat
0 milligrams cholesterol	20 milligrams cholesterol
10 grams total carbohydrates	11 grams total carbohydrates
7 grams sugar	112 grams sugar
7 grams protein	8 grams protein

Source: *[19,20]*.

- *Miso* is characterized as cheeselike, earthy, fruity, salted, savory or sweet in flavor. Miso is used for glazes, marinades for pickling vegetables and meats, sauces, spreads, and as an essential ingredient in Japanese *dashi* soup with its umami-rich flavor with its umami-rich flavor.
- *Red miso* has a full-bodied flavor that makes it suitable for marinated, simmered and stir-fried dishes with other strongly flavored ingredients. *White miso* is less salty and sweeter than red miso. It is flavorsome in dressings, marinades and sauces along with other mildly flavored ingredients. Only 1 to 2 tablespoons of either type of miso are normally needed in recipes.
- High temperatures and extended heat may destroy the healthful microorganisms in miso, so it should be cooked quickly with moderate heat. In recipes that require high heat, such as miso soup, miso should be added toward the end of cooking. It should first be blended with a small amount of the cooking liquid so it completely dissolves. Miso can be refrigerated, but it should not be frozen.
- *Seitan* can be served baked, deep-fried, marinated, oven-braised, pressure-cooked, raw, simmered, steamed or stuffed. Each method produces a different-textured result. Braised and simmered seitan is chewy; baked seitan is light; pressure-cooked seitan is soft; and fried seitan is oily and slippery.
- Seitan can be flavored by using a traditional broth of garlic, ginger, kombu (seaweed) and soy sauce. Poultry seasoning or chicken-flavored broth granules can be used for a poultry-like flavor, or a combination of cayenne, fennel, garlic, Italian seasoning and paprika can be blended for a sausage-like flavor for use in luncheon-style "meats."
- *Soy creamer* does not whip like whipping cream, but it can be used in puddings and pie fillings. Add a little less soy creamer than the recipe requires, plus about ¼ cup of cornstarch to help the mixture thicken. Whisk the mixture well before using it in recipes.
- *Soy flour* is a good substitute for 10 to 30 percent of the wheat flour in sweet and rich baked goods, such as cookies, soft yeast breads and quick breads. This is because soy flour has a significant fat content. The fat in soy flour can become rancid, so both soy flour and baked goods that contain it should be refrigerated. Defatted soy flour is also available.
- Soy flour is often used to increase the protein in baked goods. Since soy flour is gluten-free, it cannot replace all the wheat or rye flour in yeast-raised breads because it does not provide enough structure. A preferred ratio of flours in yeast-raised breads is about 50 percent soy flour with about 50 percent other gluten-free flour or starch.
- Soy flour can also be used in cookies, muffins, pancakes, quick breads and waffles. Soy flour can replace up to one-fourth the total amount of flour in a recipe. For each cup of all-purpose flour, use ¼ cup soy flour and ¾ cup all-purpose flour. Avoid packing soy flour when measuring.
- Dough with soy flour tends to brown faster than dough with wheat flour—particularly if too much is used. The oven temperature should be lowered about 25 degrees to help prevent overbrowning. Soy flour can be lightly "toasted" in a dry fry pan to enhance its nutty flavor before using.
- One tablespoon of soy flour plus 1 tablespoon of water can replace one egg in some baked good recipes. Soy flour can also be used to thicken gravies and sauces.
- *Soy milk* can be substituted for dairy milk in many recipes. Make sure that the soy solids are evenly dispersed. If soy milk is overheated, it may scorch and form a skin similar to that of dairy milk. While soy milk can be frozen, it is not recommended because freezing may adversely affect the consistency and flavor.
- *Soy yogurt* is prepared with soy milk, yogurt bacteria and sometimes a sweetener, such as raw sugar. It is commercially available in plain and fruited varieties. Soy yogurt tastes like dairy yogurt with a slight soy aftertaste, and it can be used in recipes that call for dairy yogurt or sour cream. The amount of fat in soy yogurt depends on the amount of fat in the soy milk that is used in its production.
- *Tempeh* must be cooked unless the package states that it is ready-to-use. The flavor of tempeh ranges from nutty and subtle to smoky and tangy. Tempeh can be baked, boiled, braised, broiled, fried, grilled, pan-fried, poached, sauteed, simmered or steamed. Boiling, braising or poaching tempeh in flavorful liquid serves to soften it. Dredging tempeh in cornmeal, flour or ground nuts before cooking adds texture. If ready-to-use, tempeh can be directly added to casseroles, chili, sandwiches or soups.
- *Textured vegetable or soy protein (TVP)* can be reconstituted with boiling water in the ratio of 1 cup of TVP to 1 cup of boiling water. This mixture needs to soak 5 to 10 minutes to yield about 2 cups. One pound of TVP will reconstitute into about three pounds of ground meat substitute. It can be used on its own in recipes or combined with ground meat or poultry in a 1:3 ratio of rehydrated TVP to ground

meat. TVP will take on the flavor of other foods that are cooked with it. The taste varies, depending on the type of TVP.

- *Tofu* has little flavor or aroma on its own, but it easily absorbs the flavors and aromas of seasonings and marinades. Tofu can be used in savory or sweet recipes. It can be baked, barbecued, boiled, braised, broiled, fried, grilled, pan-fried, pureed, sauteed, simmered, steamed or eaten "as is."
- Tofu is available in two forms: fresh, packed in water, and silken, packed in aseptic packaging. Water-packed tofu should be refrigerated until used. Once opened, the water should be changed daily, and the tofu should be used within a few days.
- Use fresh tofu in recipes when tofu needs to hold its shape, such as in baking, barbecuing, boiling, broiling, grilling, sauteing or steaming. To intensify the flavor and texture of fresh tofu, first cover it with a clean towel and a heavy weight; then discard the liquid, slice and use, or freeze. Freezing may alter the color and texture of fresh tofu and cause sponginess, but it can still be crumbled and added to casseroles, chili, lasagna, soups or stews.
- Silken tofu has been processed into a creamy texture that can be pureed into desserts, dressings and sauces. Silken tofu can be substituted for sour cream or cream cheese in some recipes. Some Japanese-type silken tofu is shelf-stable up to nine months.
- *Whole soybeans* should be presoaked before cooking. Use 3 cups of water for each 1 cup of soybeans. Soak soybeans 8 hours or overnight at room temperature. Discard the soaking water and replace it with fresh water. Dry soybeans contain an enzyme inhibitor that makes them difficult to digest.
- One cup (½ pound) of dry soybeans will expand when cooked to about 2¼ to 2½ cups of cooked soybeans. Do not add salt or acidic ingredients, such as tomatoes or peppers, until just before the soybeans complete cooking. They may cause the skins to harden.

Recipe: Tofu Cheesecake

*The recipe for **Tofu Cheesecake** in The recipe for Tofu Cheesecake in the **Recipe file** which is located within the* Culinary Nutrition *website at www.culinarynutrition.elsevier.com, uses silken tofu with its creamy texture to replicate the texture of traditional cheesecake without the cholesterol. While tofu might be an acquired taste for some, the silken tofu in this recipe is enhanced by semisweet chocolate, almond and vanilla extracts and a nutty crust that is made from chopped hazelnuts and toasted graham cracker crumbs. One serving of **Tofu Cheesecake** provides 5 grams of protein. In general, both tofu and tempeh provide 5 grams of protein per 1 ounce.*

Soybeans in Health and Disease

Besides high-quality protein, vitamins and minerals, soybeans contain *isoflavones*, plant chemicals with presumed health-promoting benefits. The major soy isoflavones are *genistein*, *daidzein* and *glycitein.* These isoflavones, along with soy protein, reportedly reduce the risk of cardiovascular disease and certain cancers, enhance bone health, decrease menopausal symptoms and regulate blood sugar. Each of these conditions and its relationship to soybeans is now discussed, with attention to ongoing controversies regarding their use.

CARDIOVASCULAR DISEASE

Soy protein and isoflavones may help to lower blood cholesterol, which may help decrease cardiovascular disease. Also, if soy replaces animal protein in the diet, saturated fat and cholesterol intake should decrease, which should benefit cardiovascular disease and overall health.

The FDA has approved the following health claims about soy protein and cardiovascular disease:

> *Twenty-five grams of soy protein a day, as part of a diet low in saturated fat and cholesterol, may reduce the risk of heart disease. A serving of [name of food] supplies _____ grams of soy protein.*

> or

> *Diets low in saturated fat and cholesterol that include 25 grams of soy protein may reduce the risk of heart disease. One serving of [name of food] provides _____ grams of soy protein. [21]*

The amount of isoflavones that may be effective in reducing cardiovascular disease is about 25 to 40 milligrams daily. This amount can be obtained by consuming any of the following: 4 ounces of edamame,

1½ ounces of soy nuts, 2 cups of soy milk, 4 ounces of tempeh or tofu, or one soy burger. Twenty-five to 40 milligrams of isoflavones daily may also be effective in reducing certain cancers, improving bone health and managing blood sugar.

CANCER

Isoflavones are anticarcinogens, particularly **genistein.** Genistein may help inhibit the growth of cancer cells. Miso and tofu have been used to reduce the risks of breast and prostate cancers in Japanese diets. However, some research has shown that soy foods actually *increase* certain cancers, particularly breast cancer, unless they have been consumed earlier in life. For this reason, increasing soy foods consumption may not be warranted for those with a family history of certain cancers. It is best to consult first with a health care provider [22].

MENOPAUSE

Soybeans and soy products contain **phytoestrogens**, plantlike substances that act like a weak form of estrogen in the human body. When these phytoestrogens are consumed during menopause, they behave like estrogen and may decrease headaches, insomnia and other menopausal symptoms and may protect a woman's heart and bones. These conclusions are not all borne out by clinical studies, and the effectiveness of phytoestrogens in menopause management remains controversial [23].

DIABETES

Soybeans and soy products may have a role in the management of blood sugar and be helpful in the control of diabetes. This may be due to their dietary fiber, high-quality protein, complex carbohydrates, isoflavones, phytoestrogens, protein and low Glycemic Index value. The protein and fiber in soybeans are particularly important in keeping blood sugar levels controlled.

ALLERGIES

A reason to *exclude* soybeans and soy products in the diet is the potential for food allergy. Soy is one of the main food allergens, common in infants and young children. Soy is challenging to avoid, since it is present in many processed foods, including cereals, infant formulas and salad dressings.

Just a little bit of soy can cause a host of allergic reactions that may affect the skin, respiratory and/or gastrointestinal systems. A person can be tested for a soy allergy by a skin or blood test or a supervised food challenge. If a soy allergy is confirmed, then all forms of soy should be eliminated from the diet.

QUESTIONS ABOUT SOYBEANS AND HEALTH

Since the heart-healthy claims of soy protein and the relationship of isoflavones, certain cancers and menopause have been challenged, it is wise to consider the pros and cons of soybeans for disease prevention and/or management. It may be that soybeans are beneficial to health because of other factors than soy protein, isoflavones or phytoestrogens, such as their low saturated fat content or their high content of polyunsaturated fats, fiber, vitamins and minerals.

SOYBEANS AND BIOTECHNOLOGY

The majority of soybeans and corn that is grown in the United States has been genetically modified in some way. This means that their DNA has been adapted by **biotechnology**, the science of **genetically engineered or modified foods**, for a variety of reasons—usually to help make crops stronger and microbe-resistant, impart different or better tastes, enhance nutrients, increase yield, curtail food spoilage and/or increase shelf life.

While biotechnology serves to provide long-term benefits to consumers, producers and the environment, questions about **biodiversity**, the alteration of life forms in an ecosystem, have been raised. Genetically engineered crops may replace natural weeds and challenge natural ecosystems, since gene transfer may produce new and resistant pathogens.

Other arguments against genetically modified foods center on genetically modified organisms (GMOs) that have undergone specific changes in their DNA through genetic engineering. Concern exists about the effects of ingesting foods and beverages with altered DNA. For instance, undesirable genetic mutations may lead to allergens in crops that normally do not contain allergens and negatively affect some nutritional values.

After scientific review, regulatory agencies in the United States, including the EPA, FDA and USDA, have confirmed that approved crop varieties, such as soybeans, that have undergone biotechnology are safe for consumers and the environment. The FDA's guidelines state that foods made from new crops, including those that are produced through biotechnology, must be specially labeled if they differ in composition, nutritional profile, or safety from similar crops that have not undergone biotechnology. This allows consumers to make educated and personalized food choices [24,25].

Legumes

While soybeans are the only legume with complete high-quality protein, other legumes can be complemented with dairy products, eggs, grains, nuts, seeds or vegetables to improve their protein profiles. *Legumes* are classified as *immature* and *mature*. Green beans, peas and lentils are considered immature legumes. Mature legumes are dried seeds inside pods. They contain protein, fiber, complex carbohydrates and some fat. Peanuts are mature legumes, not nuts. Other mature legumes include black beans, black-eyed peas, chick peas (garbanzos), fava beans, kidney beans, lima beans, Northern beans, mung beans and pinto beans, among others.

Legumes supply a good source of the B vitamin folic acid, as well as vitamins B1 (thiamin) and B2 (riboflavin); the minerals calcium, iron, phosphorus, potassium and selenium; and antioxidants. Because of their fiber content, legumes do not cause a rise in blood glucose, so they are considered to be low–Glycemic Index foods.

Morsel "Red beans and ricely yours." —Louis Armstrong's signature (American jazz singer and trumpeter, 1901–1971)

One-half cup serving of cooked legumes contains about 8 grams of protein, which is equal to the amount of protein in 1 ounce of cooked meat. Other nutrient comparisons between legumes and animal products are shown in Table 5-6.

210

LEGUMES IN COOKING AND BAKING

Most dried legumes require soaking in room-temperature water about 6 to 8 hours or overnight before cooking. They can also be covered with water in a pot, boiled for two minutes, and then soaked for about one hour before cooking. Soaking breaks down oligosaccharides, which are the indigestible sugars in legumes that cause intestinal distress.

TABLE 5-6 Nutrient Comparisons of Legumes to Animal Products	
Legumes	**Comparison to Animal Products**
Black beans	About as much magnesium as oysters: 60 milligrams /½ cup cooked versus 73 milligrams/4 ounces
Black-eyed peas	Highest source of folate: 179 micrograms
	More zinc than cheddar cheese: 1.32 milligrams /½ cup cooked versus 1.10 milligrams /1 ounce
Green peas	As much thiamin as salmon: .23 milligrams /½ cup cooked versus .24 milligrams /4 ounces
Lima beans	More potassium than fat-free dairy milk: 485 milligrams /½ cup cooked versus 407 milligrams /1 cup
Navy beans	Three-fourths as much phosphorus as tuna: 143 milligrams /½ cup cooked versus 185 milligrams/4 ounces
	Three-fourths as much iron as hamburger: 2.3 milligrams/½ cup cooked versus 3.13 milligrams/4 ounces
Peanut butter	Two-thirds as much niacin as turkey: 4.29 milligrams/2 tablespoons versus 6.17 milligrams /4 ounces

If legumes are labeled "quick-cooking," they have been presoaked. Canned legumes should be rinsed to remove the sodium that is added during processing. Additional guidelines for cooking legumes are included in Chapter 2. Some common uses of legumes in cooking are shown in Table 5-7.

TABLE 5-7 Common Uses of Legumes in Cooking

Types of Legumes	Common Names	Uses in Cooking
Adzuki beans	Field peas, red Oriental beans	Asian cuisine, rice dishes
Anasazi beans	Jacob's cattle beans	Southwestern cuisine, refried beans
Black beans	Turtle beans, Black Spanish beans	Mexican, Central, South Venezuelan, American cuisines, rice and bean dishes, soups, stews
Black-eyed peas	Cowpeas, cherry beans, frijoles, China and Indian peas	Southern US cuisine, bean cakes, casseroles, curries, fritters, salads
Chickpeas	Ceci, garbanzo beans	Spanish cuisine, bean spreads, casseroles, soups, stews
Fava beans	Broad beans, horse beans	Mediterranean cuisine, casseroles, side dishes, soups, stews
Lentils	French green, brown, red, dal (split)	Indian and Pakistan cuisines, salads, side dishes, soups, stews
Lima beans	Butter, Madagascar beans	Casseroles salads, sides, soups, succotash
Red kidney beans	Common bean	Cajun cuisine, casseroles, chili, salads, stews

Source: [26].

Food Allergies and Sensitivities

While protein is such a necessary component of the diet, certain proteins can be harmful to allergic and sensitive individuals. Food allergies and sensitivities can range from skin eruptions and stomachaches to difficulty breathing and even death. It is essential for food and culinary specialists to understand what causes food allergies, how they affect the body, and what actions can be taken to guard against allergic reactions to certain foods and beverages or ingredients.

The term *food allergy* is often used interchangeably for food sensitivity or intolerance. A true food allergy is an adverse reaction to a substance that involves the immune system. An example of a food allergy is a life-threatening allergic reaction to peanuts.

A *food sensitivity or intolerance* is an adverse reaction to food that does not involve the immune system. Like a food allergy, a food intolerance can be localized in a specific area of the body. For example, lactose or gluten intolerance specifically affects the gastrointestinal tract. If a person avoids a certain food but is not truly allergic to it, he or she may have a *food aversion*. For example, a wheat allergy is determined through medical testing, yet some people avoid wheat without this diagnosis.

An *adverse reaction* includes both food allergies and food sensitivities or intolerances. There are four common sites in the body where adverse reactions may occur, shown in Table 5-8.

A *food allergen* is a substance in foods or beverages that causes an allergic response by the body's immune system. Food allergens are usually harmless proteins that are perceived by the body as harmful. There are eight foods that have been determined as true food allergens: eggs, fish, milk, nuts, shellfish, soy and wheat.

TABLE 5-8 Body Sites of Food Allergies and Sensitivities with Adverse Reactions

Body Sites	Adverse Reactions
Mouth	Itching and swelling of the lips and tongue
Skin	Eczema, hives and rashes
Respiratory system	Asthma, breathing problems and wheezing
Digestive system	Cramps, diarrhea, nausea and vomiting

Antibodies or *immunoglobulins* are found in the blood and other bodily fluids. They function to recognize and neutralize allergens and other invaders, such as bacteria and viruses. When an allergic person comes into contact with a food allergen, he or she will produce the antibody *immunoglobulin E (IgE)* to combat the food allergen. IgE is specific to certain foods, such as the eight true food allergens. When activated by one of these allergens, IgE attaches to a specific cell called a *mast cell.* These mast cells store *histamines*, which are released during allergic reactions, at one or more of the common allergic sites (mouth, skin, airways or digestive tract). Histamines are compounds that the body releases in response to allergens. They trigger inflammatory responses, from itchy skin to *anaphylaxis.*

Anaphylaxis is a severe allergic reaction that affects more than one body part. It can occur within seconds and may include difficulty breathing, pale skin, low blood pressure, weak and rapid pulse, loss of consciousness, and sometimes death. Eggs, fish and shellfish, peanuts and tree nuts (almond, cashews and walnuts) are mainly associated with this potentially fatal condition.

Food and nutrition specialists should also be aware of cross reactions in food handling. *Cross reactions* are reactions to foods with similar food family characteristics. For example, if someone is allergic to cow's milk, he or she might also be allergic to goat's or sheep's milk. Other cross reactions include chicken eggs and eggs from other types of poultry, peanuts and soybeans, green beans and green peas, cod and mackerel or herring, shrimp and other shellfish, wheat and other grains such as barley and rye, pollen, almonds, corn, green apples, hazelnuts, kiwis, peaches, rye, tomatoes and wheat.

IDENTIFICATION AND TREATMENT OF FOOD ALLERGIES

True food allergies can be inherited. Cow's milk, chicken eggs and peanuts are common food allergies in children. They should be avoided in allergy-prone families, and the advice of a health care practitioner should be sought.

In 2006, the FDA updated the Food Allergen Labeling and Consumer Protection Act that requires food labels to state if food products contain any amount of the eight true food allergens. However, food allergens can come into contact with food during processing and cause *cross contamination* [27].

The use of biotechnology in our food supply may also increase the risk of exposure to food allergens, since genes are spliced onto other genes in foods that may not normally contain allergens. For example, a seafood gene can be spliced onto a tomato gene to improve the tomato's qualities. But this procedure may expose an allergic individual to the seafood gene if they eat this genetically modified tomato. This is one of the opposing arguments against the value of biotechnology.

There are no medicines or treatments to eliminate food allergies. Pharmaceuticals are available that help control the symptoms, and epinephrine is available in syringe form to help counter anaphylactic reactions.

Food allergies are on the rise in the United States, particularly in children. It is speculated that this might be the result of their immature immune systems that permit allergens to enter the bloodstream and initiate allergic reactions. Breastfeeding right after birth is recommended, especially in allergy-prone families. Colostrum, or early breastmilk, contains protective factors and helps to stimulate the immature digestive tract of children.

In highly allergic families, the eight true food allergens should be delayed or avoided until a child's immature immune system develops. Since this varies greatly, medical guidance should be sought. More information on infant and childhood feeding is found in Chapter 11.

Allergy-Free Food Service Considerations

Making a recipe from scratch does not guarantee that it is free of allergens. This is because allergens can be present in microscopic amounts in ingredients or equipment. Countless new products enter the US food supply with undetected allergens, such as nut and seed oils in salad dressing (walnut or sesame); desserts with almond paste (marzipan or frangipane) or hazelnuts (praline); sauces with gluten; and ethnic dishes with soy or peanut flour and nut and seed pastes.

212

To avoid these and other allergens, read all labels and contact the FDA with any questionable foods, beverages or ingredients. Ingredients should be stored in tightly sealed containers to prevent cross-contamination. Keep ingredient information along with the ingredients. Make sure that brands remain the same if you replace any ingredients. Work surfaces and equipment should be thoroughly sanitized, and personal sanitation should be carefully followed. More information about allergies and food sensitivity prevention in food service can be found in "Hungry for More?" at the end of this chapter.

FOOD BYTE

Color in meats and poultry is influenced by the age of the animal, diet, exercise, gender and species. The meat from older animals is darker in color because myoglobin, a muscle protein contained in tissues, increases with age. Myoglobin is purple in color, but when mixed with oxygen, it becomes bright red. Exercised muscles are darker in color, also due to myoglobin. Some hemoglobin (the iron-containing protein in red blood cells) may also appear in animal tissues after slaughter. Storage may also cause some changes in the color of meat and poultry. If safely stored, most color changes are normal [28].

Bite on This: handling protein foods safely

All foods require safe food handling to ensure the health and well-being of the consuming public. Foods with animal protein require exceptional attention to prevent contamination from foodborne illnesses that are unique to animal products. Direct contamination is attributed to direct contact with environmental contaminates, while cross-contamination is due to the transport of contaminants, generally by food handlers.

Contaminates can be biological, chemical or physical. Biological contaminants include bacteria, fungi, parasites and viruses, which can cause illness by infection, intoxication or toxin-mediated infection.

The most common bacterial foodborne pathogens are *Campylobacter jejuni*, *Escherichia coli (E.coli)*, *Listeria*, *Salmonella*, *Staphylococcus* and *Streptococcus*. *Botulism* is caused by intoxication, or poisoning by a toxic substance; Salmonella is caused by an infection, and *Clostridium* and *E. coli* are caused by toxin-mediated infections.

Chemical contaminates can be from polluted air, soil or water. Agrochemicals, animal drugs, dioxins, PCBs, pesticides and toxic metals may pose risks.

Physical contaminates include objects that mix with food during processing or handling, such as bones, hair or jewelry. Physical contamination can also occur when physical conditions are not ideal.

The conditions that foster bacterial intoxication and infections are acid/alkali balance, atmosphere, moisture, temperature and time. High-protein foods are considered potentially hazardous foods.

Simple guidelines should be followed at each stage of protein procurement, storage, preparation and cleanup to help prevent the conditions that promote bacteria from initiating and spreading, including the following:

- *Handling:* Hand washing is considered the most effective way to help prevent the spread of foodborne illness. The hands should be washed with warm soapy water for about 20 seconds before handling any protein food. Ready-to-eat food should not be handled with bare hands. Rather, disposable gloves, tongs or other clean and contaminant-free utensils should be used. Disposable gloves should be changed regularly to prevent cross-contamination.
- *Refrigeration:*
  1. Follow the *time-and-temperature principle* with foods that require refrigeration, particularly protein foods. This means keeping cold foods cold. Bacteria that cause foodborne illness thrive between 60 °F and 120 °F (16 °C and 49 °C). This is referred to as the *temperature danger zone.* The less time that high-protein foods are in this danger zone, the safer they will be to eat.
  2. Refrigerate foods at 40 °F (4 °C). Do not expose protein foods to room temperature for more than two hours, especially in warmer climates.

213

3. Avoid crowding foods; this will help to decrease cooling time and prevent possible cross-contamination.
4. Use containers that are less than 2 inches deep to decrease cooling time.

- *Freezing and thawing:*
   1. Freeze foods that are freezer-safe at 0 °F (−18 °C). Fruits and vegetables should stay freezer-safe about eight months; fish and shellfish six months; hard cheese four months; meat, poultry and medium-fat soft cheese such as curd cheese three months; fruit yogurt three months; natural yogurt two months; and homogenized milk and full-fat soft cheese such as cream cheese up to one month.
   2. Follow the expiration dates on packaged items. Discard anything that smells or tastes off-flavor.
   3. Thaw frozen foods in the refrigerator. Place on a plate or platter on a low shelf. Do not let any liquid spill onto other foods to prevent cross-contamination.
   4. Thaw frozen foods in the microwave, but cook them immediately. Microwave-thawed foods promote more bacterial growth than refrigerator-thawed foods due to warmer temperatures.
   5. Do not refreeze defrosted foods because their texture and flavor may suffer.

- *Preparation:*
   1. Use a clean cutting board and knives. Wash the cutting board and knives with hot, soapy water and then rinse with hot, clear water after use. As an alternative, wash the cutting board and knives in a dishwasher (if they are both dishwasher safe) and dry at a hot temperature.
   2. Bacteria require a specific amount of moisture to multiply. This is measured by **water activity** or **Aw**. Water activity is based on a scale of 0 to 1.0. Usually products that contain a low percentage of moisture have lower water activity. A water activity of 0.85 or greater provides the medium for bacteria to multiply. Distilled water, meat, poultry, raw bacon and soft cheese are all above this level; dry milk, dried pasta and flour are below. To prevent moisture from breeding bacteria, keep dry foods dry; refrigerate or freeze most foods that have some moisture.
   3. Foods with acid, such as citrus juice, tomatoes, vinegar or wine, have a low pH and inhibit, but do not destroy, bacteria. When using an acidic marinade with fresh meats, it is best to refrigerate the dish; then discard the marinade before cooking.

- *Cooking:*
   1. Follow the time-and-temperature principle when cooking foods: Keep hot foods hot.
   2. Heat the smallest quantity of food possible.
   3. Cook in close proximity to service time.
   4. Use a food thermometer to ensure correct temperatures.
   5. Thoroughly cook all high-protein foods.
   6. To reheat foods, heat rapidly to 165 °F (74 °C). Do not mix with fresh, uncooked food.

- *Storage:*
   1. Some bacteria need air **(aerobic bacteria)**, while others thrive without air **(anaerobic bacteria).** Some bacteria can survive in both conditions.
   2. Place leftovers into 2-inch shallow pans and cool before refrigerating or freezing.
   3. Loosely cover leftovers to allow heat to escape and to protect from accidental contamination. Cover tightly when cooled.
   4. Wrap for refrigerator or freezer.
   5. Use refrigerated foods in one or two days; freeze for longer storage [29].

FOOD BYTE

Six ounces of lean beef supply an excellent amount of protein. This amount approximates the 50 gram Daily Value for protein, based upon a 2,000-calorie diet. The suggested serving size for meats is about 3 ounces, which means that two servings of beef will meet the protein DV. Obtaining this amount of protein from nonmeat sources requires 1.38 pounds of white bread, 1.14 pounds of wheat bread, 1.6 pounds of tofu, 1.25 pounds of black beans, or 3.36 pounds of corn [30].

Bite on This: healthy protein choices

It is relatively easy to make healthy protein choices armed with some protein know-how. Choose leaner protein foods, such as select or choice grades of beef that are trimmed of fat; lean game, lamb, pork or veal; skinless white meat poultry; canned, fresh or fresh frozen fish and shellfish; egg whites; cheese with 3 grams of fat or less per ounce; and vegetable protein substitutes most of the time.

Medium- and higher-fat protein foods tend to have more calories, total fat, saturated fats and cholesterol, which may be unhealthy in excess. Here are some general guidelines for healthy protein choices:

- *Read the label.* Ground or chopped meats and poultry products, with or without seasonings, must carry mandatory food labeling, as do the major cuts of single-ingredient raw meat and poultry. As of 2010, the USDA Food Safety and Inspection Service requires that when ground or chopped products do not meet the regulatory criteria for low-fat, a lean and fat percentage statement may be included [31].
- A comparison of calories, protein and total fat in ground meat, along with the percentage of lean (protein) and fat, is shown in Table 5-9. Note that when total fat and calories increase, protein decreases. Use the leanest ground beef for the most protein.

TABLE 5-9 Comparison of Calories, Total Fat and Protein in Cooked Ground Beef

Cooked Ground Beef (3-ounce serving)	Calories (kcal)	Total Fat (grams)	Total Protein (grams)
95% lean/5% fat	145	6	22
90/10	184	10	22
85/15	197	12	21
80/20	209	14	20

- A meat processor can use a "lean" claim on the package if the contents are less than 10 grams of fat, 4.5 grams or less of saturated fat, and less than 95 mg of cholesterol per 100 grams. An "extra-lean" claim can be used if the contents are less than 5 grams of fat, 2 grams or less of saturated fat, and less than 95 mg of cholesterol per 100 grams [32].
- *Choose the leanest cuts of meat and poultry when possible.* Select meats with the least visible fat most of the time, either around the perimeter or marbled throughout the meat. USDA prime meats are well marbled and covered by thick, firm fat. USDA choice has less fat than prime but is still tender and juicy. USDA select or standard has even less fat and lacks the flavor and tenderness of choice or prime. These cuts will require more flavoring and tenderizing in preparation.
- Select or choice grades of beef include ground round, roast (chuck, rib, rump) round, sirloin, steak (cubed, flank, porterhouse, T-bone) and tenderloin. Lean pork choices include pork rib or loin chop/roast, ham or tenderloin. Lean game meats include buffalo, ostrich, rabbit and venison. Lean lamb includes chop, leg or roast. Lean veal includes loin chop and roast. While organ meats are classified as lean, they may be high in cholesterol. Processed sandwich meats and sausages with 3 grams or fewer of fat per ounce are considered lean, but they may be high in sodium.
- *Trim away most visible fat from meats and poultry before cooking*, including the skin on poultry. The exception is when roasting a whole chicken or turkey, since the skin prevents the bird from drying out during cooking. Remove the skin before eating.

FOOD BYTE

The color of chicken skin varies—just like the color of eggs that hens produce. Chicken skin can range from cream-colored to yellow. This comes from the type of feed the chickens eat and is not an indication of fat content, flavor, nutritional value or tenderness of the chicken. Growers use the type of feed that produces a desired color, which is dependent on different areas of the United States [33].

- *Substitute lower-fat ground turkey or chicken for some ground meat in recipes.* If lean ground poultry replaces all of the ground meat in a recipe, the final product may be too dry. Add a liquid ingredient to increase moisture, such as dairy milk or tomato juice. Do not add more fat or oil, since this will increase the total fat in the recipe. Skinless poultry is a versatile substitute for lean beef in some recipes, especially if they contain liquid, such as soups or stews.

Recipe: Chicken or Turkey Soup with Corn on the Cob

*The recipe for **Chicken or Turkey Soup with Corn on the Cob** in the **Recipe file** which is located within the Culinary Nutrition website at www.culinarynutrition.elsevier.com, uses lean, skinless chicken or turkey. This robust soup looks like a bunch of leftover Thanksgiving vegetables replete with succulent poultry, but a lean cut of pork or beef or even firm tofu could be easily substituted. While this soup contains the classic trilogy of carrots, celery and onions, other root vegetables may be substituted. In the summer, use fresh herbs; in the winter, dried ones will do, and the soup will take on a different character. The finished dish is shown within the centerfold **Photo file** in Plate 5.2.*

- *Use lower-fat marinades* to help tenderize meats, poultry and fish. Marinades also contribute moistness and impart flavor. Typically, lower-fat marinades have a greater percentage of acidic ingredients, such as citrus or vegetable juice, vinegar, or wine, than oil. To compensate, garlic, shallots, herbs and spices are often added.
- *Use lower-fat cooking methods,* such as baking, broiling, dry-sauteing, grilling or roasting so fat can drip away and be discarded. **Satay**, from Indonesia, yakitori from Japan, and shish kebab from Turkey are examples of dishes that are prepared in this manner. For very low-fat diets, ground meat can be rinsed and then blotted with paper towels before adding to other ingredients.
- *Cook meats in advance whenever possible* and then refrigerate. The fat should rise to the surface so it can be removed easily and discarded. Chili, soups and stews that are cooked with meat or poultry can benefit from this technique.
- *Control serving sizes.* To reduce total fat, calories, cholesterol and saturated fats, reduce the portion sizes of meats, poultry and fish. Use a 3-ounce portion of cooked animal protein, which is about the size of a deck of cards. This amounts to about half of a boneless, skinless chicken breast, one skinless chicken leg and thigh, or two slices of lean meat. Higher-fat protein foods can occasionally be consumed or used in smaller quantities. Use more vegetables or whole grains to fill out the plate

Morsel *"Rice and fish are as inseparable as mother and child."* —Vietnamese proverb

FOOD BYTE

Fish is "fast food" in terms of speed—but not in terms of calories, fat, sugar or sodium. Cooking time for fish is 10 minutes for every inch of thickness, whether it is baked, broiled, grilled or poached. If fish is frozen and unthawed, the cooking time should be doubled to 20 minutes for every inch, but it should be watched carefully in case it cooks quicker. Fish should flake in the thickest part when it is done. Let fish stand about 3 to 4 minutes to finish cooking [34].

Bite on This: cooking fish and seafood

Recommendations by the USDA, American Heart Association (AHA), and other associations suggest that fish, with its lean protein and healthful omega-3 fats, be consumed two to three times a week. The *2010 US Dietary Guidelines* recommended two (4-ounce) portions or 8 ounces for most adults and 12 ounces in total for women who are pregnant or breastfeeding [35].

Some fish contain methyl mercury, which may be harmful to the still-developing nervous system of unborn babies and young children. Large fish, such as albacore tuna, king mackerel (golden bass), shark, swordfish, and tilefish, are of particular concern. Pregnant women should not exceed 6 ounces of albacore tuna weekly.

Fish and seafood, like other animal protein foods, must be safely handled to prevent illness. Fish should be refrigerated in its original package immediately after purchase and used in one to two days. Fresh fish should be packaged for freezing and stored at 0 °F or colder.

Fish and seafood can be thawed in the refrigerator. They take about 18 to 24 hours per pound to defrost. Unwrapped packages can be placed in a bowl of cold water in the refrigerator for quicker thawing. They will take about one to two hours to defrost. Frozen fish can be cooked frozen; the defrosting stage can be skipped. They will take additional cooking time. If a recipe calls for breading or stuffing, the fish should be defrosted first. Prebreaded fish and seafood should be cooked without defrosting.

Fish and shellfish are generally classified as crustaceans, mollusks, oily fish and white fish. There are two types of white fish that are characterized by white, firm flesh: *round*, such as cod, halibut and sea bass, and *flat*, such as dover sole and tilapia, which are delicate and should be carefully handled. Mackerel and haddock are examples of oily fish. Crustaceans include crab, crawfish, lobsters and prawns. Mollusks include mussels, oysters and scallops.

Recipe: Mixed Tomato and Onion Salad with Grilled Shrimp

*Little shrimp have big taste and nutritional appeal. Four ounces of shrimp supply just 112 calories, 23.7 grams of protein (47.4% of the DV), 11.02 grams of total fat, 2.95 grams of saturated fat, and 221.13 milligrams of cholesterol. (Shrimp have actually decreased in cholesterol over the last few years.) The recipe for **Mixed Tomato and Onion Salad with Grilled Shrimp** in the **Recipe file** which is located within the* Culinary Nutrition *website at www.culinarynutrition.elsevier.com, merges their briny umami taste with tomatoes and their acidic, salty, sweet and umami tastes. Grilling adds another taste dimension. Onions add crunch and brightness to this eye-appealing dish. The finished dish is shown within the centerfold* **Photo file** *in Plate 5.3.*

217

Fish should be marinated or cooked to tenderize the connective tissue, which assists in its digestion. Cooking also enhances the flavor of fish. Suggested cooking methods include baking, broiling, microwaving, poaching and steaming. If fish is cooked too long or at temperatures that are too high, the texture and flavor can be altered. It could dry out and be tasteless.

Baking fish seals its natural juices and creates a flavorful coating. Additional fats do not have to be used; the fish stays intact and does not have to be turned, and a quantity of fish can be prepared this way.

Broiling lean fish generally requires some moisture to prevent it from drying. Butter, citrus or vegetable juice, oil, vinaigrette, wine, or some combination of ingredients can be used. The pieces of fish should be about the same size for even broiling. It is recommended that thick fish be broiled about 5 minutes per side. Thin fish may not have to be turned.

Microwaving can be used for fish fillets or steaks. To promote even heat transfer, microwave fish in a single layer. One pound of half-inch fish fillets should take about 5 to 7 minutes to cook. They should be turned about halfway through cooking.

It is best to let fish rest about 2 minutes after microwaving before serving because it continues to cook. Scallops and shrimp can be cooked by microwave until opaque in color. Cut the shellfish into the same size to promote uniform cooking. One pound of seafood may take 5 to 9 minutes of microwaving; turn after 3 to 4 minutes, and then let rest about 3 minutes before serving.

Pan-frying fish can be done with a little bit of fat or oil in a single layer to promote even cooking. Some fish can be carefully turned during pan-frying. Delicate fish should be cooked on one side only.

An option to pan-frying delicate fish is to cook it in parchment paper or foil to retain moisture, concentrate flavor, and protect its delicate flesh. Parchment paper can be used in an oven or Dutch oven; aluminum foil can also be used in the oven or on a grill.

The healthful benefit of steaming fish is that no fat or sauce is required. Fish is placed on a rack above steaming liquid that does not come in contact with the fish. The cooking liquid can be clam juice, fish broth, milk, water, wine or a combination of these liquids with citrus peel, garlic, herbs and/or spices. The flavor permeates the fish through the steam. Poached or steamed fish can be used as an appetizer or entree or as a versatile ingredient in salads, soups or casseroles.

FOOD BYTE

The bloom, or cuticle, in eggs is a waxy coating or covering that seals the eggshell's pores, prevents bacteria from getting inside the eggshell, reduces moisture loss and preserves freshness. Thousands of microscopic pores are distributed under the bloom and over the surface of the egg, with more at the larger end. These pores let moisture and carbon dioxide leave the egg and allow air to enter the egg, When eggs are washed and sanitized, the bloom dries and flakes off or is lost [36].

Bite on This: cooking eggs

Most of the protein in an egg is located inside the egg white, which changes in structure when it is beaten, heated, or mixed with acids or salts. Egg white proteins are long and compacted into spherical shapes. They are weakly held together by chemical bonds. When heat is applied, the proteins are agitated, which breaks these bonds. The long strands of protein unfold, and new bonds form into a web that captures water. With high, sustained temperature, this web becomes rubbery. Remember the last time you ate an overcooked fried egg? The egg white was probably chewy.

The reason this chemical reaction takes place is important to cooking. The protein in egg whites both attracts and repels water. Think of egg white proteins as little batteries, with one side of the egg white protein molecule that is positive and one side of the egg white protein that is negative.

Now think of these batteries all stuck together into a complex maze due to their positive and negative forces. When heated water comes into contact with these charged protein molecules, the molecules capture the water and new bonds occur. The bonds hold the cooked egg proteins together.

When egg whites are whipped for a meringue or soufflé, air is incorporated into this protein and water web, much like what happens when egg whites are heated. This increased air volume causes the egg's protein bonds to unwind and recreate a complex structure that inflates, stays intact and supports the meringue or soufflé.

While the egg white contains much of the protein, the egg yolk contains much of the fat—and some protein, too. Egg yolks are responsible for creating emulsions—suspensions of one substance within another that do not normally mix, such as oil and water.

Emulsifiers help to blend sauces, such as hollandaise and mayonnaise, into smooth consistencies. The proteins inside of egg yolks act as emulsifiers. They have the same magnetic qualities as the proteins in egg whites to hold substances together.

If eggs are eliminated in recipes, the magnetic capabilities of both egg white and egg yolk proteins may be lost. While egg replacers mimic the action of eggs, they do not replace their magnetic character.

Recipe: Spinach Pancakes

Pan "cakes," such as the recipe for **Spinach Pancakes** in the **Recipe file** which is located within the Culinary Nutrition website at www.culinarynutrition.elsevier.com, can act as a side dish for meats, poultry or fish, or hold their own for brunch or as a light entree. While two whole eggs are called for in this recipe, one whole egg may be replaced with two egg whites plus 1 teaspoon of neutral-flavored vegetable oil, such as canola, to eliminate cholesterol. Other piquant greens can be substituted for the spinach, and the chopped red pepper can be added to the batter. The finished dish in shown within the centerfold **Photo file** in Plate 5.4.

FOOD BYTE

The shelf life of dairy milk is determined by several factors, including how the dairy milk was handled and exposed to temperature changes before consumers use it. If in doubt, check with the grocer. Assuming that dairy milk is stored at 40 °F and refrigerated continually, it should last about 7 days beyond the sell-by date on the container. It is always best to smell milk before using it, and if questionable, discard it immediately [37].

Bite on This: cooking with dairy products

Dairy products have specific and important functions in cooking and baking, much like eggs. If you eliminate or substitute dairy products, the final products may lose their structure, taste and/ or texture. Knowing the food science behind dairy products in cooking and baking helps illustrate their vital roles in recipes.

Milk scorches easily if it is heated to high temperature due to its milk sugar content. It also forms a skin over the surface, which can be eliminated if it is heated quickly or lightly foamed. Whole milk or low-fat milk with 2% fat can be used for sauces because there is enough fat for creaminess. Nonfat and skim milk are too low in fat to create and hold a smooth sauce together.

Both **condensed milk** and **evaporated milk** are concentrated with some of their water removed. Condensed milk is usually sweetened and is useful in making fudge and toffee. Evaporated milk is usually unsweetened and is useful in creamy recipes, such as puddings or pie fillings. Goat's and sheep's milk have a fat content that is similar to or greater than cow's milk. They are not reliable alternatives for people with lactose intolerance, nor can they replace cow's milk in some recipes due to their taste. Coconut "milk" is a nut beverage with distinctive flavor and texture. It is higher in fat than dairy milk, but a reduced-fat variety is available. The saturated fat in coconut milk is mostly lauric acid, which may have some beneficial cardiovascular effects [38].

Cream, with its high fat content, is easier to whip than reduced-fat cream. It is also more stable and is less likely to curdle when heat is applied. Reduced-fat cream can be used to create some dessert toppings, enrich soups and add body to some sauces, but the final product may collapse. If either cream is overwhipped, it can turn into butter.

Crème fraiche is a higher-fat cream that is also slightly acidic. It has been treated with a bacterial culture similar to the production of yogurt. Because crème fraiche does not easily curdle, it can be added to warm dishes, such as casseroles, sauces, soups and stews.

Sour cream is also cultured and is lower in fat than crème fraiche (18 percent versus 39 percent), but more sour. Like crème fraiche, sour cream can be used in soups and stews. Sour cream is used in some sponge cake recipes along with cream of tartar for lightness. It lends tanginess to cheesecake and balances the sweet chocolate flavor in brownies.

Milk and cream are pasteurized by heat to kill bacteria. Unpasteurized or raw dairy milk and cream are available from local farms, but they may carry bacteria, such as *Salmonella*, *Campylobacter* or *E. coli*. Raw milk advocates maintain that raw milk contains beneficial bacteria, enzymes, immunoglobulins and vitamins that are heat sensitive and lost in pasteurization with ultra-high temperatures.

Cheese is heat-sensitive. It burns easily, and its protein can become rubbery, like egg whites. If too much heat is applied, cheese can separate into curds and whey, with a solid mass and oily residue. Cheese should be wrapped lightly and stored away from meats so as not to cross-contaminate or pick up aroma. Remove cheese about 30 minutes before serving for maximum flavor.

Pay close attention to the "use-by" dates on bottles, cartons or packages of dairy products. Some can be frozen, but the flavor and texture may be affected. Once frozen, they are best used as ingredients that are not essential to the appearance or texture of the finished dishes.

Bite on This: cooking texturized vegetable protein

Texturized soy or **vegetable protein (TVP)**, which is made from soy flour, is 50 to 70 percent protein. TVP duplicates the taste and texture of meat in recipes. It is an economical and nutritious substitute. TVP adds a significant amount of protein without cholesterol. It also supplies fiber, calcium, magnesium and potassium. A reason to be wary about TVP is a soy allergy.

If a recipe calls for one pound of ground beef, TVP can be used for all or part of it. TVP has a milder and meatier taste than tofu and readily absorbs the flavors of other foods that are cooked with it. It is particularly versatile in ground beef dishes, such as casseroles, chili, soups and stews.

Dry TVP needs to be hydrated with water or other liquid before use. Combine about $7/8$ to 1 cup of hot liquid with 1 cup of TVP. Hydration will take about 5 to 10 minutes if warmer liquid is used. Broth, fruit or vegetable juice, stock or wine can be used for all or part of the liquid. Expect the TVP to double in volume after hydration, which means for each cup of TVP and liquid, you can expect 2 cups of rehydrated TVP. If you are adding TVP to stews or soups with a lot of liquid, you can add it dry, but it will reduce the total liquid in the recipe. You may have to add additional liquid to compensate.

Dry TVP is found in bulk commercially and in some specialty food stores and supermarkets. It can also be purchased rehydrated with some seasonings and nutrient fortification. Rehydrated TVP may be found in the refrigerated or frozen sections of specialty stores.

Bite on This: proteins from the sea

Seaweed is an important part of the Asian diet. It is also consumed in the British Isles, Iceland and Scotland. *Carrageenan* and *agar-agar* are two types of seaweed that are often used in US food production. Carrageenan is made from *Irish moss*, a red algae that is also used in Irish cuisine. Carrageenan is used as a thickening agent in cottage and cream cheese, ice cream and salad dressing.

- **Agar-agar** contains a high proportion of plant-based gelatin, which makes it useful in vegetarian diets. Agar-agar thickens vegetable or fruit aspics, custards and pie fillings. It is also used to make **kanten**, a fibrous ingredient in Japanese recipes.
- **Alaria** is an olive-brown kelp (see following) with a rhubarb-like taste. It can be added to rice or pasta dishes, chopped like celery into salads, cooked in soups or stews, used as a "bed" for fish, or wrapped around seafood before steaming. Alaria becomes a uniquely bright green color when cooked.
- **Arame** is the most mild-tasting seaweed. It is easy to prepare, quick-cooking, and versatile because it does not need cooking. Arame can be used in salads, sauteed vegetable dishes and soups. It is slightly chewy.
- **Dulse** is used for salads, soups and stir-fry dishes. Dried dulse is consumed as a snack, like beef jerky. Powdered dulse can be used as a garnish or fried into chips.
- **Egregia** is a brown kelp that turns vibrant green when cooked. It can be used raw and chopped into salads or in stir-fry cooking.
- **Fucus** helps thicken broths and is sometimes added to herbal teas.
- **Hijiki** acts as a cold side dish or garnish. It has a distinguishable stringiness, and is very chewy, with a strong ocean-like taste. The color, texture and taste of hijiki pair well with delicate foods, such as fish, noodles or rice with their soft textures and lightly sweet flavors.
- **Kelp** flakes are used as a tenderizer and flavor enhancer.
- **Kombu** is made from kelp, which is consumed in Japan as a vegetable. Kombu is also processed into powders or flakes and used in braises, legumes and soups. It has a mild, ocean-like flavor.
- **Nori**, or **laver** in Irish and Welsh cuisines, is thin, dried seaweed sheets that are used in condiments, rice balls, snacks and sushi dishes. Nori adds flavor and nutrients when sprinkled over grains and vegetables. Nori flakes are about 40 percent protein and 36 percent dietary fiber.

Sea lettuce is green alga. *Ulva* sea lettuce is light green and almost transparent. It is used in breads, side dishes, soups and stews and stir-fry cooking. Because ulva is so delicate, it is added near the end of cooking.

Wakame is a type of kelp that is used in noodle dishes, soups and stir-fry cooking. In Japanese cuisine, wakame is used in miso soup and sunomono salads. It is somewhat salty, with a strong flavor of the sea.

SERVE IT FORTH

Food science continues to push the limits of the global food supply by refining existing foods and food products and creating new ones. Hundreds of years ago, eggs were whole and not liquified as they are today. Beef was featured as steaks and roasts, not formulated into patties and hot dogs. Cereals were whole grains, not formed into comical shapes and sprayed with vitamins and minerals. Today, eggs, beef and cereals are produced in countless forms with numerous ingredients. As up-and-coming nutrition, food science and culinary professionals, let your food science sides solve the following three new food challenges:

1a. Create an Allergy-Free Egg Product

Eggs have been consumed as far back as 3200 BC, first in India and then in China, Egypt and the Roman Empire, where they were eaten whole and used as thickening agents [39]. Throughout the years, nutrition, food science and culinary professionals have preserved eggs, scrambled eggs with an acidic ingredient like fruit juice to make curds, dried eggs into powder, processed eggs into portable liquids, and enhanced eggs with omega-3 fats and vitamins D and E, among other food science achievements.

While eggs are nutritious and versatile, some people restrict egg yolks due to their cholesterol content and others are allergic to the protein in egg whites. In this exercise, the challenge is to create an allergy-free egg product so allergic people can tolerate it, much like lactose-free milk can be digested by people who are lactose intolerant and gluten-free bread can be eaten by people who are gluten sensitive.

221

Some of the impressive nutrients in one large raw egg are shown in Table 5-10. Other nutrient information about eggs can be found at the Egg Nutrition Center at http://www.enc-online.org/.

TABLE 5-10 Egg Nutrition			
Nutrients in One Large Raw Egg	**Whole Egg**	**Egg White**	**Egg Yolk**
Calories (kcal)	72	17	55
Protein (grams)	6.29	3.6	2.7
Carbohydrate (grams)	0.39	0.21	0.61
Total fat (grams)	4.97	0.06	4.51
Saturated fat (grams)	1.55	0	1.624
Cholesterol (milligrams)	212	0	210
Vitamin A (International Units)	244	0	245
Vitamin D (International Units)	18	0	18
Vitamin E (milligrams)	0.48	0	0.44
Vitamin B6 (milligrams)	0.071	0.002	0.059
Vitamin B12 (micrograms)	0.65	0.03	0.33
Folate (micrograms)	24	1	25
Calcium (milligrams)	26	2	22
Sodium (milligrams)	70	55	8
Potassium (milligrams)	67	54	19
Phosphorus (milligrams)	96	5	66
Iron (milligrams)	0.92	0.03	0.46

Source: *[40]*.

Eggs function in two main roles in recipes: They bind ingredients, or hold them together, and in baked goods, eggs are used to leaven, or sometimes both to bind and leaven. The following substitutes for one large raw egg can be used to bind ingredients:

- 3½ tablespoons of gelatin blend, made from 1 cup of boiling water plus 2 teaspoons of unflavored gelatin

or

- 1 tablespoon of ground flaxseeds plus 3 tablespoons of warm water; let set about 1 minute before using

The following substitute for one large egg can be used to leaven ingredients:

- 1½ tablespoons of vegetable oil plus 1½ tablespoons of water and 1 teaspoon of baking powder, mixed well

Replacing multiple eggs in recipes is more complicated. A commercial egg replacer may be warranted. A resource for egg replacers can be found in "Hungry for More?" in this chapter. Suppose you were given the task to create an allergy-free egg product that replicates one large raw egg. Answer the following questions:

- Describe which ingredients could be used in an allergy-free egg product.
- How do the nutrients in these ingredients compare to one whole large egg?
- Consider the roles of eggs in cooking and baking. How should recipes be adjusted to accommodate for this allergy-free egg product? Support all of your comments.

2a. Create Better Beef

Laura's Lean Beef is a natural lean beef company in Kentucky that has been producing lean beef since the mid-1980s. Not only is Laura's Lean Beef lean, but it is healthful and environmentally conscious because it is raised by sustainable farming practices.

Laura's Lean Beef is produced from lean, heavily muscled cattle breeds without additives, antibiotics, fillers, growth hormones, salt or water. The beef achieves its leanness through a feed program that is based on grazing on natural grains and grasses.

Many healthful foods, like beef, are enriched and fortified today. For example, orange juice is fortified with calcium and vitamin D, and some breads and cereals are fortified with folic acid and extra fiber. The nutrients in Laura's Lean Beef are provided in Table 5-11 in comparison with other cuts of beef.

TABLE 5-11 Nutrients in Laura's Lean Beef in Comparison to Other Beef Cuts

Laura's Lean Beef 4 ounces (112 grams) uncooked	Calories (cal)	Total Fat (grams)	Saturated Fat (grams)	Cholesterol (milligrams)	Protein (grams)	Carbohydrates (grams)	Sodium (milligrams)
96% lean ground round	140	4.5	2	60	24	0	85
96% lean ground sirloin	140	4.5	2	60	24	0	85
Sirloin steak	145	5	2	65	24	0	70
In comparison							
92% lean ground beef	160	9	4	60	21	0	70
Top round	135	4	1.5	55	25	0	65
Eye of round	135	4	1.5	50	25	0	75
Rib eye steak	175	9	3.5	60	24	0	60
Strip steak	150	5	2	55	26	0	70
Flank steak	140	5	2	55	24	0	85
Tenderloin filet	145	5	2	55	25	0	80

Source: *Nutrition information submitted by Laura's Lean Beef (2012). Healthy beef nutrition facts from Laura's Lean Beef. [accessed 3.06.08]. from http://www.laurasleanbeef.com/healthy-beef [41].*

TABLE 5-12 Nutrients in Quinoa and Amaranth (½ Cup Cooked)		
Nutrients	**Quinoa**	**Amaranth**
Calories (kcal)	120	102
Total fat (grams)	2	2
Carbohydrate (grams)	21	19
Total dietary fiber (grams)	3	2
Protein (grams)	4	4
Riboflavin (milligrams)	0.1	0
Folate (micrograms)	42	22
Potassium (milligrams)	172	135
Calcium (milligrams)	17	47
Phosphorus (milligrams)	152	148
Magnesium (milligrams)	64	65
Sodium (milligrams)	7	6
Iron (milligrams)	1.5	2.1
Zinc (milligrams)	1.1	0.9
Copper (milligrams)	0.2	0.2

Source: [15].

Answer the following questions:

- While lean beef is such a good source of high-quality protein, what can be added or removed from lean beef such as Laura's to make it "Better Beef"?
- Would "Better Beef" need different grazing, feeding and/or production procedures and techniques? If so, why and which ones?
- What cooking methods and equipment would "Better Beef" require?
- What other recipe adaptations would be needed to tastefully prepare "Better Beef"?

3a. Create New Uses for Ancient Grains

The cereal grains amaranth and quinoa contain all of the essential amino acids like animal proteins. Aside from their use in hot and cold cereals and breadstuffs, amaranth and quinoa are not as commonly consumed in the United States as they are in other parts of the world. If amaranth and quinoa were more prevalent in the US food supply, they could supply high-quality protein with less fat and cholesterol than some animal products. The nutrients in amaranth and quinoa are shown in Table 5-12.

1. How could these ancient grains be incorporated into common recipes to increase their appeal, nutritional value and use? Be specific.
2. Suggest innovative uses of amaranth and quinoa in appetizers, soups, salads, entrees and desserts.
3. How do the innovative uses of amaranth and quinoa in #2 affect the nutritional values of these courses? Incorporate the nutritional information in Table 5-12 in your responses.

Three additional activities can be found within the *Culinary Nutrition* website at www.culinarynutrition. elsevier.com

WHAT'S COOKING?

1. **The properties of egg whites**
   Objectives
   - To gain knowledge about the proteins in egg whites
   - To discover how texture and consistency affect food preparation
   - To apply the characteristics of egg whites in cooking and baking
   Materials
   3 eggs at room temperature, water, bowl, 3 glasses, container with lid, flashlight, measuring spoons, egg beater or whisk, magnifying glass (optional)

Procedure

1. Separate the egg whites from the egg yolks. (Only the egg whites are needed. The yolks can be put into the container and refrigerated; place the whites into the bowl.)
2. Pour about one-third of the egg whites into a glass to a depth of about 2 inches.
3. Shine a beam of light from the flashlight through the egg whites; record what you see.
4. Fill the second glass with water. Add a teaspoon of egg whites and stir it into the water. Shine a beam of light from the flashlight through the egg white mixture; record what you see.
5. Whisk or beat the remaining egg white in the bowl until it foams but is not firm. Fill the third glass with water. Add 1 teaspoon of egg white foam to the water. Shine a beam of light from the flashlight through the egg white mixture; record what you see. You can use a magnifying glass for each of these observations.

Evaluation

Egg white is 87 percent water and 9 percent protein, with some vitamins and minerals. The shape of the proteins in the egg white affects how they react in cooking and baking. The proteins are very compacted until they are beaten or whisked, and then they unwind, or denature.

When heat and acid are applied to egg whites, they also denature. The purpose of the flashlight is to show the size of the protein molecules. They are large and remain in suspension. It is impossible to restore denatured egg whites to their original form.

Compare and contrast your recorded observations to these characteristics of egg white proteins. Did you arrive at the same conclusions? If not, assess the issues. What procedures could be done to test for the effects of heat and acid on egg white proteins?

Culinary applications

How can this information be applied to new product or recipe development?

2. **Coagulating protein with heat**

   Objectives

   - To see how liquid proteins transform into solids
   - To prepare egg custard and test the cooking times
   - To apply the characteristics of whole eggs to cooking and baking

   Materials

   Measuring cups and spoons, hand beater or whisk, bowl, ½ cup sugar, ⅛ teaspoon salt, 1 tsp vanilla, 2 cups 2% milk, 3 eggs, 4 ovenproof cups, one 9×13-inch baking pan, boiling water, oven

   Procedure

   1. Preheat oven to 325 °F.
   2. Mix sugar, salt, vanilla and milk in bowl.
   3. Add eggs; beat well.
   4. Divide egg mixture among each of the 4 ovenproof cups. Place the cups into the baking pan.
   5. Carefully fill the baking pan with 1 to 2 inches of boiling water.
   6. Place the baking pan with the custard cups on the middle rack in the preheated oven.
   7. Remove the first custard cup after 30 minutes of baking, the second after 40 minutes, the third after 50 minutes, and the fourth after one hour of baking.

   Evaluation

   When proteins coagulate, foods change from a raw to a cooked state.
   Meat, poultry, and fish firm, and baked goods change from a liquid batter to a solid form, created by weblike protein structures.

   When eggs coagulate, their proteins unravel and their colorless egg whites band together into a white solid. This band of eggs whites traps water or other liquid, such as milk. Overheating causes egg whites to toughen. They are then unable to hold any more water. When custard is cooked at the correct temperature and time, it will become semisolid, smooth and shiny. There will not be any liquid remaining.

   Compare and contrast each custard cup to the characteristics of properly made custard: semisolid, smooth and shiny. What was the effect of time and heat on each custard cup? Based on your observations, what factors in the preparation of custard are ideal?

   Culinary applications

   How can this information be applied to new product or recipe development?

3. Denaturing protein with acid

Objectives
- To separate milk into solid and liquid components
- To apply the characteristics of milk to cooking and baking

Materials
2 small jars, 2 cups whole milk, measuring spoons, vinegar, lemon juice

Procedure
1. Fill each jar with 1 cup of milk.
2. Add 2 tablespoons of vinegar to the first jar and stir.
3. Let the mixture stand for 2 to 3 minutes; note what happens.
4. Add 2 tablespoons of lemon juice to the second jar and stir.
5. Let the mixture stand for 2 to 3 minutes; note what happens.
6. Compare and contrast the two mixtures.
7. Stir the mixtures again. Does stirring affect either mixture in any way?

Evaluation
Protein can be denatured, or unwound by using acidic ingredients such as vinegar or lemon juice. Milk is a *colloid*, which is a mixture of liquids and small particles that are dispersed throughout a liquid. Both vinegar and lemon juice, which are acidic, can cause the dissolved particles to clump together and form curds. The watery liquid is called the whey. Once the milk protein is denatured and curds form, the curds cannot dissolve. Additional stirring should not make a difference.

Compare and contrast the appearance of the milk on its own, with the addition of vinegar and agitation, and with the addition of lemon juice and agitation. Compare and contrast the effects (if any) of letting the mixtures stand and stirring the mixtures again. What other combinations of ingredients may produce similar effects? How can the results of *each* of these experiments be applied to other cooking and baking conditions?

Culinary applications
How can this information be applied to new product or recipe development?

OVER EASY

The next time a hamburger or chicken breast is grilled or a bean taco or tofu stir-fry are prepared, keep in mind their foundations: protein, and how it is essential for growth, repair and maintenance. Protein is fundamental. It plays a central role in antibody, enzyme and hormone production; fluid and acid-base balance; the ability to transport substances throughout the body; and energy production, if essential.

While protein is indispensable to every living cell, remember that it is present in many foods, both animal and vegetable. It is almost impossible not to have enough protein, except in malnutrition. If you eat meat, the protein is complete, with all of the essential amino acids. If you are vegetarian, most vegetable proteins have an incomplete protein profile. It is recommended that they be complemented with other vegetable proteins to match the quality of animal protein, except for soy, quinoa and amaranth. This does not have to be at the same meal. Well-planned vegetarian diets can meet nutritional needs, particularly with the help of soy products and texturized vegetable proteins. Particular care needs to be paid to vitamins D and B12 and the minerals calcium, iron and zinc.

When protein is digested, it denatures, or changes in structure, and is broken down into its building blocks, amino acids. These amino acids rebuild into other substances or are metabolized into energy. Cooking protein by applying heat or by adding acids, such as lemon juice or vinegar, helps to break it down, much like digestion.

Too much or too little protein can be detrimental to health. Too much protein can burden the kidneys, and too little protein can lead to muscle weakness and wasting. Protein's role in disease, such as food allergies and sensitivities, is significant. Nutrition and culinary specialists must make accommodations for lactose and gluten intolerance.

Protein needs are based on body weight. Generally, the larger the individual, the more protein is required. The USDA Recommended Daily Allowance for protein based on a 2,000-calorie diet is 50 grams. This amount of protein can be translated into protein-rich foods, guide recipe and menu development, and assist label comparisons in grocery shopping.

Higher-protein and lower-carbohydrate diets are popular to help lose and maintain weight. Some of the more poorly designed higher-protein diets may result in rapid water and nutrient loss. While lean protein is very diet-friendly, too much of any one nutrient may throw off sensitive body systems. Paying attention to the right serving sizes of protein may serve one better in the long term.

New insights into higher-protein diets, raw food diets, sea proteins, irradiation and genetic engineering demonstrate that there is still much to be learned about the role of protein in health and disease.

CHECK PLEASE

1. The daily need for protein is based on:
 a. body size
 b. body frame
 c. body weight
 d. body fat
 e. body muscle
2. Lactose intolerance is a(n):
 a. allergy
 b. allergen
 c. antibody
 d. sensitivity
 e. antigen
3. Gluten intolerance is a(n):
 a. allergy
 b. allergen
 c. antigen
 d. antibody
 e. sensitivity

Essay Question

1. Which five nutrients are critical in vegetarian diets, and what are five vegetarian sources of these nutrients? Describe a meal that contains each of these food sources.

For additional questions, please see the *Culinary Nutrition* website at www.culinarynutrition.elsevier.com

HUNGRY FOR MORE?

Asthma and Allergy Foundation of America   http://www.aafa.org
Celiac Sprue Association   http://www.csaceliacs.org
Centers for Disease Control and Prevention   http://www.cdc.gov
Ener-G-Foods, Inc. (Egg Replacers)   http://www.ener-g.com
FDA Center for Food Safety and Applied Nutrition   http://vm.cfsan.fda.gov
National Cattlemen's Beef Association   http://www.beefusa.org
National Dairy Council   http://www.nationaldairycouncil.org
National Digestive Diseases Information Clearinghouse   http://digestive.niddk.nih.gov
National Fisheries Institute   http://www.aboutseafood.com
Peanut & Tree Nut Processors Association   http://www.ptnpa.org
USDA Food Safety and Inspection Service   http://www.fsis.usda.gov
USDA/FSIS Meat and Poultry Hotline   mphotline.fsis@usda.gov
US Poultry and Egg Association   http://www.poultryegg.org
US Soy Foods Director   www.soyfoods.com
The Vegetarian Resource Group   www.vrg.org

TAKE AWAY
Raw Food Diets

A *raw food diet* is based on foods that have not been heated above 115 °F (46 °C). Raw foods are often, but not always, unprocessed, unpasteurized and organic. Raw foods include some cheeses, eggs, fish, fresh herbs, fruits, meats, nuts, fresh spices, seaweeds, seeds, sprouts, vegetables and yogurt. A limited amount of processed foods may be included as long as they have not been processed at high temperatures. These may include cold pressed oils; dried fruits and vegetables; fermented foods such as kimchee, miso and sauerkraut; pure maple syrup; vinegar and foods cured in vinegar; and raw soy sauce.

> **Morsel** "The nearer the bone, the sweeter the flesh."
> —Fourteenth-century proverb

Raw foods have been consumed for thousands of years, since before the discovery of fire. There simply were no other options. Today, some raw food advocates believe that a raw foods diet is healthier than consuming cooked foods. The belief is that foods cooked above 115 °F have lost a significant amount of nutritional value and are harmful to the human body.

The reasons given for choosing a raw foods diet are disease prevention, health enhancement and weight management. Some raw food supporters believe that raw foods contain enzymes that assist digestion and improve immunity and that too much heat destroys these enzymes. Foods that have lost their natural enzymes are perceived as unhealthy and the cause of chronic disease, obesity and toxicity.

Aside from salivary amylase, most of the enzymatic action that takes place in the digestive system occurs in the stomach and small intestine. These enzymes are then denatured, or broken down, as they pass through the stomach's powerful hydrochloric acid—much like other proteins. So enzymatic digestion is only supported by a raw foods diet up to the stomach.

In addition, the shape of each enzyme uniquely determines its use in specific chemical reactions, much like the pieces of a puzzle that have only one configuration. Increasing the amount or availability of enzymes might not cause them to work harder or better if they do not fit into the right chemical reactions.

Consuming a raw foods diet requires thoughtful planning. People need the right amount of calories to maintain their ideal body weight, with enough protein, carbohydrates, lipids, vitamins, minerals and water to supply their nutrient needs.

227

A blender, dehydrator, food processor and juicer are useful pieces of equipment for preparing recipes and retaining nutrients. Some foods may still need minimal processing for healthy digestion. For example, rice needs to be sprouted to be digestible. Sprouted rice activates the enzymes and deactivates the enzyme inhibitors. Some phytochemicals can be enhanced when cooked, such as lycopene in tomatoes.

A raw food diet may not be best for people with specialized nutritional needs, such as children, pregnant and nursing women, and the elderly. Any time that a diet is restrictive, fewer nutrients may be available for increased periods of growth and repair. Additionally, heat kills some potentially fatal microorganisms. People with immature or compromised immune systems, for example, should not drink unpasteurized milk.

The benefits of a raw food diet should be weighed against the warnings, particularly for people with special nutritional and health needs. The benefits should also be weighed against the drawbacks, and one of the most important drawbacks is time. As modern life accelerates, a diet that was originally based on prehistory may be difficult to integrate into today's busy lifestyles [42–46].

Food Irradiation

Food irradiation is used in food processing to help ensure food safety. In food irradiation, ionizing radiation uses electricity, x-rays and gamma rays to destroy microorganisms, such as bacteria, viruses or insects in food. Irradiation also delays ripening, improves rehydration, increases juice yield and inhibits sprouting, which helps preserve foods and/or keeps them at their peak.

Ionizing radiation damages the microorganisms' DNA or makes them incapable of reproducing. While these effects may be mutually beneficial to consumers and the food industry, the level of radiation and the alteration of DNA in our food supply are concerns.

Irradiation does not make food radioactive. The amount of energy that is used in effective food irradiation is low compared to cooking. Processing food by ionizing radiation can split food molecules beyond what can be achieved by heating.

However, in the process of food irradiation, **unique radiolytic products** form that do not occur naturally. Concerns over their health risks have been raised, as have the potential of nutrient losses. Neither concern has been fully validated in extensive testing. However, human exposure to radiation from food processing continues to be a matter of apprehension.

Other methods besides irradiation to reduce pathogens include the gas ethylene oxide, high temperature processing, pasteurization and ultraviolet (UV) radiation. Some opponents to these methods suggest that there be better agriculture processes to help curb disease.

Food irradiation in the United States is mostly regulated by the FDA because irradiation is considered a food additive. The FDA has approved the irradiation of citrus fruits, flours, fresh and frozen meats, mushrooms, onions, potatoes, poultry, spices, strawberries, tropical fruits and wheat.

Other US agencies that regulate certain aspects of food irradiation include the US Department of Agriculture (USDA), which oversees meat and poultry products and fresh fruit; the Nuclear Regulatory Commission (NRC), which oversees the safety of processing facilities; and the Department of Transportation (DOT), which oversees the safety in transporting radioactive substances. Packaging materials must also undergo FDA approval.

An internationally recognized symbol called the **Radura logo** (Figure 5-2) must be present on all irradiated foods in the US food supply, as regulated by the FDA. Unpackaged, irradiated meat must contain this logo and the statement "Treated with irradiation" or "Treated by irradiation" at the point of sale. This logo does not have to appear on restaurant menus.

A number of international health-related organizations have approved food irradiation to control foodborne diseases. These include the World Health Organization (WHO) and the Food and Agriculture Organization (FAO) of the United Nations.

Many US supermarkets carry irradiated food products, but certain supermarkets prefer not to sell them for a variety of reasons, but mostly due to consumer perception. Food irradiation is currently permitted in many countries worldwide. Some global opponents of food irradiation claim that it affects the ecological balance, with more dependence on foreign versus locally grown foods [48–50].

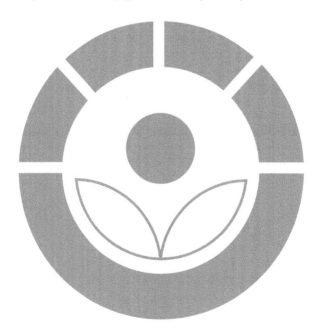

FIGURE 5-2
The Radura Logo [47].

References

[1] Perrett D. From "protein" to the beginnings of clinical proteomics. Proteomics Clin Appl 2007;1(8) 720–38.

[2] Reynolds JA, Tanford C. In: Nature's robots: a history of proteins. New York: Oxford University Press; 2003.

[3] Lappe FM. In: Diet for a small planet. Balantine Books; New York, NY 1981.

[4] National Pork Producers Council. <http://www.nppc.org>; [accessed 3.06.08].

[5] University of Wisconsin-Extension. Facts & figures about swine. <http://www.uwex.edu/ces/animalscience/swine/about.cfm>; [accessed 3.6.2008.]

[6] Institute of Medicine, Food and Nutrition Board. In: Dietary Reference Intakes for energy, carbohydrate, fiber, fat, fatty acids, cholesterol, protein, and amino acids. Washington, DC: National Academy Press; 2010.

[7] http://www.iom.edu/Global/News%20Announcements/~/media/C5CD2DD7840544979A549EC47E56A02B.ashx

[8] US Department of Agriculture (USDA). Profiling food consumption in America. http://www.usda.gov/factbook/chapter2.pdf>; [accessed 3.06.08].

[9] Condrasky M, Ledikwe JH, Flood JE, et al. Chefs' opinion of restaurant portion sizes. Obesity 2007;15:2086–94.>; [accessed 3.6.08].

[10] US Census Bureau. <http://2010.census.gov/2010census/>; [accessed 2.2.10].

[11] SelfNutritionData. Know what you eat. <http://nutritiondata.self.com/>; [accessed 3.3.12].

[12] US Food and Drug Administration (FDA). Additional requirements for nutrient content claims. <http://www.fda.gov/Food/GuidanceComplianceRegulatoryInformation/GuidanceDocuments/FoodLabelingNutrition/FoodLabelingGuide/ucm064916.htm>; [accessed 3.06.08].

[13] Snowdon DA. Animal product consumption and mortality because of all causes combined, coronary heart disease, stroke, diabetes, and cancer in Seventh-Day Adventists. Am J Clin Nutr 1988;48:739–48.

[14] Vegetarian Resource Group. Vegetarian nutrition. <http://www.vrg.org/nutrition/>; [accessed 3.06.08].

[15] US Department of Agriculture (USDA). Search the USDA National Nutrient Database for standard reference. <http://www.nal.usda.gov/fnic/foodcomp/search/>; [accessed 3.06.08].

[16] United Soybean Board. <http://www.unitedsoybean.org/>; [accessed 3.06.08]

[17] Soyinfo Center. <http://www.soyinfocenter.com>; [accessed 3.06.08].

[18] United Soybean Board. Soy lecithin fact sheet. <http://www.soyconnection.com/soyfoods/pdf/Soy-Lecithin-Fact-Sheet.pdf>; [accessed 3.06.08].

[19] US Department of Agriculture (USDA).< http://www.nal.usda.gov/fnic/foodcomp/Data/SR18/reports/sr18page.htm>; [accessed 3.06.08].

[20] US Department of Agriculture (USDA).< http://www.nal.usda.gov/fnic/foodcomp/Data/SR18/nutrlist/sr18list.html>; [accessed 3.06.08].

[21] United Soybean Board. Health claim guide for food manufacturers. <http://www.soyconnection.com/health_nutrition/heart_health/health_claim_guide.php>; [accessed 3.06.08].

[22] Messina MJ, Wood CE. Soy isoflavones, estrogen therapy, and breast cancer risk: analysis and commentary. Nutr J 2008;7:17.

[23] Creighton University Medical Center. <http://altmed.creighton.edu/SoyProtein/Scientific%20Evidence.htm>; [accessed 3.06.08].

[24] Food and Agricultural Organization of the United Nations. Agricultural biotechnology: will it help? <http://www.fao.org/english/newsroom/focus/2003/gmo1.htm>; [accessed 3.06.08].

[25] US Food and Drug Administration (FDA). <http://www.fda.gov/food/guidancecomplianceregulatoryinformation/guidancedocuments/foodlabelingnutrition/ucm059098.htm>; [accessed 2.02.08].

[26] Centers for Disease Control and Prevention (CDC). Vegetable of the month: beans. <http://www.fruitsandveggiesmatter.gov/month/beans.html>; [accessed 17.03.11].

[27] US Food and Drug Administration (FDA). Food allergen labeling and consumer protection act of 2004 questions and answers. <http://www.fda.gov/food/labelingnutrition/foodallergenslabeling/guidancecomplianceregulatoryinformation/ucm106890.htm>; [accessed 3.06.08].

[28] US Department of Agriculture (USDA). The color of meat and poultry. <http://www.fsis.usda.gov/FactSheets/Color_of_Meat_&_Poultry/index.asp>; [accessed 3.06.08].

[29] Garden-Robinson J. Food safety basics: A reference guide for foodservice operators. <http://www.ag.ndsu.edu/pubs/yf/foods/fn572.pdf>; [accessed 5.05.11].

[30] Beef.org. <www.beef.org/uDocs/Factoid%20Fighter%20Revisions%2011-03-03.doc>; [accessed 3.06.08].

[31] US Food and Drug Administration (FDA). Ingredient lists. <http://www.fda.gov/food/guidancecomplianceregulatoryinformation/guidancedocuments/foodlabelingnutrition/foodlabelingguide/ucm064880.htm>; [accessed 3.06.08].

[32] Food Safety and Inspection Service. <http://edocket.access.gpo.gov/cfr_2003/pdf/9CFR317.363.pdf

[33] FoodReference.com. <http://www.foodreference.com>; [accessed 3.06.08].

[34] Washington State Department of Health. <http://www.doh.wa.gov>; [accessed 3.06.08].

[35] US Department of Agriculture (USDA). Dietary guidelines for Americans, 2010. <http://www.cnpp.usda.gov/DGAs2010-PolicyDocument.htm>; [accessed 3.06.08].

[36] Incredible egg. <http://incredibleegg.org>; [accessed 3.06.08].

[37] Moomilk: how long after purchase will milk keep in the refrigerator? <http://www.moomilk.com/faq/2-milk-faqs/27-how-long-after-purchase-will-milk-keep-in-the-refrigerator>; [accessed 3.06.08].

[38] Mensink RP, Zock PL, Kester AD, et al. Effects of dietary fatty acids and carbohydrates on the ratio of serum total to HDL cholesterol and on serum lipids and apolipoproteins: a meta-analysis of 60 controlled trials. Am J Clin Nutr 2003;77:1146–55.

[39] Katz SH, Weaver WW. In: Encyclopedia of food and culture. New York: Charles Scribner; 2003.

[40] US Department of Agriculture (USDA). <http://www.ars.usda.gov/SP2UserFiles/Place/12354500/Data/SR23/nutrlist/sr23a421.pdf>; [accessed 3.06.08].

[41] Freedman, L. Nutrition facts, Laura's Lean Beef. <http://www.laurasleanbeef.com/nutrition-facts>; [accessed 3.06.08].

[42] Koebnick C, Garcia AL, Dagnelie PC, et al. Long-term consumption of a raw food diet is associated with favorable serum LDL cholesterol and triglycerides but also with elevated plasma homocysteine and low serum HDL cholesterol in humans. J Nutr 2005;135:2372–8.

[43] Garcia AL, Koebnick C, Dagnelie PC, et al. Long-term strict raw food diet is associated with favourable plasma beta-carotene and low plasma lycopene concentrations in Germans. Br J Nutr 2008;99:1293–300.

[44] Fontana L, Shew JL, Holloszy JO, et al. Low bone mass in subjects on a long-term raw vegetarian diet. Arch Intern Med 2005;165:684–9.

[45] Cunningham E. What is a raw foods diet and are there any risks or benefits associated with it?. J Am Diet Assoc 2004;104:1623.

[46] American Dietetic Association. Position of the American Dietetic Association and Dietitians of Canada: vegetarian diets. J Am Diet Assoc 2003;103:748–65.

[47] US Food and Drug Administration (FDA). <http://www.cfsan.fda.gov/~dms/opa-fdir.html>; [accessed 3.03.12].

[48] Wood OB, Bruhn CM. Position of the American Dietetic Association: food irradiation. J Am Diet Assoc 2000;100:246–53.

[49] Mindfully.org. Food irradiation: position of ADA. <http://www.mindfully.org/Food/Irradiation-Position-ADA.htm>; [accessed 3.06.08].

[50] US Environmental Protection Agency (EPA). Food irradiation. <http://www.epa.gov/radiation/sources/food_irrad.html>; [accessed 3.06.08].

CHAPTER 6

Lipids Basics: Fats and Oils in Foods and Health
Healthy Lipid Choices, Roles and Applications in Nutrition, Food Science and the Culinary Arts

OBJECTIVES

1. Explain why the term *lipids* is a comprehensive term for fats, oils, phospholipids and sterols
2. Describe the sources and functions of lipids in the human body
3. Explain how lipids are digested and metabolized by the human body
4. Identify how lipids are used in cooking and baking
5. Know how to decipher fat and cholesterol information on food labels

Culinary Nutrition. DOI: http://dx.doi.org/10.1016/B978-0-12-391882-6.00006-6

6. Evaluate lipid controversies
7. Understand the roles of lipids in coronary heart disease and how diet may provide prevention and reduction
8. Describe how to reduce total fat, saturated fat and cholesterol in cooking and baking
9. Clarify fat substitutes and their uses in cooking and baking
10. Discover the role of lipids in global cuisines

INTRODUCTION: FATS, OILS, PHOSPHOLIPIDS AND STEROLS

Fats and oils belong to the class of organic compounds called "lipids" that are fatty acids or their derivatives. Aside from fats and oils, lipids also include phospholipids, such as lecithin that is found in egg yolk, cholesterol and other sterols.

There are many types of lipids, including HDL and LDL cholesterol, essential fatty acids, lecithin, mono- and polyunsaturated fatty acids, omega-3 fatty acids, phospholipids, saturated fatty acids, sterols, trans fats, triglycerides and more.

Lipids have been both implicated in disease and praised for their roles in disease protection and management. In excess, lipids contribute to obesity, but some lipids are essential to the diet and defend the human body against disease. One of the goals of this chapter is to set the record straight about the roles of lipids in nutrition, health and disease. Another goal is to understand to apply this information to cooking and baking.

It is both challenging and inspiring for nutrition, food science and culinary professionals to understand where lipids come from in the diet; how they are digested, absorbed, metabolized and stored by the body; what happens if too much or too few lipids are consumed; the relationship of lipids to health and disease; how lipids are used in cooking and baking; and how lipids can be incorporated into healthy cooking and baking.

Cooking and baking depend on lipids for texture and flavor. Perfectly emulsified cream sauce, custard or mayonnaise; well-executed whipped toppings; succulent steaks and chops; rich and flavorful pastries; and delectable nuts, olives and avocadoes would simply not be as delicious without fats and oils. But a little fat or oil goes a long way, because fats and oils are so concentrated in calories and flavor.

Reduced-fat and cholesterol-free cooking and baking are tricky for both professionals and consumers. This is because fats and oils impart texture and flavor in recipes and provide functions that are challenging to duplicate. This chapter contains information about which ingredients and techniques can be utilized to replicate the flavors, functions and textures of fats and oils, and which fat and oil substitutes can be used successfully in recipes.

A solid foundation of lipid digestion and metabolism is essential to grasp the complex journey that lipids take within the body. The term *lipids* will mostly be used throughout the chapter, unless specified. Certain lipids will be highlighted for their roles in cooking and baking and their functions in the body.

MAIN COURSE
What Are Lipids?

Lipids are an all-encompassing term for a family of fats, oils, phospholipids such as lecithin and sterols such as cholesterol that are found in animals and plants. The exception is cholesterol, which is only found in animals.

Fats are solid at room temperature. Animal fats are found in foods such as bacon and sausage, butter, cheese, eggs, ice cream and meats. Vegetable fats are found in foods such as avocado, coconut, margarine, nuts, olives, peanut butter and seeds. *Oils* are liquid at room temperature. Oils include cooking oils such as canola, corn,

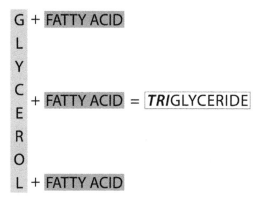

FIGURE 6-1
A triglyceride with glycerol backbone and three fatty acids.

olive, peanut, soy and vegetable; and flavoring oils, such as hazelnut, sesame, olive and walnut. *Phospholipids*, such as lecithin, are lipids that also contain the mineral phosphorus. *Lecithin* is naturally found in egg yolk, nuts and seeds and soybeans, and it is also made commercially. *Sterols* occur naturally in animal foods as *cholesterol* and in plant foods as *phytosterols*; they can also be made commercially.

Triglycerides are the main form of lipid (fat) that is found in the body and in food. A triglyceride is made of a molecule of *glycerol*, which provides the "backbone" structure for three *fatty acids.* This configuration is shown in Figure 6-1.

The fatty acids in a triglyceride can be **unsaturated** or **saturated**. **Unsaturated fatty acids** have one or more gaps within their chemical structures that are unsaturated, which means that their chemical bonds are not saturated or filled. This is a good feature, since the unsaturated fatty acid can break down at these points, which is desirable for digestion and overall health. If there is one point of unsaturation, this is called a *monounsaturated fatty acid.* If there are many points of unsaturation, this is called a *polyunsaturated fatty acid.* Monounsaturated fatty acids are more stable than polyunsaturated fatty acids.

Monounsaturated fatty acids are mostly found in vegetables oils, such as canola, olive, and peanut, and avocadoes, nuts and olives. Polyunsaturated fatty acids are mostly found in vegetable oils, such as safflower, soybean and sunflower, and fatty fish and nuts. Both mono- and polyunsaturated fatty acids have specific roles in health and disease.

As opposed to monounsaturated and polyunsaturated fatty acids, the chemical bonds in **saturated fatty acids** are all saturated or filled. As a consequence, saturated fatty acids are more difficult to undo during digestion and are a risk factor in cardiovascular and other diseases. Saturated fatty acids are mostly found in animal foods, but they are also found in foods that contain tropical oils, such as coconut or palm oil.

Trans fatty acids (or trans fats) are formed when oils are hydrogenated, or changed into saturated solid fats, such as stick margarine. Unsaturated fatty acids become saturated with the addition of hydrogen through *trans bonds.* This process of *hydrogenation* makes fatty acids with trans fats difficult for the body to eliminate. Trans fats have been implicated as a risk factor in cardiovascular disease. As of January 1, 2006, trans fatty acids must be listed on US food labels along with saturated fatty acids, total fat and cholesterol, as mandated by the FDA [1,2].

Essential fatty acids cannot be made by the body in needed amounts, so they must be consumed in the diet. They are classified as *omega-3* and *omega-6* fatty acids. Omega-3 fatty acids are found mainly in fish and fish oils, and omega-6 fatty acids are abundant in plants and plant oils.

Omega-3 fatty acids have distinct health benefits. They help reduce inflammation in the body, which is associated with disease. Some omega-6 fatty acids tend to promote inflammation. A balance of omega-3 and omega-6 fatty acids is recommended.

233

Linolenic acid is an example of an omega-3 fatty acid, and *linoleic acid* is an example of an omega-6 fatty acid. While the US diet is filled with an abundance of omega-6 fatty acids from fried foods, greater fish consumption is encouraged by the *2010 US Dietary Guidelines*.

Phospholipids, such as lecithin, serve to emulsify, or help break down, other lipids. They also provide the major structural component within cell membranes. Phospholipids are found in egg yolks, liver, peanuts, soy beans and wheat germ. A summary of lipids is shown in Table 6-1.

TABLE 6-1 Summary of Lipids

Types of Lipids	Descriptions
Fats	Lipids that are solid at room temperature
Oils	Lipids that are liquid at room temperature
Triglyceride	The major form of dietary lipids; made of glycerol and three fatty acids
Unsaturated fatty acid	A fatty acid with one or more points of unsaturation
Monounsaturated fatty acid	A fatty acid with one point of unsaturation
Polyunsaturated fatty acid	A fatty acid with many points of unsaturation
Saturated fatty acid	A fatty acid that is fully saturated
Phospholipid	A dietary lipid that is similar to a triglyceride; also contains phosphorus
Sterol	A dietary lipid with a structure that is similar to cholesterol
Trans fatty acid	A fatty acid that is formed during hydrogenation
Essential fatty acid	A fatty acid that cannot be made by the body in sufficient quantity

Bite on This: trans fatty acids

Scientific research has demonstrated that saturated fatty acids, *trans* fatty acids and dietary cholesterol raise low-density lipoprotein (LDL), which increases the risk of cardiovascular disease. Since 1993, the FDA has required that total fat, saturated fat and dietary cholesterol must be listed on food labels. Since January 1, 2006, the presence of *trans* fatty acids is also required on food labels, regulated by the FDA [1,3–6].

Prior to 2006, the average daily trans fatty acid intake was about 6 grams, or about 3 percent of total daily calories. This was roughly one-third of the amount of saturated fatty acids that were recommended in the daily diet. On the average, Americans were consuming this amount of trans fatty acids in addition to saturated fatty acids, which were already implemented with increased blood cholesterol and cardiovascular risk.

At this time, about 40 percent of trans fatty acids in the US diet were from bread, cakes, cookies, crackers and pies; 21 percent from animal products; 17 percent from margarine; 8 percent from fried potatoes; 5 percent from potato chips, corn chips and popcorn; 4 percent from vegetable shortening; 3 percent from salad dressing; 1 percent from breakfast cereal; and 1 percent from candy. Many of these products depended on trans fatty acids for flavor, texture and shelf life [7].

Research since 2006 associates trans fatty acids with increased blood cholesterol and cardiovascular disease. It suggests that the unhealthy effects of trans fatty acids are principally due to the **hydrogenation** process and that trans fats that are naturally found in foods, such as tropical oils, may not carry similar health risks.

The process of hydrogenation converts unsaturated fatty acids into saturated fatty acids by bonding hydrogen atoms and either partially hydrogenating or fully hydrogenating them. In hydrogenation, a liquid oil can be converted into a tub of soft margarine or a solid stick of margarine.

The bonds can be one of two configurations: "cis" or "trans." The trans configuration "costs" less energy and was prevalent in the food industry until its roles in increased blood cholesterol and cardiovascular disease were identified [8–10].

The food industry is investigating alternatives to trans fatty acids. Some options include animal fats, butter, coconut oil, fully hydrogenated vegetable oil, interesterification, liquid vegetable oils from advanced oil seeds, nonfats, palm oil and traditional liquid vegetable oils.

Animal fats do not all contain saturated fatty acids. For example, lard contains nearly equal amounts of mono-unsaturated and saturated fatty acids. Plus, lard is very low in myristic acid, a saturated fatty acid that has been implicated with increased LDL-cholesterol and risk of cardiovascular disease [11].

Butter contains small amounts of the saturated fatty acid lauric acid, which is also found in coconut oil and mother's milk. Butter is also a good source of conjugated linoleic acid (CLA), a natural polyunsaturated trans fat (see "Bite on This: trans fatty acids" in this chapter).

Coconut oil is also a good source of lauric acid, medium chain fatty acids, and antioxidants with anti-inflammatory properties. Medium chain fatty acids do not require energy for absorption, utilization or storage, so they are useful for people who have digestive problems.

Fully hydrogenated vegetable oils are fully saturated through conversion into solid or semisolid fats, but they do not contain trans fat. The main fatty acid in these oils is usually stearic acid. Stearic acid is associated with lowered LDL cholesterol. Fully hydrogenated vegetable oils can be blended with unhydrogenated vegetable oils to yield desirable properties [12]. Interesterification rearranges the fat molecules of oils without adding hydrogen, so very few trans fats are produced.

Selective breeding changes plants and the seeds they produce so the resulting products have desirable characteristics. Selective breeding is not genetic modification. An example of selective breeding is soybeans that have been bred with a very low level of alpha-linolenic acid (ALA). At this low level, hydrogenation is not required.

Nonfats have texture and mouthfeel that replicate fat and imitate some of its physical properties. As a result, some nonfats may be able to replace some or all of the fat in a food product.

Palm oil, like coconut oil, contains natural saturated fatty acids; particularly palmitic acid. Its role in cardiovascular disease is controversial [13,14].

Liquid vegetable oils, such as canola/rapeseed, corn, olive or soy oil, might provide some beneficial options; however, canola/rapeseed and soy oils may contain up to 5 percent trans fatty acids formed during the processing of alpha-linolenic acid.

While the food industry continues to grapple with trans fatty acid alternatives, it is important to read the Nutrition Facts Panel on food labels for foods with the least total fat, saturated fats and cholesterol that still deliver the flavor and texture that consumers desire [15–21].

235

Bite on This: essential fats: omega-3 and omega-6 fatty acids

Omega-3 Fatty Acids

Omega-3 fatty acids came to the forefront in food and nutrition about 1970. Studies of native Greenland Inuits demonstrated their very low rates of coronary heart disease despite their high fat consumption. High amounts of the essential fatty acids *eicosapentaenoic acid (EPA)* and *docosahexaenoic acid (DHA)* were present in their blood. Both are mainly found in oily, cold-water fish, such as herring, mackerel, salmon and sardines. These essential fatty acids may protect the brain, eyes and heart, and are important in normal growth and development [22].

Other than oily, cold-water fish, few foods are naturally high in omega-3 fatty acids. Eggs laid by chickens that are fed a diet of fish oils, greens or insects may be higher in omega-3 fatty acids than grass-fed beef or lamb. Canola oil, dried cloves and oregano, flaxseeds and mustard seeds, green leafy plants, red and black currant seeds, soybeans, walnuts and wheat germ contain the essential fatty acid *alpha-linolenic acid (ALA)*.

Humans can convert alpha-linolenic acid into EPA and DHA, but the ability to do this varies. Up to 80 percent of the fatty acids in leafy green plants are in the form of ALA, but leafy greens do not contribute a significant amount of ALA to the US diet. Flaxseed is the richest source of ALA. To optimize its availability to the body, flaxseed should be crushed [23].

Because the ability to convert ALA into EPA and DHA varies, essential fatty acids may be fortified in a variety of food products. But EPA and DHA are vulnerable to oxidation, which can affect the nutrient value, smell, stability and taste of food. Improved processing techniques have been used to add EPA and DHA into cookies, juices, peanut butter and yogurt and avoid oxidation issues.

The content and sources of omega-3 fatty acids are not required on food labels because there is no Recommended Daily Intake (RDI). However the FDA allows one qualified health claim for cardiovascular risk reduction by foods that contain EPA and DHA, which reads:

> Supportive but not conclusive research shows that consumption of EPA and DHA omega-3 fatty acids may reduce the risk of coronary heart disease. One serving of ____ provides ___ grams of EPA and DHA.

The contents of the food product must also meet heart-healthy nutrient values, such as low total fat, saturated fat and cholesterol.

The Accepted Intakes (AIs) of omega-3 fatty acids are 1.6 g/day for men and 1.1 g/day for women [24–26]. The American Heart Association recommends the consumption of fish at least twice a week. The AHA also recommends the consumption of tofu and other forms of soybeans; flaxseed, canola and soybean oils; and flaxseeds and walnuts with alpha-linolenic acid.

TABLE 6-2 Food Sources of Omega-3 Fatty Acids

Fish	Serving Sizes	Amount Omega-3 Fatty Acids (grams)
King mackerel	3 ounces	0.36 g
Chinook salmon	3 ounces	1.48
Herring	3 ounces	1.3–2
Atlantic wild salmon	3 ounces	0.09–1.56
Sardines	3 ounces	0.98–1.7
Oysters	3 ounces	0.75
Rainbow farmed trout	3 ounces	0.98
Halibut	3 ounces	0.60–1.12
Swordfish	3 ounces	0.97
Shrimp	3 ounces	0.4
Snapper	3 ounces	0.22
Scallops	3 ounces	1.17
Tuna, yellow fin	3 ounces	0.25
Tuna, canned light		0.26
Tuna, canned white		0.73
Cod	3 ounces	0.32
Flounder	3 ounces	0.2
Tilapia	3 ounces	0.1
Nuts and seeds		
Flax seeds	¼ cup	7
Walnuts	¼ cup	2.27
Oils		
Flaxseed/linseed oil	1 tablespoon	7.3
Walnut oil	1 tablespoon	1.4
Canola oil	1 tablespoon	1.3
Soybean oil	1 tablespoon	0.9
Other		
Soybeans	1 cup	1
Tofu	4 ounces	0.36
Kidney beans	1 cup	0.3
Winter squash	1 cup	0.3
Cloves	2 teaspoons	0.2

Source: [30].

The *2010 US Dietary Guidelines* encourages Americans to eat more fish and recognizes the role of omega-3 fatty acids in the prevention of heart disease. Two (4-ounce) servings per week in place of red meat or poultry are recommended.

The *Mediterranean Food Guide* includes fish and nuts in addition to green leafy vegetables in its recommendations. This may be one of the reasons why it is considered to be so heart-healthy [27–29]. Common sources of omega-3 fatty acids are shown in Table 6-2.

Omega-6 Fatty Acids
Omega-6 fatty acids are also essential fatty acids. They are polyunsaturated fatty acids that function to maintain bone health and the reproductive system, regulate metabolism, and stimulate hair and skin growth.

Ideally, the human body should have 2:1 ratio of omega-3 fatty acids to omega-6 fatty acids. The typical American diet, however, contains much more omega-6 fatty acids than omega-3 fatty acids. This may be problematic, since omega-3 fatty acids help to reduce inflammation, while some omega-6 fatty acids tend to promote inflammation and may lead to disease. Omega-6 fatty acids are prevalent in meats, poultry, eggs, salad dressings and fried foods.

A Mediterranean-type diet, higher in omega-3 fatty acids from fish, fresh fruits and vegetables, garlic, olive oil and whole grains, has a healthier balance of omega-3 fatty acids and omega-6 fatty acids. Those who adhere to a Mediterranean-type diet are less likely to develop coronary heart disease [31–33].

Roles of Lipids in the Body

Lipids have many important functions in the human body in health and disease. Lipids are found in every cell membrane. They serve to cushion the body and protect it from injury. They insulate the body to help keep it warm or cool as needed. Lipids help to keep the skin and hair lubricated. They transport the essential fat-soluble vitamins A, D, E and K and essential fatty acids. One of the most important functions of lipids is the provision of energy. Each gram provides 9 calories—more than twice that of carbohydrates or protein. Lipids also provide a storage form of energy for times of need.

Of particular importance to nutrition and culinary specialists is that lipids provide satiety, or satisfaction, through their aroma, taste and texture. When fats and oils are eliminated in cooking and baking, the final products can be tasteless and unsatisfying. The solution is to find the balance between function and excess: how much fat or oil is necessary for a recipe to be successful without overwhelming the palate and contributing excessive calories. Learning about the journey that lipids take in the body shows how the fats and oils in foods and beverage affect health and disease.

Lipid Digestion, Absorption, Metabolism and Storage

Butter, mayonnaise, poultry skin, nut butter, salad dressing and sausage most likely get their delicious mouthfeel from fat or oil. From the moment these buttery, creamy and fatty foods are consumed, their complex digestion begins. In general, the harder the fat, the more difficult it is for the body to process.

LIPID DIGESTION

Lipid digestion starts in the mouth, where it is mostly physical. The teeth tear apart fatty foods, and the temperature in the mouth melts some of the fats. Then the residue passes through the esophagus into the stomach, where it is churned with stomach acid and water. Some stomach acid serves to breaks down a small portion of the lipid residue, but the majority heads to the small intestine still intact.

Most of the lipids in foods are in the form of triglycerides, which must be broken down into glycerol and fatty acids for absorption. The process tends to be slow. As a result, lipids linger in the stomach, contributing to fullness or satiety. That's why a rich meal is so filling and a fat-free meal can seem so unsatisfying.

Once inside the small intestine, the smallest fatty acids, called *short-chain*, and glycerol are able to pass through the intestinal wall into the bloodstream. They are transported to the liver, where they are stored or converted into other substances.

237

The larger triglycerides are broken down by *bile* in the small intestine. Bile is an emulsifier that is made in the *liver* and stored in the *gallbladder*. Bile emulsifies lipids; it mixes lipids with watery digestive secretions and readies them for additional breakdown by enzymes. The *pancreas* then secretes the digestive enzyme *pancreatic amylase* into the small intestine, which breaks down the emulsified triglycerides into glycerol and fatty acids.

LIPID ABSORPTION

Long-chain fatty acids, phospholipids and cholesterol cannot easily travel in the bloodstream or in the *lymph*, which is watery body fluid that carries the products of fat digestion. This is because they are large molecules, and fat and water do not mix, much like vinegar and oil salad dressing.

To compensate, these lipids reform into triglycerides and are packaged inside a protein "shell" for their journey throughout the body. These protein packages are called *lipoproteins* (lipids plus protein). There are four types of lipoproteins: *low-density lipoproteins (LDL); high-density lipoproteins (HDL); very-low-density lipoproteins (VLDL);* and *chylomicrons*. Most of the lipids that are consumed in fats and oils are absorbed into the blood as lipoproteins and into the lymph as chylomicrons.

The greater the density of lipoprotein, the fewer lipids there are in the protein package. HDL contains the most protein and the least lipids; LDL are mostly cholesterol; and VLDL and chylomicrons are mostly triglycerides.

High-density lipoproteins carry cholesterol to the liver to be recycled or for disposal. For this reason, HDLs are considered to be the "good lipoproteins." *Low-density lipoproteins* carry cholesterol to the body cells. A high blood cholesterol level is usually indicative of high LDL in the blood. For this reason, LDLs are considered to be the "bad lipoproteins." *VLDLs* carry other lipids, especially triglycerides, which are made by the liver, to body tissues. *Chylomicrons* transport newly digested fat (which is mostly triglycerides) from the small intestine through the lymph and blood. What is not used by the body is returned to the liver for recycling, disposal or storage. A summary of these lipoproteins and their roles in the body is shown in Figure 6-2. To summarize:

238

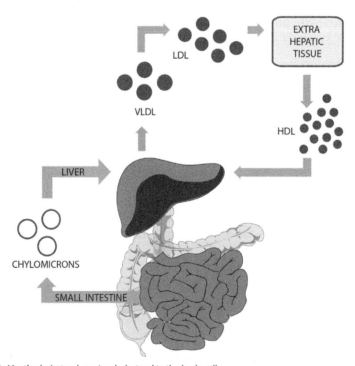

LDL: Mostly cholesterol; carries cholesterol to the body cells
HDL: Mostly protein; carries cholesterol back to the liver for recycling or disposal
VLDL: Mostly triglyceride; carries fat from the liver to the body tissues
Chylomicron: Mostly triglycerides; carries newly digested fat from the intestine through the blood and lymph

FIGURE 6-2
Lipoproteins and their roles in the body.

LIPID METABOLISM

Lipolysis is the breakdown of lipids to produce energy. When the body needs energy, stored lipids are broken down by enzymes to release glycerol and fatty acids into the bloodstream. When these fatty acids reach the muscle cells to be metabolized into energy, they enter into the mitochondria of the cell, which is the cell's powerhouse.

In the mitochondria, energy is removed from the fatty acids to produce ATP energy. ATP (*adenosine triphosphate*) is a coenzyme that transports chemical energy within the cells for metabolism. Carbon dioxide and water are also produced.

Lipids supply twice the amount of energy for ATP production than carbohydrates or protein: 9 calories per gram compared to 4 calories per gram. That is why fats and oils are so calorie-dense.

Another type of lipid metabolism, called **ketosis**, occurs in the absence of carbohydrates, which are the body's preferred energy source. Ketosis can occur in prolonged starvation or in high-protein diets that greatly reduce carbohydrate intake. Ketosis utilizes **ketones**, the by-products of stored fat, rather than glucose for energy in these special circumstances.

LIPID STORAGE

Fat cells store small droplets of fat molecules when the concentration of fatty acids in the blood rises, such as after a high-fat meal. An increase in fatty acids in the blood triggers an enzyme called **lipase**, located in fat tissue, to convert the fatty acids into triglycerides for storage in fat cells.

The majority of stored fat in the human body is under the skin, or **subcutaneous fat**. A high percentage of subcutaneous fat surrounds the breasts, buttocks, hips and waist in females. In males, most subcutaneous fat is distributed around the abdomen, buttocks and chest. There is also fat around the kidneys, liver and inside muscles.

When there is too much fat in a meal, the amount of fat in the blood rises. Unless this fat is used for body functions or energy, it can increase fat stores. Thus, too much fat in the diet can increase body fat. To help curb obesity and obesity-related diseases, nutrition and culinary specialists should familiarize themselves with ways to reduce fat in recipes and meals.

239

Another type of lipid, dietary cholesterol, also affects circulating lipids in the bloodstream and has significant effects on health and disease. Cholesterol is another important consideration in healthy cooking and baking.

Cholesterol

Cholesterol is a sterol in the lipid family. Sterols have specific bodily functions. Some of the steroid hormones, such as estrogen and testosterone, are sterols. So are *phytosterols*, which are found in plant foods, including legumes, nuts, seeds and whole grains

Cholesterol is only found in animal products, but it can be made by the body from lipids and other substances. Cholesterol has essential roles in the human body. It is an important component of cell membranes in brain and nerve cells and of bile, which helps to emulsify fats. Cholesterol helps to make the sex hormones estrogen and testosterone. A substance that resembles cholesterol in the skin is converted to a form of vitamin D when it is exposed to sunlight.

Besides its many functions, cholesterol has some drawbacks. Cholesterol can be deposited inside the walls of arteries, which contributes to the buildup of plaque. *Plaque* is a combination of calcium, cells, fibrous connective tissue, debris and lipids (cholesterol and fatty acids) that can block the arteries and lead to cardiovascular disease.

DIETARY CHOLESTEROL

Dietary cholesterol that is found in animal foods is digested and absorbed like other lipids. It is carried by lipoproteins through the bloodstream to the body cells and the liver. Low-density lipoproteins (LDLs) mainly carry cholesterol. These lipoproteins are associated with increased risk of cardiovascular disease. For this reason, LDL cholesterol is considered "bad cholesterol."

High-density lipoproteins (HDLs) carry proportionally more protein than cholesterol. They carry cholesterol in the blood back to the liver to be recycled or for disposal. For this reason, HDL cholesterol is considered "good cholesterol."

The USDA, American Heart Association and other health agencies recommend that dietary cholesterol intake be less than 300 milligrams daily. It is easy to exceed this amount by consuming a typical US diet. The amount of cholesterol in common foods is shown in Table 6-3. A person can decrease his or her intake of dietary cholesterol by eating less of some of these foods or by decreasing their portion sizes.

A 2,000-calorie diet is shown in Table 6-4. Less than 30 percent of total calories are from fat, with fewer than 20 grams (5 percent) from saturated fatty acids, and fewer than 200 milligrams of cholesterol.

TABLE 6-3 Cholesterol in Common Food and Beverages

Food and Beverages	Cholesterol (milligrams)
3 ounces pan-fried beef liver	324 mg
1 whole large egg	211
6 to 8 breaded, fried shrimp	200
3 ounces cooked salmon	74
4 ounces 80% lean broiled ground beef	77
3 ounces roasted skinless white meat turkey	58
3 ounces roasted skinless white meat chicken	73
3 ounces roasted pork leg (ham)	80
4 ounces raw oysters	56
4 ounces canned tuna in water	48
2 slices lean ham	32
1 tablespoon unsalted butter	31
1 ounce cheddar cheese	29
1 cup whole milk	24
1 ounce mozzarella cheese, part skim	18
1 cooked pork sausage link	18
1 slices beef bologna	16
1 cup plain, low-fat yogurt	14
1 cup low-fat cottage cheese	11
1 cup dairy skim milk	5
1 egg white	0

Source: [34].

TABLE 6-4 A 2,000-Calorie Total Fat, Saturated Fat and Cholesterol-Controlled Diet

Breakfast	Lunch	Dinner
½ cup grapefruit	1 cup vegetable soup	½ cup V-8 juice
1 cup whole-grain cereal	3 ounces lean hamburger	3 ounces skinless broiled chicken breast
½ medium banana	1 whole-grain hamburger bun	½ cup cooked bulgur
¼ cup cooked egg substitute	1 cup salad with deep green leafy lettuce, tomato, onions	½ cup cooked broccoli
1 slice whole-grain bread	1 tablespoon olive oil vinaigrette	1 whole-grain dinner roll
2 teaspoons margarine	½ cup fresh fruit cup	1 teaspoon margarine
1 tablespoon fruit spread	1 small oatmeal cookie	½ cup cabbage slaw with low-fat dressing
1 cup dairy skim milk	1 cup dairy skim milk	½ cup frozen yogurt
		1 cup dairy skim milk

SERUM OR BLOOD CHOLESTEROL

According to the US government and prominent health associations, total blood cholesterol should be less than 200 milligrams/deciliter, with a higher percentage of HDL cholesterol than LDL cholesterol. A total blood cholesterol level of 200 to 239 mg/dL is considered to be borderline high, while a total blood cholesterol level of 240 mg/dL and above is considered high blood cholesterol. High blood cholesterol is a risk factor in cardiovascular disease [35,36].

HDL cholesterol should be greater than or equal to 60 mg/dL for coronary heart disease protection. A HDL cholesterol level of less than 40 mg/dL is considered to be low and is a risk factor for coronary heart disease.

HDL cholesterol is more affected by a person's activity level, gender, obesity and smoking than diet. Activity helps to increase HDL cholesterol, while smoking and obesity tend to decrease it. Women tend to have higher HDL cholesterol than men due to the hormone estrogen. When estrogen decreases postmenopause, a woman is at a greater risk of cardiovascular disease. Fish and soy foods may increase HDL cholesterol, as may moderate alcohol consumption, which is considered to be two drinks per day for men and one drink per day for women.

LDL cholesterol should be less than 100 mg/dL. An LDL cholesterol level of 190 mg/dL or above is considered to be very high and a risk factor for coronary heart disease. Dietary cholesterol, saturated fat, total fat, trans fat and excess calories are some of the dietary factors that increase LDL cholesterol. Obesity, inactivity and smoking are lifestyle factors that are likely to increase LDL cholesterol.

Triglycerides should be less than 150 mg/dL. A triglyceride level of 500 mg/dL or above is considered to be very high and a risk factor for coronary heart disease. Factors that contribute to elevated triglycerides include excess alcohol consumption, inactivity, obesity and very high carbohydrate intake, as well as disease and genetic disorders.

In high-risk individuals with a family history of cardiovascular disease, these goals are even more stringent. For example, an LDL cholesterol level below 100 mg/gm/dL is recommended and a level of 70 mg/dL may be even more prudent.

A diet with less than 300 milligrams of dietary cholesterol daily may help to normalize blood cholesterol levels, while 200 milligrams of dietary cholesterol or less may be even more helpful for people with a history or risk of cardiovascular disease. Strategies to reduce blood cholesterol through diet and other means are discussed in Chapter 9 [37]. A summary of the optimal values for dietary and blood lipids as recommended by the American Heart Association is shown in Table 6-5.

241

TABLE 6-5 Optimal Daily Values for Dietary and Blood Cholesterol	
Dietary Cholesterol	**Recommendations**
Total fat	Should not exceed 30% of total calories
Saturated fats and trans fats	Should not exceed 10% of total calories
Polyunsaturated fatty acids	Should not exceed 10% of total calories
Monounsaturated fatty acids	Should not exceed 20% of total calories
Dietary cholesterol	Should not exceed 300 milligrams
Blood Cholesterol	**Recommendations**
Total blood cholesterol	Should not exceed 200 milligrams/deciliter
LDL cholesterol	Should not exceed 100 milligrams/deciliter
HDL cholesterol	Should be equal to or greater than 60 milligrams/deciliter
Triglycerides	Should not exceed 150 milligrams/deciliter

Bite on This: cholesterol controversies

The idea that lipids cause *atherosclerosis*, or hardening of the arteries, is far from a modern thought. It was originally proposed in the 1850s, when it was suggested that there was a connection between blood cholesterol and cardiovascular disease.

When cholesterol and other lipids accumulate in the artery walls, they can obstruct blood flow to the heart and its vessels. This hypothesis was further supported in the 1950s when saturated fats and cholesterol were implicated as major risk factors for cardiovascular disease.

In 1984 the National Institutes of Health (NIH) concluded that lowering blood cholesterol, specifically LDL cholesterol, reduces the risk of heart attacks that are caused by coronary heart disease. Some scientists continued to question the soundness of this conclusion [38].

This is when the *"cholesterol controversy"* unofficially began. Studies with *statins*, which are cholesterol-lowering drugs, supported the hypothesis that when blood cholesterol is reduced, there is less heart disease mortality. It was established that dietary cholesterol increased blood cholesterol levels. Current statin studies question this association. Subsequently, other factors beside dietary cholesterol have been identified that can lead to elevated blood cholesterol, such as trans fatty acids.

To help understand the cholesterol controversy, it is important to revisit what happens to dietary cholesterol once it is consumed. While animal foods contain cholesterol, the liver also manufactures cholesterol. If a person reduces dietary cholesterol, this action should help to reduce blood cholesterol and in turn coronary heart disease and the danger of a heart attack. In some individuals, this is not the case; the liver produces cholesterol over and beyond what is needed by the body, and cardiovascular disease may still develop.

Therefore, dietary cholesterol does not predict a heart attack. While dietary cholesterol can be used as a measure for those who might be at greater risk, cardiovascular disease and heart attacks are also dependent on such factors as age, diet, exercise, gender, genetics, medication, stress and other lifestyle considerations. Though there is no official proof of the association between dietary cholesterol and CHD, there is hope that dietary changes may be beneficial. Reducing hydrogenated fats, saturated fats, total fat and trans fats; incorporating mono- and polyunsaturated fats; switching to more of a plant-based diet; and undergoing weight loss to help better manage blood lipids are also sensible.

What does this controversy suggest to nutrition and culinary specialists? Lighten up! Decrease the amount of fats and oils that are used in recipes, menus and diets. Practice moderation, not deprivation, so food still tastes good.

Reducing total fat, saturated fat and cholesterol may help to decrease calories. Weight management is a preventative measure in cardiovascular disease. Incorporating more plant-based foods and meals into menus should help to decrease dietary cholesterol and calories. Using mono- and polyunsaturated fats and oils should help to improve blood lipids.

Because cardiovascular disease is multifactorial, one or two of these nutrition and culinary strategies is a start, but they may not be enough. Until the cholesterol controversy is fully answered, using a variety of these strategies in recipe development, menus and diet planning may be sensible. The relationship between dietary cholesterol and disease is discussed further in Chapter 9 [39].

Dietary Recommendations for Lipids in the Diet

The USDA Acceptable Macronutrient Distribution Range (AMDR) for total fat in the daily diet is 20 to 35 percent of total calories. The American Heart Association guideline for total fat in the daily diet is *less than* 25 to 35 percent of total calories. Based on a daily 2,000-calorie diet, this approximates:

- 400 to 700 calories from fats and oils:
  2,000 calories × .20 = 400 calories to 2,000 calories × .35 = 700 calories or ...

- 44 to 78 grams from fats and oils:
  400 calories/9 calories per gram = 44.4 grams to 700 calories/9 calories per gram = 77.7 grams [40,41]

To show how quickly this fat "allowance" can be exceeded, consider this example: One tablespoon of butter or margarine roughly contains 100 calories. To meet the daily total fat allowance of 400 to 700 calories, 4 to 7 tablespoons ($4 \times 100 = 400$ calories or $7 \times 100 = 700$ calories) could be consumed. However, the American diet is filled with high-fat animal products and fried foods. Fats and oils that are used in cooking and baking also contribute to total daily fat intake. It is easy to see how quickly daily fat intake can surpass what is recommended.

The AHA also recommends the following:

- Saturated fats should not exceed 10 percent of total daily calories.
- Trans fats should not exceed 1 percent of total daily calories.
- Any remaining fat should be obtained from monounsaturated and polyunsaturated fats from fish, nuts, seeds and vegetable oils.
- Dietary cholesterol should not exceed 300 milligrams daily.
- Higher-risk individuals should limit their saturated fat intake to no more than 7 percent of total calories and their dietary cholesterol intake to less than 200 milligrams daily.

Based on a 2,000-calorie diet, this approximates:

- No more than 200 calories from saturated fats
- No more than 20 calories from trans fats

or …

- 200 calories/9 calories per gram = 22 grams of saturated fats
- 20 calories/9 calories per gram = 2.2 grams of trans fats [42]

The foods in Table 6-6 provide about 22 grams of saturated fatty acids, 22 grams of polyunsaturated fatty acids, and 44 grams of monounsaturated fatty acids. No one food is all saturated or monounsaturated fat, but a combination.

243

TABLE 6-6 Sources of Saturated, Monounsaturated and Polyunsaturated Fatty Acids That Meet AHA Recommendations

Sources	Saturated Fatty Acids (grams)
1 ounce of cheddar cheese	6.0 g
1 cup whole milk	4.6
½ cup ice cream	4.9
3 ounces regular ground beef (25% fat)	6.1
Total saturated fatty acids	21.6

Sources	Monounsaturated Fatty Acids (grams)
2 tablespoons peanut butter	7.6 g
1 tablespoon margarine	5.4
½ cup almonds	12.2
or	
1 oz. extra-virgin olive oil	20
Total monounsaturated fatty acids	20–25.2

Sources	Polyunsaturated Fatty Acids
½ cup walnuts	23 g
or	
¼ cup mayonnaise	22
or	
4 tablespoons sesame oil	24
Total polyunsaturated fatty acids	22–24

TABLE 6-7 Daily Allowances of Total Fat and Saturated Fat at Different Calorie Levels Compared to the Daily Value

Calories	30% Total Fat		10% Saturated Fat	
	Calories	Grams	Calories	Grams
1,200	360 cal	40 g	120 cal	13 g
1,500	450	50	150	17
1,800	540	60	180	20
2,000	600	67	200	22
2,500	750	83	250	28
3,000	900	100	300	33

TABLE 6-8 A Sample Total Fat and Saturated Fat-Controlled Diet That Meets the Daily Values

Breakfast	Morning Snack
1 medium bran muffin 2 tablespoons reduced-fat cream cheese 1 cup mixed berries 1 cup dairy skim milk	6 dried apricots ¼ cup almonds

Lunch	Afternoon Snack
3 ounces lean ham 1 ounce reduced-fat Colby or cheddar cheese ¼ cup grilled onions ¼ cup grilled mushrooms 2 slices multigrain bread 2 tablespoon reduced-fat mayonnaise 1 ounce pretzels 4 each carrot, celery, bell pepper strips	1 low-fat granola bar with oats, dried fruit and nuts 1 cup dairy skim milk

Dinner	Evening Snack
1 cup romaine lettuce 2 ounces lean ground beef 1 ounce reduced-fat Colby or cheddar cheese ¼ cup diced tomatoes ¼ cup each chopped red onions and green peppers 1 ounce baked tortilla chips 2 tablespoons nonfat plain yogurt 2 tablespoons reduced-fat vinaigrette salad dressing	1 cup frozen yogurt

The daily allowances of total fat and saturated fat at different calorie levels are shown in Table 6-7. The Daily Values (DVs) are highlighted. A sample fat-controlled diet that approximates the Daily Values at 2,000 calories, with 67 grams of total fat and 22 grams of saturated fat is shown in Table 6-8.

Lipids in Health and Disease

Dietary lipids are essential to well-being, but the amount and types of lipids that are consumed matter. Needing essential dietary fats is not a license to overeat fatty foods.

The concentrated amount of calories in lipids is designed to supply energy, especially during times of need when carbohydrates are not available. When people labored all day and expended the calories they consumed, they made good use of dietary lipids. With today's labor-saving devices, there is far less need for excess lipid calories.

Lipids function as the body's thermostat. The subcutaneous layer of lipids keeps humans warm or induces perspiration for cooling, and cushions the body from shock. Lipids contribute to steroid hormones, cell membranes and bile acids, and help to regulate fluid balance. Too many or too few lipids in the diet may influence each of these delicate balances.

As we gravitate from a plant-based diet toward an animal-based diet, the composition of lipids switches to more saturated fatty acids, which are known for their relation to cardiovascular disease. Incorporating more plant-based foods and beverages into one's diet helps maintains a healthier proportion of lipids and fatty acids for good health.

LIPIDS AND LIFESTYLE

The connection among dietary fats and oils and blood fats has been established. Greater intake of saturated fatty acids and cholesterol has a direct bearing on the types and amounts of lipoproteins and cholesterol in the bloodstream.

Genetics and lifestyle factors may also affect the types and amounts of lipoproteins and cholesterol in the bloodstream. Factors that may increase LDL cholesterol include age, diabetes, family history, high blood pressure, male gender, obesity and physical inactivity.

Factors that may increase HDL cholesterol are female gender, physical activity, red wine consumption and antioxidants. Moreover, consuming foods that are high in antioxidants from fruits, vegetables and whole grains may help prevent LDL cholesterol from injuring the artery walls.

LIPIDS AND DISEASE

Besides cardiovascular disease, excess lipids are associated with cerebral vascular disease, certain cancers, diabetes, obesity and metabolic syndrome. These conditions are discussed in Chapter 9. Many risk factors that are identified with metabolic syndrome are linked to dietary lipids.

245

Bite on This: metabolic syndrome

Metabolic syndrome is a set of risk factors that predispose a person to disorders of metabolism. Metabolism is the total of chemical reactions that function to support life in living organisms. Metabolic syndrome can lead to cardiovascular disease and diabetes, among other conditions.

Many of the risk factors involved in metabolic syndrome involve dietary lipids and blood lipids, including the following:

- Abnormal abdominal obesity
- Blood clots
- Elevated blood fats, including high LDL cholesterol and triglycerides
- Elevated blood pressure
- Inflammation
- Insulin resistance or glucose intolerance
- Low HDL cholesterol
- Plaque buildup in the arteries

Abnormal abdominal obesity and insulin resistance are also precursors of diabetes.

The American Heart Association and the National Heart, Lung and Blood Institute have identified that three or more of the following risk factors increase the risks of metabolic syndrome:

- Elevated blood pressure (which may lead to hypertension): Men and women—equal to or greater than 130/85 mm Hg
- Elevated fasting blood glucose (which may lead to diabetes): Men and women—equal to or greater than 100 mg/dL
- Elevated triglycerides (which may lead to cardiovascular disease): Men and women—equal to or greater than 150 mg/dL

- Elevated waist circumference (which may lead to obesity): Men—equal to or greater than 40 inches (102 cm) Women—equal to or greater than 35 inches (88 cm)
- Reduced HDL cholesterol (which may lead to cardiovascular disease): Men—less than 40 mg/dL Women—less than 50 mg/dL

Aging, hormonal imbalance and physical inactivity are nondietary risk factors of metabolic syndrome. Goals for risk factor reduction of metabolic syndrome include weight loss to reach and maintain desirable weight (BMI less than 25 kg/m^2); at least 30 minutes of moderate-intensity activity most days; and dietary control of total fat, saturated fat, dietary cholesterol, carbohydrates and sodium [43].

The Role of Nutrition, Food Science and Culinary Professionals

At least two risk factors in metabolic syndrome—elevated waist circumference and poor insulin response—have dietary connections. Nutrition, food science and culinary professionals should team to develop products, recipes and menus that are decreased in total fat, saturated fat, dietary cholesterol, carbohydrates and sodium. These efforts may help to decrease obesity and adult-onset diabetes and halt this progressive and devastating syndrome.

One particularly important step is decreasing portion sizes. Rich protein foods can be less of a focus on the plate. Recipes can be made with less total fat, saturated fat and dietary cholesterol by using the tips and techniques found in this chapter. Refined carbohydrates can be reduced and/or replaced with whole grains, fresh fruits and vegetables to increase fiber. Sodium can be reduced and replaced by fresh and dried herbs and spices to restore flavor.

An important start in this direction is the ability of nutrition, food science and culinary professionals to purposely read food labels and apply this information in ingredient selection, cooking and baking.

Lipids on the Nutrition Facts Panel and Food Label

The FDA requires that food labels display a Nutrition Facts Panel with the Daily Values (DVs) for total fat, saturated fat and cholesterol *per serving*, based on a 2,000-calorie diet. These DVs are 65 grams of total fat, 20 grams of saturated fat, and 300 milligrams of cholesterol. This information allows the consumer to compare and contrast food products for total fat, saturated fat and cholesterol, in addition to other nutrients.

A Nutrition Facts Panel for a generic package of macaroni and cheese is shown in Figure 6-3. The following information can be determined about this product that can be compared to other brands:

- One cup of prepared macaroni and cheese has 250 calories, with 110 calories from fat.
- The total fat per serving is 12 grams, which is 18 percent of the DV.
  The number of calories of total fat is equal to 108 calories (12 grams of total fat × 9 calories/gram = 108 calories).
- The amount of saturated fat per serving is 3 grams, which is 15 percent of the DV.
  The number of calories of saturated fat is equal to 27 calories (3 grams of saturated fat × 9 calories/gram = 27 calories).
- The percentage of total fat per serving compared to total calories is 44 percent (110 calories of total fat/250 total calories × 100% = 44%). This means that almost half of one serving of macaroni and cheese is from fat.
- The percentage of saturated fat compared to total fat per serving is 24.5 percent (27 calories of saturated fat/110 calories of total fat is 24.5%). This means that almost one-fourth of the serving of macaroni and cheese is from saturated fat.
- The amount of cholesterol in one serving is 30 milligrams, which is 10 percent of the DV for cholesterol (30 milligrams of cholesterol/300 milligrams of cholesterol recommended/day=.10 × 100 = 10%). This means that 90 percent of a serving of macaroni and cheese is cholesterol-free.

Remember that this is just one food product that will be consumed over the course of a day. Aim to stay well under 100 percent of the DV for total fat, saturated fat and cholesterol. By using Nutrition Facts Panels such

Nutrition Facts

Serving Size 1 cup (228g)
Servings Per Container 2

Amount Per Serving

Calories 250	Calories from Fat 110

	% Daily Value*
Total Fat 12g	18%
Saturated Fat 3g	15%
Trans Fat 1.5g	
Cholesterol 30mg	10%
Sodium 470mg	20%
Total Carbohydrate 31g	10%
Dietary Fiber 0g	0%
Sugars 5g	
Protein 5g	

Vitamin A	4%
Vitamin C	2%
Calcium	20%
Iron	4%

* Percent Daily Values are based on a 2,000 calorie diet. Your Daily Values may be higher or lower depending on your calorie needs:

FIGURE 6-3
Nutrition facts panel for macaroni and cheese. [44]

as the one in Figure 6-3, new and revised products, recipes and menus can be devised to meet FDA and health association recommendations for good health and disease prevention.

LIPIDS ON THE FOOD LABEL

Aside from the Nutrition Facts Panel, the FDA regulates other nutritional statements on food labels, including the following:

- **Free:** A *free* food has negligible amounts of fat, saturated fat, trans fat and cholesterol.
- **Low-fat:** A *low-fat* food contains 3 grams or fewer of fat per serving. The exception is 2% milk: although it contains 5 grams of fat per serving, it can still be called low-fat.
- **Low–saturated fat:** A food that is *low in saturated fat* contains no more than 1 gram of saturated fat per serving.
- **Lean:** Lean meat, poultry, seafood or game meat that contains fewer than 10 grams of total fat; fewer than 4 grams of saturated fat; and fewer than 95 milligrams of cholesterol per 100 grams can be called *lean*.
- **Extra-lean:** Meat, poultry, seafood or game meats with fewer than 5 grams of total fat; fewer than 2 grams of saturated fat; and fewer than 95 milligrams of cholesterol per 100 grams can be called *extra-lean*.
- **Light or lite:** *Light or lite* foods are nutritionally altered, and contain one-third fewer calories than a comparable product, or they contain half of the fat of a comparable product. The food label must specify the comparable product. If *light* is used to describe the color, smell or taste of a food, it must be clearly stated.
- **Percent fat-free:** *Percent fat free* indicates the amount of a food that is "fat-free" by weight, not calories.
- **Fat-free:** *Fat-free* foods contain 0.5 grams of fat or fewer per serving, and they do not contain any added fat or oil.
- **Reduced-fat:** A *reduced-fat* food has been nutritionally altered. It contains 25 percent less of a nutrient, such as fat or calories.

- **Low-cholesterol**: *Low-cholesterol* foods contain no more than 20 milligrams of cholesterol and no more than 2 grams of saturated fat per serving.
- **Cholesterol-free**: *Cholesterol-free* foods contain 2 milligrams or fewer of cholesterol per serving and no more than 2 grams of saturated fat per serving [45,46].

HEALTH CLAIMS AND QUALIFIED CLAIMS FOR LIPIDS ON THE FOOD LABEL

Health claims that meet significant scientific agreement (SSA) and qualified health claims can appear on food labels along with their qualifications as long as they meet FDA qualifications. *Health claims* are claims that are made on food labels or dietary supplements that specifically represent or imply a relationship between a substance and a disease or health-related condition. *Qualified health claims* are claims for conventional foods and dietary supplements that are based on less scientific evidence than the standards of SSA as long as these claims do not mislead consumers. The following are examples of claim requirements, required terms and model claims among lipids and diseases:

- Health claim requirements/required terms: *"A diet low in saturated fat and cholesterol and reduced risk of coronary heart disease (CHD)."* To carry a health claim for this association, a food must meet the definitions for "low–saturated fat," "low cholesterol" and "low fat," or if it is fish or game meat, for "extra lean." It may mention the link between reduced risk of CHD as a result of lower saturated fat and cholesterol intake.

  Model claim: *"While many factors affect heart disease, diets low in saturated fat and cholesterol may reduce the risk of this disease."*
- Health claim requirements/required terms: *"Low-fat diet and reduced risk of cancers."* To carry a health claim for this association, a food must meet the nutrient content claim requirements for "low-fat" or, if it is fish or game meat, for "extra-lean."

  Model claim: *"Development of cancer depends on many factors. A diet low in total fat may reduce the risk of some cancers."*

In 2003, the FDA approved the first qualified health claim for almonds, hazelnuts, pecans, pistachios, walnuts, and peanuts.

  Model claim: *"Scientific evidence suggests but does not prove that eating 1.5 ounces per day of most nuts, as part of a diet low in saturated fat and cholesterol, may reduce the risk of heart disease."*

A 1.5-ounce serving of nuts is about one-third of a cup or a small handful.

After evaluating the research on two essential fatty acids (EPA and DHA), the FDA released the following qualified health claim to acknowledge their potential beneficial effects in reducing the risk of coronary heart disease.

  Model claim: *"Supportive but not conclusive research shows that consumption of EPA and DHA omega-3 fatty acids may reduce the risk of coronary heart disease. One serving of [name of food] provides [x] grams of EPA and DHA omega-3 fatty acids."*

The food label and Nutrition Facts Panel are powerful tools for nutrition and culinary specialists because they can guide purchasing decisions, recipe development and menu design. Reduced-fat foods may be teamed with higher-fat ingredients and vice versa so the final products are moderate in fat and calories. Understanding the roles of fats and oils in cooking and baking provides a framework for reducing, substituting and eliminating excessive lipids in the diet [47].

Fats and Oils in Cooking and Baking

Morsel "My dear boy, when curds are churned, the finest part rises upward and turns into butter. So too, dear boy, when food is eaten, the choice parts rise upward and become mind." —Chandogya Upanishad (ancient source of principal fundamentals of Vedanta [Hindu] philosophy)

Fats and oils are invaluable in cooking and baking. They provide flavor, richness, smoothness and tenderness, but also crispness. Fats and oils prevent foods from drying out; allow liquids to be heated above the boiling point of water; and dissolve in each other, but not in water. One of the greatest attributes of fats and oils in cooking and baking is their ability to create satiety or satisfaction. An overview of these characteristics precedes an in-depth look at various fats and oils.

SATIETY

Because fats and oils provide satiety or satisfaction beyond capacity, when they are absent in cooked or baked recipes, the finished products may be unsatisfactory. That is because fats and oils carry tasteful and aromatic compounds with luxurious mouthfeel. Finding comparable substitutes is challenging.

SOLUBILITY

The fact that fats and oils do not mix with water is one of their handiest features in cooking and baking. Fats and oils are large molecules that float on water due to their protective cell membranes. This makes it easy to remove fat or oil during and after cooking. Also, these large molecules have some weak bonds that allow them to stick and hold ingredients together.

CONSISTENCY

Fats and oils have consistency or uniformity, which is a valuable feature in *emulsions*. Certain lipids can *emulsify* ingredients, or create a creamy consistency between fat and liquid ingredients.

Classic emulsions are mayonnaise and hollandaise sauce. In both of these sauces, lecithin, a *phospholipid* that is found in egg yolks, acts like a group of tiny magnets that hold the fat and liquid together in a stable suspension.

Just like real magnets, imagine that these tiny magnets have different charges at their poles. Phospholipids are water-soluble at one pole and fat-soluble at the other pole, so they can hold both fat and water in suspension. Well-made mayonnaise and hollandaise sauces will stay in suspension unless they are subjected to high temperatures or stand too long. Phospholipids are also used commercially in cake mixes, margarines and salad dressings among other food products.

FUNCTIONALITY

The types of fatty acids in fats and oils affect their functions in cooking and baking. Most foods are combinations of monounsaturated, saturated and polyunsaturated fatty acids. On the whole, animal fats are about one-half saturated fatty acids and one-half unsaturated fatty acids. Beef and lamb have more saturated fatty acids than poultry or pork. Vegetable oils are about 85 percent unsaturated fatty acids, with a range of saturated fatty acids, depending on the oil source.

> **Morsel** "If you pour oil and vinegar into the same vessel, you would call them not friends but opponents." —Aeschylus (Greek playwright c. 525–456 BC)

Heat melts solid fats, and cold solidifies oils. Ingredients will melt at different rates due to their fatty acid composition. This will affect their cooking or baking times. Smoke points also vary depending on fatty acid composition. The *smoke point* is the temperature at which a fat or oil decomposes into glycerol and free fatty acids, smokes and/or burns, and produces an undesirable taste and smell.

RANCIDITY

Unsaturated fatty acids are less stable than saturated fatty acids. This makes them more vulnerable to rancidity. *Rancidity* is the oxidation of fats that is caused by hydration (water), oxidation (oxygen), metallic atoms or microbes. Rancidity often produces unusual odor and/or taste.

Some unsaturated fatty acid fragments created by oxidation give food unique volatile qualities. Consider the aroma of crushed greens, cucumbers and deep-fried foods. Antioxidants, such as beta-carotene, and vitamins C and E, can be used to prevent oxidative damage in fats and oil. So can BHA and BHT, two preservatives. Proper wrapping and storage of foods that contain fats and oils are also advised.

HYDROGENATION

Since unsaturated fatty acids are so prone to rancidity, products that contain them tend to have short shelf lives. To combat this problem, food manufacturers may chemically alter unsaturated fatty acids through a process called *hydrogenation*. Hydrogenation strengthens the chemical bonds by adding hydrogen at the points of unsaturation. The completed chemical structures closely resemble saturated fats.

The two types of chemical bonds that are used in hydrogenation are *cis* (Latin for "on this side of") and *trans* (Latin for "across from"). Both bonds firm unsaturated fatty acids so they are able to withstand atmospheric oxygen. The reformed structures are similar to saturated fatty acids. Those made with trans bonds act like saturated fatty acids in the body and cause blood lipids to rise. They can also make blood platelets sticky and can lower high-density lipoproteins (HDL), both of which increase the risk of cardiovascular disease.

The degree of hydrogenation influences the trans fat content of unsaturated fats. Partially hydrogenated fats are the main source of trans fats. They are mostly found in vegetable oils that are used for commercial baking, fried foods, and hardened margarines. This is because they are more stable at higher temperatures and have to be replaced less frequently in commercial deep fryers.

While trans fats have had wide usage in the food industry, their health issues have been under significant scrutiny (see "Bite on This: trans fats on the food label"). The limitation of trans fats in the US diet may be a significant step in cardiovascular disease reduction. The challenge to the food industry is to find practical, serviceable and healthful replacements for trans fats, which is currently underway.

Bite on This: trans fats on the food label

Until 2006, US consumers could not directly determine the presence or quantity of trans fats in food products. On July 11, 2003, the Food and Drug Administration issued a regulation that requires food manufacturers to list trans fat on the Nutrition Facts Panel of foods and some dietary supplements, which became mandatory on January 1, 2006.

While scientific reports have confirmed the relationship between trans fat and increased risk of CHD, there is not a recommended amount of trans fat that the FDA could use to establish a Percent Daily Value (%DV). This is why the US FDA does not approve nutrient content claims such as "trans fat free" or "low trans fat." Trans fat levels of less than 0.5 grams per serving can be listed as 0 grams trans fat. There is no requirement to list trans fats on institutional food packaging.

There is, however, a Percent Daily Values (%DV) shown on the Nutrition Facts Panel for saturated fat and cholesterol. To choose foods low in saturated fat and cholesterol, use the general rule of thumb that 5 percent of the DV or less is low, and 20 percent or more is high [6,48].

The Nutrition Facts Panel in Figure 6-3 includes trans fat. There are 1.5 grams of trans fat, 3 grams of saturated fat (15 percent of the DV), 12 grams of total fat (18 percent of the DV) and 30 milligrams of cholesterol (10 percent of the DV) per serving of macaroni and cheese.

To find the healthiest products, combine the number of grams of trans fat *and* saturated fat. In this product, it is 4.5 grams (1.5 grams of trans fat *plus* 3 grams of saturated fat = 4.5 grams).

Also look for the DV cholesterol. In this product it is 10 percent DV. Compare the total trans fat and saturated fat with the %DV for cholesterol. Try to find the lowest possible scores to control trans fat, saturated fat and cholesterol.

Because fat is so important for flavor, a product may need some palatable additions. A touch of sharp grated cheese right before serving may give the illusion that the macaroni and cheese is richer than it appears.

MELTING POINT

The **melting point** of fats is determined by their saturated fatty acid content. Fats melt or soften gradually over a range of temperatures, which softens their entire structure. Fats eventually turn into liquids and then gases at very high temperatures.

SMOKE POINT

The **smoke point** of fats is usually somewhere under their melting point. The smoke point occurs when fat breaks down into visible gas. In some instances, the smoke point restricts the usefulness of fats in cooking and baking. For example, canola oil has a high smoke point, which makes it excellent for frying, whereas olive oil has a lower smoke point, which makes it better for quick sautes. If an oil or fat smokes, it can affect the flavor (especially taste and smell) and appearance of a food. The smoke points of common fats and oils are provided in Chapter 2.

Overall, the more free fatty acids in a fat or oil, the lower the smoke point. This is because free fatty acids are less stable than bound fatty acids. There are more free fatty acids in refined and old vegetable oils than in unrefined fresh oils.

Refined vegetable oils are suitable for heat at 500°F (280°C) or above. These include high-oleic safflower or sunflower oils. Refined corn oil, peanut oil or soy oil can handle heat around 450°F (230°C), while fresh vegetables oils will smoke around this level. Unrefined vegetable oils should be used at temperatures below 225°F (105°C). These include canola, flaxseed, safflower and sunflower. In comparison, vegetable shortening will smoke at about 325°F (163°C); butter at about 350°F (176°C); and lard between 360°F and 400°F (182°C and 204°C).

The smoke point of margarine depends on the oil that is used in hydrogenation. Margarine made with canola, high-oleic safflower or sunflower, or soybean oil will likely have higher smoke points, while margarine made with sunflower oil may be more suitable for medium heat.

If fats or oils contain emulsifiers, preservatives or nutrients, such as proteins or carbohydrates, their smoke points may be lowered. A tall, narrow pot will decrease the amount of fat or oil that is exposed to oxygen and help to slow the fat or oil from breaking down. Reusing oil, which is sometimes done in deep-fat frying, also lowers the smoke point.

> **Morsel** "Good oil, like good wine, is a gift from the gods. The grape and the olive are among the priceless benefactions of the soil and were destined, each in its way, to promote the welfare of man."
> —George Ellwanger (author and culinarian 1848–1906)

TYPES OF FATS AND OILS

251

Recipe: Olive Oil Cake

Most cakes rely on solid fat, such as butter, margarine or shortening, to coat gluten molecules so they cannot combine and toughen the finished product. Fat also carries flavor and contributes mouthfeel. The fat in this **Olive Oil Cake** *in the* **Recipe file** *which is located within the Culinary Nutrition website at www.culinarynutrition.elsevier.com, is liquid instead of solid. The cake is moist, tender and rich-tasting from the monounsaturated fatty acids. A very small piece is very satisfying. Serve with fresh or dried fruits, as it is commonly paired in Italy. The finished dish is shown within the centerfold* **Photo file** *in Plate 6.1.*

VEGETABLE OILS

Vegetable oils are blends of oils, often made with corn, palm, soybean or sunflower oils. They can be flavored with dried or fresh herbs. Fresh vegetables, garlic and onions should be avoided, since they can promote the growth of *Clostridium botulinum*, bacteria that can lead to botulism. Botulism is a rare but life-threatening condition that can lead to paralysis.

Vegetable oils are sensitive to exposure to oxygen, heat and light. They are best stored in a cool, dark place or in the refrigerator. Refrigeration can cause oils to cloud and thicken, but this state should normalize at room temperature.

Refined oils with monounsaturated fatty acids, such as canola, olive or peanut, may be safe to use for a year or longer, as demonstrated by some high-quality extra-virgin olive oils. Oils that are high in polyunsaturated fatty acids, such as corn or safflower oil, may be safe for about six months, since they may break down faster.

The fatty acid contents of common oils and their uses in cooking and baking follow:

- *Canola oil* is made with 6 percent saturated fatty acids, 62 percent monounsaturated fatty acids and 32 percent polyunsaturated fatty acids. It primarily is used for baking, frying and salad dressings.

- *Coconut oil* is made with 92 percent saturated fatty acids, 6 percent monounsaturated fatty acids and 2 percent polyunsaturated fatty acids. It is mainly used for commercial baking, confections, frying, nondairy coffee creamers, salad dressings, shortening and whipped toppings.
- *Corn oil* is made with 13 percent saturated fatty acids, 25 percent monounsaturated fatty acids and 62 percent polyunsaturated fatty acids. It is mostly used for baking, frying, margarine, salad dressings and shortening.
- *Cottonseed oil* is made with 24 percent saturated fatty acids, 26 percent monounsaturated fatty acids and 50 percent polyunsaturated fatty acids. It is largely used for frying, margarine, salad dressings, and shortening.
- *Grape seed oil* is made with 12 percent saturated fatty acids, 17 percent monounsaturated fatty acids and 71 percent polyunsaturated fatty acids. It is generally used for all-purpose cooking, margarine, and salad dressings.
- *Olive oil* is made with 14 percent saturated fatty acids, 73 percent monounsaturated fatty acids and 11 percent polyunsaturated fatty acids. Extra-virgin olive oil is used for appetizers, dips, salads, and vegetables. Virgin olive oil is used for all-purpose cooking, margarine and salad dressing. Refined and extra-light olive oil is used for sauteing and stir-frying because it can withstand more heat than extra-virgin olive oil.

Olive oil can be used for poaching firm foods, such as halibut, which is noted for its dense and firm texture. While the fish does pick up some oil, it is mostly comprised of monounsaturated fatty acids.

Bite on This: infused oils

An *infusion* is an extract that is prepared by soaking the leaves of a plant in a liquid. When herbs and spices are soaked in oils, some of their compounds infuse into the oils. This is because herbs and spices contain essential oils with aromatic compounds. These aromatic compounds are fat soluble so they can infuse into oils and release their aromas.

Oils for infusions should have relatively neutral flavors, such as canola or safflower. Olive oil tends to have a distinct taste and become rancid quicker. Use fresh, whole leaves of herbs or spices. Ground spices should be strained through cheesecloth before bottling the oils so that they remain clear.

Make sure that herbs are washed and perfectly dried before adding to oils. This can be done by using a food dehydrator, an oven set at low temperature, or sunlight. Another option is to preserve the herbs and/or spices in a brine (salt) or vinegar solution to help prevent bacterial growth.

Do not put anything into oil that has a trace of water or other moisture. Some ingredients to avoid include fresh garlic, lemon or lemon peel, and/or fresh peppers. The water or moisture in these ingredients supports bacterial growth. Botulism bacteria spores can grow in environments such as infused oils—even if the bottles are tightly sealed.

There are two basic methods for preparing infusions: with heat and without. For the hot method, combine about 4 to 4½ cups of flavorless oil and about 1 cup of herbs and/or spices in a nonreactive saucepan over medium heat. Heat the mixture at 140°F for about 5 minutes. Remove from heat and transfer the contents to a bowl to cool; then strain the ingredients and pour the oil into bottles with airtight seals. Refrigerate.

For the cold method, gently bruise whole herbs and/or spices to release their flavors. Place into bottles and add warm oil; cool, then cover tightly and refrigerate. The oil may cloud from refrigeration, but it should return to normal at room temperature. If properly prepared, infused oils may last one to two months unless they become cloudy or odorous.

The bottles of infused oils shown in Plate 6.2 in the centerfold **Photo File**, contain basil, oregano, tarragon, rosemary and thyme. They make a herbaceous base for marinades, sauces or salad dressings. Use the stronger infusions, such as basil, oregano or rosemary, in assertive dishes. Use the delicate infusions, such as tarragon or thyme, in milder preparations.

- *Palm oil* is made with 52 percent saturated fatty acids, 38 percent monounsaturated fatty acids and 10 percent polyunsaturated fatty acids. It is chiefly used for all-purpose cooking, as well as shortening and vegetable oils and to impart flavor.

- *Peanut oil* is made with 18 percent saturated fatty acids, 49 percent monounsaturated fatty acids and 33 percent polyunsaturated fatty acids. It is principally used for frying and all-purpose cooking in addition to margarine and salad dressings.
- *Safflower oil* is made with 10 percent saturated fatty acids, 13 percent monounsaturated fatty acids and 77 percent polyunsaturated fatty acids. It is predominately used for all-purpose cooking, besides margarine and salad dressings.
- *Sesame oil (unrefined)* is made with 14 percent saturated fatty acids, 43 percent monounsaturated fatty acids and 43 percent polyunsaturated fatty acids. It is often used for deep-fat frying and in all-purpose cooking. Semirefined sesame oil has a higher smoke point than unrefined sesame oil.
- *Soybean oil* is made with 15 percent saturated fatty acids, 24 percent monounsaturated fatty acids and 61 percent polyunsaturated fatty acids. It is frequently used for all-purpose cooking, plus margarine, salad dressings, shortening and vegetable oil.
- *Sunflower oil* is made with 11 percent saturated fatty acids, 20 percent monounsaturated fatty acids and 69 percent polyunsaturated fatty acids. It is commonly used for all-purpose cooking, along with margarine, salad dressings and shortening.

BUTTER VERSUS MARGARINE

Whether to use butter or margarine has been an ongoing question since margarine was first introduced into US markets in the 1800s. Even then there were color bans and issues about margarine labeling. The decision about which spread to use in baking, cooking and spreading is many-sided. It is dependent on such factors as nutrition, performance (including smoke point) and taste.

> **Morsel** "As for butter versus margarine, I trust cows more than chemists." —Joan Dye Gussow (author, food policy expert, environmentalist, gardener and professor, 1928–)

Calorie compared to calorie, butter and margarine are close in range, but butter contains cholesterol, since it is an animal product. Margarine only contains a trace of cholesterol from dairy milk solids. Butter is a natural product, while margarine is "man-made." Most culinary professionals expound the flavor and versatility of butter. Some margarine is flavorsome as a spread and suitable in some cooking and baking applications. A comparison of these two fats offers more insights about their use.

253

Margarine

Margarine was invented by a French chemist in 1869, when fats and oils were scarce in Western Europe. It was originally an extract from animal fat, but today margarine is mostly made from vegetable oils, including corn, cottonseed, safflower, soy and sunflower.

Today, margarine comes in many forms, from a hardened stick that resembles a stick of butter to a variety of softened products in tubs and other containers. One tablespoon of stick margarine contains about 100 calories per tablespoon, 11 to 12 grams of total fat, 2 to 3 grams of saturated fat, 3 to 4 grams of polyunsaturated fat, 5 to 6 grams of monounsaturated fat and no cholesterol. It may be fortified with vitamins A and E and omega-3 (EPA) fatty acids.

As seen, most of the fat in margarine is from polyunsaturated and monounsaturated fatty acids, which vary according to the oils that are used in their production. While margarine has less saturated fatty acids than butter, it does not have the healthy saturated fatty acids, butyric acid and myristic acid, that butter does.

Margarines are chemically created during hydrogenation which, until January 1, 2006, relied upon trans fats to solidify their vegetable oils. Food companies have been exploring options for replacing trans fat in partially hydrogenated margarine.

Generally, the more solid the margarine, the more hydrogenated fat it contains, and the softer or more liquified the margarine, the less hydrogenated fat. Partially hydrogenated margarine tends to have more water or liquid vegetable oil. A growing number of tub and liquid margarines with varying amounts of partially hydrogenated vegetable oil are available.

TABLE 6-9 Comparison of Lipids in Butter and Margarine

Butter and Margarine (1 tablespoon)	Total Fat (grams)	Saturated Fat (grams)	Trans Fat (grams)	Calories (calories)	Cholesterol (milligrams)
Butter	10.8 g	7.2 g	0.3 g	108 cal	32 mg
Margarine, stick (82% fat)	11.4	2.3	2.4	101	0
Margarine, stick (68% fat)	9.5	1.6	1.8	87	0
Margarine, tub (80% fat)	11.2	1.9	1.1	101	0
Margarine-like, tub (40% fat)	7	1	0.5	46	0

The FDA has established a standard of identity for a product to be called "margarine." Margarine must contain not less than 80 percent edible fat of animal or vegetable origin; water, dairy milk or milk products; suitable edible protein; and vitamin A [49].

Some *vegetable oil spreads* that do not qualify to be called margarine contain *phytosterols*, natural plant compounds that act like sterols in the body. Phytosterols have been shown to reduce LDL cholesterol when they are consumed in the recommended amounts on the food label [50,51].

Today many margarine products contain less total fat, saturated fat and no trans fat as compared to earlier margarines. These changes have occurred in response to consumer and health professional demand to reformulate products that are reduced in total fat, saturated fat, trans fat and calories.

Butter

Butter is a dairy product that is made by churning fresh or fermented cream or buffalo, cow, goat, sheep or yak milk until the mixture solidifies. One tablespoon of butter averages 100 calories, 11 to 12 grams of total fat, 7 to 8 grams of saturated fat, 0.4 grams of polyunsaturated fat, 3 grams of monounsaturated fat, and 31 milligrams of cholesterol with vitamins A and E. Butter contains two blood cholesterol-raising substances: dietary cholesterol and saturated fat.

As described, all saturated fat is not bad, particularly short- and medium-chain saturated fatty acids. Butter has both of these fatty acids. *Butyric acid* is short chain, and *myristic acid* is medium chain. Both of these saturated fatty acids have health benefits. For example, they are easier to transport and absorb. They also help to supply flavor. In contrast, long-chain saturated fatty acids, *stearic acid* and *palmitic acid*, also found in butter, may be risk factors in cardiovascular disease in high amounts. A comparison of the nutrients in margarine and butter is shown in Table 6-9.

MARGARINE AND BUTTER IN COOKING AND BAKING

> **FOOD BYTE**
>
> *Margarine* is white, not yellow. From the late 1800s to the late 1900s, margarine that was produced in the United States looked white—its natural color—to distinguish it from butter. Most of the ingredients in margarine are colorless to white. These include a small amount of animal or dairy fat, flavorings, dairy milk solids, vegetable oil and water. A variety of colorants are now used, including beta-carotene, a natural pigment. The color of margarine today is sometimes indistinguishable from some types of butter.

Margarine in Cooking and Baking

Margarine is available in most markets in one-pound packages: four (4-ounce) sticks; two (8-ounce) tubs; one (16-ounce) tub and other containers. Stick and tub margarines have been formulated to act and spread like butter. Color and flavor extracts give margarine the appearance and aroma of butter. Some margarine contains beef tallow for flavor and functionality, but it is not used in vegetarian and vegan products. Lecithin is often added to help stabilize the liquid and reduce spattering.

Margarine readily absorbs flavors, so it should be wrapped airtight after use. It can be refrigerated up to two months or frozen up to six months.

Many different forms of margarine affect its use in cooking and baking. In general, the more oil in the product, the more total fat, and the less oil, the less total fat, which may affect texture and browning. A product with 60 percent or more oil can be used the same as butter. Products with 50 to 59 percent oil can be used for sauteing, spreading and topping. If products have 49 percent or less oil, they are best used for spreading and topping to add texture and flavor. Some of these products include the following:

- *Butter-margarine blends* are about 60 percent margarine and 40 percent butter. They provide the flavor of butter and some of its versatility in cooking and baking, without all of the cholesterol and saturated fats.
- *Cholesterol-lowering margarines* are typically made from a blend of oils, such as canola, olive, palm or soybean, and plant-based sterols and sterol esters that block the absorption of cholesterol. However, they tend to be expensive and are not substitutes for cholesterol-lowering drugs to lower blood cholesterol and decrease the risk of cardiovascular disease. It is not recommended for cooking or baking because the sterols break down with heat and the water content is too high.
- *Fat-free margarine* contains less than ½ gram of fat per serving. It may contain gelatin, lactose or rice starch stabilizers. The first ingredient on the food label of fat-free margarine is water, so it cannot be substituted for regular margarine in cooking and baking. Besides being watery, most fat-free margarine does not melt, and some scorch.
- *Light/lower fat margarine* contains no more than 40 percent oil, which is a 50 percent or more reduction in fat from regular (stick) margarine. These products should not be used in baking if precise amounts of fat and moisture are required, as in pastry crusts.
- *Liquid margarine* is soft and squeezable when cold. It is handy for basting and for quick applications, such as corn on the cob or pancakes, when a soft spread is desired.
- *Regular (stick) margarine* contains 80 percent fat with 20 percent liquid in addition to additives, coloring, flavoring and solids. It is available in salted and unsalted varieties. It can be substituted in general cooking for stick butter, which is also about 80 percent fat. Stick margarine can be creamed like butter to make frostings.
- *Reduced-fat margarine* contains no more than 60 percent oil, which is a 25 percent reduction in fat and calories from regular (stick) margarine. At 60 percent oil, reduced-fat margarine can be used in recipes that require a specific amount of fat and moisture.
- *Soft margarine* is made with all vegetable oils. It is soft and spreadable when cold, but it is too soft to cream. It is best for spreading or topping.
- *Whipped margarine* has air (as much as half of the volume) beaten into it. It is light in texture and spreadable. It cannot be substituted for regular margarine in baked goods, and it is not suitable for frying.

Morsel "Butter is life." —Indian proverb

Butter in Cooking and Baking

Butter is useful to the cook or baker as a garnish, in sauces, and as a spread, as well as for coating pans, frying and sauteing. The saturated fats in butter hold up to heat and do not gum like unsaturated fats do, but its milk solids may burn, which is why butter is clarified.

Clarified butter has been purified to separate the milk solids and water from the butterfat. It is typically produced by heating butter until the fat, milk solids and water separate by density. Clarified butter is clear when heated. In India, clarified butter is called **ghee**, which has a high smoke point and is ideal for frying and sauteing. Other types of butter include the following:

- *Cultured butter* is made from cream that has undergone some fermentation of its milk sugar. Lactic acid bacteria stimulate fermentation and create a sharp "cultured" taste. Cultured butter is the preferred butter in most of Europe.
- *Pasteurized butter* is characteristic of most butter that is available in the United States. It is made from cream that has undergone pasteurization, which kills naturally occurring bacteria. This makes it unlike cultured butter in taste.
- *Preserved butter*, such as Moroccan *smen*, is fermented, aged, and sometimes seasoned with herbs and spices.

255

- *Raw-cream butter* is made from farm-fresh, unpasteurized cream with a clean cream taste. It has a shorter shelf life than pasteurized butter.
- *Salted butter* is available in both cultured and uncultured varieties. Salted butter that contains sea salt, such as French *fleur de sel*, is used more as a condiment than for general cooking or baking.
- *Specialty butters* are made for baking and pastry. They are almost pure butterfat.
- *Sweet cream butter* is made from fresh, pasteurized cream. It is smooth, neutral in flavor, and an excellent choice for baking if it is unsalted.
- *Whipped butter* is whipped with nitrogen gas after it has been churned. It is soft at cool temperatures. Because whipped butter is low in density, it is a poor choice for cooking and baking and is best used as a spread.

Whichever fat is used in baking, cooking or consuming as a topping or a spread, consider form, function and flavor. While the content of total fat, saturated fat, trans fat and cholesterol vary, so does taste as fats and oils are altered. Plan ahead, and keep all of these considerations in mind.

> **FOOD BYTE**
>
> Schmaltz is a rich and flavorful cooking fat that is made from rendered chicken, goose or pig fat. Chicken schmaltz is common in traditional Jewish cuisine because Jewish dietary laws forbid frying meat in butter or lard. Schmaltz is used in quick sauteing and to enrich savory dishes. Schmaltz is also spread on hearty bread the same as butter and is often salted. There are vegetarian versions of schmaltz. The taste and texture are similar to chicken schmaltz, but the saturated fatty acid content may be lower.

OTHER FATS IN COOKING AND BAKING

Fat that is used for cooking from cattle or sheep is known as *suet* or *tallow*. Cooking fat from chickens, ducks or geese is known as schmaltz. Bacon grease is sometimes used in culinary applications for its rich and smoky flavor and texture. *Confit* is a process by which foods (typically poultry and meats) are slowly cooked and immersed in their own rendered fat. It is also the name of the finished product. Vegetarians can choose cooking fats from vegetarian suet, palm oil (with a comparable fatty acid ratio to lard) and pure vegetable shortening.

> **FOOD BYTE**
>
> Confit is a French method of slowly cooking meat or poultry in its own fat until it is tender. It is then covered with fat and stored. Confit has been used to preserve salt-cured duck, goose and pork. The resultant taste is salty, and the texture is moist and delicate. Confit is often paired with foods with sweet or sour tastes in stews and cassoulets, or accompanied by blander foods such as legumes, potatoes and rice. Confit also describes a process of slowly cooking onions and garlic in oil. This produces a very flavorful, reduced mixture with no cholesterol and few saturated fats.

Lard and Vegetable Shortening

Lard is fat from pigs. It has been an important ingredient for years in countries where pork is a staple food, such as in many Asian and Latino cuisines. Today, lard is popular in British, central European, Chinese and Mexican cuisines. It is used in Christmas puddings, fish and chips, lardy cake and mince pies in British cuisine; dripping or schmalz sandwiches in central European cuisines, and mixed with rice in Mexican and in Chinese cuisines. In the Jewish Orthodox and Muslim cultures the consumption of pork is prohibited by the dietary laws of *kashrut* and *halal*, respectively.

Lard has been scorned due to its saturated fat content. However, by weight, lard has less saturated fat, more unsaturated fat, and less cholesterol than an equal amount of butter as shown in Table 6-10. Beef tallow (fat) is provided for comparison.

TABLE 6-10 Comparison of Lard to Butter and Beef Tallow

Nutrients/100 grams	Lard	Butter	Beef Tallow
Carbohydrates (grams)	0	0	0
Protein (grams)	0	1	0
Total fat (grams)	100	81	100
Saturated fat (grams)	39	51	50
Monounsaturated fat (grams)	45	21	42
Polyunsaturated fat (grams)	11	10	4
Cholesterol (milligrams)	95	215	109
Calories (calories)	902	717	902

Source: [34].

Lard is available in both rendered (extracted or melted) and unrendered forms for cooking and baking and as a spread. Its flavor and culinary applications are dependent on where lard is located within the pig.

Lard is generally found in concentrations of fatty tissue. *Leaf lard* is the highest quality of lard. It is found in the "flare" deposit of fat that surrounds the kidneys, and inside the loin. *Fatback*, the next highest grade of lard, is the hard fat between the back skin and flesh. *Caul fat* is the lowest grade of lard. It surrounds the digestive organs, such as the small intestine. Caul fat is sometimes used to wrap lean meat for roasting and in pâtés.

Lard may be rendered by *wet* or *dry rendering*. *Wet rendering* is similar to braising, where the fat can be skimmed off the surface and removed. *Dry rendering* is like frying bacon; some fat can also be discarded. Wet rendered lard has a light color, neutral flavor and high smoke point. Dry rendered lard is brown in color and smoky in flavor, with a low smoke point. A by-product of dry-rendered lard is *cracklings*, which are deep-fried meat, skin and membrane tissue.

The lard that is sold in supermarkets is mostly rendered from a mixture of high- and low-quality lards. It may be bleached, deodorized, emulsified, hydrogenated or treated with antioxidants to be shelf stable.

Unlike some vegetable shortenings and margarines, unhydrogenated lard does not contain trans fat. Beef tallow is sometimes substituted for lard in baking to supply mouthfeel. While it eliminates the religious restrictions of pork, it is not suitable for vegetarians.

Due to its saturated fat content, lard has a relatively high smoke point, which makes it very useful in cooking. Its umami-like taste adds meatiness to savory dishes. Its large fat crystals help make flakier piecrusts than butter. When lard is mixed with butter in baking, it helps to create both flaky and flavorful piecrusts. Vegetable shortening in combination with butter has similar effects.

Vegetable Shortening

Vegetable shortening was developed in the early 1900s as a more economical and nutritional alternative to animal fat. It also provided a vegetable-based fat that vegetarians and people with religious dietary restrictions could use in cooking and baking.

Vegetable shortening is a semisolid fat that is mostly solid at room temperature. It is named for the "short" or crumbly texture that it produces in cooking and baking applications, particularly in shortbread, piecrusts and puff pastry. Vegetable shortening inhibits the formation of long, tough strands of gluten in dough and contributes a light texture.

Vegetable shortening is typically made from hydrogenated and partially hydrogenated vegetable oils, such as corn, cottonseed or soybean. It has a higher smoke point than butter and margarine, and is 100 percent fat (compared to butter and margarine that contain milk solids). One tablespoon of vegetable shortening has about 113 calories, 13 grams of total fat, 3 grams of saturated fat, and 0 milligrams of cholesterol. Some vegetable shortening contains 2 grams of trans fats.

The fat content of vegetable shortening makes it useful for frying and for recipes that require pure fat. It is more economical than butter or lard; does not require refrigeration (it may last up to one year in an airtight container); and can extend the shelf life of some foods and baked goods.

Some vegetable shortening contains tiny bubbles filled with nitrogen. These bubbles are useful in recipes that require leavening. These vegetable shortenings may also contain emulsifiers that help stabilize the gas-filled bubbles and disperse the fat.

When vegetable shortening is used in cookies instead of butter, the cookies may have a fluffy texture but lack flavor. If half butter and half vegetable shortening are used, both texture and flavor may improve. If butter must be excluded for religious or dietary reasons, butter flavoring or ground nuts could be added to the batter for their rich flavor and for the granular texture of nuts.

NUTS AND SEEDS

Nuts are the dry seed or fruit of plants. They are filled with protein; lipids (especially mono- and polyunsaturated fatty acids and omega-3 fatty acids); insoluble fiber; and vitamins and minerals, especially vitamin E and the B vitamins magnesium, manganese, phosphorus and zinc.

Nuts can be found fresh or dried in their shell; shelled and whole; flaked or ground; in nut butters, such as almond or cashew; and in nut oils, such as hazelnut or walnut. Nut butters can be added to soups or stews for flavor, richness and thickening, and nut oils can be mixed into salad dressings and added to baked goods for flavor and mouthfeel.

The nutrients in nuts may have protective cardiovascular benefits. In particular, the fatty acids profiles of almonds and walnuts may be helpful in lowering certain blood lipids. In addition, nuts have low Glycemic Index (GI) values, which may be useful for diabetics with insulin resistance [52,53].

Two disease-related concerns of nuts in the diet are nut allergies and aflatoxins. Tree nuts are among the most common food allergens, which were described in Chapter 5. *Aflatoxins* are poisonous substances that are formed by molds that grow on nuts, particularly in the tropics and subtropics. High levels of aflatoxins can be harmful to the liver.

If nuts have changed in appearance, odor or texture, they probably should not be consumed. That is because nuts can easily become rancid due to their high fat content. Purchase nuts in small amounts whenever possible, and store them in an airtight container in a cool, dry place away from light. Refrigerating or freezing nuts may help prevent or delay rancidity, but there might be changes in quality.

Nuts have numerous cooking and baking applications in many cuisines, including the ones that follow. The nutrient content of nuts often drives their use: fattier nuts and seeds may replicate the mouthfeel of animal fats, while drier nuts and seeds may be useful for texture and garnish.

Almonds

Almonds originated in the Middle East and are now grown in the Mediterranean region, Western Asia, California, South Australia and South Africa. Bitter almonds are used to make almond oil. Sweet almonds are used to make macaroons, marzipan, nougat and nut crusts. Almonds are also used in many savory dishes as a thickening agent and to add texture, such as in Spanish *Romesco* sauce, French *Trout Almandine*, and Indian *Chicken Korma*.

A half cup (100 grams) of almonds contains: 575 calories, 22 g carbohydrates, 12 g fiber, 21 g protein, 49 g total fat, 4 g saturated fat, 31 g monounsaturated fat, 12 g polyunsaturated fat, 0 mg cholesterol

Brazil Nuts

Brazil nuts are native to South America. They are high in fat and become rancid easily. Brazil nuts are used in baking and are especially tasty with chocolate. Their tender, mild flavor provides a rich addition to savory dishes, such as pork or beef roast.

A half cup (100 grams) of Brazil nuts contains: 656 calories, 12 g carbohydrates, 8 g fiber, 14 g protein, 66 g total fat, 15 g saturated fat, 25 g monounsaturated fat, 21 g polyunsaturated fat, 0 mg cholesterol

Cashew Nuts

Cashew nuts are native to America and are now grown in India and East Africa. Cashews are used in Asian stir-fries, curries and noodle dishes, among others. They are often matched with chicken, and they lend creaminess to sweets. Cashew butter is a rich alternative to peanut butter.

A half cup (100 grams) of cashew nuts contains: 553 calories, 33 g carbohydrates, 3 g fiber, 18 g protein, 44 g total fat, 8 g saturated fat, 29 g monounsaturated fat, 8 g polyunsaturated fat, 0 mg cholesterol

Chestnuts

Chestnuts are native to Southern Europe; especially Spain. Since chestnuts have a high starch content, they are frequently used in soups, stews and stuffing. Chestnuts are also ground into flour for cakes and fritters and preserved in syrup, called *marrons glaces*. Chestnuts should not be consumed raw because of their high level of tannic acid. In excess, tannic acid can cause ulceration of the mouth, esophagus, and gastrointestinal tract.

A half cup (100 grams) of chestnuts contains: 245 calories, 53 g carbohydrate, 5 g fiber, 3 g protein, 2 g total fat. 0.4 g saturated fat, 0.8 g monounsaturated fat, 0.9 g polyunsaturated fat, 0 mg cholesterol

Coconuts

Coconuts are common in tropical areas throughout the world. Unripe coconuts contain coconut milk, which is used in curries and soups. The nutmeat from coconuts can be found creamed, dried and fresh. Coconut is used in sweet dishes, such as ice cream or rice pudding, and in savory dishes, both as an ingredient and as a garnish. Coconut oil is used in the production of baked goods and confectionery items, margarine, and as frying oil.

A half cup (100 grams) of fresh coconut contains: 354 calories, 15 g carbohydrates, 9 g fiber, 3 g protein, 33 g total fat, 30 g saturated fat, 1.4 g monounsaturated fat, 0.4 g polyunsaturated fat, 0 mg cholesterol

Hazelnuts

Hazelnuts are common in Europe, particularly in Britain, and in Asia, particularly in Turkey. They are available flaked, ground and whole, and are also made into oil and nut butter. Hazelnuts can be used in sweet recipes such as praline, and they pair well with chocolate. They are also tasty in nut crusts, salads, specialty butters and vegetables.

A half cup (100 grams) of hazelnuts contains: 628 calories, 17 g carbohydrates, 10 g fiber, 15 g protein, 61 g total fat, 4 g saturated fat, 45.7 g monounsaturated fat, 7.9 g polyunsaturated fat, 0 mg cholesterol

Macadamia Nuts

Macadamia nuts are native of northeast Australia and are now commonly grown in Hawaii. They taste like fine hazelnuts, with smoother texture and richer taste. Macadamia nuts are used in cookies and ice cream. They have a particular affinity for coconut and white chocolate.

A half cup (100 grams) of macadamia nuts contains: 718 calories, 14 g carbohydrates, 9 g fiber, 8 g protein, 76 g total fat, 12 g saturated fat, 58.9 g monounsaturated fat, 1.5 g polyunsaturated fat, 0 mg cholesterol

Pecans

Pecans are native to North America. They are used chopped, ground or whole in brownies, cakes, confectioneries, cookies, ice cream, nut breads and pies, and in chicken and fish coatings, salads and stuffing. The flavor and texture of pecans are close to mild, sweet walnuts.

A half cup (100 grams) of pecans contains: 753 calories, 15 g carbohydrates, 10 g fiber, 10 g protein, 78 g total fat, 7 g saturated fat, 44.5 g monounsaturated fat, 23.6 g polyunsaturated fat, 0 mg cholesterol

Pine Nuts

Pine nuts are native to the Middle East and the Mediterranean region. They have a distinct, delicate, buttery taste and creamy texture. Pine nuts are used in Italian *pesto* sauce; French *salade landaise*; Italian *pignoli* cookies and other baked desserts; Middle Eastern *kibbeh* and *sambusek*, and in pine nut coffee.

A half cup (100 grams) of pine nuts contains: 673 calories, 15 g carbohydrates, 10 g fiber, 10 g protein, 78 g total fat, 7 g saturated fat, 44.5 g monounsaturated fat, 23.6 g polyunsaturated fat, 0 mg cholesterol

Pistachios

Pistachios are native to central Asia, the Mediterranean region and the Middle East, and they are now cultivated in the southern United States. They are used in sweets, such as Middle Eastern *baklava*, and Asian *seera* and in ice cream. They also have savory uses in chicken, meat loaf and rice dishes and are a common snack food plain or salted.

A half cup (100 grams) of shelled pistachios contains about: 357 calories, 17 g carbohydrates, 10 g fiber, 15 g protein, 44 g total fat, 5 g saturated fat, 23.3 g monounsaturated fat, 13.5 g polyunsaturated fat, 0 mg cholesterol

Recipe: Cherry Pistachio Biscotti

*The green pistachios in the recipe for **Cherry Pistachio Biscotti** in the **Recipe file** which is located within the Culinary Nutrition website at www.culinarynutrition.elsevier.com, are interspersed among the burgundy cherries and golden-crusted biscotti for a visual treat. While dry (since biscotti are twice baked), pistachios lend their monounsaturated fats for little bursts of richness. These biscotti offer just enough sweetness for a savory and sweet bread basket, snack, or after-meal finale. The pistachios can be swapped for pine nuts, and the cherries can be replaced with snipped apricots for another colorful and tasty combination. The finished biscotti are shown within the centerfold **Photo file** in Plate 6.3.*

Walnuts

Walnuts are native to southeast Europe and western and central Asia, and are now grown in California, China and the United Kingdom. English walnuts are used in *Waldorf salad* and other salads, sauces, soups and stews. Walnuts have an umami-like flavor that pairs well with cheese, particularly blue cheese. Walnut oil adds a strong and nutty flavor to beef, pasta, salads and baked goods.

A half cup (100 grams) of walnuts contains: 654 calories, 14 g carbohydrates, 7 g fiber, 15 g protein, 65 g total fat, 6 g saturated fat, 8.9 g monounsaturated fat, 47.2 g polyunsaturated fat, 0 mg cholesterol

SEEDS

Seeds are composed of storage nutrients surrounded by a seed coat. They provide fiber, phytonutrients, and concentrated calories in the form of lipids, protein and some carbohydrates. Seeds are used in cooking oils such as sesame and sunflower, spices and food additives.

Pumpkin Seeds

Pumpkin seeds are also known as *pepitas*. They are common in Mexican and Native American cuisines. Today, the leading commercial producers of pumpkin seeds include China, India, Mexico and the United States. Pumpkin seeds are used in both raw and cooked forms in savory and sweet dishes, including cereal, granola, salads and vegetables.

A half cup (100 g) of pumpkin seeds contains: 541 calories, 18 g carbohydrates, 4 g fiber, 25 g protein, 46 g total fat, 9 g saturated fat, 14.3 g monounsaturated fat, 20.9 g polyunsaturated fat, 0 mg cholesterol

Sesame Seeds

Sesame seeds are of African origin, but they are now grown throughout Asia. Sesame seeds come in black, brown, ivory, red and yellow varieties. Darker sesame seeds have the most flavor, which can be heightened by toasting.

Sesame seeds are used in savory recipes and as a garnish for breadstuffs, and in sweet recipes and as a garnish for cakes, confectionery and pastries. In Asian, African, Mediterranean and South American dishes, sesame seeds are used in main dishes with chicken and other meats; in salads as a garnish and in salad dressing; and in rice dishes, stir-fries and vegetables. Ground sesame seeds are used to make *tahini*, a smooth paste that is common in Middle Eastern cuisine. Sesame oil is distinct, aromatic and flavorful, and is primarily used to finish dishes.

A half cup (100 grams) of sesame seeds contains: 573 calories, 23 g carbohydrates, 12 g fiber, 18 g protein, 48 g total fat, 7 g saturated fat, 18.8 g monounsaturated fat, 21.8 g polyunsaturated fat, 0 mg cholesterol

> ## Recipe: Sugar Snap Peas and Tofu Salad with Tahini Dressing
>
> *The combination of tofu, fresh sugar snap peas and tahini has an Asian-Mediterranean appearance and flavor, as captured in this recipe for **Sugar Snap Peas and Tofu Salad with Tahini Dressing**, found in the **Recipe file** which is located within the Culinary Nutrition website at www.culinarynutrition.elsevier.com. Additional salad dressing is not required because the sesame-based tahini dresses and binds the salad ingredients. One (3.5-ounce) serving of tofu contains about 5 grams of total fat, 1 gram of saturated fat, 0 cholesterol, 228 milligrams of omega-3 fatty acids and 2,019 milligrams of omega-6 fatty acids. Typically, softer tofu has a lower fat content. One tablespoon of tahini contains about 7 grams of total fat, 1 gram of saturated fat, 0 cholesterol, 54.4 milligrams of omega-3 fatty acids and 3,099 milligrams of omega-6 fatty acids. The finished dish is shown within the centerfold **Photo file** in Plate 6.4.*

Sunflower Seeds

Sunflower seeds originated in either North America or Mexico. They are now primarily consumed in China, Israel, Spain, Turkey and the southeastern United States. Sunflower seeds can be added to breads, cakes, candies, cookies, granola, salads and soups. Sunflower seed oil is used in margarine.

A half cup (100 grams) of sunflower seeds contains: 584 calories, 20 g carbohydrates, 9 g fiber, 21 g protein, 51 g total fat, 4 g saturated fat, 18.5 g monounsaturated fat, 23.1 g polyunsaturated fat, 0 mg cholesterol

LOWERING TOTAL FAT, SATURATED FAT, AND CHOLESTEROL IN COOKING AND BAKING

> ### FOOD BYTE
>
> A **fat separator** is also called a **degreasing pitcher** or **gravy separator**. It is usually made of glass or heat-resistant plastic, with a long neck or spout. When gravy or drippings are poured into a fat separator and allowed to settle, the fat or oil will rise. This is because fat tends to be lighter than other liquids. The design of the fat separator allows the heavier gravy or liquid to be poured from the spout and the fat or oil to remain for discarding.

Decreasing total fat, saturated fat and cholesterol in cooking and baking requires cutting back ingredients with fats and oils, although not cutting them out altogether. Since fats and oils are so satisfying and function in many reactions, their elimination may cause recipes to fail. Try some of these ideas to help preserve the flavor and functionality of reduced-fat recipes:

- Use good-quality nonstick pots and pans that do not require extra fat, or pots and pans that have been "seasoned" to create nonstick surfaces. *Seasoning* is a process that fills the pores of cookware, blocks the oxidation process, and prevents pitting, rusting and sticking.
- Trim away almost all visible fat. This includes the fat that surrounds meat and the skin of poultry and firm fish. The exception is when broiling or roasting poultry, since removing the skin before cooking tends to dry out poultry. Place seasonings under the skin before cooking; then remove the skin before serving or eating.
- Use dry heat cooking methods where fat can drip away and be discarded. These include baking, broiling, grilling, microwaving, roasting and stir-frying. A wire rack should be used whenever possible to facilitate this process.
- Skim the fat as it rises to the surface when preparing braises, soups and stews.
- Utilize quick-chill methods for removing fat or oil from soups, stews or stocks. These include placing soup or stock in a shallow pan, then freezing it for a short amount of time to solidify the fat or oil; or dropping ice cubes into hot soup or stock, and skimming the fat or oil as it floats to the surface. This may thin the soup or stock and dilute the flavor.

- Remove any large pieces of meat from the cooking liquid when a dish has finished cooking. Meat that is cooled in cooking liquid may reabsorb some of the fat. Then cool the dish, and remove as much congealed fat as possible.
- Avoid deep-fat frying. Shallow frying is preferred with a minimal amount of oil.
- Sweat vegetables instead of cooking them in fat or oil. *Sweating* is a process where vegetables are cooked over low heat in a little fat or none at all to draw out moisture, weaken and soften the cell walls, and build flavor.
- Use 1 to 2 tablespoons of defatted broth, hot water, juice, or wine in place of fats or oils for sauteing.

REDUCING AND SUBSTITUTING FATS AND OILS IN COOKING
Butter

- Protein foods that contain some fat can be basted with a combination of butter and natural juices, broth, stock, vegetable juice or wine. This will cut the amount of butter and retain moistness.

> **FOOD BYTE**
>
> *Basting* is a technique that adds color, flavor and moisture via liquid to foods such as whole chicken or turkey, pork loin or standing rib roast. Flavorful liquid, such as beer, broth, fruit juice, stock, vegetable juice or wine, can be mixed with a little fat or oil and brushed, poured or spooned over food during cooking. A bulb or metal baster may also be used. Basting helps to prevent foods from drying out too quickly by adding moisture to the surface. The fallacy of basting is that meat cannot absorb moisture during cooking.

262

- Reduced-fat butter can replace the solid fat in some recipes. It works best in recipes that do not require cooking because the fat is replaced in this product by water and/or air. In recipes that require heat, the extra water may cause food to burn or alter the final texture.
- Reduced-fat butter can be used as a spread or topping in recipes with little to no heat.

Cheese

- Reduced-fat and fat-free cheeses do not melt smoothly. Finely shred and then toss with a small amount of arrowroot, cornstarch or flour before adding to sauces or soups. Use reduced-fat cheese within casseroles, lasagna, hot sandwiches or pizzas, or as a topping. Slightly undercook reduced-fat cheese when used as a topping to prevent hardening.
- Two percent extra-sharp cheese can replace mild cheese in some cheese sauce recipes to sharpen flavor with less fat.

Chocolate

- Cocoa powder is low in saturated fat and can be used in some recipes as a chocolate substitute in this proportion:

    3 tablespoons dry cocoa powder *plus* 1½ teaspoons neutral oil (such as canola) = 1 ounce (or square) of unsweetened chocolate
- Add ½ to 1 teaspoon of instant coffee granules to cocoa powder for an intense chocolate flavor.

Coconut

- Lite coconut milk is available as a substitute for full-fat coconut milk. Full-fat coconut milk contains about 552 calories per cup, with 57 grams of total fat and 51 grams of saturated fat. Lite coconut milk contains about 180 calories per cup, with about 16 grams of total fat and 12 grams of saturated fat.
- Use ½ cup of coconut plus 1 teaspoon of coconut flavoring in place of 1 cup of shredded coconut. The other dry ingredients in the recipe may need to be adjusted.

Cream

- Use evaporated dairy skim milk or 2% milk in recipes to replace cream where texture and function are not issues. Evaporated skim milk can be substituted for whipping cream in ice cream, but puddings may set softer. Skim milk and nonfat milk products do not have enough fat to produce desired consistencies.
- To create a velvety vegetable soup without cream, puree the vegetables directly in the pot with a handheld immersion blender, or transfer some of the mixture to a blender or food processor and then blend. Cooked potatoes or potato flakes that have been reconstituted in some of the soup stock can be added for thickening.

Crust

- For a healthy savory crust on baked meats, fish and sturdy vegetables, drizzle with oil, then rub on ground nuts, whole-grain crumbs, herbs and/or spices. Cook as directed.
- For a healthy sweet crust, mix 1 to 2 tablespoons of melted light butter with 1 cup of graham cracker crumbs; then add a little light corn syrup or honey to hold the mixture together, and press into a prepared baking pan. Bake as directed.
- Lightly brush phyllo dough with oil or an oil/light butter mixture to brown with less fat.

> **Morsel** "No clever arrangement of bad eggs ever made a good omelet."
> —C. S. Lewis (British novelist and scholar, 1898–1963)

Eggs

- Egg substitutes are discussed in Chapter 5. In general, use two egg whites plus 1 tablespoon of vegetable oil for one whole egg. The egg whites will provide structure, and the vegetable oil will preserve moistness. Because egg substitutes do not contain yolks, they do not function as emulsifiers in sauces and custards. Without yolks, custards lose their smoothness and creaminess.
- In savory dishes, try pureed cauliflower, mushrooms or potatoes to replace eggs for thickening.

263

Recipe: "Cream" of Mushroom Soup with Truffle Oil

*The **"Cream" of Mushroom Soup with Truffle Oil** in the **Recipe file** which is located within the Culinary Nutrition website at www.culinarynutrition.elsevier.com, uses vegetable broth and reduced-fat milk thickened with a little flour instead of higher-fat cream for body, taste and flavor. Other mild-flavored vegetables can be substituted for mushrooms, such as cauliflower, celery or onions, but this may sacrifice the umami taste of the mushrooms. Truffle oil contains the essence of truffles (underground fungus) in an olive oil or grapeseed oil base. True truffle oil may be prohibitive in price.*

Frosting

- Dust with cocoa, cinnamon, nutmeg or powdered sugar.
- Dribble frosting; then top with shaved chocolate, coconut curls or slivered nuts. The idea is to trick the eye and the palate that there is more frosting.

Meat

- Substitute 1 cup of lightly sauteed finely grated potato, or cooked bulgur, couscous, legumes or rice for one-quarter to one-half pound of ground meat in some recipes. One to two tablespoons of neutral oil, such as canola, may need to be added for moisture.
- Replace smoked meats and sausages with poultry or soy sausage where appropriate. Cholesterol and saturated fat may lessen, but sodium may remain high.

Dairy Milk

- Evaporated skim milk may be substituted for whole milk in some casseroles, sauces and soup recipes in this proportion:
    ½ cup evaporated skim milk *plus* ½ cup water *plus* 2 teaspoons liquid oil *equals* 1 cup of whole milk

- Evaporated skim milk can be whipped until stiff, and a little sweetening and flavoring can be added for dessert toppings. Serve immediately, as the structure may deflate.

Nuts and seeds

- Toast nuts, seeds and spices in a dry pan over moderate heat or on a baking sheet in a 350°F oven. Stir frequently for even toasting and to prevent burning. Once cooled, chop finely and mix well to distribute flavor.

Oil

- In general, less oil is required in cooking than butter or solid shortening:
  ¾ cup liquid oil *equals* about 1 cup butter or solid shortening
- There is no standard replacement for solid fats with oil in baked products. This is because oil is 100 percent fat; butter, margarine and solid shortenings often have other ingredients, such as milk solids, and are lower in fat on a volume-for-volume basis.
- Oil does not "cream" like solid fats. Solid fats help to incorporate air into batter, especially when it is whipped with other ingredients such as sugar and eggs. This procedure is called "creaming." If ingredients are creamed with oil, baked products may be compacted and oily.
- Plain or flavored oil can be used to pan-fry fish or poultry and to saute vegetables. It can also be added to whipped or scalloped potatoes, pancake and waffle batter, and to soups or stews for a touch of richness and body.
- A pump bottle filled with vegetable oil can be used to spray a little oil on baked goods, casseroles or meats for browning.
- Substitute up to one-third of the oil in vinaigrette with broth, fruit juice, defatted-vegetable juice, stock or tomato juice. Apple, orange, mango, pineapple, or white grape juice will add a sweet touch of flavor, while herbs and spices will add savory undertones. This reduced-fat vinaigrette can be used as a flavorful salad dressing or to baste protein foods during broiling.

264

Recipe: Avocado, Orange and Red Onion Salad with Shallot Dressing

*The combination of smooth, tangy and sharp in the **Avocado, Orange and Red Onion Salad** in the **Recipe file** which is located within the Culinary Nutrition website at www.culinarynutrition.elsevier.com, equates with fresh, tasteful and unified. The monounsaturated fats in the avocado serve to balance the other assertive tastes. A little avocado is all that is needed. One-quarter of a ripe avocado (the amount in one serving) contains about 56 calories, 5 grams of total fat, 0.75 grams of saturated fat, 3.3 grams of monounsaturated fat, and 0.6 grams of polyunsaturated fat.*

Sour Cream

- Instead of 1 cup of sour cream in recipes, use about ¾ cup of drained plain nonfat yogurt with about ¼ cup sour cream.
- Fat-free sour cream does not have enough rich texture or flavor in recipes, but can be used to top dishes.
- Evaporated skim milk or fat-free cottage cheese can be used in place of sour cream in some recipes in these proportions:
  1 can of chilled and whipped evaporated skim milk *plus* 1 teaspoon of lemon juice
  or
  1 cup of pureed fat-free cottage cheese *plus* 1 tablespoon of lemon juice

Thickeners

- Whole-grain breadcrumbs are a quick, fiber-rich thickener for darker-colored casseroles, sauces, soups and stews.
- Toast high-fiber white bread and crumb; then use in lighter-colored dishes, such as macaroni and cheese or broiled white fish.

FOOD BYTE

Mayonnaise is an emulsion that functions as a base or thickener for many sauces and dressings. One tablespoon of mayonnaise contains about 100 calories and 11 grams of total fat—similar to butter. The following types of mayonnaise vary by just a few ingredients. Most of them can be lightened in fat and calories.

Type of Mayonnaise	Additional Ingredients
Aïoli	Olive oil and garlic
Rouille	Aïoli with red pepper or paprika
Tartar sauce	Pickled cucumbers and onions
Russian dressing	Tomato sauce or ketchup
Thousand Island dressing	Chili sauce or sweet pickle relish
Fry sauce	Hot sauce
Mayonesa	Lime
Rémoulade	Anchovies, capers, chervil, gherkins, mustard, parsley and tarragon
Ranch dressing	Buttermilk or sour cream and minced green onions

---

REDUCING AND SUBSTITUTING FATS AND OILS IN BAKING

A general rule of thumb to reduce fat in baking is to decrease the total fat in a recipe by about 30 percent. A significant percentage of fat still remains for flavor and function. One of the major failures in reduced-fat baking is overbaking. Cakes, cookies or quick breads may look moist with shiny surfaces, but they can be dry from the inside out. Check for doneness at the beginning of a recipe's time range. For example, if a recipe reads, "Bake 30–40 minutes," check for doneness after about 30 minutes. The surface should spring back when gently pressed in the center, and the edges should be lightly browned and slightly pulled away from the sides of the pan.

Most reduced-fat baked products will keep for a few days at room temperature if they are wrapped tightly with aluminum foil. Plastic wrap holds in moisture. In addition, some reduced-fat baked goods that are made with fruit purees will form droplets of moisture.

The exception is reduced-fat cookies, which keep best in zip-tight plastic bags. Reduced-fat baked goods can be refrigerated or frozen if wrapped in aluminum foil and placed in zip-tight plastic bags. They are best served at room temperature

Yeast Breads

Yeast breads are naturally low in fat. If butter is used purely for flavor and not for texture, it may be replaced with butter-flavored granules. Switching from bread flour to cake flour where possible may produce a more tender product. Rather than scooping the measuring cup into the flour and packing it to the brim, lightly spoon the flour into the measuring cup; then level it with the backside of a knife.

Cakes

Butter has three functions in cake recipes. First, butter helps to make cakes light and delicate by holding air bubbles in suspension. These air bubbles are produced by leavening agents such as eggs, baking powder or baking soda. Second, butter helps to make cakes tender by coating the protein in the flour and limiting gluten formation. Third, butter helps to make a cake flavorful by transporting rich flavors. Stick margarine and vegetable shortening have similar characteristics but fewer flavors. Vegetable shortening is aerated, so it can help create tenderness. But a margarine spread that is soft at room temperature is not a good butter substitute.

Check cakes, muffins and quick breads a minute or two before the finished baking time, or at the earlier time in a given time range. With less fat, these baked items may lose moisture and dry out quickly.

Cookies

Cookies present challenges for decreasing fat and maintaining desired texture and flavor. Cookies made with butter tend to spread during baking, which causes them to be thin. Decreasing the amount of butter in a recipe may limit their spread. The cookies may become chewy or fudgy. A small amount of applesauce, egg white or plain yogurt may help provide crispness. Also, a little corn syrup can be added to the cookie recipe. Part vegetable shortening will limit the spread and create a puffy cookie that maintains its softness.

Some butter in cookies and cakes can be replaced with reduced-fat cream cheese. Margarine will not reduce the total fat or calories, but it will reduce the cholesterol. The same holds true for oil: substituting oil for butter will not reduce the calories. It will eliminate the cholesterol and provide more polyunsaturated fatty acids than saturated fatty acids.

Bake reduced-fat cookies one baking sheet at a time in the center of the oven. The hot air should circulate to brown the cookies evenly. The cookies should be lightly browned around the edges when done, and the centers should firm upon cooling. If the cookies cool and harden quickly, return the baking sheet to the oven just until the cookies soften.

Pies

Piecrusts that are made with vegetable oil may be hard to roll out and may bake into a tough and mealy crust. Vegetable shortening, lard or margarine in combination with butter may be better choices.

Use one crust, not two, which will save both calories and fat, or eliminate the crust in some recipes where appropriate. Coat the pie dish with nonfat cooking spray; then press about ½ cup of graham cracker or gingersnap crumbs onto the sides and bottom of the dish for a sweet filling or with whole-grain cracker crumbs for a savory filling. Check for doneness at the beginning of the time range.

Piecrusts should be baked until just golden brown to prevent drying. If a piecrust overbrowns before the filling is finished, cover the crust with aluminum foil, and then finish baking.

Quick Breads and Muffins

Many quick bread and muffin recipes can be reduced in fat to 1 ounce (30 grams) of fat per 4 ounces (120 grams) of flour. When combining the wet and dry ingredients in a recipe, do not overmix; simply stir until just moistened.

Fruit purees, such as prune, banana and apricot, lend color, taste and texture to quick bread and muffin recipes.

In general, try to match the flavor of the fruit puree with the desired flavor of the quick bread. The dark color of prune puree is masked in chocolate recipes. Banana puree will add flavor and specks of banana to recipes, but these may not be desirable in light-colored products. Apricot puree supplies more flavor than pumpkin or squash. All yield a yellowish-orange finished product.

FAT SUBSTITUTES

Fat substitutes are substances that look, feel and/or taste like fat. Some have calories, while others are low in calories or are calorie-free. The three main categories of fat substitutes are *carbohydrate, protein* and *fat-based.*

Carbohydrate-based fat substitutes, such as starches and gums, have many unique properties. They hold water, impart a creamy texture, and add form and structure that are similar to fat. They cannot be used for cooking or frying. Carbohydrate-based fat substitutes are used to replace the fat in baked foods, cake and cookie mixes, dairy products, frostings, frozen desserts and salad dressing.

Common carbohydrate-based fat substitutes include carrageenan (a type of seaweed); cellulose or starch-based gels; cornstarch; fruit purees (like apricot or prune); guar gum; Oatrim (with oat fiber) and Z-trim (with insoluble fiber); maltodextrins (corn-based); polydextrose; and xanthan gum.

Protein-based fat substitutes, such as egg white, milk and whey, are blended to trap water, and to create a creamy liquid that is similar to fat. They contribute less total fat and fewer calories than the fat they replace.

Protein-based fat substitutes cannot be used for baking or frying, since heat causes a change in their structure. It causes them to gel and lose their creaminess. Protein-based fat substitutes are used to replace the fat in baked goods, butter, cheese, dairy products, ice cream, mayonnaise, salad dressings and sour cream.

Common protein-based fat substitutes include egg white protein; microparticulated protein (as *Simplesse* used in ice cream); milk protein; whey protein concentrate; and whey protein.

Fat-based fat substitutes, with more fatty acids than triglycerides, are too large to be digested, so they do not contribute fat or calories. Large amounts of fat-based fat substitutes may cause a loss of fat-soluble vitamins or gastrointestinal side effects. Fat-based fat substitutes are used in baked goods, chocolate, confections, snacks and savories.

Common fat-based fat substitutes are *Caprenin* (a cocoa butter substitute); mono- and diglycerides; *Olestra* (with fat and sucrose); *Salatrim* (used in reduced-fat baking chips); and short- and long-chain fatty acids, which are partially absorbed by the body.

Each of these fat substitutes will reduce total fat and calories, but their disadvantages may affect appearance, aroma, taste, texture, cooking or baking reactions and the final products. It may be better to use less fat and oil and/or reduce the finished portion sizes before using fat substitutes unless diet and health issues dictate otherwise.

SERVE IT FORTH

1a. Fast-Food Makeovers

Three high-fat foods that make up the US diet are hamburgers, pizza and fried chicken. Food manufacturers have tried a variety of alternatives to reduce the fat and calories, such as lean beef burgers, cheeseless pizza and baked chicken tenders. Not all have survived the test of consumer acceptance because they have not tasted like the real foods they tried to replace. Consider this reaction to McDonald's reduced-fat hamburger:

> The McDonald's Corporation will discontinue its reduced-fat hamburger, McLean Deluxe, after it did little to improve the company's bottom line. The company will also discontinue its chef's salad and side salads. McDonald's introduced McLean Deluxe about five years ago. It had 10 grams of fat compared with 21 grams of fat in a Quarter Pounder [54].

- Why do you think the reduced-fat hamburger, chef's salad and side salads failed?
- Refer to the McDonald's website at http://nutrition.mcdonalds.com/getnutrition/nutritionfacts.pdf.
- Record the nutrients in one of each of the burgers, premium salads and sides.
- You are responsible for reducing the total fat, saturated fat and cholesterol in these items. What do you propose? Consider that the DVs for total fat, saturated fat and cholesterol are 65 g total fat, 20 g or fewer saturated fat and 300 milligrams cholesterol, respectively, based on a 2,000-calorie-per-day diet. Support your comments.
- If a reduced-fat hamburger, chef's salad and side salads were offered today, what do you think the reaction to each of these items would be?

2a. Better Brownies

The local chapter of the American Heart Association has hired you as an instructor to teach reduced-fat baking classes. The AHA has provided the following Chocolate Nut Brownies recipe and asked that you develop a reduced-fat version that feels, looks and tastes like a higher-fat brownie.

CHOCOLATE NUT BROWNIES

Ingredients
   Vegetable shortening
   1 cup unsalted butter
   4 (1-ounce) squares bittersweet chocolate
   2 cups granulated white sugar

4 large eggs
1 teaspoon vanilla or mint extract
1 cup enriched all-purpose flour
½ teaspoon salt
2 cups chopped pecans or walnuts

Instructions

1. Preheat oven to 350°F.
2. Prepare 9×13-inch baking pan with vegetable shortening.
3. Melt butter and chocolate together in double boiler, stirring constantly.
4. Remove from heat; stir sugar into butter-chocolate mixture. Set aside to slightly cool.
5. Beat eggs into butter-chocolate mixture one at a time; mix well. Stir in vanilla or mint extract.
6. Combine flour and salt; stir into butter-chocolate mixture.
7. Fold in walnuts or pecans. Spread batter smoothly into prepared baking pan.
8. Bake 30 to 35 minutes, or until toothpick inserted into center appears clean.
9. Cool in pan on wire rack.

Yield 12 servings.
Nutrients per serving: 508 calories, 318 calories from fat (54 percent of the DV), 35 grams total fat (72 percent of the DV), 14 g saturated fat (70 percent of the DV), 112 mg cholesterol (37 percent of the Daily Value) [55]

- What ingredients should be eliminated in these brownies to reduce the fat? Reduced? Substituted? Why?
- What ingredients should be added to improve the appearance, taste and/or texture of these brownies? Why?
- What techniques should be changed to reduce the fat and/or improve the sensory qualities of these brownies? Why?
- Create the recipe and evaluate its outcome. Support your comments.

3a. Healthier Italian Eatery Menu Options

The local Italian restaurant wants to lighten up its menu. They have hired you as a culinary professional to review their menu and recipes and suggest new options that are reduced in total fat, saturated fat and cholesterol. In addition, they have asked for one new heart-healthy item in each category.

Suggest new menu options that are reduced in total fat, saturated fat and cholesterol next to each original menu item. Add one new heart-healthy option to each category. Support each of your additions.

Original Menu Options	New Menu Options	Heart-healthy Options
Appetizers		
Antipasto		
Buffalo wings		
Mozzarella sticks		
Salads		
Caesar salad		
Chef's salad with Italian meats and cheese		
Spinach salad with bacon dressing		
Soups		
Cream of mushroom		
Chicken noodle		
Minestrone		
Burgers (with french fries)		
Hamburger		
Cheeseburger		
Portobello burger		

Pizza (meat and vegetarian)
    Sicilian
    Pan
    Calzones
Subs
    Sausage, peppers and cheese
    Meatball parmesan
    Italian sub with hot peppers
Pasta
    Spaghetti with choice of
    mushrooms, meat sauce, marinara sauce, sausage, olive oil and garlic
    Fettuccine Alfredo
    Manicotti
Seafood
    Fried shrimp
    Fish and chips
    Shrimp scampi
Combos
    Shrimp with spaghetti
    Chicken parmesan with mostaccioli
    Cheese ravioli

Three additional activities can be found within the *Culinary Nutrition* website at www.culinarynutrition.elsevier.com.

WHAT'S COOKING?

1. Find the fat
    Objectives
    ○ To discover if a food contains fat or oil
    ○ To examine for *translucency* (light that passes through a stain or spot)
    ○ To determine if water creates a translucent spot that remains after it has dried
    ○ To apply this information to cooking and baking

    Materials
    Uncooked macaroni shell, raw potato slice, potato chip, ⅛ teaspoon mayonnaise, shelled peanut, raw bacon strip, ⅛ teaspoon water, ⅛ teaspoon margarine, measuring spoons, knife and cutting board (for potato), brown paper bag, marker, ruler

    Procedure
    1. Rub each food on a flat section of the brown paper bag.
    2. Number or identify each of the spots using the marker.
    3. Allow the spots to dry about 20 minutes.
    4. Record the food and whether or not fat was present by its fatty appearance on the bag.
    5. If fat was present; measure the spot with the ruler, and record in the chart.

Foods and Beverages	Fat Present	Fat Not Present	Measurement of Spot
Macaroni shell			
Raw potato slice			
Potato chip			
Mayonnaise			
Shelled peanut			
Raw bacon strip			
Water			
Margarine			

Evaluation

In addition to completing the chart, answer the following questions based upon your observations:

○ Compare the raw potato spot to the potato chip spot. Did they test the same or differently? If a french fry was tested instead of a potato chip, what would be the results?

○ Did the peanut create a spot? How did it compare to the raw potato spot? The french fry spot? If peanut butter was used, what would be the results?

○ Did the macaroni create a spot? How did it compare to the raw potato spot? The french fry spot? The peanut spot? How much fat is in the macaroni (which is a grain) in comparison to peanuts (which are legumes) or potatoes (which are root vegetables)? If cooked macaroni was used, what would be the results?

Most of the lipids that people consume come from fats in animal foods and oils in processing. Fruits (except olives and avocados), vegetables (except some legumes like peanuts and soy) and most grains are low in fat. But low-fat foods can turn into higher-fat foods through processing. Processed potato chips and peanut butter are higher in fat than raw potatoes and peanuts.

Culinary applications

Which insights from this experiment about lipids can be applied to cooking and baking? What properties of lipids should be considered when taking the finished products into account?

2. **Handmade ice cream**

Objectives

○ To create ice cream, a semisolid foam of air bubbles that is stabilized by fat

○ To explore the three components of ice cream: ice crystals, concentrated cream and air cells

○ To compare different fat ingredients in ice cream production

○ To apply this information to cooking and baking

Materials

Four small and four large zip-lock heavy-duty freezer bags; ice cubes; 24 tablespoons salt; measuring spoons; ½ cup each whole milk, cream, liquid coffee whitener and condensed milk; 4 tablespoons sugar; 2 teaspoons vanilla; container, scoop or spoon

Procedure

1. Place ice cubes inside a large bag; fill to one-half full.
2. Add 6 tablespoons of salt.
3. Put a small bag inside the large bag.
4. Add ½ cup of whole milk, 1 tablespoon of sugar and ½ teaspoon of vanilla into the small bag.
5. Seal the small bag; then seal the large bag.
6. Shake the bags about 5 minutes or until the mixture has thickened.
7. The ice cream should be softly frozen.
8. Remove the small bag; pour or scoop the ice cream into a container.
9. Repeat the experiment with the cream, coffee whitener and condensed milk, using fresh bags and ingredients each time.
10. Record how long it took for each of the liquid ingredients to thicken, the degree of thickness and the flavor of each mixture.
11. Refer to a food composition table (http://www.nalusda.gov/fnic/foodcomp/Data/); record the total fat and saturated fat of each of the liquid ingredients.

Type of Milk/Cream	Time to Thicken	Degree of Thickness	Flavor	Total Fat	Saturated Fat
Whole milk					
Cream					
Coffee whitener					
Condensed milk					

Evaluation

○ Which milk or cream produced the quickest ice cream? The thickest? The ice cream with the most flavor?

○ Which milk or cream contains the most total fat? Saturated fat? The least?

○ What associations can be made among the type of milk or cream, thickening properties, flavor, total fat and saturated fat content?

○ Does more total fat ensure thickness and/or flavor? Does saturated fat make a difference in thickness and/or flavor?

○ What ingredients and what quantities should be used to make reduced-fat ice cream? Why?

○ Since fat provides texture and flavor, how could both qualities be enhanced in reduced-fat ice cream?

The main ingredients in ice cream are fat, milk solids, sugar, gelatin (or other stabilizer), eggs and flavoring. Gelatin and other stabilizers help to absorb water and prevent the formation of large crystals. Eggs help to create an emulsion between the fat and water, which gives the ice cream greater resistance to melting. In this experiment, neither a stabilizer nor eggs are used. So these simple ice creams may not thicken or harden.

Fat provides richness, smoothness and flavor. A variety of milk products can be used to make ice cream: cream, whole milk, coffee creamer, condensed milk, and/or instant milk powder. In this experiment, the cream and whole milk should create creamy consistencies. An equal volume of whole milk and heavy cream will also create a smooth ice cream, but the total fat content will increase. See "Tips for making ice cream."

Reduced-fat ice cream can be made by replacing some of the cream with evaporated, condensed or powdered milk. Liquid coffee whitener yields a slightly different flavor and very creamy texture. Milk powder increases the milk solid content, and adds body and protein. Sugar increases palatability and improves body and texture.

Which of these characteristics were observed in this experiment?

Culinary applications

Which insights from this experiment about ice cream can be applied to cooking and baking? What properties of ice cream are the most important in successful finished products?

TIPS FOR MAKING ICE CREAM

- If the ice cream is very soft, the ice cubes/salt mixture may not be cold enough. Add more salt to reduce the temperature.
- If the ice cream is coarse and ices in less than 20 minutes, the ice/salt mixture has become too cold too quickly. Too much salt has been added to the ice cubes.
- Use crushed ice.
- Add fresh or dried fruit or nuts *after* the ice cream is made and before it is frozen.
- Make the ice cream mixture the day before it is to be served for a smoother finished product, *or*
- Freeze the ice cream at least 3 hours before it is to be served.

---

3. Fat content in milk products

Objectives

○ To observe the fat in various milk products

○ To compare the nutrients in various milk products

○ To apply this information to cooking and baking

Materials

Dairy skim milk with milk solids, 2% white milk, 2% chocolate milk and whole milk in single-serving cartons with the lids cut off (or four wide-mouthed glasses), food coloring, vegetable oil, droppers

Procedure

1. Cut the lids off each of the cartons of milk, or put each sample of milk into a wide-mouth glass.

2. Place one drop of food coloring in the corner along the side of each of the cartons or glasses of milk.

3. Place a drop of vegetable oil in the middle of the drop of food coloring in each of the cartons or glasses of milk.

4. Be careful not to move the glass or carton or shake the surface where the cartons or glasses are set. The milk samples must not be disturbed for the experiment to work properly.

After a short amount of time, the colors should mix. Gently pick up each of the glasses or cartons and swirl the contents. Record the appearance of each of the contents, the total fat and saturated fat content (which can be obtained from the Nutrition Facts Panels), the speeds of the color-mixing reactions, and the patterns of color mixing.

Type of Milk	Appearance	Total Fat	Saturated Fat	Speed of Reaction	Pattern of Reaction
Skim milk with milk solids					
2% milk					
2% chocolate milk					
Whole milk					

Evaluation

○ Does the total fat and saturated fat contents of the milks affect or not affect the patterns and rates of mixing? If so, which ones and what effects?
○ Do the milk solids in the skim milk and the chocolate flavoring and coloring have any effects on the patterns and rates of mixing? If so, what effects?

Oil causes the food coloring to circulate throughout the milk and make the swirls of color possible. Milk is mostly water and some fat. The oil is only soluble within the fat of the milk. The oil creates a current which causes the colors to circulate throughout the milk.

The fat content of the milk should affect both the speed of the reaction and the pattern and rate of the swirling. The milk solids and chocolate coloring and flavoring may have some effects because this means there is less fat in each of these milks.

Culinary applications

Which insights from this experiment about milk can be applied to cooking and baking? If ingredients are low in fat, how would this affect their functionality in recipes?

OVER EASY

Animals and plants are filled with many different kinds of lipids with a myriad of functions. Likewise, the lipids that are consumed in foods and beverages—some natural and some manmade—defy the imagination.

Lipids are essential to health and well-being. They are a component of every cell; lipids cushion and insulate the body and keep it lubricated, furnish essential fat-soluble vitamins and essential fatty acids, provide satiety, and supply energy. From a food scientist and chef's standpoint, lipids are crucial for aroma, taste and texture.

But too many lipids in the diet can lead to obesity and disease. Understanding the roles of lipids in the diet and their relationship to health and disease is complicated and ongoing. The best way to master lipids—fats, oils, phospholipids and sterols—is to review which foods and beverages contain fats and oils and in what quantities. Then examine the nutritional attributes of these foods and beverages in context with the rest of the diet. Study their effects on the body in health and disease. Then revisit lipid-containing foods and ingredients from a standpoint of how they can be reduced—not eliminated from the diet. Review how recipes and meals can be modified for reduced-fat cooking and baking, and note what accommodations must be made to restore aroma, taste and texture.

Using the lipid information on food labels and the Nutrition Facts Panel is essential in this process. There are a myriad of terms and values that are designed to assist purchasing and use. The FDA is the gatekeeper of this information. Knowing how to determine the percentage of fat in a serving of food and the weight of fat or oil in grams is important for translating these ingredients into recipe development and dietary advice.

Understanding the differences and uses of fat substitutes is important in expanding one's culinary and baking repertoire. Learning how to reduce and substitute lower-fat ingredients helps transform reduced-fat dishes into delicious alternatives.

This chapter is a resource for sorting out all of these challenges of dietary lipids, including controversies about cholesterol, essential fatty acids, trans fatty acids and tropical oils. Many of these controversies involve other nutrients: carbohydrates, protein, vitamins and minerals, so they should be viewed holistically in terms of food production, health and taste. And like other nutrients, one should not be viewed with more or less favor than the others.

CHECK PLEASE

1. A lipid that is solid at room temperature is called a(n):
   a. oil
   b. phospholipid
   c. fat
   d. sterol
   e. omega-3 fatty acid

2. A lipid that is liquid at room temperature is called a(n):
   a. fat
   b. sterol
   c. trans fat
   d. omega-3 fatty acid
   e. oil

3. A lipid that is only found in animal foods is called a(n):
   a. phospholipid
   b. cholesterol
   c. fat
   d. oil
   e. omega-3 fatty acid

Essay Question

1. Which three lipids should be reduced in the diet to help decrease blood cholesterol and cardiovascular disease? Support each response. Which foods or beverages contain these lipids? Which foods can be substituted to reduce each of these lipids?

For additional questions, please see the *Culinary Nutrition* website at www.culinarynutrition.elsevier.com.

HUNGRY FOR MORE?

American Heart Association   http://www.heart.org/HEARTORG
International Nut and Dried Fruit Foundation   http://www.nutfruit.org
National Association of Margarine Manufacturers   http://www.butteryspreads.org
National Dairy Council   http://www.nationaldairycouncil.org
National Heart, Lung, and Blood Institute   http://www.nhlbi.nih.gov
North America Olive Oil Association   http://naooa.org/aboutoliveoil
The Best Light Recipe, Editors of *Cook's Illustrated Magazine*,
America's Test Kitchen, 2006
American Heart Association. *The New American Heart Association Cookbook*, 7th ed. New York, NY: Clarkson Potter Publishers, 2004.
McCullough F. *The Good Fat Cookbook*. New York, NY: Scribner, 2003.

TAKE AWAY
Tropical Oils

Tropical oils include *coconut oil, palm kernel oil* and *palm oils*. Unlike other plant oils that contain mostly mono- and polyunsaturated fatty acids, tropical oils contain a greater proportion of saturated fatty acids. Coconut oil contains about 92 percent saturated fatty acids; palm kernel oil contains around 82 percent; and palm oil contains approximately 50 percent. Tropical oils are found mostly in commercial cakes, cookies and snack foods. They create a rich taste and aroma and palatable mouthfeel.

Coconut oil is also known as coconut butter. It has the consistency and appearance of vegetable shortening. Coconut oil mainly comes from Australia, East Africa, Indonesia, Malaysia, the Philippines and Sri Lanka, where it is used for frying foods and flavor.

One tablespoon of coconut oil contains 116 calories, 13.5 grams of total fat, 11.7 grams of saturated fat, 0.8 grams of monounsaturated fats, and 0.2 grams of polyunsaturated fats.

The fatty acids in coconut oil are primarily medium-chain triglycerides (MCTs). MCTs are shorter than long-chain triglycerides that are found in other fats and oils and more easily metabolized. This is the reason why MCTs are used in some infant formulas and supplements to nourish hospital patients. Some animal studies have concluded that MCTs raise metabolism and promote weight loss, but preliminary human studies are not supportive at this time.

MCTs either do not affect total cholesterol, or they may raise HDL cholesterol and may improve the ratio of HDL (good) to LDL (bad) cholesterol. However, there is currently not enough evidence to correlate this relationship with reduced risk of heart attack or stroke due. Do not mistake virgin coconut oil for partially hydrogenated coconut oil in packaged goods, since any reported benefits are associated with virgin coconut oil.

Palm oil originated in western Guinea and is now cultivated in other tropical countries. Mostly it is obtained from the fruit of the African palm. Palm oil is orange-red in color due to its beta-carotene content. It is used in cooking oil, margarine, and rich-tasting processed foods. If the oil is boiled, the carotenoid content may be destroyed, and the oil may become colorless. One tablespoon of palm oil contains 119 calories, 13.5 grams of total fat, 6.7 grams of saturated fat, 5 grams of monounsaturated fats, and 1.3 grams of polyunsaturated fats.

Palm kernel oil is extracted from the seeds of the palm. Palm oil is healthier than palm kernel oil because it has less saturated fat and higher antioxidant activity from its significant amount of vitamin E. Because palm kernel oil must be extracted from the seeds, it cannot be obtained organically. One tablespoon of palm kernel oil contains 116 calories, 13.5 grams of total fat, 11.0 grams of saturated fat, 1.5 grams of monounsaturated fats, and 0.2 grams of polyunsaturated fats.

About 20 years ago, tropical oils were implicated with coronary heart disease, heart attack and stroke due to their saturated fatty acid content. They were removed from the US food supply. To replace their taste, aroma and mouthfeel, the food industry used partially hydrogenated fatty acids with trans bonds. Since trans fats have come under such criticism due to their relationship with elevated saturated fatty acids in the bloodstream, alternative oils and fats, including tropical oils, have been reexamined.

It is important to note that tropical oils have been used in food processing for decades. While nonhydrogenated vegetable oils have better lipid profiles than tropical oils, they are not as useful in food processing. Tropical oils are both functional and somewhat interchangeable with lard in savory food processing. Palm kernel oil is particularly useful in chocolates and frostings.

Though controversial, the ingestion of tropical oils in moderation may not be harmful and may prove to be beneficial. Their saturated fatty acid content is indisputable. However, they contain health-promoting nutrients such as phytonutrients, including carotenoids; antioxidants, including vitamin E; phenolic acids; and flavonoids—and MCTs. Like other debatable food sources, tropical oils should be viewed in context of the entire diet—not just their fatty acid compositions. And they should be used in moderation like other natural fats and oils.

The French Paradox

The *French Paradox* is both an experience and a contradiction. One does not need to travel to France to experience a typical French meal. Many fine US restaurants serve its many courses, from a starter or appetizer, to soup, fish, sorbet, entree, dessert and cheese course. A baguette and butter are common additions. Less scrutiny is paid to the amount of fat or oil in a dish. Flavor reigns.

French people have little coronary heart disease, despite higher fat and cholesterol intake than in the United States. This is a contradiction. In the United States, a high-fat and high-cholesterol diet reportedly increases the risk of cardiovascular disease—*but does it always* [56–58]?

The French Paradox suggests that a higher-fat diet coupled with red wine consumption may lower blood lipids and cardiovascular disease. Red wine consumption is suggested as a protective factor in coronary heart disease. This is because red wine is a source of antioxidants, particularly *flavonoid phenolics*. The most prominent is *resveratrol*, found in grape skins and seeds, which is thought to increase HDL cholesterol and prevent blood clots. Some research suggests that moderate drinkers may be less likely to suffer heart attacks than abstainers or heavy drinkers.

The French Paradox has been disputed since it first appeared in the US media in the 1990s. Some researchers now question the validity of the statistics that were then gathered by the World Health Organization (WHO). They believe that the number of French people with CHD was greatly underreported and that in some areas of France, CHD is higher and diet related.

Overweight in France has increased appreciably since the French Paradox was first identified. Like in the United States, regional differences exist. There is higher saturated fat intake in the north of France concurrent with increased heart attacks and death than there is in the south of France, where a more Mediterranean-type diet is followed. It has been speculated that the southern French diet and other lifestyle factors may alter the effects of cholesterol and saturated fat in the causation of coronary heart disease.

The French consume more saturated fats in the form of butter, cheese and pork than people in the United States, who consume more vegetable oils, and, until 2006, more trans fats. The French diet also includes smaller portions of food; higher amounts of whole foods—especially fruits, vegetables and whole grains with protective antioxidants and fiber; higher quantities of fish with protective omega-3 fatty acids; and lower quantities of refined carbohydrates.

The French also have a lower incidence of snacking between meals and slower, more relaxed mealtimes as compared to Americans. While a higher percentage of French people smoke than US residents, and smoking is known to increase metabolism, it does not seem to be a major factor in the French Paradox.

What may be a more important factor in the French Paradox than smoking is physical activity. Walking is more common in France than it is in the United States due to less urban sprawl. Walking after meals is known to increase metabolism and help burn some of the calories that are consumed. People who undergo increased physical activity tend to be leaner and manage their calories better than sedentary individuals. Inactivity is a risk factor in cardiovascular disease.

Physical activity; a Mediterranean-type diet with an abundance of fruits, vegetable and whole grains; and moderate red wine consumption may all contribute to cardiovascular health. So may a partiality to smaller portion sizes, but a wide array of all foods, sparing few. French women, in particular, have been exemplified for their modest portion sizes [59].

References

[1] Mozaffarian D, Katan MB, Ascherio A, et al. Trans fatty acids and cardiovascular disease. N Engl J Med 2006;354:1601–13.

[2] U.S. Food and Drug Administration (FDA). Trans fatty acids in nutrition labeling, nutrient content claims, and health claims, <http://www.fda.gov/Food/GuidanceComplianceRegulatoryInformation/GuidanceDocuments/FoodLabelingNutrition/ucm053479.htm>; [accessed 17.05.08].

[3] Howard BV, Van Horn L, Hsia J, et al. Low-fat dietary pattern and risk of cardiovascular disease: the women's health initiative randomized controlled dietary modification trial. JAM 2006;295:655–66.

[4] Kratz M. Dietary cholesterol, atherosclerosis and coronary heart disease. Handb Exp Pharmacol 2005;170:195–213.

[5] <http://www.fda.gov/food/labelingnutrition/consumerinformation/ucm078889.htm>

[6] <http://www.fda.gov/food/labelingnutrition/ConsumerInformation/ucm109832.htm>

[7] U.S. Food and Drug Administration (FDA). Guidance for industry: trans fatty acids in nutrition labeling, nutrient content claims, health claims; small entity compliance guide, <http://www.fda.gov/Food/GuidanceComplianceRegulatoryInformation/GuidanceDocuments/FoodLabelingNutrition/ucm053479.htm>; [accessed 17.05.08].

[8] Collier A. Deadly fats: why are we still eating them? <http://www.independent.co.uk/life-style/health-and-families/healthy-living/deadly-fats-why-are-we-still-eating-them-843400.html>; [accessed 16.06.08].

[9] Associated Press. New York City passes trans fat ban, <http://www.msnbc.msn.com/id/16051436/#.TwDYudQV2Vo>; [accessed 17.05.08].

[10] Astrup A, Dyerberg J, Elwood P, et al. The role of reducing intakes of saturated fat in the prevention of cardiovascular disease: where does the evidence stand in 2010? Am J Clin Nutr 2011;93:684–8.

[11] Agriculture and Consumer Protection, <http://www.fao.org/docrep/V4700E/V4700E0e.htm>.

[12] Hunter JE, Zhang J, Kris-Etherton PM. Cardiovascular disease risk of dietary stearic acid compared with trans, other saturated, and unsaturated fatty acids: a systematic review. Am J Clin Nutr 2010;91:46–63.

[13] Joint WHO/FAO Expert Consultation. Diet, nutrition and the prevention of chronic diseases, <http://www.who.int/hpr/NPH/docs/who_fao_expert_report.pdf>; [accessed 17.05.08].

[14] French MA, Sundram K, Clandinin MT, Cholesterolaemic effect of palmitic acid in relation to other dietary fatty acids. Asia Pac J Clin Nutr 2002;11:S401–407; [accessed 17.05.08].

[15] Soyatech. Trans fat facts, <http://www.soyatech.com/trans_fats.htm>; [accessed 17.05.08].

[16] American Oil Chemists' Society, <http://www.aocs.org>; [accessed 17.05.08].

[17] American Palm Oil Council, <http://www.americanpalmoil.com>; [accessed 17.05.08].

[18] European Society for the Science and Technology of Lipids, <http://www.eurofedlipid.org>. [accessed 17.05.08].

[19] Institute of Shortening and Edible Oils, <http://www.iseo.org>; [accessed 17.5.08].

[20] National Sunflower Association. <http://www.sunflowernsa.com>; [accessed 17.05.08].

[21] United Soybean Board, <http://www.soybean.org>; [accessed 17.05.08].

[22] Lee KW, Lip GY. The role of omega-3 fatty acids in the secondary prevention of cardiovascular disease. QJM 2003;96:465–80.

[23] Cunnane SC. The contribution of α-linolenic acid in flaxseed to human health. In: Muir AD, Wescott ND, editors. Flax: the genus linum. Westcott: CRC Press; 2003.

[24] U.S. Food and Drug Administration (FDA). FDA announces qualified health claims for omega-3 fatty acids, <http://www.fda.gov/SiteIndex/ucm108351.htm>; [accessed 17.05.08].

[25] U.S. Food and Drug Administration (FDA). Food labeling: nutrient content claims; alpha-linolenic acid, eicosapentaenoic acid, and docosahexaenoic acid omega-3 fatty acids, <http://www.fda.gov/Food/LabelingNutrition/FoodLabelingGuidanceRegulatoryInformation/RegulationsFederalRegisterDocuments/ucm073457.htm>; [accessed 17.05.08].

[26] Nutri-Facts: Essential Fatty Acids, <http://www.nutri-facts.org/Intake-Recommendations.411 + M54a708de802.0.html>; [accessed 17.05.08].

[27] American Heart Association (AHA). Fish and omega-3 fatty acids, <http://www.heart.org/HEARTORG/General/Fish-and-Omega-3-Fatty-Acids_UCM_303248_Article.jsp>; [accessed 17.05.08].

[28] Kris-Etherton PM, Harris WS, Appel LJ, et al. Omega-3 fatty acids and cardiovascular disease: new recommendations from the American heart association. Arterioscler Thromb Vasc Biol 2003;23:151–2.

[29] Harvard School of Public Health, <http://www.hsph.harvard.edu/nutritionsource/what-should-you-eat/dietary-guidelines-2010/index.html>; [accessed 17.05.08].

[30] Kris-Etherton P, Harris WS, et al. AHA scientific statement: fish consumption, fish oil, omega-3 fatty acids and cardiovascular diseases. Circulation 2002;106:2747–57.

[31] National Cancer Institute. Risk factor monitoring and methods, <http://riskfactor.cancer.gov/diet/foodsources/fatty_acids/table2.html>; [accessed 17.05.08].

[32] Kris-Etherton PM, Taylor DS, Yu-Poth S, et al. Polyunsaturated fatty acids in the food chain in the United States. Am J Clin Nutr 2000;71(1 Suppl):179S–88S.

[33] Weaver KL, Ivester P, Seeds M, et al. Effect of dietary fatty acids on inflammatory gene expression in healthy humans. J Biol Chem 2009;284(23):15400–15407.

[34] US Department of Agriculture (USDA), <http://www.nal.usda.gov/fnic/foodcomp/Data/SR21/nutrlist/sr21w303.pdf>; [accessed 17.05.08].

[35] US Department of Agriculture (USDA), <http://www.health.gov/dietaryguidelines/dga2010/DietaryGuidelines2010.pdf>; [accessed 17.05.08].

[36] American Heart Association (AHA). What your cholesterol levels mean, <http://www.heart.org/HEARTORG/Conditions/What-Your-Cholesterol-Levels-Mean_UCM_305562_Article.jsp>; [accessed 17.05.08].

[37] Mayo Clinic. Cholesterol levels: what numbers should you aim for?, <http://www.mayoclinic.com/health/cholesterol-levels/CL00001/NSECTIONGROUP=2>; [accessed 17.05.08].

[38] National Institute of Health (NIH) Lowering blood cholesterol to prevent heart disease. JAMA 1985;253:2080–6.

[39] <http://www.nejm.org/doi/full/10.1056/NEJMp0805953>

[40] Food and Nutrition Board. Macronutrients and healthful diets, <http://www.nap.edu/openbook.php?record_id = 10490&page = 769>; [accessed 17.05.08].

[41] American Heart Association (AHA). Know your fats, <http://www.heart.org/HEARTORG/Conditions/Cholesterol/PreventionTreatmentofHighCholesterol/Know-Your-Fats_UCM_305628_Article.jsp>; [accessed 17.05.08].

[42] Mayo Clinic. Dietary fats: know what types to choose, <http://www.mayoclinic.com/health/fat/NU00262/NSECTIONGROUP=2>; [accessed 17.05.08].

[43] Grundy SM, Brewer Jr HB, Cleeman JI, et al. Definition of metabolic syndrome, report of the National Heart, Lung, and Blood Institute/American heart association conference on scientific issues related to definition. Circulation 2004;109:433–8.

[44] U.S. Food and Drug Administration (FDA). How to understand and use the nutrition facts label, <http://www.fda.gov/Food/ResourcesForYou/Consumers/NFLPM/ucm274593.htm>; [accessed 17.05.08].

[45] U.S. Food and Drug Administration (FDA). Definitions of nutrient content claims, <http://www.fda.gov/Food/GuidanceComplianceRegulatoryInformation/GuidanceDocuments/FoodLabelingNutrition/FoodLabelingGuide/ucm064911.htm>. [accessed 17.05.08].

[46] U.S. Food and Drug Administration (FDA). Additional requirements for nutrient content claims, <http://www.fda.gov/Food/GuidanceComplianceRegulatoryInformation/GuidanceDocuments/FoodLabelingNutrition/FoodLabelingGuide/ucm064916.htm>; [accessed 17.05.08].

[47] U.S. Food and Drug Administration (FDA). Claims, <http://www.fda.gov/Food/GuidanceComplianceRegulatoryInformation/GuidanceDocuments/FoodLabelingNutrition/FoodLabelingGuide/ucm064908.htm>; [accessed 17.05.08].

[48] FDA Consumer Magazine. September–October 2003, <http://www.fda.gov/FDAC/features/2003/503_fats.html>.

[49] US Department of Agriculture (USDA). USDA specifications for vegetable oil margarine, <http://www.ams.usda.gov/AMSv1.0/getfile?dDocName=STELDEV3004553>; [accessed 17.05.08].

[50] Berger A, Jones PJ, Abumweis SS. Plant sterols: factors affecting their efficacy and safety as functional food ingredients. Lipids Health Dis 2004;3:5.

[51] Katan MB, Grundy SM, Jones P, et al. Efficacy and safety of plant stanols and sterols in the management of blood cholesterol levels. Mayo Clin Proc 2003;78:965–78.

[52] Kris-Etherton PM, Hu FB, Ros E, et al. The role of tree nuts and peanuts in the prevention of coronary heart disease: multiple potential mechanisms. J Nutr 2008;138:1746S–1751S.

[53] Jenkins DJ, Hu FB, Tapsell LC, et al. Possible benefit of nuts in type 2 diabetes. J Nutr 2008;138:1752S–1756S.

[54] Bloomberg Business News. Fast food restaurants bring home the bacon, <http://articles.baltimoresun.com/keyword/fast-food-restaurant/recent/3>; [accessed 17.05.08].

[55] Adapted from allrecipes.com at <http://allrecipes.com/Recipe/Fudge-Brownies-I/Detail.aspx\>.

[56] Lippi G, Franchini M, Favaloro EJ, et al. Moderate red wine consumption and cardiovascular disease risk: beyond the "French paradox.". Semin Thromb Hemost 2010;36:59–70.

[57] Renaud S, de Lorgeril M. Wine, alcohol, platelets, and the French paradox for coronary heart disease. Lancet 1992;339:1523–6.

[58] Artaud-Wild SM, Connor SL, Sexton G, et al. Differences in coronary mortality can be explained by differences in cholesterol and saturated fat intakes in 40 countries but not in France and Finland. A paradox. Circulation 1993;88:2771–9.

[59] Ducimetière P, Lang T, Amouyel P, et al. Why mortality from heart disease is low in France. Rates of coronary events are similar in France and southern Europe. J BMJ 2000;320:249–50.

CHAPTER 7

Vitamin and Mineral Basics: The ABCs of Healthy Foods and Beverages, Including Phytonutrients and Functional Foods

Healthy Vitamin and Mineral Choices, Roles and Applications in Nutrition, Food Science and the Culinary Arts

279

Culinary Nutrition. DOI: http://dx.doi.org/10.1016/B978-0-12-391882-6.00007-8

OBJECTIVES

1. Identify the significance of vitamins and minerals in the human body
2. Discriminate among the different types of vitamins, minerals and substances that function like vitamins and minerals
3. Recognize the importance of vitamins and minerals in health and disease
4. Distinguish the food groups that supply each vitamin and mineral
5. Describe the pathways of digestion, absorption and utilization of each vitamin and mineral
6. Identify the benefits of antioxidants, phytonutrients, functional foods, prebiotics and probiotics
7. Detect the benefits and warnings of medicinal herbs
8. Identify and correct for vitamin and mineral losses in cooking and baking
9. Create plant-based recipes, meals and menus
10. Increase the prominence of fruits and vegetables in cooking and baking

INTRODUCTION: THE IMPORTANCE OF VITAMINS AND MINERALS THROUGHOUT HISTORY

Like carbohydrates, protein and lipids, vitamins and minerals are essential nutrients and are indispensable for optimal health. While most vitamins and minerals can be obtained through the diet, some can be made by the body or other sources.

Vitamins and minerals and their roles in health and disease are some of the most dynamic issues in nutrition today. Perhaps it is because the discoveries of vitamins and minerals are relatively young in relation to other breakthroughs in nutrition.

Fruits and vegetables, the carriers of *phyto (plant) nutrients*, have been around since antiquity. Understanding the roles of fruits and vegetables in the diet is central for recognizing their importance in health and disease. Knowing the roles of vitamins and minerals from proteins and lipids helps to establish their place in a healthy diet.

Cooking and baking can have major impacts on vitamin and mineral retention. This chapter features techniques for identifying potential vitamin and mineral losses, tips for replacing vitamin and mineral losses with nutrient-rich ingredients, and cooking and baking techniques for treating foods with vitamins and minerals with care.

Vitamins and Minerals Throughout History

Vitamins and minerals have been used by trial and error throughout history. It was not until it was realized that their absence in the human diet caused disease that their identities were named and categorized. Ancient Egyptians were thought to have used liver to cure *night blindness*. Night blindness, the inability to see acutely at night or in poor light, is partially caused by a vitamin A deficiency. Beef liver is high in vitamin A, among other nutrients.

In the 1700s, citrus foods were thought to cure *scurvy*, a disease that is marked by poor wound healing, bleeding gums, severe pain and even death. Citrus foods are high in vitamins A and C—two vitamins that are associated with healthy tissues and repaired damage.

In Asia during the 1800s, a debilitating disease called *beriberi* was widespread. One of the contributing factors of beriberi is the lack of vitamin B1 or thiamin. During this time, Asians consumed polished rice (without nutrient-rich bran or germ). Christiaan Eijkman, a Dutch physician and pathologist, discovered that feeding unpolished rice to chickens helped prevent beriberi. Laboratory research such as this has helped to solve similar conditions in humans. Today, whole grains with the germ, endosperm and bran intact are recommended for healthy diets.

Frederick Hopkins, a British biochemist, suggested that some foods contained "accessory factors" in addition to proteins, carbohydrates and lipids, and that these accessory factors were necessary to life. In the 1900s, Polish biochemist Kazimierz Funk isolated a complex of micronutrients, and suggested that it be named "vitamine" (*vita-amine*, or "essential to life"). This term became interchangeable with the term "accessory factors."

As time went on, it was discovered that vitamins were more than accessory factors and that they were indeed essential to life. Throughout the early 1900s, elimination studies helped scientists to isolate and identify more vitamins and their importance. Elimination studies eliminate certain foods and note the reactions. As a result of these studies, vitamin D in fish oil was shown to treat *rickets*, a bowlegged disease in children; vitamin K and its relationship to blood clotting was identified; and vitamin C and its "antiscorbutic" activity was confirmed. This is how the alternative name for vitamin C, "ascorbic acid," was established.

Like vitamins, the necessity of minerals naturally found in the earth's rocks, soil and water was discovered only in the last few hundred years. The iron that travels in the bloodstream, called *serum iron*, was identified in the early 1700s, and the calcium that is found in bones and teeth was recognized in the late 1700s. Fifteen minerals have since been found to have distinct bodily functions; without them, the body is unable to accomplish its many roles.

Understanding the food sources and bodily functions of vitamins, minerals and phytonutrients is essential for today's nutrition and culinary specialists. This is because their minute chemicals help food taste and smell so delicious and appear to have significant effects on health and disease.

The way foods are procured, prepared and stored can influence the *bioavailability* of vitamins and minerals— the extent to which they are absorbed and used by the body. This chapter focuses on vitamin and mineral retention at every stage of the food-to-table process. It also serves to integrate the nutritional science behind vitamin and mineral-containing foods with culinary artistry so that their nutritional and sensory characteristics can be maximized for optimal taste and health [1–3].

281

MAIN COURSES
The Importance of Vitamins in the Human Body

The significance of vitamins to the human body and health and wellness should not be taken lightly. Vitamins are as indispensible to daily functions as they are to disease prevention. Skimp on certain vitamins, and your body will pay the cost. Instead, open your eyes to their rainbow of colors and functions.

The Vitality of Vitamins

While vitamins, like protein, carbohydrates and lipids, are essential nutrients in the diet, they are needed in very small quantities by the human body. This is why vitamins are often referred to as **micronutrients** (*micro* meaning very small). Vitamins are needed in the majority of body processes, either to promote or regulate chemical reactions. They help to build bones, connective tissue, teeth and blood; defend the body and help it to heal; promote growth and reproduction; and maintain the central nervous system, among other functions. While vitamins do not supply calories or energy, they are responsible for helping carbohydrates, protein and lipids produce energy.

Though fruits and vegetables contain a small amount of calories, they are major contributors of vitamins and minerals. In total, fruits and vegetables supply about all of the vitamin C required daily, about one-half of the vitamin A, and a substantial amount of folic acid, necessary for proper growth and development. Other contributors of vitamins are whole grains and foods that contain carbohydrates, protein and lipids. Ordinary drinking water does not contain vitamins, but fortified water may contain both vitamins and minerals.

The Classification of Vitamins: Fat-Soluble and Water-Soluble

Vitamins can be classified as *fat-soluble* or *water-soluble*. **Fat-soluble vitamins** are obtained through the diet from foods and beverages that contain some type of fatty substance as a carrier, such as butter or nuts. They include vitamins A, D, E and K. Each of these vitamins has distinct sources and functions. Some fat-soluble vitamins can be obtained from sources other than foods or beverages, such as sunlight.

Water-soluble vitamins are obtained through the diet in foods and beverages that contain some type of liquid as a carrier, such as dairy milk or watermelon. They include all of the B vitamins and vitamin C. Some water-soluble vitamins can be obtained from other sources than foods or beverages, such as supplements, or they can be made inside the body. Like fat-soluble vitamins, water-soluble vitamins also have distinct sources and functions.

Fat-Soluble Vitamins

Fat-soluble vitamins A, D, E and K are needed in very small amounts by the human body. Unused fat-soluble vitamins are stored in the liver and in fat tissue. As a result, deficiencies of fat-soluble vitamins are rare, and excesses may be toxic.

A typical US diet should prevent both excesses and deficiencies of fat-soluble vitamins. Vitamin supplements can create the greatest risk of fat-soluble vitamin toxicity because more can be ingested than used. Fat-soluble vitamin deficiencies can be caused by extreme dieting, disease or genetic disorders.

A characteristic of fat-soluble vitamins is that they are *insoluble* in water, which means that they do not mix with body fluids and need assistance in moving around the body. This feature also affects the way that fat-soluble vitamins react in cooking and baking.

The groups of fat-soluble vitamins that work together for good health include, but are not limited to:

282

- Vitamin A (beta-carotene precursor) and vitamin E function as antioxidants.
- Vitamins A, D and K support bone health.
- Vitamins A, D, E and K assist growth and development.
- Vitamins E and K support blood formation and maintenance.

FOOD BYTE

Carrots can be categorized as Eastern or Western carrots. Eastern carrots may have been domesticated in Afghanistan around the tenth century. They were purple or yellow, with branched roots. The purple color came from colorful anthocyanin pigments—known today for their antioxidant properties. Some Eastern carrots are still available.

Western carrots likely grew in the Netherlands around the fifteenth or sixteenth century. They were orange in color from bright beta-carotene pigments. Orange carrots were an emblem of the House of Orange and represented Dutch independence. Western carrots were valued then as they are today for their carotenoids—antioxidants and immunity boosters.

VITAMIN A

Vitamin A is known as the "eyesight" vitamin because of its relationship to vision. Vitamin A is actually a family of compounds that include *retinol (preformed vitamin A)*, an active form of vitamin A that is only found in animal foods, and *carotenoids (vitamin A precursors or pro-vitamins)* that are found in plants. Carotenoids are called "precursors" because the body can convert some carotenoids into retinol.

The *retina* is a light-sensitive tissue in the back of the eye. It receives images and sends them to the brain for interpretation by way of the optic nerve. There is a pigment in the retina that contains *retinal*, an active form of vitamin A.

Rhodopsin is a protein in the eye that contains a retinal compound. Rhodopsin helps to change the light that enters the eye into nerve impulses. These nerve impulses are sent to the brain to create visual images.

Rhodopsin can only be synthesized if vitamin A is supplied by the diet. Without rhodopsin, vision may be impaired, and a condition called *night-blindness* may occur. An inability to see in dim light and a slow recovery to bright light at night are early signs of night-blindness.

The best animal sources of preformed vitamin A are beef liver, eggs, fortified dairy products and margarine. Carotenoids are found in dark green and brightly colored orange, red and yellow fruits and vegetables. The most common carotenoid is *beta-carotene*, which has powerful antioxidant properties. Fruits and vegetables particularly rich in beta-carotene include broccoli, oranges, spinach, sweet bell peppers and tomatoes.

Other than eyesight, vitamin A has other important functions in the human body. It helps to maintain the skin and epithelial tissues (one of the main tissues of the skin), provides immunity, and supports growth, development and reproduction.

Once absorbed from food, vitamin A is transported to the liver, where a protein complex picks it up and transports it through the bloodstream. About 90 percent of vitamin A is stored in the liver. That is why beef liver supplies so much vitamin A.

Too much vitamin A can cause liver disorders and birth defects in a developing fetus. Too much beta-carotene, after it is converted to vitamin A, can build up in fat tissue and cause the skin to discolor and look golden yellow.

Besides night-blindness, too little vitamin A may lead to *xerophthalmia*, an abnormal dryness of the eyeball that is characterized by *conjunctivitis*, an inflammation or infection of the membrane that lines the eyelids. Insufficient vitamin A may also lead to *keratinization*, a reduction of cells in the lining of the gastrointestinal tract.

> **Morsel** "An apple is an excellent thing—until you have tried a peach." — George du Maurier (Author and cartoonist, 1834–1896)

Sources of vitamin A:
- **Retinol**—eggs, fortified dairy products, liver, margarine
- **Beta-carotene**—acorn squash, apricots, broccoli, cantaloupe, peaches, pumpkin, spinach, sweet potatoes

Roles in body: eyesight, immunity, reproduction and growth, skin and epithelial cells
Deficiency: night-blindness, keratinization, xerophthalmia
Toxicity: discoloration of skin creating yellow hue, liver disorders

Cooking Foods with Carotenoids

In some instances, cooking can improve the bioavailability of some carotenoids, such as beta-carotene. For example, lightly steaming carrots or spinach may improve the body's ability to absorb their beta-carotene. However, prolonged cooking of carrots and spinach decreases the bioavailability of beta-carotene. It changes the shape of carotenoids from their natural *trans* form to a *cis* form (much like trans and cis fatty acids). Fresh carrots contain 100 percent trans beta-carotene; canned carrots contain only 73 percent. Trans beta-carotene is the preferred form.

The Dietary Reference Intake (DRI) for vitamin A is 900 micrograms per day (3,000 IU) for men and 700 micrograms per day (2,300 IU) Retinol Activity Equivalents (RAE) for women ages 19 years or older.

Sources of Vitamin A	Amount (micrograms RAE)*
3 ounces beef liver (preformed vitamin A)	6,582 mcg RAE
½ cup fresh carrots (beta-carotene)	971
½ cup raw butternut squash (beta-carotene)	532
½ cup cooked spinach (beta-carotene)	472
½ cup fresh cantaloupe (beta-carotene)	444
1 cup fortified dairy milk (preformed vitamin A)	150

*Retinol Activity Equivalents (mcg RAE).
Retinol Equivalent is a unit used for quantifying the sources of vitamin A, including preformed retinoids in animal foods and precursor carotenoids in plant foods. It is defined as 3.3 International Units (IU) of vitamin A. Retinol Activity Equivalents (RAE) reduces by half the vitamin A activity of the carotenoids.

> **Recipe: Butternut Squash Soup**
>
> *Orange soup? It depends on the color of butternut squash, from golden yellow to auburn. This* **Butternut Squash Soup** *in the* **Recipe file** *which is located within the Culinary Nutrition website at www.culinarynutrition.elsevier.com, is filled with the beta-carotene-rich vegetable, thickened by pureeing the squash itself, without the help of other thickeners. Equally bright garnishes add texture. One-half cup of raw butternut squash contains 12 grams of carbohydrates, 2 grams of fiber, 1 gram of protein, only 0.10 gram of fat, and 532 micrograms of vitamin A. The finished dish is shown within the centerfold* **Photo file** *in Plate 7.1 [4, 5].*

VITAMIN D

Vitamin D is known as the "sunlight" vitamin. The ultraviolet rays of the sun help to convert a vitamin D precursor in the skin into the active form of vitamin D. This ability makes vitamin D distinct from other vitamins because it does not have to be supplied by the diet.

Vitamin D can also be obtained by consuming animal products, such as egg yolks, fatty fish, fortified dairy products and liver, and through supplements. Vitamin D in animal products is called *cholecalciferol.* Vitamin D in plant-based products, such as margarine and fortified cereals, is called *ergocalciferol.*

The roles of vitamin D in the body cannot be overstated. Its roles in human nutrition are indispensable. This vitamin is essential for bone growth and maintenance. Vitamin D helps to make the minerals calcium and phosphorus available to the bones for absorption and improved bone density.

Vitamin D also normalizes calcium in the bloodstream, which helps to regulate the heartbeat. In this capacity, vitamin D acts like a powerful hormone. When calcium is needed by the body, vitamin D can withdraw calcium from the bones into the bloodstream and increase its absorption in the intestinal tract. It also influences the kidneys to recycle calcium rather than excrete it.

Vitamin D deficiency may result in a condition called *rickets* in children, which is marked by low blood calcium and abnormal bone development. Bowed legs and growth retardation are characteristics of rickets in children. Adult rickets is known as *osteomalacia*, which is characterized by weakening of the bones and rounding of the spine. Osteomalacia often leads to bone fractures.

Extreme dieting can lead to a vitamin D deficiency. Since vitamin D is fat-soluble, a diet that is extremely low in fat may cause a reduction in the ability to absorb dietary fat and a vitamin D deficiency.

Too much vitamin D can be toxic because it can build up and affect the soft tissues of the body. Toxicity is mostly caused by vitamin D supplements in excess of the requirement. The gastrointestinal tract absorbs excess vitamin D from the bloodstream, which causes a release of calcium from the skeleton and potential cardiovascular and kidney damage.

Many factors contribute to the amount of vitamin D that is absorbed from sunlight. These include climate, clothing, pollution, skin color and sun block solutions. Aging, decreased dairy product intake, inactivity and increased use of sun protection increase the risks of skeletal disorders.

Optimal serum concentrations for bones and general health have not been established. However, vitamin D research has escalated in importance and scope. While vitamin D supplements were once cautioned for their potential liver toxicity, they can augment poor vitamin D intake and uptake factors, especially in women. Advice should be sought from a health care provider regarding their use.

> **Sources of vitamin D:** eggs, fortified dairy products, liver, sardines
> **Roles in body:** bone and teeth mineralization
> **Deficiency:** abnormal growth and development, osteomalacia, rickets
> **Toxicity:** increase in kidneys and liver, elevated calcium in bloodstream leading to calcification of soft tissues, kidney stones and irregular heartbeat

Cooking Foods with Vitamin D

Vitamin D tends to be stable. Cooking and long-term storage do not appear to significantly reduce the levels of vitamin D in food.

The Dietary Reference Intake (DRI) for vitamin D is 600 IU (15 micrograms) for both men and women aged 19 years or older [6, 7].

Sources of Vitamin D	Amount (International Units)	Amount (micrograms)
3 ounces cooked salmon	447 IU	11.2 mcg
3 ounces canned tuna in water	388	9.7
1 cup fortified dairy milk	115–124[a]	2.9–3.1
1 tablespoon fortified margarine	60	1.5
2 sardines, canned in oil	46	1.2
1 large egg	41	1.0

[a]Varies according to fat content.

> ## Recipe: Barbecue Salmon with Sweet and Spicy Sauce and Wilted Arugula
>
> *The flesh of fatty fish, such as mackerel, salmon and tuna, and fish liver oils, such as cod liver oil, are some of the highest food sources of vitamin D. This recipe for **Barbecue Salmon with Sweet and Spicy Sauce and Wilted Arugula** in the **Recipe file** which is located within the Culinary Nutrition website at www.culinarynutrition.elsevier.com, provides a significant amount of vitamin D per serving (596 IU or 14.9 micrograms). The natural fattiness of the salmon balances the bitterness of the wilted arugula, and their colors are also brightly harmonious. Salmon pairs equally well with the piquancy of the sauce. The finished dish is shown within the centerfold **Photo file** in Plate 7.2.*

VITAMIN E

Vitamin E is often referred to as the vitamin of "vitality" or youth. This is because it has so many vital functions that are associated with cellular longevity, such as cellular reproduction and healthy skin. Like beta-carotene, vitamin E functions as an antioxidant and protects the cells from destruction due to oxygen-free radicals.

The scientific name of vitamin E is *tocopherol*, which, loosely translated, means "to life." There are four biologically active forms of tocopherol: *alpha, beta, gamma* and *delta*. *Alpha-tocopherol* is the most abundant and active form. It helps to prevent the potentially harmful oxidation of polyunsaturated fatty acids (PUFA), nicotine, smog and other pollutants. Alpha-tocopherol also serves to protect the cell membranes from infections and to keep blood flowing smoothly through the blood vessels.

No disease is associated with a deficiency of vitamin E. This is because it is common in the US food supply, with all the margarine, shortening and salad dressings that are consumed. Vitamin E is naturally found in higher-fat foods such as avocadoes, nuts, olives and soy products. It is also positioned within vegetable oils and products that contain them, such as cheese products, fried foods and nut butters.

A vitamin E deficiency may cause red blood cells to rupture and become dysfunctional. It may also cause nerve tissues to fail and lead to eyesight and neuromuscular disorders, including impaired vision. These symptoms may be seen with prolonged low-fat dieting and in *cystic fibrosis*, a malabsorption disorder in premature infants.

Vitamin E toxicity could result from supplementation and may cause problems with normal blood clotting. People who consume a large amount of polyunsaturated fatty acid–rich vegetable oils may have increased needs for vitamin E.

> **Sources of vitamin E:** dark green leafy vegetables, nuts, polyunsaturated fruit and vegetable oils, seeds, wheat germ, whole grains
> **Roles in body:** antioxidant, cell membrane integrity
> **Deficiency:** anemia, skin disorders, red blood cell rupture, weakness
> **Toxicity:** increased bleeding, reduced blood clotting

Cooking Foods with Vitamin E

The vitamin E content of food can be damaged by exposure to air and commercial processing. To help protect vitamin E in vegetable oils, keep the bottles tightly capped and away from direct light and heat.

In extracted wheat flour, which is used to make most of the baked goods, breads and pastas in the United States, the alpha-tocopherol content significantly drops when the germ is extracted. Whole grains preserve more vitamin E, but they must be refrigerated or frozen.

The RDA for adult men and women older than 14 years of age is 15 milligrams (mg) or 22.5 International Units (IU) daily [8].

Sources of Vitamin E	Amount (milligrams)
2 tablespoons sunflower seeds	8.5 mg
2 tablespoons dry-roasted almonds	6.8
1 tablespoon safflower oil	6.0
2 tablespoons peanut butter	3.0
1 avocado	2.8
1 mango	2.4

VITAMIN K

Vitamin K is known as the "anticlotting" vitamin because its major role in the body is to help blood coagulate or thicken. It accomplishes this with the help of several proteins, the most important being *prothrombin*. Prothrombin is made by the liver; it is a precursor to *thrombin*, which forms a mesh and traps the blood to clot.

Vitamin K is also responsible for producing bone proteins and assisting minerals to bind to these proteins, making the bones stronger. In this process, vitamin K helps to prevent *osteoporosis*, a brittle-bone disease.

Vitamin K is found in both animals and plants. The animal form of vitamin K is called *menaquinone.* It can be found in eggs, liver, meats and dairy milk. It can also be synthesized by bacteria in the intestine, but this amount can be inadequate for bodily needs. The plant form of vitamin K is called *phylloquinone*. It is found in cruciferous and dark green leafy vegetables, such as broccoli and spinach.

Many factors can contribute to a vitamin K deficiency. It is mainly due to poor vitamin K intake or when fat is malabsorbed. Fat malabsorption limits bile production, which in turn limits the absorption of vitamin K. Antibiotics can destroy the vitamin K–producing bacteria in the intestine. Anticoagulant medication, used to treat heart attacks and strokes, may also interfere with the effectiveness of vitamin K. The vitamin K content of human breast milk is low. Newborn infants are sometimes given injections of vitamin K at birth so that their immature intestinal tract can produce enough of their own supply of vitamin K.

Vitamin K toxicity is generally not a problem, but supplementation and drug interactions could increase the possibilities. Vitamin K toxicity could lead to *anemia* from hemorrhages in the red blood cells; *jaundice* from *bilirubin*, a yellow pigment that surfaces right under the skin; or brain damage.

> **Sources of vitamin K:** dark green leafy vegetables, soybeans, vegetable oils
> **Roles in body:** bone mineralization, synthesis of blood-clotting proteins
> **Deficiency:** bone-demineralization, hemorrhages
> **Toxicity:** anemia, brain damage, jaundice

Cooking Foods with Vitamin K

Vitamin K is more stable during processing than other vitamins. Some naturally occurring vitamin K can be found in oils that are resistant to heat and moisture during cooking, but it is diminished by acids, bases, light and oxidizers. Freezing may decrease the level of vitamin K. Vitamin K is sometimes added to food as a preservative to control fermentation.

There is no RDA for vitamin K, since there is inadequate information for the USDA to create a standard. An Adequate Intake (AI) has been established, which is based on observations and experimental evidence. The daily AI for vitamin K is 90 mcg for women and 120 mcg for men aged 19 years and over [4, 9].

286

Sources of Vitamin K	Amount (micrograms)
¼ cup raw parsley	246 mcg
1 cup cooked broccoli	220
1 cup raw spinach	145
1 cup raw shredded green leafy lettuce	62.5
1 tablespoon soybean oil	25
1 tablespoon canola oil	16.6

Water-Soluble Vitamins

The *water-soluble vitamins* include all the B vitamins, called the **B-complex**, plus vitamin C. They are found in beverages and foods with liquid content and are located throughout the body in its watery components.

The body excretes any water-soluble vitamins that are in excess, so toxicities are rare. Deficiencies are more common and can affect the blood, central nervous system, metabolism, immunity and other important bodily functions.

There are eight B-complex vitamins: thiamine (B1), riboflavin (B2), niacin (B3), folate (folacin, folic acid), B6, B12, pantothenic acid and biotin. These B vitamins function as coenzymes in the body by binding to enzymes to speed up reactions.

While these B vitamins do not supply energy, they assist in energy production. Thiamin, riboflavin, niacin, pantothenic acid and biotin have specific energy-related functions. Folate and vitamin B12 are active in synthesizing new cells, delivering nutrients, and keeping the blood healthy. Vitamin B6 is involved in amino acid metabolism and is directly related to protein intake.

Each of these B vitamins works closely with other vitamins and related compounds in an interdependent web of biological and chemical activities. That is why it is important to consume a well-balanced diet to obtain adequate amounts of each of these vitamins.

287

The groups of water-soluble vitamins that work together to help maintain good health include, but are not limited to, the following:

- Thiamine, riboflavin, niacin, pantothenic acid and biotin, *plus* vitamins B6 and B12 are important for energy production.
- Vitamin B6 (pyridoxine), folate (folic acid, folacin) and vitamin B12, *plus* vitamin C are involved in amino acid metabolism.
- Folate (folic acid, folacin) and vitamin B12, along with riboflavin, vitamin B6, vitamin C and choline, are responsible for blood formation.
- Vitamin C (ascorbic acid, ascorbate) *plus* beta-carotene, vitamin E and selenium function as antioxidants.

Toxicity from foods and beverages is generally uncommon, but it could happen from oversupplementation. A dose 100 times the normal level could disrupt cell function. The RDAs for these vitamins vary, as shown following.

FOOD BYTE

Blood or Sicilian oranges are hybrids of ancient origin. They probably originated in Sicily. Blood oranges are possibly a combination of the pomelo and the tangerine. They have red to crimson, blood-colored flesh due to their colorful anthocyanin pigments. This pigmentation is dependent on light, temperature and variety. Blood oranges are smaller than common oranges and they have pitted skin. The juice is semisweet, with less acidity than common oranges. Blood oranges can be used to make marmalade, gelato and Italian soda. Blood oranges can also be used in salads and entrees for their vibrant color and tangy taste.

WATER-SOLUBLE VITAMINS AND ENERGY PRODUCTION

The water-soluble vitamins thiamine, riboflavin, niacin, pantothenic acid and biotin, *plus* vitamins B6 and B12 are important for *energy production* in the human body.

VITAMIN B1—THIAMINE (THIAMIN)

Thiamine was the first water-soluble vitamin to be discovered. That is why it was named vitamin B1. Thiamine functions as a coenzyme in the release of energy from carbohydrates. It is also involved in nerve function and appetite regulation.

While thiamine is found in a variety of foods, fortified cereals, pork chops, salmon, sunflower seeds, watermelon and whole grains have some of the highest amounts. Alcoholics are at risk for thiamine deficiency, since thiamine is required in the metabolism of alcohol. A severe thiamine deficiency could result in *beriberi*, a debilitating disease that may cause edema, an enlarged heart, irregular heartbeats, muscle wasting and sometimes paralysis. Thiamine toxicity is rare, since it is water soluble.

> **Sources of thiamine:** nuts, legumes, pork, poultry, whole grains
> **Roles in body:** appetite regulation, central nervous system function, coenzyme participation, energy release
> **Deficiency:** beriberi, edema, heart irregularities, impaired growth and development, weakness
> **Toxicity:** not documented

Cooking Foods with Thiamine

To retain the thiamine content in vegetables, chop vegetables into pieces with minimal exposed surfaces, and cook vegetables in a minimum amount of water. Some thiamine can be lost in cooking liquids because it is water soluble.

Use enriched or whole-grain pasta or rice. Do not wash it before cooking or rinse it after cooking (the boiling liquid should destroy microorganisms). Roast meat and vegetables at a moderate temperature, and cook them only until done, as overcooking at high temperature destroys thiamin. Storage losses of thiamine are small.

The RDA for thiamine for adult women aged 19 years and older is 1.1 micrograms and 1.2 micrograms for men.

Sources of Thiamine	Amount (milligrams)
3 ounces cooked lean pork	0.72 mg
1 cup cooked black beans	0.42
1 cup cooked green peas	0.41
1 cup cooked lentils	0.33
1 cup cooked whole-grain oats	0.26
2 tablespoons pecans	0.20
1 cup cooked bulgur wheat	0.11

Bulgur wheat is a recognized whole grain by the USDA and Wheat Foods Council. Bulgur can be substituted with other whole grains for their taste and texture. However, not all nutrients in whole grains may be equal, including thiamine. One-half cup of cooked bulgur contains 0.10 milligrams of thiamine [10].

RIBOFLAVIN

Riboflavin, like thiamin, is a coenzyme that helps to release energy from carbohydrates. In addition to carbohydrates, riboflavin helps prepare amino acids and fatty acids for breakdown. A riboflavin deficiency is rare, but it can cause severe skin problems, particularly around the eyes, mouth and tongue. Toxicity is also rare; few to none have been documented.

Riboflavin is yellow to yellow-orange in color. In food processing, riboflavin is used as a food coloring and to fortify some baby foods, breakfast cereals, energy and fruit drinks, dairy milk products, pasta and processed cheese.

Almonds, dark green leafy vegetables, fat-free dairy milk, fortified cereals, low-fat yogurt and meats, especially pork chops, are high in riboflavin. Riboflavin is sensitive to light, so these foods should be purchased from and stored in protective containers.

Sources of riboflavin: enriched breads and cereals, dark green leafy vegetables, dairy milk and fortified dairy products, whole grains
Roles in body: coenzyme, healthy skin, normal vision
Deficiency: eye and skin disorders (including hypersensitivity to light), sores around the mouth, nose and eyes
Toxicity: none documented

Cooking Foods with Riboflavin

Loss of riboflavin from cooking and storing is typically less than 25 percent. Heat and air do little damage to riboflavin, but light is a concern. High-riboflavin foods should be cooked in covered pots and stored in opaque containers. With prolonged exposure to light, riboflavin loss could occur.

The RDA for riboflavin is 1.3 milligrams (mg) daily for men and 1.1 milligrams daily for women aged 19 years and older [4, 11].

Sources of Riboflavin	Amount (milligrams)
1 cup fortified breakfast cereal	0.59–2.27 mg[a]
1 cup fortified nonfat dairy milk	0.34
1 large cooked egg	0.27
2 tablespoons almonds	0.23
½ cup cooked spinach	0.21
3 ounces broiled pork chop	0.20

[a]*Average fortification.*

NIACIN

Niacin is a coenzyme, like thiamine and riboflavin, that is responsible for energy release from carbohydrates. A niacin deficiency can lead to *pellagra*, a disabling disease with symptoms that may be characterized by four "Ds": depression, diarrhea, delirium and dementia.

Niacin is found in fortified breads and cereals. Protein foods, such as eggs, fish, meat, dairy milk and poultry, are naturally rich in niacin. They are also plentiful in the amino acid *tryptophan*, which can be synthesized into niacin by the liver. Chicken breast, ground beef, halibut, tuna and turkey are particularly good sources of tryptophan. In the vegetable kingdom, asparagus, baked potatoes and cantaloupe have significant amounts of tryptophan.

Niacin has been used to lower LDL cholesterol and raise HDL cholesterol when administered as a drug under medical guidance. In heavy doses, niacin has been known to cause a *"niacin flush"* due to the capillaries increasing in size. This condition can lead to fatigue and even liver damage. Caution should be used if one is taking niacin or B-complex supplements.

Sources of niacin: eggs, fish, legumes, meats nuts, peanuts, poultry, pork
Roles in body: coenzyme, digestive and nervous system functions, healthy skin
Deficiency: appetite loss, confusion, fatigue, flaky skin, indigestion, pellagra
Toxicity: cramping, flushing, headaches, irregular heartbeat, irritated ulcers, liver dysfunction

Cooking Foods with Niacin

Niacin is one of the more stable water-soluble vitamins and is minimally at risk for destruction by air, heat or light.

The adult RDA for niacin is 14 to 16 milligrams of niacin equivalents (NE) daily [4, 12].

Sources of Niacin	Amount (milligrams Niacin Equivalents [NE])[a]
3 ounces canned white tuna in water	11.30 mg NE
3 ounces skinless chicken breast	7.3
3 ounces skinless turkey breast	5.8
1 cup fortified breakfast cereal	5–7[b]
2 tablespoons dry-roasted peanuts	3.8
1 cup cooked lentils	2.1

[a]Niacin Equivalents (NE) are units that are used to express the niacin content of food. They represent preformed niacin plus tryptophan equivalents. 1 mg NE = 60 mg of tryptophan = 1 mg niacin.
[b]Average fortification.

PANTOTHENIC ACID AND BIOTIN

Pantothenic acid and biotin are two B vitamins that synthesize coenzymes for many reactions in the human, ranging from cellular growth to energy production. Their functions include DNA synthesis and blood glucose maintenance.

Bacteria in the large intestine (colon) can make pantothenic acid, but the human body may not be able to absorb it in significant amounts. Both pantothenic acid and biotin are widely available in food. Carrots, chicken breast, eggs, orange juice and oatmeal are particularly rich sources.

> **Sources of pantothenic acid and biotin:** many foods; principally carrots, chicken breast, eggs, orange juice, oatmeal
> **Roles in body:** coenzyme in energy metabolism, fat synthesis, glycogen production
> **Deficiency:** appetite loss, depression, fatigue, muscle pain, nausea, skin rash, sleep disorders
> **Toxicity:** none documented

Cooking with Pantothenic Acid and Biotin

Pantothenic acid is relatively unstable in food. Significant amounts can be lost in commercial processing, packaging, cooking and freezing.

Biotin is relatively stable when exposed to heat, light or oxygen. Strongly acidic conditions can denature biotin. Biotin is bound to a sugar-protein molecule in raw eggs. It cannot be absorbed unless eggs are cooked, which allows biotin to separate from this protein.

The Food and Nutrition Board of the Institute of Medicine has established AI levels for pantothenic acid and biotin based on estimated dietary intakes of healthy people. The AI for pantothenic acid is 5 milligrams (mg) daily for adults 19 years of age and older. The AI for biotin is 30 micrograms (mcg) daily for adults 19 years of age and older [13,14].

Sources of Pantothenic Acid and Biotin	Pantothenic Acid Amount (milligrams)	Biotin Amount (micrograms)
1 cup plain nonfat yogurt	1.60 mg	
1 medium cooked sweet potato	0.88	
1 large cooked egg	0.61	13–25 mg
½ cup cooked peas	0.58	
½ cup chopped raw mushrooms		0.52
3 ounces cooked pork	2–4	
3 ounces cooked salmon	4–5	
½ avocado	1–3	
1 ounce Cheddar cheese	0.4–2	

WATER-SOLUBLE VITAMINS AND AMINO ACID METABOLISM

The water-soluble vitamins B6 (pyridoxine), folate (folic acid, folacin) and B12, *plus* vitamin C are involved in *amino acid metabolism* in the human body. *Vitamin B6*, also called *pyridoxine*, is a coenzyme that plays vital roles in protein and fat metabolism. The more protein a person consumes, the greater their vitamin B6 requirement.

A vitamin B6 deficiency contributes to conditions including insomnia, irritability, increased risk of heart disease, poor immune response and weakness. Vitamin B6 is sometimes used to treat premenstrual syndrome (PMS) disorders. Toxicity from vitamin B6 supplements may lead to nervous system disorders.

Vitamin B6 must be obtained from the diet because the human body cannot synthesize it. Baked potatoes, bananas, chicken breast, figs, pork chops and salmon are particularly rich sources of vitamin B6.

VITAMIN B6 (PYRIDOXINE)

Sources of vitamin B6: deep green leafy vegetables, fish, meats, poultry, soy, whole grains
Roles in body: antibody formation, converts the amino acid tryptophan into niacin, fat and protein metabolism, red blood cell formation
Deficiency: central nervous system disorders, kidney stones, rashes, weakness
Toxicity: depression, fatigue, headaches, numbness and nerve damage, poor coordination

Cooking Foods with Vitamin B6

Vitamin B6 is easily lost during processing and cooking. This includes canning fruits and vegetables, freezing fruits, and processing grains and meats into by-products.

The acidity of food is a factor to consider in the loss of vitamin B6. In general, the more acidic the food, the more B6 is lost in food processing and cooking. Freezing can result in about a one-third to one-half loss of vitamin B6.

The RDA for vitamin B6 is 1.3 milligrams (mg) daily for adult men and women 19 years of age and older [15, 16].

Sources of Vitamin B6	Amount (milligrams)
1 baked potato with skin	0.70 mg
1 banana	0.68
3 ounces cooked salmon	0.48
3 ounces cooked skinless chicken breast	0.51
1 cup cooked spinach	0.44
3 ounces lean pork loin	0.42

THE WATER-SOLUBLE VITAMINS AND BLOOD FORMATION

The water-soluble vitamins: folate (folic acid, folacin) and vitamin B12, along with riboflavin, vitamin B6, vitamin C and choline are responsible for blood formation in the human body.

FOLATE (FOLIC ACID, FOLACIN)

Like thiamin, riboflavin and niacin, *folate* is a coenzyme. It is essential for DNA synthesis and red blood cell formation. Folate deficiency can lead to *megaloblastic anemia* (also called *pernicious anemia*). In this type of anemia, red blood cells are malformed, which affects their oxygen-carrying capacity, and fewer red blood cells are produced in the bone marrow. Symptoms such as appetite loss, fatigue, headache and/or weakness may follow.

Folate is especially important during pregnancy because it reduces the risk of *neural tube defects*, which may cause *spina bifida* in infants. Spina bifida is characterized bifida is characterized by the incomplete closure of the bony casing around the base of the spinal cord. This may lead to partial paralysis and a condition called *anencephaly*, where major parts of the brain are deformed.

To help prevent neural tube defects, young women of childbearing age are encouraged to consume foods that are fortified with folate or take a folate supplement in addition to a folate-rich diet. The RDA for folic acid for this group of women is 600 micrograms of folic acid daily. Supplementation may be warranted under medical care.

To help meet this amount, the US Food and Drug Administration (FDA) has required that all enriched grain products be fortified with folate. As approved by the FDA, nutrition labels may read "Adequate intake of folate has been shown to reduce the risk of neural tube defects." To carry this claim, the food must meet or exceed the criteria for a good source of folate. This amounts to 40 micrograms of folate per serving, or at least 10 percent of the Daily Value for folate.

Folate toxicity is rare, other than as a result of supplements. Too much folate in the diet may mask a vitamin B12 deficiency. Alcohol ingestion interferes with folate absorption. Folate is abundant in foliage, such as green leafy vegetables like spinach and broccoli; fortified breads and cereals; legumes; and orange juice. Asparagus, black-eyed peas, lentils and oatmeal are other significant sources of folate.

FOOD BYTE

Asparagus The consumption of *asparagus* is a reported treatment for kidney and bladder disorders and urinary infections. Nevertheless, asparagus contains a high level of purines—substances that are found in all body cells that help provide chemical structure for genes. In excess, purines may build up crystals of uric acid and lead to a painful condition called gouty arthritis in the joints, tendons and tissues of susceptible people. Certain chemicals in asparagus emit a distinctive smell to the urine when they are metabolized. This phenomenon is due to various sulfur-containing by-products that are produced, including ammonia. When tolerated, *asparagus* is low in calories and very low in sodium; contains no fat or cholesterol; and is a good source of folic acid, dietary fiber and potassium.

VITAMIN: FOLATE (FOLIC ACID, FOLACIN)

Sources of folate: dark green leafy vegetables, enriched breads and cereals, legumes, liver, melons, oranges
Roles in body: cell division, new cell formation, red blood cell production
Deficiency: anemia, depression, diarrhea, heartburn, increased risk of certain cancers and heart disease, megoloblastic (pernicious) anemia, neural tube defects, poor growth
Toxicity: conceals vitamin B12 deficiency, diarrhea, insomnia, irritability

Cooking Foods with Folate

Processed grains and flours may lose a significant amount of folate during processing. This is one of the reasons why grains and flours are fortified with folate. The folate in animal foods appears to be relatively stable to cooking, unlike the folate in plant foods, which can lose up to 40 percent of the folate during cooking. This is because folate is lost whenever high temperatures or large amounts of water are used. Microwave cooking appears to destroy more folate than other cooking methods.

The RDA for folate is expressed as Dietary Folate Equivalent (DFE) to account for differences in absorption. The RDA for folate is 400 micrograms DFE for adult men and women 19 years of age and older [17, 18].

Sources of Folate	Amount (micrograms of DFE)
1 cup fortified breakfast cereal	200–400 mcg DFE[a]
½ cup cooked lentils	179
½ cup cooked garbanzo beans	141
½ cup cooked asparagus	134
½ cup cooked spinach	132
6 ounces orange juice	83
⅓ cup peanuts	71

[a]Average fortification.

Recipe: Roasted Asparagus with Parmesan "Crackers" and Eggs

*This recipe for **Roasted Asparagus with Parmesan "Crackers" and Eggs** in the **Recipe file** which is located within the Culinary Nutrition website at www.culinarynutrition.elsevier.com, showcases folate-rich asparagus, topped with a sweet and tart aged balsamic vinegar dressing, poached eggs and Parmesan cheese that has been browned into "crackers." It makes an ample meal, especially when teamed with whole-grain bread and soup, such as the Cream of Tomato Basil soup that is featured in Chapter 11. The finished dish is shown within the centerfold **Photo file** in Plate 7.3.*

VITAMIN B12 (COBALAMIN)

The chief role of *vitamin B12*, also known as *cobalamin*, is to maintain a healthy central nervous system. Vitamin B12 deficiency can cause nerve degeneration and permanent nerve damage. Vitamin B12 also works with folate to help manufacture red blood cells. Like folic acid deficiency, insufficient vitamin B12 can cause anemia, which is characterized by large, immature and dysfunctional red blood cells.

Vitamin B12 is only found in foods of animal origin. That is why vegetarians and vegans run the risk of deficiency. Chicken liver, cottage cheese, ground beef, sardines and tuna are good sources of vitamin B12.

There are vegetarian sources of vitamin B12, such as fortified soy foods and beverages and breakfast cereals. Some breakfast cereals contain vitamin B12, with high bioavailability for vegetarians. But foods vary in their formulations, so it is important to read food labels for added nutrients [19,20].

The absorption of Vitamin B12 is dependent on a compound called the *intrinsic factor* that is produced in the stomach. Certain groups of people are born without it, thus requiring vitamin B12 supplementation.

Vitamin B12 is best absorbed when the stomach is acidic. Some elderly develop a condition known as *atrophic gastritis* that prevents them from producing enough acid for vitamin B12 absorption. Once again, vitamin B12 supplements may be warranted.

> **Sources of vitamin B12:** animal products, including dairy products; eggs; fish; red meat; poultry; pork; seafood; some fortified plant products, such as vitamin B12–fortified soy foods and cereals (fortification varies)
> **Roles in body:** red blood cell formation, central nervous system maintenance, DNA synthesis
> **Deficiency:** anemia, central nervous system degeneration, fatigue, paralysis
> **Toxicity:** not documented

Cooking Foods with Vitamin B12

Vitamin B12 is fairly well retained in animal foods under most cooking conditions. Retention of vitamin B12 in plant-based foods after cooking is not well documented.

The RDA for vitamin B12 is 2.4 micrograms daily for men and women aged 14 years and older [19, 21].

Sources of Vitamin B12	Amount (micrograms)
3 ounces steamed clams	84.0 mcg
3¼ ounces sardines	8.22
4 ounces broiled Chinook salmon	3.25
4 ounces broiled beef tenderloin	2.92
1 cup plain nonfat yogurt	1.39
1 whole large egg	0.60

THE WATER-SOLUBLE VITAMIN AND ANTIOXIDANTS

The water-soluble vitamin C (ascorbic acid, ascorbate), *plus* beta-carotene, vitamin E and selenium function as *antioxidants* in the human body.

VITAMIN C (ASCORBIC ACID, ASCORBATE)

In contrast to other mammals, humans cannot make their own vitamin C, so it must be obtained by the diet. *Vitamin C* is responsible for producing and maintaining *collagen*, the protein that is found in bones, connective tissues, skin, teeth and tendons. Vitamin C also functions as an antioxidant; it protects the human body from oxidative damage due to factors such as environmental pollutants, ozone, radiation and ultraviolet light.

Vitamin C is essential in the immune process; it fights infections and illnesses from the common cold to certain cancers and cardiovascular disease. While vitamin C may not prevent colds, it may help to decrease their severity and duration—especially if it is started at the onset of symptoms.

293

Vitamin C may also help the human body rebound from physical stress, such as from strenuous physical exertion or extreme temperatures. Vitamin C studies, which assess its relationship to cancers, cardiovascular disease, diabetes, hypertension, and other stressful conditions, are ongoing.

Vitamin C is abundant in fruits and vegetables, particularly bell peppers, broccoli, cantaloupe, grapefruit, kiwifruit, oranges and papaya. These foods and their juices contain many other health-enhancing phytonutrients beside antioxidants.

A vitamin C deficiency may develop in people who do not consume enough fruits or vegetables. A classic example of vitamin C deficiency occurred in the 1700s when British sailors developed *scurvy*, a potentially fatal disease that is characterized by bleeding, bruising, hair and tooth loss, joint pain and swelling. These symptoms are related to weakened blood vessels, bones and connective tissues, since the disease affects collagen formation. While scurvy is rare today in developed countries, cases of scurvy in undeveloped countries and in some children and the elderly who follow very restricted diets have been reported. Taken in excess in supplements, vitamin C may cause gastrointestinal distress.

> **Sources of vitamin C:** berries, citrus fruits, cruciferous vegetables, dark green leafy vegetables, melons, potatoes, tomatoes, tropical fruits
> **Roles in body:** antioxidant, collagen formation, immunity, promotes iron absorption, wound healing
> **Deficiency:** anemia, bleeding gums, bone weakening, depression, hemorrhages, infections, poor wound healing, scurvy, muscle wasting
> **Toxicity:** abdominal pain, diarrhea, kidney stones, nausea

Cooking Foods with Vitamin C

Vitamin C is very sensitive to air, temperature and water. The longer the time that fruits and vegetables are exposed to any of these factors, the greater the potential loss of vitamin C. Vitamin C can also decrease during blanching, freezing and/or unthawing.

To preserve vitamin C, store raw, cut fruits and vegetables in airtight containers and refrigerate. Do not soak or store fruits and vegetables in water for extended periods of time. Refrigerate juices, and then store them only 2 to 3 days. Simmer or steam foods in a very small amount of water, or microwave for a short time. Cook potatoes in their skins.

The RDA for vitamin C is 75 milligrams (mg) daily for females and 90 milligrams (mg) for males aged 19 years and older. The RDA for smokers is 110 milligrams of vitamin C for woman and 125 milligrams of vitamin C for men aged 19 years and older [22–24].

Sources of Vitamin C	Amount (milligrams)
1 cup whole strawberries	85 mg
1 orange	70
½ cup sweet bell pepper	65
½ cup cooked broccoli	51
½ medium grapefruit	38
1 medium tomato	16

FOOD BYTE

Limes are tarter than lemons. Limes come in two varieties: the larger, greener Persian lime and the smaller, yellow key or Mexican lime. "Key lime" is an American creation. Limes are valued in Mexican, southwestern United States, and Thai cuisines for their acidity and zest. Common culinary uses of limes include key lime pie, a traditional Floridian dessert; limeade, a refreshing citrus beverage; and ceviche, a raw seafood dish that relies on acidic ingredients, such as lime juice, to break down the protein fibers. The leaves of the Kaffir lime are used in Southeast Asian cooking. Dried limes are used as flavoring in Persian cuisine. The tartness of limes can be tempered by a little bitters, cream, salt or sugar.

Nonvitamins

Nonvitamins are also called "vitamin-like" substances. Nonvitamins *do not* remedy diseases as vitamins do. Vitamin-depletion studies have demonstrated the essential nature of vitamins. In the absence of vitamins, vitamin deficiencies and diseases often follow. This is not always the case with nonvitamins. However, nonvitamins are known to have vitamin-like effects on the body, and some are quite important.

For example, *choline*, which helps form lecithin and other molecules, is a nonvitamin that is considered "conditionally essential" to the human body. A *conditionally essential nutrient* is fundamental for proper body functioning. The human body can only synthesize a small amount of choline, so it is required through food. Choline is primarily found in butter, cauliflower, egg yolk, flaxseeds, lentils, oats, peanuts, potatoes, sesame seeds and soybeans.

Inosotol, is another nonvitamin that is important in cell membranes. Inosotol can be synthesized by the body. It is mainly found in substances with high bran content and in bananas, brewer's yeast, brown rice, cantaloupe, legumes, liver, nuts, oats, oranges, raisins, unrefined molasses, vegetables and wheat germ.

Carnitine is also considered a nonvitamin because under normal circumstances, the body can make both inosotol and carnitine in sufficient amounts. Carnitine is produced by the liver and kidneys and stored in the brain, heart, muscles and sperm. Carnitine is essential in cellular activities. It helps to convert lipids into energy. Dairy products and red meat, especially lamb, are excellent sources of carnitine. Other sources include asparagus, avocadoes, fish, peanut butter, poultry, tempeh and wheat.

Other nonvitamins, including some that have been added to vitamin and mineral supplements, include bioflavonoids (such as vitamin "P" and coenzyme Q10), PABA (para-aminobenzoic acid), vitamin B15 and vitamin B17.

It may be that these nonvitamins and other yet unidentified substances are classified as vitamins in the future as research unveils. Until then, it is best to review all the evidence when contemplating their usage and not take any substance in excess.

The Classification of Minerals: Major Minerals and Trace Minerals

Just like vitamins, *minerals* are essential nutrients. They are also required in very small amounts and can become toxic in higher quantities. Also, like vitamins, minerals do not contain calories, but some are involved in energy production. Other minerals have structural or regulatory functions in the human body, such as maintaining fluid balance and acid-base balance. While vitamins are considered organic compounds (meaning they contain carbon), minerals are considered inorganic. They are composed of matter other than plants or animals. Most minerals occur naturally in the earth's crust, such as iron or copper.

Minerals, like vitamins, are grouped into two main categories: *major minerals* and *trace minerals.* The main difference between major minerals and trace minerals is the quantity that is found in the human body.

Major minerals are found in quantities that are greater than 5 grams, while trace minerals are found in quantities that are less than 5 grams. The major minerals include calcium, chloride, magnesium, phosphorus, potassium, sodium and sulfur. The trace minerals include chromium, copper, fluoride, iodine, iron, manganese, molybdenum, selenium and zinc.

On the whole, animal foods contain more calcium, iron and zinc than plant foods, plus the bioavailability of these minerals is higher. *Bioavailability* is the extent that the digestive tract can absorb a nutrient and how well the human body uses it. Overall, the more a food is processed, the fewer minerals that are available. Enrichment helps to put minerals and other nutrients back into processed foods, and fortification helps to add even more minerals and other nutrients. Such is the case when cereal grains are enriched and fortified. Even tap water is a source of minerals, but bottled water may be devoid of certain minerals or very concentrated in others.

Mineral research, similar to vitamin research, is ever changing. The bioavailability of minerals in foods and beverages, the functions of minerals in the human body, and the functions of minerals in disease prevention are still being questioned.

Mineral deficiencies and excesses are of equal concern. Though vitamin and mineral supplements are convenient, they are easy to overdose. That is why it is important to consume an array of foods with minerals to meet daily needs.

The Importance of Minerals in the Human Body

Comparable to vitamins, groups of minerals work together to help maintain good health. These groups include, but are not limited to, the following:

- Calcium, phosphorus and zinc support growth and development.
- Calcium, copper, fluoride, iron, magnesium, phosphorus and zinc are essential for bone and teeth mineralization.
- Calcium, chromium, copper, iron, iodine, magnesium, manganese, phosphorus and zinc help cellular metabolism.
- Calcium, copper, and iron promote blood formation and blood clotting (along with vitamin K).
- Calcium, chloride, potassium and sodium are important for the transmission of nerve impulses.
- Chloride, magnesium, phosphorus and potassium are critical in fluid balance.

Major Minerals

Major minerals are called "major" because they are required in the daily diet in quantities that are greater than 100 milligrams. Since bones make up such a sizeable proportion of the human body, it is not surprising that the major bone minerals are needed in significant amounts. Likewise, since water makes up 60 percent of the human body, it follows that the major minerals that are found in body fluids are also needed in abundance.

Calcium

Calcium is the most plentiful mineral in the human body. The majority of calcium is found in bones and teeth. A small percentage of calcium is found in blood and other fluids. The roles of calcium in the body include bone development and maintenance, body fluid balance, blood clotting, blood pressure, enzyme activation, muscle contraction and nerve transmission. A calcium deficiency can lead to poor growth and development, and *osteoporosis*, a brittle-bone disease (see "Bite on This: osteoporosis"). Calcium toxicity can be caused by calcium supplements, hormonal disorders and conditions that prevent calcium excretion, such as kidney dysfunction.

Dairy products, dark green leafy vegetables, fish with small bones, and fortified beverages and soy products are good sources of calcium. Examples of these foods include plain low-fat and nonfat yogurt; bok choy, broccoli and kale; sardines and shrimp; and calcium-fortified orange juice and tofu.

Dairy products commonly contain the most calcium per serving, plus they contain vitamin D, which aids calcium absorption. Vitamin D helps absorb calcium from the small intestine into the bloodstream and helps to maintain normal blood calcium, which is essential to cardiac function.

Though green leafy vegetables are good sources of calcium, they also contain *oxalic acid*, which tends to bind calcium and prevents its absorption. High-fiber foods may interfere with calcium absorption, as well as phosphorus, a mineral that is found in soft drinks in the form of phosphoric acid.

It has been estimated that humans absorb around 25 percent less of the calcium that is available from foods and beverages. This factor should be considered in recipe and menu development and diet planning.

Sources of calcium: dairy products, dark green leafy vegetables, fish with small bones, fortified beverages, soy products
Roles in body: blood pressure and blood clotting, bone and teeth formation and maintenance, fluid balance, muscle contraction, nerve transmission
Deficiency: osteoporosis, central nervous system disorders, coronary disorders, poor growth and development
Toxicity: central nervous system disorders, coronary disorders

296

Cooking Foods with Calcium

The amount of calcium in foods does not seem to be affected by cooking or long-term storage.

The RDA for calcium is 1,000 milligrams for women and men aged 19 to 50 years and 1,200 milligrams daily for women aged 51 years and older.

Sources of Calcium	Amount (milligrams)
1 cup plain low-fat yogurt	415 mg
6 ounces calcium-fortified orange juice	378[a]
1½ ounces part-skim mozzarella cheese	253
½ cup calcium-fortified tofu	138[a]
3 ounces sardines in oil	324
½ cup cooked spinach	123

[a]Average fortification.

Bite on This: osteoporosis—the bone-breaker disease

Osteoporosis is a disease that affects the skeletal structure of the body. The term *osteoporosis* literally means "porous bones," which are filled with holes, and not a solid matrix or web as dense, healthy bones.

Porous bones are more prone to fractures than dense bones, in part due to lower bone mineral density. Since the minerals calcium, phosphorus and magnesium and the vitamins A, C, D and K all contribute to healthy bones, one or more of these vitamins or minerals may be deficient in osteoporosis.

Many factors predispose a person to osteoporosis. Osteoporosis is more common in women than in men, mostly due to poor calcium intake, less peak bone mass after puberty, and menopause, which deprives women of estrogen and its bone-protective effects. Men can also become osteoporotic due to smoking, alcohol ingestion, poor calcium intake, steroid use, and other factors.

A family history of osteoporosis increases the risk of this disease, as does ethnicity. People of British, Chinese, Japanese, Mexican American, and Northern European descent are at the greatest risk. African Americans tend to have thicker bones and less risk. Smaller-framed individuals with less bone mass are more vulnerable.

In addition to family history, ethnicity and body frame size, inactivity may increase the risk of osteoporosis. Weight-bearing exercises such as walking, running or dancing place a healthy stress on the large bones of the torso.

Medical conditions, such as asthma, organ transplants, rheumatoid arthritis, seizures, thyroid disorders and Type I diabetes can increase the risk of osteoporosis because the drugs that are necessary in their management may accelerate bone loss, decrease calcium absorption, and reduce bone formation.

Diets that are high in phosphorus, sodium and protein may contribute to bone loss because the body seeks to have a balance of nutrients in the bloodstream for *homeostasis*, or equilibrium. Calcium may be drawn from its stores within the skeletal system to maintain this homeostasis. This condition is one of the concerns about high-protein diets.

A diet that provides enough potassium and magnesium, through ample fruit and vegetable intake, may improve bone density—especially in older people. Perhaps the phytochemicals in these foods help to protect the skeletal system in some yet unconfirmed ways.

A careful assessment of calcium intake should be the first line of action in preventing osteoporosis. Table 7-1 summarizes the daily calcium requirements based on age and gender. Recommended Dietary Allowances have not been established for infants from birth until 12 months of age. Instead, AI levels of 200 milligrams for infants aged 0 to 6 months and 260 milligrams for infants 7 to 12 months have been established.

TABLE 7-1 Daily Calcium Requirements

Age in Years	Daily Calcium Requirement (milligrams)
1 to 3	700 mg
4 to 8	1,000
9 to 13	1,300
14–18	1,300
19–50	1,000
51–70	1,000 men; 1,200 women
71 *plus*	1,200
14–18 pregnancy or lactation	1,300
19–50 pregnancy or lactation	1,000

Source: [25].

If the level of calcium is not met during pregnancy, the fetus will draw calcium from the mother's calcium stores. A person over 71 years of age requires 1,300 milligrams of calcium daily because most bone fractures occur in people of this age and older. Calcium absorption is less efficient throughout aging, coupled with lower vitamin D intake and sun exposure.

The topmost dietary sources of calcium include the following:

- Dairy milk and plain low-fat yogurt, at around 300 milligrams per cup
- Calcium-fortified soy and other beverages, at 300 to 350 milligrams of calcium per cup
- Cheese, at 250 to 300 per 1½ ounces
- Blackstrap molasses, at 180 milligrams per tablespoon
- Cooked legumes, such as pinto beans or white Northern, at 50 to 115 milligrams per cup
- Green leafy vegetables, at 35 to 80 milligrams per ½ cup

Oranges (74 mg per one large), figs (22 mg per one large), and cooked rhubarb (174 mg per ½ cup) also have respectable amounts of calcium per serving.

The best dietary sources of calcium may not be enough to prevent osteoporosis in osteoporosis-prone individuals. Roughly one-quarter less calcium is absorbed from foods and beverages, and calcium absorption may be poorer in people who take medications for disease complications. This is where supplements may fill the gap.

Common calcium supplements include calcium carbonate and calcium citrate. Calcium carbonate is the least expensive, most available and most commonly consumed calcium supplement. Antacids contain calcium carbonate for relatively low cost.

Calcium carbonate should be consumed with meals, ideally with a source of calcium, such as dairy milk, to improve its absorption. This may be problematic in populations that are lactose intolerant. Calcium carbonate also requires an acidic medium for best absorption. Older people tend to have less gastric acid, so they may require a different calcium supplement to improve absorption.

Calcium citrate tends to be more expensive than calcium carbonate, but absorption is better because it does not require an acidic medium. Other calcium supplements include calcium gluconate, malate, lactate and phosphate, with varying degrees of absorption.

Calcium absorption from supplements is also dependent on the amount consumed. It is best to keep dosages at 500 milligrams or fewer. Some people might experience side effects from calcium supplements, such as bloating, constipation and/or gas. In general, calcium citrate may be better tolerated.

If calcium supplements are used to supplement dietary intake, then one should follow the guidelines that are shown in Table 7-1. Calcium intake that exceeds the RDA should be first discussed with a health care provider.

Despite genetic predisposition to osteoporosis, some steps can be taken for its prevention and control. Eat plenty of calcium-containing foods, especially before peak bone mass forms during adolescence; exercise; do not smoke; drink alcohol in moderation; and consider supplements if any of these factors are not attainable. More information about calcium, osteoporosis and disease prevention can be found in Chapter 9.

PHOSPHORUS

Phosphorus is the second most abundant mineral in the human body. As much as 85 percent of phosphorus is found with calcium in bones and teeth. Phosphorus is also a part of DNA and RNA, the genetic code of every cell, which makes it essential for cellular growth and development. Another role of phosphorus is in energy metabolism, similar to the B vitamins. Also, phospholipids, like lecithin, rely on phosphorus in their structure.

A natural source of phosphorus is animal protein because phosphorus is contained in every cell. Carbonated beverages contain phosphorus in the form of phosphoric acid. Excess phosphorus can affect the level of calcium in the body and cause calcium excretion. For this reason, diets that are abundant in animal protein and carbonated beverages should be balanced by ample intake of calcium-rich foods.

Phosphorus toxicity can lead to gastrointestinal disorders and calcification of nonskeletal tissues, such as the kidneys, and lead to kidney damage. Phosphorus deficiency can lead to bone pain and muscle weakness. Excellent sources of phosphorus include canned salmon, cottage cheese, pork, sirloin steak and yogurt.

Sources of phosphorus: carbonated beverages, dairy products, fish, meats, poultry, processed foods
Roles in body: acid-base balance, bone and teeth formation, development and maintenance, energy metabolism
Deficiency: bone pain, general lethargy, muscle weakness
Toxicity: calcium imbalance in blood, bones and teeth, leading to calcium deposits in nonskeletal tissues, gastrointestinal disorders, kidney damage

Cooking Foods with Phosphorus

Phosphorus is lost in cooking some foods, even under the most careful conditions. To retain phosphorus, cook foods in a minimal amount of water for the shortest cooking time. Roast or broil lamb, pork, poultry and veal. Beef appears to retain phosphorus despite the cooking method.

The RDA for phosphorus is 700 milligrams (mg) daily for women and men aged 19 years and older [26, 27].

Sources of Phosphorus	Amount (milligrams)
1 cup plain nonfat yogurt	385 mg
3 ounces cooked salmon	252
1 cup dairy skim milk	247
3 ounces cooked beef	173
1 large cooked egg	104
1 slice whole wheat bread	57

MAGNESIUM

Magnesium, like calcium and phosphorus, is a mineral that is important in bone and teeth mineralization. Magnesium also functions in the protein synthesis of the heart, liver, muscle and soft tissue cells and is critical in their metabolism. Magnesium helps muscles to contract and relax, and nerves to transmit impulses.

The human body only absorbs about 40 to 60 percent of magnesium that is consumed from foods and beverages, unless there is a deficiency, in which case more is absorbed. Magnesium deficiency can be caused by alcoholism, inadequate intake, protein malnutrition, severe vomiting or diarrhea. It may lead to confusion, growth failure, muscle spasms and overall weakness.

Magnesium toxicity may cause unusually low blood pressure, coordination disorders and fatality. Toxicity can result from magnesium-based antacids, laxatives or supplements. The elderly are of particular concern if they mistakenly take too much magnesium with their medications.

Top sources of magnesium include almonds, cashews, fortified cereals, spinach, tofu, and oysters. Good sources include chocolate, dark green leafy vegetables, legumes, nuts and seafood. Dark leafy greens are high in chlorophyll, a green pigment that contains magnesium. Refined grains are generally low in magnesium unless they are fortified, since their nutrient-rich germ and bran are removed in processing. Hard water is a good source of magnesium, like calcium.

> **Sources of magnesium:** chocolate, dark green leafy vegetables, fortified cereals, legumes, nuts, seafood, whole grains
> **Roles in body:** protein synthesis, muscular contraction and relaxation, nerve transmission, teeth and bone mineralization
> **Deficiency:** confusion, failure to grow, muscle spasms, weakness
> **Toxicity:** coma, coordination difficulties, unusually low blood pressure, death

Cooking Foods with Magnesium

Cooking and processing can affect the magnesium content of foods, which can vary greatly. Some magnesium is water-soluble, so blanching or steaming can lead to magnesium loss. When spinach is blanched, magnesium loss is about one-third of the content of fresh spinach, and when legumes are cooked, they may lose about two-thirds of their magnesium content. There is very little magnesium loss in processing almonds and/or peanuts.

The RDA for magnesium is 310 milligrams (mg) daily for women and 400 milligrams daily for men aged 19 to 30 years, and 310 milligrams daily for women and 420 milligrams daily for men aged 31 years and older. During pregnancy, the RDA for magnesium is 350 milligrams daily for women aged 19 to 30 years, and 360 milligrams daily for women aged 31 years and older. During lactation, the RDA for magnesium is 310 milligrams daily for women aged 19 to 30 years, and 320 milligrams daily for women 31 years and older [28, 29].

Sources of Magnesium	Amount (milligrams)
2 tablespoons almonds	90 mg
2 tablespoons dry-roasted peanuts	50
½ cup cooked spinach	75
1 baked potato	50
½ cup cooked brown rice	40
1 medium banana	30

SODIUM

Sodium, like potassium and chloride, is an **electrolyte**. Electrolytes are dissolved substances that maintain the human body's fluid balance both inside and outside the cells. They carry positive and negative charges, much like a battery, so they are attracted to or repelled from each other.

Sodium (Na^+) and chloride (Cl^-) are the most abundant electrolytes outside of the cells in extracellular fluid. Potassium (K^+) is the most abundant electrolyte inside of the cells in intracellular fluid. The human body is capable of diffusing, or moving, electrolytes throughout the cells to keep these electrically charged minerals in balance. But when electrolytes are "off," meaning too high or too low in concentration, major body systems may be affected.

Sodium also helps to maintain acid-base balance, muscular contraction and nerve transmission. Too little sodium can cause appetite loss, mental confusion, muscular cramping, and, in extreme conditions, stroke or heart failure. Excess sodium can increase blood pressure and place undue stress on the brain, heart, kidneys and other organs.

The richest sources of sodium are common table salt, cured foods such as anchovies and pork products, pickled foods such as olives and pickles, processed foods, and soy sauce and other condiments. A sodium deficiency is generally rare because sodium is found in so many processed foods. Animal foods tend to be higher in sodium than plant foods because sodium is found in animal tissues. Green leafy vegetables, root vegetables and tomatoes are some of the plant foods that contain high levels of sodium.

The physiological need for sodium in the human body ranges from 220 to 500 milligrams daily. The average consumption of sodium in the United States may be as much as 10 times this amount. Ordinary table salt contains about 2,300 milligrams of sodium per teaspoon, or 40 percent sodium (60 percent chloride). Some kosher salt contains about 1,920 milligrams of sodium per teaspoon, while some sea salt contains about 1,320 milligrams of sodium per teaspoon. While these are preferred in many cooking and baking applications, they are still significant sources of sodium.

Sources of sodium: condiments, cured foods, pickled foods, processed foods, table salt
Roles in body: maintenance of normal fluid balance and acid-base balance, nerve impulses
Deficiency: appetite loss, mental disorientation, muscle cramps
Toxicity: high blood pressure, stress on organ systems, death

Cooking Foods with Sodium

Sodium loss in cooking is usually not a nutritional concern because it can be compensated by condiments or sauces. If there is too much sodium in a recipe (usually the result of too much salt), add a cut potato or slice of bread with the crust removed, which acts like a sponge to soak up the salt (discard the potato or bread afterward). A teaspoon each of sugar and vinegar may balance the saltiness in a dish. This is because sweetness lessens saltiness, and sourness enhances sweetness and counteracts saltiness. Extra ingredients can also be added to recipes to lower the sodium, such as water or low-sodium broth to dilute soups or stews.

The RDA for sodium is 2,300 milligrams daily for women and men aged 19 to 50 years, or the equivalent of about 1 teaspoon of table salt daily. For adults over 50 years of age, African Americans, and people who have been diagnosed with chronic kidney disease, diabetes or hypertension, the RDA is established at 1,500 milligrams of sodium daily. These groups are considered to be more sodium sensitive [30–33]. Common foods with their sodium content are shown in Table 7-2.

Bite on This: reducing sodium in the diet

The current average daily intake of sodium in the United States has been trending upward for the past 40 years, despite public health efforts to reduce sodium consumption. While a certain amount of sodium is safe, makes food palatable, and is valued in food manufacturing, recipe development, and food preservation, too much sodium is detrimental to human health.

Sodium recommendations are driven by scientific research and public health. High blood pressure (hypertension) and prehypertension are prevalent in the United States, along with rising obesity, which are all expected to increase and burden the US health care system and economy. Reduced hypertension could save health care costs from fewer strokes and heart attacks and lower the risks of some cancers.

While most people may benefit from cutting back sodium consumption, those who have hypertension or those who have a genetic predisposition for hypertension may benefit even more. An intake of 2,300 milligrams of sodium daily is preferred for most healthy US adults. People who are 51 years of age and older, African American, diabetic, prehypertensive or have chronic kidney disease should consume no more than 1,500 milligrams of sodium daily (about ⅔ teaspoon of salt).

Lowering sodium in the food supply while maintaining flavor will help people adjust to less. If the food supply is too low in sodium, people will not favor lower-sodium foods. A 10 to 25 percent reduction of sodium may still be perceived as flavorful as long as flavor-enhancement techniques are used to maintain flavor.

Ethnic cuisines are good examples of how to incorporate a little bit of higher-sodium foods to give the perception that foods are saltier. A touch of soy sauce (Asian), salted fish (Scandinavian), and/or salty cheese and olives (Mediterranean) can give the illusion that a food is salty, but the total sodium content may be lower than sodium-rich fast foods that monopolize the US diet.

Like other nutrients, sodium should be viewed in moderation, not elimination. Sodium has many valuable functions, and diets would be tasteless and tiresome without it. Tips for reducing sodium while preserving palatability can be found in "Bite on This: decreasing the sodium in foods, cooking and baking" and in Chapter 9.

TABLE 7-2 Sodium Content of Common Foods and Beverages

Sources of Sodium	Amount (milligrams)
½ cup canned kidney beans	435 mg
½ cup cooked dried or frozen navy beans without salt[a]	2
1 cup ready-to-eat breakfast cereal	0–300
½ cup unsalted cooked breakfast cereal[a]	0–5
½ cup canned corn	280
½ cup cooked fresh corn kernels[a]	4
½ cup stewed tomatoes	282
½ cup fresh chopped tomatoes[a]	8
½ cup applesauce	4
1 fresh apple[a]	0
1 cup low-fat dairy chocolate milk	153
1 cup nonfat dairy milk[a]	127
1 cup skim milk yogurt	175
1 cup low-fat yogurt with fruit[a]	132
1 ounce pasteurized processed cheese	405
1 ounce part-skim mozzarella cheese[a]	150
2 tablespoons salted dry-roasted peanuts	230
2 tablespoons unsalted dry roasted peanuts[a]	2
3 ounces cured ham	1,128
3 ounces roast pork[a]	54
3 ounces canned pink salmon	471
3 ounces cooked sockeye salmon[a]	56
1 ounce salted potato chips	168
1 ounce unsalted potato chips[a]	2
1 tablespoon blue cheese–type salad dressing	167
1 tablespoon homemade vinegar and oil salad dressing (without salt)[a]	0

Source: [34,35].
[a]Lower sodium choices.

Bite on This: decreasing the sodium in foods, cooking and baking

Alternatives to Table Salt: Kosher and Sea Salts

A wide variety of kosher and sea salts are marketed as alternatives to table salt. Many food developers and chefs instinctively know how kosher and sea salt crystals flavor foods and beverages. This is because of the taste, tactile and visual qualities of kosher and sea salts, which convey where they should be mixed into a formula or recipe and how much should be used.

What makes kosher salt distinctive is that it is a pure mineral combination of sodium and chloride and that it has a unique size and shape. Kosher salt is produced by an alteration in the evaporation process that causes the crystals to be larger and more irregular than table salt. In general, kosher salt lacks the anticaking additives and whitening agents of table salt. Many cooks prefer kosher salt because its larger crystals are convenient and practical in certain recipes and types of food preparation.

Kosher salt was initially devised for the "koshering" of meats, which is a critical process that is specified in the dietary laws of many religions—especially in Judaism. For meats to be considered Kosher, all of the blood must be thoroughly removed. Because kosher salt has a large crystal size, it tends to dissolve more slowly in the curing process of meats, and it more meticulously removes any traces of blood.

Sea salt contains several calcium, magnesium, potassium and zinc compounds that contribute flavor and some minerals to the diet. These compounds may comprise as much as 60 percent of the total composition of some varieties.

Some sea salts may range from 40 to 70 percent less sodium than standard table salt. They may be free of any chemicals or artificial flavors, but brands vary. Like kosher salt, many sea salt crystals are larger and more irregular in shape than table salt, so they are preferred for their wide range of culinary applications.

Finishing sea salts, plain or flavored, may provide lasting and memorable opportunities for the food developer or chef to balance flavor and enhance texture.

Newer Technologies

Newer technologies have produced substances to help reduce the amount of sodium in food products. Compounds that activate the calcium receptors on the tongue may enhance the flavor of low-salt and low-sugar foods and reduce the need for extra flavoring. Some calcium and potassium compounds have salty flavors, but they may also have some undesirable off-flavors, such as metallic or bitter tastes. Potassium chloride may replace up to 30 percent of sodium chloride in some foods; anything over that level may become unpalatable. Bitter blockers that are used to reduce objectionable flavors in salt substitutes and low-salt foods are being studied.

Decreasing sodium in foods, cooking and baking is the mutual responsibility of food developers, chefs and consumers. Simple consumer actions such as label reading, using less salt in cooking, and avoiding salt at the table are prudent. More aggressive actions by food manufacturers and the food service industry may be warranted. Lowering sodium in foods, cooking and baking could have a profound intake on disease prevention and health enhancement [36,37,38,39,40,41].

CHLORIDE

Chloride is an electrolyte, like potassium and sodium. It is the main *negatively* charged electrolyte outside of cells, where it partners with sodium. Along with sodium outside of the cells and potassium inside of the cells, chloride helps to keep fluids in balance. Because chloride has the ability to cross the cell membranes, it helps to transport nutrients inside the cells where they are needed, and waste products outside the cells for disposal.

In addition to fluid balance, chloride functions to maintain the acid-base balance in the body. Chloride is a part of hydrochloric acid in the stomach, which is essential for protein digestion. The majority of chloride comes from table salt, or **sodium chloride**. It is also found in condiments and processed foods and naturally in many vegetables, especially celery, lettuce, tomatoes and seaweed.

A chloride deficiency may be caused by diarrhea, diuretics, excessive sweating or vomiting. It may lead to apathy, appetite loss, growth failure in children or muscle cramps.

Chloride toxicity may lead to gastrointestinal disturbances or hypertension because of its association with sodium.

> **Sources of chloride:** condiments, processed foods, rye, seaweed, sea salt and table salt, fruits and vegetables, especially celery, lettuce, olives, tomatoes
> **Roles in body:** acid-base balance, fluid balance, protein digestion
> **Deficiency:** apathy, appetite loss, growth failure, muscle cramps
> **Toxicity:** altered acid-base balance, fluid retention, hypertension

Cooking Foods with Chloride

Chloride generally accompanies sodium in table salt (sodium chloride, or NaCl). A pinch of table salt helps to keep vegetables green when cooking; it raises the boiling point of water so that vegetables cook faster, prevents vegetables from getting soggy, and enhances their flavor.

Calcium ($CaCl_2$) and potassium chloride (KCl) are two salt substitutes that are used to reduce sodium in food and beverage production. Calcium chloride is used in canned tomatoes, sport drinks and tofu as a firming agent. Potassium chloride is used in artificially sweetened jellies, foods that contain the seaweed carrageenan, and chocolate milk as a firming agent.

The AI level for chloride is 2.3 grams daily for women and men aged 14 to 50 years; 2.0 grams daily for women and men aged 51 to 70 years; and 1.8 grams for women and men aged 71 years and older [42, 43].

Sources of Chloride	Amounts (milligrams)
2 teaspoons Parmesan cheese	1,110 mg
3 ounces canned salmon	880
½ cup roasted, salted peanuts	660
(½ cup raw peanuts = mg)	
½ cup celery	180
½ cup fresh carrots	70
½ cup fresh tomatoes	50

FOOD BYTE

Cruciferous vegetables are members of the Brassica family. Some have a "cross" on their stem end. They have a characteristic odor and bitterness and are filled with an impressive array of minerals (especially potassium and selenium), phytonutrients, protein, and vitamins (especially vitamins C and K). A little sourness lessens the perception of bitterness, such as a squirt of lemon juice. So does a little saltiness and umami, such as a few bacon bits. Cruciferous vegetables include broccoli, broccoflower, broccoli romanesco, Brussels sprouts, cabbage, canola/rapeseeds and greens, Chinese broccoli, Chinese cabbage, collard greens, daikon, flowering cabbage, garden cress, horseradish, kohlrabi, kale, mustard seeds and greens, napa cabbage, radish, rapini (broccoli rabe), rutabaga, rocket, Siberian kale, turnip roots and greens, wasabi, and watercress.

POTASSIUM

Potassium, like chloride and sodium, is an electrolyte. It is the principal *positively* charged electrolyte inside of the cells. Potassium plays a major role in the fluid balance throughout the body. It is also critical in the regulation of the heartbeat. If the amount of potassium is disturbed in the human body, then irregular heartbeats and death could result. Potassium imbalance may be caused by diuretics, extreme diarrhea, fad dieting, fasting, sweating or vomiting. If brain cells are affected, a potassium deficiency can cause a stroke.

The best sources of potassium are fish, fruits and vegetables, poultry, meats and whole grains. Top choices among these categories include baked potato, banana, cantaloupe, lima beans, orange juice, tea and yogurt. While a potassium deficiency is unlikely unless there is unusual fluid loss, potassium supplements may be toxic, upsetting fluid balance and potentially causing death.

Supplementary potassium is sometimes prescribed along with blood pressure medication, since it acts as a diuretic. The kidneys typically regulate potassium, as long as it passes through the gastrointestinal tract. If potassium ever bypasses the GI tract or is too high in the bloodstream, it may cause the heart to stop beating. Supplementary potassium should be supervised by a health care provider.

> **Sources of potassium:** fresh fruits and vegetables, legumes, meats, poultry, whole grains
> **Roles in body:** acid-base balance and fluid balance, heartbeat regulation, muscle contraction, nerve transmission, protein synthesis
> **Deficiency:** appetite loss, confusion, constipation, increased excretion of calcium, muscle cramps
> **Toxicity:** heart failure, muscular weakness, death

Potassium in Cooking and Baking

Some food additives contain potassium, such as potassium iodate, which is used in bread baking. In general, potassium losses from cooking and processing can be considerable. This is because potassium tends to leach into cooking liquids. After spinach is blanched, the potassium content may drop by as much as half of its raw state.

This characteristic of potassium can also be beneficial. For example, parsley contains a respectable amount of potassium. When it is dried and seeped into tea, parsley tea becomes a good source of potassium. To decrease potassium loss in cooking, use minimal amounts of water. Steam or microwave foods whenever possible.

The AI level for potassium is 4,700 milligrams daily for women and men aged 19 years and older [44, 45].

Sources of Potassium	Amount (milligrams)
1 baked potato	926 mg
1 cup plain low-fat yogurt	573
½ cup lima beans	485
1 banana	422
3 ounces pork chop	382
6 ounces orange juice	372

Morsel *"It's no use boiling your cabbage twice."* —Irish proverb

SULFUR

Sulfur is associated with protein foods with amino acids, such as dairy products, eggs, fish, meat, poultry and seafood. Sulfur helps these amino acids maintain their shapes so that they can perform their roles in the human body.

Sulfur helps to make cells rigid, such as those that are found in the hair, nails and skin. There is no RDA for sulfur because it is so abundant in the US food supply. Nor are there risks of sulfur deficiency, unless there is extreme protein deprivation, or toxicity, unless protein supplements with sulfur are consumed in excess. Sulfur has a very characteristic rotten-egg smell that can be detected in some protein supplements.

Sources of sulfur: cabbage, eggs, dairy products, fish, garlic, legumes, meats, nuts, onions, raspberries, soft water, wheat germ
Roles in body: component of some amino acids, biotin, insulin and vitamin B1 (thiamine)
Deficiency: no known; except during protein deficiencies
Toxicity: depressed growth from excessive intake of amino acid supplements with sulfur

Sulfur in Cooking

Dark green rings around hard-cooked egg yolks are characteristic of sulfur. If these rings form, the eggs were probably cooked too long and at temperatures that were too high. To help prevent sulfur rings, eggs should be placed into cold water and then quickly brought to a boil over high heat. The eggs should immediately be taken off the heat, covered, and allowed to stand for about 11 minutes. Then the eggs should be removed to a bowl that is filled with ice water to cool.

Cabbage and its relatives in the cruciferous family (broccoli, cauliflower and Brussels sprouts) do not lose all of their sulfur compounds after cutting or cooking. This is because much of the sulfur is either attached to proteins or other compounds. Additionally, more sulfur-containing molecules may be formed when cruciferous vegetables are cooked. Some of these molecules may have cancer-prevention properties. There is no RDA for sulfur [46].

Sources of Sulfur	Amount (milligrams)
½ cup raw cabbage	90 mg
½ cup cooked Brussels sprouts	80
1 cup dairy skim milk	60
½ cup raw onions	50
½ cup cooked kidney beans	50

Trace Minerals

Trace minerals are called "trace" because they are needed in very small amounts in the human body. They include chromium, copper, fluoride, iron, iodine, manganese, molybdenum, selenium and zinc. Trace minerals have only been distinguished for their importance in human nutrition and health about 50 years. Like major minerals, trace mineral research is mounting. Also, like major minerals, the bioavailability of trace minerals varies, and some are greatly affected by cooking and baking

Morsel *"Spinach is the broom of the stomach."* —French proverb

305

IRON

Iron is a trace mineral that is required in minute amounts in the human body, yet it has major functions. Iron is a component of both *hemoglobin* and *myoglobin*. **Hemoglobin** is a protein that is found in red blood cells and is what gives blood its red color. It transports oxygen to the tissues for energy metabolism and carbon dioxide away from the tissues for excretion. *Myoglobin* is a protein that is found in muscle cells. It controls oxygen uptake from the red blood cells. If iron is lacking in the diet, iron-deficiency anemia may result, which may lead to decreased concentration and energy and increased susceptibility to infection.

Iron-deficiency anemia is common around the world, particularly in iron-poor, grain-dependent countries. It is characterized by small, pale red blood cells and low hemoglobin. Conditions that create serious blood loss, such as extreme menstrual blood losses, serious intestinal diseases, or severe physical injuries, may increase the prevalence of anemia.

Pregnancy increases the need for iron, since a woman's blood supply expands to meet both her iron needs and those of the growing fetus. Iron-deficiency anemia during pregnancy can lead to premature birth, a low-birth-weight infant, and even death of the mother and fetus. Iron-deficient infants may not develop normally, and they may have serious mental and motor function disabilities. Furthermore, a heavily dairy milk–based diet during infancy may worsen iron deficiency, since dairy products are such a poor source of iron. Vegetarian children may be at particular risk.

Iron is lost daily in the feces, intestinal tract, skin, urine, and during menstruation. That is why it is important to regularly consume iron-rich foods in the diet. There are two types of iron that are found in foods: *heme iron*, which is found in fish, meats and poultry, and *nonheme iron*, which is found in plant foods. More heme iron is absorbed from the intestinal tract than nonheme iron, which is why vegetarians may have a harder time obtaining enough iron from their diet. Iron-fortified cereals, dried fruits, lentils, soybeans and spinach contain appreciable amounts of iron.

Some plant foods with nonheme iron, such as spinach or kale, contain *oxalates* that bind iron and make it less available to the human body. Only about 5 to 15 percent of dietary iron is normally absorbed in the intestinal tract, so oxalates may decrease iron absorption even more. Other binders that may interfere with iron absorption include *phytates* that are found in whole grains, and *tannins* that are found in chocolate, coffee, red wine and tea. A vegetarian diet that is rich in these foods may be compromised in iron.

Vitamin C–containing foods, such as citrus fruits or juice or tomatoes, will enhance the absorption of foods with nonheme iron. For example, if orange juice is consumed with iron-fortified cereal iron, then iron absorption should improve. Another technique for improving iron absorption is cooking nonheme iron foods in cast-iron cookware. For example, if minestrone soup with legumes and greens is cooked in a cast-iron pot, then some of the iron fillings may leach into the soup. This is called *contaminated iron*, which may be desirable, unless the body absorbs too much iron, as in *iron overload.*

Iron overload, or *hemochromatosis*, is a condition that can cause tissue damage and infections. Men are particularly prone to iron overload, which is one of the reasons why their RDA for iron is lower than a woman's daily iron requirement. Vitamin and mineral supplements with iron and iron supplements should be taken with caution; liver toxicity is of particular concern.

The best heme sources of iron include clams, fish, liver, meats, oysters and shrimp. The best nonheme sources of iron include dark green leafy vegetables such as collards, kale and spinach; dried fruits; enriched and fortified breads and cereals and whole-grain breads and cereals; legumes; and potatoes.

> **Sources of iron:** dark green leafy vegetables, dried fruits, eggs, fish, enriched and fortified cereals, legumes, poultry, red meat and shellfish
> **Roles in body:** energy generation and use, hemoglobin and myoglobin formation, immunity
> **Deficiency:** anemia (small, pale red blood cells and low hemoglobin), concentration problems, headache, intolerance to cold, paleness, reduced immunity, weakness
> **Toxicity:** acidosis, infections, injury to the liver, shock, death

Iron in Cooking

The milling of grain, which removes the bran and germ, eliminates about three-quarters of the naturally occurring iron in whole grains. Refined grains are often enriched and fortified with iron, such as breadstuffs, iron-fortified cold and hot breakfast cereals, pasta and rice. Cooking with cast-iron cookware adds iron to food. Care should be taken so that the food does not take on a metallic taste. This can be accomplished by "seasoning" cast-iron cookware before use by washing with mild soap and water, coating with oil, heating about 30 minutes, and wiping dry.

Cooking iron-rich foods with foods that are high in vitamin C increases its bioavailability, such as legumes with tomatoes in soup or clams with tomatoes in Manhattan clam chowder.

The RDA for iron is 18 milligrams (mg) daily for women aged 19 to 50 years, and 8 milligrams of iron daily for women aged 51 years and older. Pregnant women of all ages require 27 milligrams of iron daily. Lactating women aged 14 to 18 years require 10 milligrams of iron daily; those over 18 years of age require 9 milligrams of iron daily. Men aged 19 years and older require 8 milligrams of iron daily [47–49].

Sources of Iron	Amount (milligrams)
3 ounces steamed clams	23.80 mg
¼ cup enriched breakfast cereal	1.80–21.1
1 tablespoon blackstrap molasses	3.50
½ cup cooked spinach	3.20
3 ounces chuck roast	3.13
¼ cup prune juice	2.25

ZINC

Zinc is a trace mineral that supports many enzymes and proteins. Zinc is essential in DNA synthesis, growth and development, immunity and wound healing. People have increased zinc requirements during periods of growth, development and repair. In regions of the world where animal food is limited and grain-based diets are common, zinc deficiency is common. Zinc deficiency is characterized by delayed sexual maturity and stunted growth, particularly in young men. Unleavened whole-grain bread, as consumed in many undeveloped countries, is high in *phytates* and *fiber*, two substances that interfere with both zinc and iron bioavailability. Yeast breads reduce the binding effects of phytates and fiber and improve zinc and iron bioavailability.

Too much iron or copper in the diet also affects the bioavailability of zinc because they are so intricately connected. Alcoholics are at risk for zinc deficiency because alcohol interferes with its absorption and increases its excretion. People with chronic diarrhea or other digestive tract disorders, and breastfed babies may also be prone to zinc deficiency.

When physical needs are high, as in wound healing, the body is actually able to absorb more zinc, which is stored by the liver. But zinc supplements should only be taken under medical supervision. Zinc toxicity can reduce "good" HDL cholesterol and cause decreased copper and iron absorption and metabolism, depressed immunity, diarrhea, nausea and vomiting.

The most common zinc-containing foods are enriched and fortified breads and cereals, legumes, meats, poultry and whole grains. Baked beans, beef, crabmeat, oysters and soybeans are particularly high.

> **Sources of zinc:** dairy products, fish, legumes, meats, nuts, poultry, shellfish, whole grains
> **Roles in body:** enzymes (such as insulin), fetal development, genetic material, immunity, insulin, sperm production, vitamin A transport, wound healing
> **Deficiency:** decreased wound healing, delayed sexual maturation, failure to grow and thrive in children
> **Toxicity:** decreased HDL cholesterol, depressed immune function, diarrhea, kidney failure, nausea, reduced copper and iron absorption, vomiting

Zinc in Cooking

The zinc content of foods may greatly vary due to cooking and processing. In some foods where zinc is found in water-soluble form and there is water used in cooking, high losses can occur. For instance, legumes like black-eyed peas or black beans may lose as much as half of their zinc content after cooking. In 60 percent extraction wheat flour, used to make most of the baked goods, breads, and pastas in the United States, almost three-quarters of the original zinc is lost in processing before enrichment.

The RDA for zinc is 8 milligrams (mg) daily for women and 11 milligrams daily for men aged 19 years and older. Pregnant women aged 19 years of age and older also require 11 milligrams of zinc daily and 12 milligrams of zinc daily during lactation [50, 51].

Sources of Zinc	Amount (milligrams)
3 ounces cooked oysters	28.3 mg
3 ounces cooked beef shanks	8.9
3 ounces cooked pork tenderloin	2.5
½ cup baked beans	1.7
1 cup low-fat yogurt with fruit	1.6
2 tablespoons dry-roasted almonds	1.0

IODINE

Iodine is a trace mineral that plays an essential role in thyroid hormones that regulate growth, reproduction, temperature and metabolism of every cell in the human body. An iodine deficiency may lead to *simple goiter*, an enlarged thyroid gland. This condition may cause injury to the thyroid gland, coupled with weariness and weight gain. Severe thyroid malfunction during pregnancy may lead to an infant born with *cretinism*, a condition that may cause debilitating mental and physical retardation.

The amount of iodine that is present in food is greatly dependent on the iodine quality of the soil where plants are grown or animals graze. At one time, US coastal fields were higher in iodine than interior fields. However, many of the iodine-deficient conditions that were common in the central United States in the mid-1900s have been reduced today. Still, the iodine in older fields that are more exposed to erosion may be leached.

Iodine is a component of iodized salt, which is abundant in processed foods. Diets that exclude iodized salt, fish, seafood or seaweed may be deficient in iodine. With the use of noniodized salts in commercial food production and cooking and the replacement of iodine-based salts with bromine salts in baking, iodine status has again become a subject of public health concern.

While iodine toxicity is rare, it can also affect normal thyroid activity and metabolism. Symptoms may include burning, diarrhea, fever, nausea, vomiting and weakness. Excessive iodized salt intake should be discouraged.

Sources of iodine: dairy products, iodized salt, processed foods, seafood
Roles in body: metabolism regulation
Deficiency: cretinism (intellect and growth impairment), simple goiter (thyroid gland enlargement)
Toxicity: decreased thyroid activity and metabolism

Iodine in Cooking

Table salt that is used in food processing can increase the iodine content in foods. When salted water is used in commercial or home cooking, because salt is *hygroscopic*, it absorbs water, and iodine leaches out. In dry-heat cooking, such as roasting, water is not necessary, so there is less iodine loss. Iodine-based dough conditioners are used in some commercial bread production, which increase the iodine content.

The RDA for iodine is 150 micrograms (mcg) daily for men and women aged 19 years and older [52–54].

Sources of Iodine	Amount (micrograms)
3 ounces cooked cod	99 mcg
1 cup plain low-fat yogurt	75
1 medium baked potato with skin	60
3 ounces cooked shrimp	35
½ cup cooked navy beans	32
1 large egg	24

SELENIUM

Selenium is a trace mineral that functions as part of an antioxidant enzyme. It can substitute for vitamin E in some of its functions. In these roles, selenium may protect the human body from certain cancers.

Selenium deficiency may occur in people with digestive disorders, which can interfere with normal absorption. Reduced selenium may depress immune function and cause eye disorders, heart failure, reduced thyroid activity and weakened red blood cells.

Selenium is generally widespread in the US food supply, but it varies regionally by the soil content in which plants grow and animals graze. Certain areas in the western United States have higher amounts of selenium that can be toxic to animals if it is ingested. Selenium supplements can cause *selenosis*, which is selenium toxicity that is marked by fatigue, hair loss, nausea, weak and brittle fingernails, unusual body odor and vomiting.

Fish, meats, nuts, and whole grains are plentiful sources of selenium. Beef, Brazil nuts, oysters, sunflower seeds, tuna, and turkey are particularly high.

> **Sources of selenium:** eggs, fish, meats, seafood, vegetables, whole grains
> **Roles in body:** antioxidant, partners with vitamin E
> **Deficiency:** cataracts, depressed immune function, failure to grow and thrive, goiter, heart failure, reduced thyroid activity, weakened red blood cells
> **Toxicity:** changes in nails and hair, nausea, nerve and liver damage, vomiting, weakness

Selenium in Cooking

The selenium content of plant foods can vary from processing and cooking, especially when these foods are exposed to water or when wheat is processed into by-products. In the case of animal foods, selenium losses from processing and cooking are mostly minimal.

The RDA for selenium is 55 micrograms (mcg) daily for men and women aged 19 years and older. Pregnant women aged 14 years and older require 60 micrograms of selenium daily, and lactating women aged 14 years and older require 70 micrograms of selenium daily [55, 56].

Sources of Selenium	Amount (micrograms)
2 tablespoons Brazil nuts	544 mcg
3 ounces light tuna canned in oil	63
3 ounces roasted light meat turkey	27
3 ounces beef chuck roast	23
1 cup cooked enriched noodles	17
1 medium egg	14

COPPER

Copper is a trace mineral that plays a role in red blood cell formation, much like iron. It also serves in collagen formation, enzymes, maintaining the covering around nerves, and wound healing,

Copper and zinc compete for absorption in the digestive tract. A diet that is high in one of these minerals may cause a deficiency in the other. Because copper plays a role in iron absorption, a copper deficiency may produce anemia-like symptoms. Chronic copper deficiency may also cause abnormal lipid metabolism, depression and sunburn. This is because copper helps make *dopamine*, a neurotransmitter that lessens depression, and **melanin**, a pigment that protects the skin. *Wilson's disease* is caused by an accumulation of copper in body tissues. It causes neurological or psychiatric symptoms and liver disease.

Rich sources of copper include avocadoes, beef or lamb liver, black pepper, blackstrap molasses, Brazil nuts, cocoa, green olives, lobster, nuts and sunflower seeds, oysters and wheat bran. Dairy milk and egg proteins block copper absorption.

> **Sources of copper:** nuts, meats, organ foods, seafood, water
> **Roles in body:** creates hemoglobin, produces enzymes, promotes iron metabolism

309

Deficiency: anemia, changes in bone formations, poor growth and development, reduced immune functions
Toxicity: central nervous system dysfunction, diarrhea, nausea, liver damage, vomiting

Copper in Cooking

If copper leaches from copper-clad pipes, then this can increase the level of copper in cooking and drinking water. Cooking in copper cookware can also increase the copper content of foods.

Foods that require longer cooking may undergo copper losses. When legumes are cooked, they may lose nearly half of their copper content. Processing whole grains into flour may also result in a decreased copper content. Some vegetables and whole grains may have less copper from soil depletion than in the mid-1900s.

The RDA for copper is 900 micrograms for men and women aged 19 years of age and older; 1,000 micrograms for women during pregnancy; and 1,300 micrograms for women during lactation [54, 57, 58].

Sources of Copper	Amount (micrograms)
3 ounces cooked clams	585 mcg
2 tablespoons dry-roasted sunflower seeds	519
1 cup cooked lentils	497
1 cup raw mushrooms	344
1 ounce semisweet chocolate	198
2 tablespoons peanut butter	185

MANGANESE

Manganese is a trace mineral that functions in many enzymes and cellular reactions. It is widespread in the food supply and is stored mainly in the liver and kidneys. A manganese deficiency may affect central nervous system functions, growth and reproduction. Manganese toxicity may also cause central nervous disturbances. Nuts, oats and teas are particularly rich sources of manganese.

Sources of manganese: widely available in food, especially legumes, nuts, oats, tea
Roles in body: partners with enzymes in many cellular processes
Deficiency: abnormal reproduction and poor growth, central nervous system disturbances
Toxicity: central nervous system dysfunction

Manganese in Cooking

Manganese can be lost in food processing, especially in the milling of whole grains to produce flour and flour-based products and in cooking legumes. As much as 60 percent of manganese loss in legumes may be due to cooking.

The RDA for manganese is 1.8 milligrams daily for women and 2.3 milligrams daily for men aged 19 years and older. Women require 2.0 milligrams of manganese daily during pregnancy and 2.6 milligrams of manganese daily during lactation [59–61].

Sources of Manganese	Amount (milligrams)
½ cup fresh pineapple	0.77 mg
½ cup cooked spinach	0.84
2 tablespoons almonds	0.65
½ cup cooked Navy beans	0.48
½ cup mashed sweet potato	0.44
1 cup brewed black tea	0.18–0.77

FLUORIDE

Fluoride is a highly protective trace mineral for emerging teeth and dental maintenance. It is also important in protecting bones from mineral loss, as in osteoporosis. Important sources of fluoride are drinking water, mouthwash, toothpaste and supplements. Daily intake of high amounts of fluoride has been associated with *fluorosis*, a discoloration and mottling of the teeth during development.

The US Department of Health and Human Services is examining the standard fluoride level that has been used since the 1960s. This is because fluorosis has become more common in US teenagers. The prevalence of fluoride-free bottled drinking water may decrease fluoride intake over time.

Sources of fluoride: drinking water, mechanically deboned poultry, mouthwash, processed cereals, seafood, seaweed, tea, toothpaste
Roles in body: formation of bones and teeth, prevention of tooth decay
Deficiency: tooth decay
Toxicity: bone deterioration, diarrhea, fluorosis (mottled or white spotted teeth), nausea, vomiting

Fluoride in Cooking

Cooking food in fluoridated water increases the level of dietary fluoride. Approximately 65 percent of US public drinking water is fluoridated. Unlike chlorine, fluoride does not enter the steam when water is boiled, so it increases in concentration. The natural food content of fluoride in food is small. Its contribution is insignificant compared to the amount of fluoride in cooking water and food processing.

The RDA for fluoride is 3 milligrams (mg) daily for women and 4 milligrams daily for men [62–64].

Sources of Fluoride	Amounts (milligrams)
3½ ounces canned sardines with bones	0.2–0.4 mg
½ cup grape juice	0.2–0.28
½ cup tea	0.1–0.6
3½ ounces chicken	0.06–0.10
3½ ounces fish	0.01–0.17

CHROMIUM

Chromium is a fairly new established trace mineral. Chromium is an important partner along with insulin in glucose metabolism, but its roles are not firmly understood. The amount of chromium in body tissues is quite low because the digestive tract can only absorb a small amount.

A chromium deficiency may show up as impaired glucose tolerance (poor blood sugar maintenance) and elevated blood cholesterol and triglycerides. Chromium deficiency may be seen in people who are on very restricted diets or in those who are severely malnourished. Chromium toxicity, like other minerals, can result from oversupplementation.

Chromium is widely available in foods; fruits and vegetables, meats, whole grains and yeast are some of the best sources. Reliable data on the chromium content of foods varies because it is dependent on the soil content, like selenium.

Sources of chromium: egg yolks, meats, mushrooms, nuts, unprocessed foods, vegetable oils
Roles in body: partners with insulin to assist in glucose metabolism
Deficiency: poor glucose metabolism
Toxicity: skin and kidney disorders

Chromium in Cooking

In general, food processing decreases the chromium in food. Since chromium naturally occurs in the bran and germ of whole grains, when whole grains are refined into flour and flour products, the majority of chromium is lost. The refinement of sugar cane and sugar beets into sugar also removes most of the naturally occurring chromium. Acidic foods, such as cabbage or tomatoes, that are cooked in stainless steel may cause some chromium to leach from the cookware and be absorbed.

The RDA for chromium is 25 micrograms (mcg) daily for women aged 19 to 50 years and 20 milligrams daily for women aged 51 years and older; 35 micrograms daily for men aged 19 to 50 years; and 30 micrograms daily for men 51 years and older. Pregnant women require 30 micrograms of chromium daily; 45 micrograms of chromium daily are required during lactation [65, 66].

Sources of Chromium	Amount (micrograms)
½ cup cooked broccoli	11 mcg
1 whole wheat English muffin	4
1 cup mashed potatoes	3
3 ounces cooked turkey breast	2
1 medium banana	1
½ cup cooked green beans	1

MOLYBDENUM

Molybdenum is a trace mineral that functions in several enzymes and their reactions. It forms compounds with carbohydrates and amino acids and assists their many functions in the human body. Molybdenum also helps to break down *purines* in the human body, which are associated with gout. *Gout* is a condition that is caused by the buildup of uric acid and is associated with joint pain and stiffness. Molybdenum is concentrated in the kidneys, liver, tooth enamel and vertebrae.

Eggs, pork, lamb, low-fat dairy milk and beef liver are significant animal sources of molybdenum, as are cereal grains, dark green leafy vegetables, green beans, lentils, sunflower seeds and wheat flour.

> **Sources of molybdenum:** cereals, dark green leafy vegetables, legumes, low-fat dairy milk, nuts, organ meats
> **Roles in body:** works with enzymes in many body processes
> **Deficiency:** central nervous system dysfunctions, poor reproduction, growth and development (mostly seen in laboratory animals)
> **Toxicity:** central nervous system dysfunctions, joint pain and swelling in legs and feet (mostly seen in laboratory animals)

Molybdenum in Cooking

Molybdenum helps prevent toxicity from excessive copper in cooking and food processing. That is why good food sources of molybdenum may be useful in copper-rich environments (see the section on copper).

The RDA for molybdenum is 45 micrograms (mcg) daily for both men and women aged 19 years and older. Pregnant and lactating women require 50 micrograms of molybdenum daily [67, 68].

Sources of Molybdenum	Amount (micrograms)
½ cup cooked black beans	64.0 mcg
¼ cup almonds	11.6
1 cup yogurt	11.3
1 cooked whole egg	9.0
½ cup cottage cheese	5.2
½ cup fresh tomatoes	4.5

Bite on This: fruits and vegetables in health and disease

America was built on an agrarian society, rich in fruits, vegetables and whole grains. A solid base of science has supported the intake of fruits, vegetables and whole grains for health promotion and disease prevention. The *2010 US Dietary Guidelines* recommend that at least one-half of the dining plate be filled with fruits and vegetables. In specific, these dietary guidelines advise the following:

- Increase vegetable and fruit intake.
- Eat a variety of vegetables, especially dark green and red and orange vegetables and beans and peas.
- Consume at least half of all grains as whole grains. Increase whole-grain intake by replacing refined grains with whole grains.

The emphasis on fruits and vegetables in these recommendations is due to the fact that they are underconsumed in the United States and that there are a number of vitamins and minerals of public health concern—namely, vitamins A and C, folate, magnesium and potassium, in addition to dietary fiber.

Certain vitamin and mineral deficiencies and conditions are linked to fruit and vegetable intake. These include iron, folic acid and vitamin B12 with anemias; calcium, magnesium and vitamin D and K with osteoporosis; sodium and other electrolytes with hypertension; B vitamins with metabolic disorders; and antioxidants and fiber with cancer, diabetes and heart disease. At least 2½ cups of fruits and vegetables daily are associated with reduced risks of heart attack and strokes.

Moreover, because most fruits and vegetables are relatively low in calories without added fats or sugars, they may help children and adults achieve a healthy weight. Normal weight may help prevent some of these diet-related conditions.

One of the most compelling associations between fruit and vegetable intake and disease was seen in the Dietary Approaches to Stop Hypertension (DASH) study. This study examined the effect of a diet rich in fruits, vegetables and low-fat dairy products on blood pressure. People with hypertension who followed the DASH diet reduced their blood pressure by almost as much as medications could achieve.

The World Cancer Research Fund and the American Institute for Cancer Research have suggested that nonstarchy vegetables, such as lettuce and other leafy greens, and fruits most likely protect against several types of cancers, including esophageal, lung, mouth, stomach, throat and larynx.

One of the conclusions of the Harvard-based *Nurses' Health Study* and the *Health Professionals Follow-up Study* concluded that the higher the average daily intake of fruits and vegetables, the lower the chances of developing cardiovascular disease.

How does the United States rate in meeting these dietary guidelines? In 2005, about 33 percent of the US adult population surveyed consumed fruit two or more times daily, and about 27 percent ate vegetables three or more times per day. Those figures represented just one-third of the US population that came close to meeting the recommendations for fruit and vegetable intake.

In 2010, very few Americans 2 years of age and older reportedly consumed the amounts of vegetables that were recommended. While most Americans aged 2 to 3 years consumed the amount of fruit recommended, those aged 4 years and older did not. Additionally, those aged 2 to 30 years consumed more than half of their fruit intake as fruit juice. Fruit juice lacks dietary fiber and can contribute excess calories.

Almost everyone can benefit from eating more fruits and vegetables, not only to prevent conditions and diseases but for daily health maintenance. The type of fruit and vegetable and variety are as important as the quantity. No single fruit or vegetable provides all of the nutrients that are needed for good nutrition and health. The solution lies in choosing a range of fruits and vegetables daily, maximizing their nutrients in cooking and baking, and serving them in quantities to equal at least one-half of the dining plate [69–74].

General Guidelines for Decreasing Vitamin and Mineral Losses in Cooking and Baking

Water-soluble vitamin loss is dependent on the amount of cooking water and the ratio of surface area to volume of foods. This means that vitamin and mineral losses will be greater when more cooking water is used or when foods are finely cut or minced. When soaking and cooking liquids remain after cooking, integrate them into low-fat gravies, sauces, soups and/or stews.

Controversy exists about using or discarding the cooking water from soaked legumes due to gas formation. Wash well; discard any irregular legumes; cook until tooth-tender; and chew well to preserve the most nutrients with the least discomfort.

Vitamin losses from boiling cereal grains may be high. This is one of the reasons why they are enriched and/or fortified. Steaming helps to retain vitamins and minerals because the hot liquid does not come into contact with the food being steamed. In stir-frying, uniformly cut food is cooked quickly over high heat, which sears the surface and locks in vitamins and minerals.

Fat-soluble vitamins are more stable than water-soluble in cooking and baking, except at high frying temperatures. The dry heat that savories and sweets experience during baking may cause some thiamine (vitamin B1) and vitamin C losses.

Vitamin losses in meats may be about 20 percent in roasting, frying, or grilling and about 20 to 60 percent in stewing and boiling. Meats are vulnerable to thiamine loss.

Calcium, potassium and sodium can leach into cooking water and be lost if it is discarded. This may be prevented if foods are steamed. Root vegetables do not undergo many vitamin and mineral losses in cooking, since the outer skins help to prevent leaching. Scrub them well, and try to avoid peeling because the skin is fiber-rich. When possible, peel *after* cooking [75].

Bite on This: vitamins, minerals and dietary supplements

With all of the foods that are necessary for good health and disease prevention, some may think that dietary supplements are an easier option. While dietary supplements are more convenient than purchasing, preparing and storing foods to maximize their nutrients, they may not guarantee the wide array of nutrients that whole foods provide.

A *dietary supplement* is defined in the US Dietary Supplement Health and Education Act that became a law in 1994. This act defines a dietary supplement as a product (other than tobacco) that is intended to supplement the diet; is filled with one or more dietary ingredients, such as amino acids, botanicals, herbs, vitamins or minerals; is meant to be consumed by mouth as a capsule, liquid, pill or tablet; and is labeled on the front of the package as a dietary supplement.

Dietary supplements are regulated by the FDA based on their intended use and the information that is supplied by the manufacturer. Dietary supplements may not claim that a product will cure, diagnose, mitigate, prevent or treat a disease. However, dietary supplements may contain health claims, nutrient claims, or structure-function claims.

A *health claim* describes a relationship between a dietary supplement and the reduced risk of a disease or condition. A *nutrient content* claim describes the relative amount of a nutrient or dietary substance. A *structure-function claim* describes how a substance affects body organs and/or systems without mention of a particular disease. Structure-function claims do not require FDA approval, but they must carry a disclaimer that the product with not cure, diagnose, prevent or treat any disease.

An example of a **health claim** that includes both vitamin D and calcium is:

> "Adequate calcium and vitamin D, as part of a well-balanced diet, along with physical activity may reduce the risk of osteoporosis."

A **nutrient content claim** claim for sodium is:

> "At least 25% less sodium per Reference Amount Commonly Consumed (RACC) than an appropriate reference food (or for meals and main dishes, at least 25% less sodium per 100 g)."

A **structure-function claim** for vitamin E may read:

> "Helps maintain cardiovascular function and a healthy circulatory system, or ... protects against the development of cancer."

Unlike drugs, the FDA does not have to approve dietary supplements for safety or effectiveness before they are purchased and/or used by consumers. However, the FDA must prove that the dietary supplements are unsafe to restrict their usage.

The labeling of dietary supplements must include the name of the product (including the phrase that the product is a supplement); amount per serving; business, distributor, manufacturer or packer information; directions for use; list of ingredients; net quantity; nondietary ingredients, such as artificial colors, flavors, binders and/or fillers; percent of Daily Value (DV); scientific name if it is a botanical; serving size; and an optional cautionary statement.

Good Manufacturing Practices (GMPs) for dietary supplements were issued by the FDA in 2007. GMPs are a set of requirements and expectations for the manufacture, preparation and storage of dietary supplements to ensure quality. Manufacturers are expected to guarantee the composition, identity, purity and strength of dietary supplements.

Standardization of dietary supplements is not required in the United States to ensure consistency, quality or uniformity. As a result, the scientific evidence that supports their efficacy varies widely. Animal experiments, history of use, laboratory investigations and population studies that include individual case reports, observational studies and clinical trials provide the most direct evidence of the effectiveness of dietary supplements on health and disease.

Moderate consumption of adequate nutrients from an array of foods is a sensible strategy for good health and disease prevention. The USDA Dietary Reference Intakes (DRIs) are wise guidelines for safe and adequate nutrient consumption. There is not sufficient long-term research to support vitamin and mineral supplements in excess of the DRIs or to maintain that vitamin and mineral supplements can successfully replace a balanced and nutritious diet.

Practically any vitamin or mineral can be toxic if consumed in excess over time. In addition, vitamin and mineral supplements and prescription drug interactions may amplify or diminish normal body functions. For example, excess iron may cause **hemochromatosis**, a condition where too much iron is absorbed into the gastrointestinal tract, which may harm the finely integrated GI organs and systems. And excess of vitamin A might be detrimental to a pregnant woman and contribute to birth defects.

Until dietary supplements can guarantee safety, effectiveness and standardization across the industry, let the buyer beware. Consider dietary supplements as medicine with potential side effects. Vitamins and minerals should support rather than replace nutritious foods and beverages. As Hippocrates, the father of modern medicine, reportedly stated over 2,000 years ago, "Let food be thy medicine and medicine be thy food" [76,77,85].

315

Recipe: Turkey Pomegranate Meatballs

*Sweet-and-sour meatballs are a popular appetizer and buffet item. Bite-sized, meaty and tangy-sweet, they are also a good accompaniment to cooked rice, other grains or pasta. Simply switch the ground beef to ground turkey and the sweet-tart Sweet and Spicy Sauce juice from cranberry to pomegranate, and this recipe for **Turkey Pomegranate Meatballs** in the **Recipe file** which is located within the* Culinary Nutrition *website at www.culinarynutrition.elsevier.com, bespeaks healthy options. Ground chicken can substitute for the turkey and cranberry juice can replace the pomegranate juice for equally tasty and nutritious results.*

SERVE IT FORTH

Cooking for people with different vitamin and mineral needs requires an understanding of the nutritional science that supports vitamins and minerals and how vitamins and minerals are affected by food procurement, preparation and storage. Also important, and sometimes overlooked, are the foods and beverages that should be consumed together or separately for maximum vitamin and mineral absorption.

SCENARIO 1A: PRIMARY SCHOOL COOK

Anemia is prevalent in African-American populations due to genetic origins and poor dietary intake of blood-building nutrients. It is wintertime, and the local southeastern school district that educates African-American children has reported a number of absences due to colds and other infections. This school district is in a "food desert," where healthy foods and beverages are difficult to procure. The 35 *plus* schoolchildren in each class have complained of headaches and poor concentration. The physical education teacher has reported that the children do not have enough energy for activities. A survey of care providers revealed that the children do not consume breakfast at home before going to school.

- What are the environmental issues (i.e., time of year, location, etc.) of this scenario? What are the nutritional issues? Which vitamins and minerals are of most concern?
- Create a meal that requires little preparation that the children could eat when they arrive at school. Which foods and beverages would you select and why?
- Some vitamins and minerals are poorly absorbed due to "binders." Which are they?
- Which foods and/or beverages should be added (or deleted) from this meal to ensure that these children absorb all of the vitamins and minerals that they consume?
- What other actions should the school district take to help reduce iron-anemia in African-American children?

SCENARIO 2A: HIGH SCHOOL COOK

It has been said that the bones that a person "wears" as a teenager are the bones that a person wears when they are older. Bone mass increases rapidly from birth during the first few years of life and adolescence, and then it peaks at about age 30. If bone mineral consumption is high throughout development, bone mass may stay high throughout adulthood, and bones may resist fracture during aging.

The local high school noticed an increase in injuries in many of their athletes, particularly the ones in contact sports, such as football and gymnastics. Reports of broken bones, pulled tendons, muscle aches and pains, and bruises were extensive.

A survey of athletes indicated dislike for dairy products, dairy allergies and intolerances. Some male athletes did not eat vegetables, and some female athletes were always on diets. Vegetarian athletes reported overall poor nutrient intake.

Your challenge is to create a lunch meal that meets teenagers' food preferences—one that they will eat and enjoy and one that will also supply the nutrients, especially vitamins and minerals, that are needed for healthy bones.

316

- Which foods and beverages should this meal include? Which nutrients do they supply?
- Identify any nutrient excesses or deficiencies, especially vitamins and minerals.
- What foods and beverages should be available à la carte and why? Which nutrients do they supply?
- What other efforts should the high school administration take to help reduce nutrition-related injuries in high school athletes?

SCENARIO 3A: SPA COOK

People frequent spas for a variety of reasons: to exercise, go on a vacation, lose weight, relax, or start a healthy eating program, among others. Many spas serve an assortment of foods and beverages: strictly organic, vegetarian-type, calorie controlled, specialized diets and more. Some are destination spas, while others are city day spas.

The national chain City Spa is planning to offer a series of healthy eating weekends that feature functional foods. It promises a different daily menu for Saturdays and Sundays with low-sugar beverages, low-fat dairy products, fish, fruits, grains, legumes, lean meats and poultry, nuts and seeds, and vegetables with nutrients that act as functional foods. Low-fat dairy products and lean meats are to be more "accents" to these meals than the "center of the plate." Mostly plant foods that are high in phytonutrients and medicinal herbs will be used in the recipes. The management is planning to market this weekend as a "jump start" for dietary changes.

- Create these two weekend menus. Use the list of vitamin- and mineral-rich foods and beverages that follow. Support your meal choices. (Consider how some vitamins and minerals complement one another, while others detract from one another.)
- Describe the health benefits of the foods and beverages in each of these menus. Support your comments.
- What actions could the spa management take to promote these City Spa menus and the healthy benefits that spa-goers may achieve? Support your comments.

VITAMIN AND MINERAL-RICH FOODS AND BEVERAGES

A. Vitamin A and beta-carotene—apricots, cantaloupe, carrots, dark green leafy vegetables, vitamin A–fortified dairy products, mangos, peaches, sweet potatoes, yams

B. Vitamin D—canned fish with bones, egg yolks, salmon, shrimp, Vitamin D–fortified dairy products

C. B vitamins—eggs, enriched breads and cereals, fish, fortified dairy products, lean meats, liver, pork, poultry, whole grains

D. Vitamin C—bell peppers, berries, broccoli, cabbage, citrus fruits, kiwifruit, melons, potatoes, tomatoes

E. Calcium—broccoli and other dark green leafy vegetables, cottage cheese and hard cheese, fortified orange juice, ice cream, dairy milk, yogurt

F. Iron and zinc—dried fruits, eggs, fortified breads and cereals, red meat, spinach and other dark green leafy vegetables

G. Functional foods—those that:
- act as *antioxidants*, including carrots, flaxseed, grapes and tomatoes
- improve *bone, cardiovascular and gastrointestinal health*, including soy products, oats and yogurt
- maintain *vision and urinary tract health*, including blueberries and cranberries
- reduce *cancer risk and blood pressure*, including broccoli and bananas

H. Phytonutrients—brightly colored plant foods from each of these categories

I. Medicinal herbs—capsicum, chamomile, dandelion, dill, garlic, ginger, lemongrass, peppermint, poppy seeds, quince, rosemary, sage

Three additional activities can be found within the *Culinary Nutrition* website at www.culinarynutrition.elsevier.com.

WHAT'S COOKING?

1. Iron bioavailability

Objectives
- To identify certain chemicals in tea that react with iron compounds and form *precipitates* (solid particles that can cloud solutions)
- To observe how this feature of tea can affect nutrient bioavailability
- To apply this information to recipe and meal development

Materials

Two cups strongly brewed tea, 6 glasses, labels, marker, canned and bottled pineapple, prune and cranberry juice, data sheet

Procedure

1. Pour one inch of tea into each of the glasses.

2. Place a label on or by each glass, marked with the type of juice (pineapple, prune and cranberry) and container (canned or bottled) to be tested.

3. Create a data sheet similar to the one below to record your results.

Data Sheet

Type of Juice	Type of Container (Canned/Bottled)	Cloudiness (Yes/No)	Precipitate (Yes/No)
Pineapple			
Prune			
Cranberry			

4. Add about one inch of juice to each of the tea-filled glasses.

5. Examine each of the tea-juice solutions for cloudiness. If a precipitate forms, note this on the data sheet. If no precipitate forms, note this as well. You may have to look closely for small changes, especially with the darker solutions. If you are unclear, compare the tea alone with the juice on its own; then note any color changes or sediment on the bottom of the glasses.

Evaluation

There are certain chemicals in tea, chocolate, coffee and other substances that act as binders and interfere with iron absorption in foods. Inside the human body, these substances will precipitate the iron out of

317

foods and beverages and make it less bioavailable for bodily functions. In tea, these chemicals are called *tannins*. In cooking, these chemicals may cloud the look of a dish or beverage and/or cause unwanted particles to form.

Based upon this experiment:

1. Which juices contained iron and precipitated the iron out when they are mixed with tea?
2. Did the canned juices contain more or less iron than the bottled juices? Rank the amount of iron that you suspect these juices contain.

The juice that contains the most iron should be the prune juice, then the cranberry juice, and finally the pineapple juice, in this order.

3. Did your results agree? If not, what may have been the causes?

Culinary applications

How can this information be applied to recipe and meal development, especially for at-risk populations who require more iron, such as anemic children or women of childbearing age?

2. **Chlorophyll and buffers**
   Objectives
   - To see color changes in vegetables due to cooking
   - To recognize what can be done to help prevent color changes
   - To apply this information to recipe development and meal planning

   Materials

   Water, measuring cups, 2 sauce pots, 1 pound fresh spinach leaves, slotted spoon, 3 white plates, baking soda, measuring spoons, dairy milk, data sheet

   Procedure
   1. Pour 1 cup of water into a saucepan.
   2. When the water begins to boil, place a few spinach leaves into the pot; cook about 4 to 5 minutes.
   3. Turn off the heat; let the spinach rest in the water for a few minutes; note the color changes on the data sheet.

   Data Sheet

Spinach Mixtures	Color Changes	Comparison A & B	Comparison A, B & C
A. Spinach and water			
B. Spinach, water and baking soda			
C. Milk and spinach			

   4. Place the spinach leaves on a white plate with a slotted spoon.
   5. Repeat with a fresh cup of water and fresh spinach leaves. Add a pinch of baking soda to the water before boiling.
   6. Turn off the heat; let the spinach rest in the water for a few minutes; note the color changes.
   7. Compare the color changes of the spinach in this test to the color changes of the spinach in the first test.
   8. Place the spinach leaves on a white plate with a slotted spoon.
   9. Put 1 cup of dairy milk into the saucepan; heat on a low flame until it simmers (do not let it boil).
   10. Place a few spinach leaves into the pot; cook about 4 to 5 minutes.
   11. Turn off the heat; let the spinach rest in the milk for a few minutes; note the color changes.
   12. Compare the color changes of the spinach to the first and second tests.
   13. Place the spinach leaves on a white plate with a slotted spoon.
   14. Compare all three spinach leaf samples for color changes with each other and the raw spinach leaves; note your observations.

   Evaluation

   Fresh spinach is rich in *chlorophyll*, which helps to color it bright green. When spinach is put into boiling water, it may actually brighten because the color may concentrate. This is because gases that are inside of the cells are forced outside the cells by the heat, which concentrates the color.

   Then the spinach may change in color from bright to dull green, or even gray. This is because cooking releases certain acids that change the color of chlorophyll. This amount of acids is quite small. If the acid is removed as quickly as it forms, the spinach may be able to retain the bright green color. This is the reason why a pinch of baking soda reacts with the acid to help neutralize it. However, vegetables that are cooked with baking soda tend to become soggy.

Instead, a buffer can be used to help absorb acids or bases and remove them from the solution before they do their damage. In the third experiment, milk acts as a buffer to preserve the color of the spinach. When all three spinach samples are compared for color, the third sample should appear the brightest. Does it?

Culinary applications

Compare and contrast your results in the data sheet to the evaluation described above.

What recommendations would you make in recipe and meal development when working with deep green leafy greens to preserve both their color and texture? Given their properties, how can you make deep green leafy greens, such as spinach, more appealing to consumers who do not like them?

3. Vitamin C in beverages

Objectives

○ To observe which beverages contain the most vitamin C
○ To compare and contrast the Nutrition Facts Panels for vitamin C content
○ To be able to discriminate which beverages are more nutritious based on their vitamin C content
○ To apply this information to cooking and baking methods and techniques

Materials

Water; measuring cups; measuring spoons; cornstarch; saucepan or microwave-proof container; heat source or microwave; eight 1-cup glass containers; eye droppers; tincture of iodine; unfortified apple, grape, orange, grapefruit, lemon and tomato juice; cola; orange soda with Nutrient Facts Panels; data sheet

Procedure

1. Gradually mix ½ cup water with 1 teaspoon of cornstarch in a saucepan or microwave-proof container.
2. Bring the mixture to a boil over medium heat or in the microwave.
3. Prepare 8 test glasses in this manner: Fill each glass with ½ cup of water. Add 1 teaspoon of the starch mixture and 1 drop of tincture of iodine. Put 1 drop of unfortified apple juice into one of the test cups; repeat with 1 drop of each of the other juices and orange soda in the remaining 7 test glasses.

Evaluation

Note how long it takes for each of the liquid solutions in the test glasses to change in color from blue to clear. It should take fewer drops of juice that are high in vitamin C to change the liquid solution in the test glasses from blue to clear. Record your observations on the data sheet.

Data Sheet

Type of Juice or Soda	Time for Solution to Change Colors	Number of Drops of Juice	Consistent with Nutrition Facts Panel?
1. Unfortified apple juice			
2. Grape juice			
3. Orange juice			
4. Grapefruit juice			
5. Lemon juice			
6. Tomato juice			
7. Cola			
8. Orange soda			

Juices and beverages that are lower in vitamin C include apple and grape juice and soda. They should require more drops of juice and soda and more time to change color. Juices that are higher in vitamin C are orange, grapefruit, lemon and tomato juice. They should require fewer drops of juice and less time to change color.

Compare these observations with the Nutrition Facts Panels on the juices and soda. Note whether or not your observations were correct, based on the vitamin C content of each beverage, which is one of the nutrients that must be included on foods and beverages that are produced in the United States.

Culinary applications

How can the information in this exercise be applied to cooking and baking methods and techniques?

OVER EASY

Vitamins and minerals are essential nutrients, like carbohydrates, protein, and lipids that are needed by the body to assist in energy production, growth and development and immunity, among other functions. Water, which is discussed in Chapter 9, is the sixth essential nutrient. Like vitamins and minerals, water is an important component of fruits and vegetables. Water provides an essential transport system for vitamins and mineral in the human body. In turn, some vitamins and minerals play critical roles in maintaining body fluid balance. It is not a surprise that all of these nutrients are so interconnected in our diet and body.

In this chapter, the vitamins and minerals known to be essential to human life are discussed. Their function, sources, roles, deficiencies and toxicity are also examined in the context of how they perform in cooking and baking. Special consideration is given to vitamin and mineral intake and its relation to disease, including different anemias; growth, developmental and metabolic disorders; bone diseases, such as osteomalacia, osteoporosis and rickets; coronary heart disease; certain cancers; neural tube defects; and more.

Antioxidants, functional foods, nutraceuticals, medicinal herbs and foods, nonvitamins, phytonutrients and pre- and probiotics have been in our food supply for ages, but they have come to the forefront in nutrition and health in recent years. This is because ongoing research is building and confirming connections between food and health, especially how vitamins, nonvitamins and other substances protect our body, repair it, and safeguard it for future generations.

Future nutrition and culinary specialists have the power to create recipes, meals and menus that are filled with these life-supporting vitamins and minerals and other protective substances. By learning how to preserve vitamins and minerals through food procurement, production and storage, food in restaurants, supermarkets and other venues can be selected and/or used with confidence.

There are a wealth of fruits and vegetables from A to Z that can protect health and combat disease, from apples and asparagus to zebra tomatoes and *zizania latifolia* (Manchurian wild rice or water bamboo). While many of the nutritious, health-enhancing properties of fruits and vegetables have yet to be confirmed, in many ways they are the medicines of the twenty-first century and hold great promise.

320

CHECK PLEASE

1. The food with the richest source of vitamin A is:
   a. apple
   b. banana
   c. potato
   d. carrot
   e. onion
2. An excellent source of folate is:
   a. fortified cereals
   b. pork
   c. tuna
   d. dark green leafy vegetables
   e. a and d
3. If a person is on a very low-fat diet, he or she may run the risk of a _____ deficiency.
   a. thiamin
   b. folate
   c. vitamin E
   d. vitamin B12
   e. iron

Essay Question

1. A teenage tennis player has broken some small bones in her arm after undergoing a fall. Name five vitamins and minerals that need to be included in her diet for bone healing and the foods or beverages that contain each of them. What advice would you give this athlete to improve the absorption of these nutrients?

For additional questions, please see the *Culinary Nutrition* website at www.culinarynutrition.elsevier.com.

HUNGRY FOR MORE?

American Cancer Society   http://www.cancer.org
Centers for Disease Control and Prevention—Fruits & Veggies Matter   http://www.fruitsandveggiesmatter.gov
International Food Information Council   http://www.ific.org
National Center for Complementary and Alternative Medicine   http://nccam.nih.gov
National Institutes of Health—Office of Dietary Supplements   http://dietary-supplements.info.nih.gov
National Osteoporosis Foundation   http://www.nof.org
United Fresh Produce Association   http://www.unitedfresh.org
University of Nebraska-Lincoln Extension—Fruit and Vegetable Fact Sheets
http://lancaster.unl.edu/nep/FruitVeggie.shtml
United States Department of Agriculture (USDA)   http://www.usda.gov
USDA Agricultural Research Service   http://www.ars.usda.gov/main/main.htm
US Department of Health & Human Services
Office of Disease Prevention and Health Promotion   http://odphp.osophs.dhhs.gov

TAKE AWAY
Antioxidants

While oxidative reactions are crucial for life, they can also damage the human body. *Oxidation* is a chemical reaction that can produce free radicals, which can damage the cells. Antioxidants are molecules that slow or prevent the oxidation of other molecules. Antioxidants block potentially damaging chemical reactions by removing free radicals and inhibiting other reactions. They are able to quickly accomplish these feats because antioxidants are reactive with extra electrons to "give away."

> **Morsel** "One must ask children and birds how cherries and strawberries taste." —Johann Wolfgang Goethe (German natural philosopher, novelist, playwright and poet, 1749–1832)

Plants and animals maintain complex systems of antioxidants. When antioxidant levels are low or inhibited, there may be oxidative stress to the body, which may cause cellular damage or demise.

This is the reason why certain antioxidants are used in dietary supplements to maintain health and prevent disease. This is also why the antioxidants in foods have developed such high interest, both in research and by consumers.

The antioxidants in fruits and vegetables may offer some benefits against certain cancers, coronary heart disease, immunity, macular degeneration and neurological diseases. These include fruits and vegetables that contain the "ACES": beta carotene (pro-vitamin **A**), vitamin **C**, vitamin **E** and Selenium.

Beta-carotene and carotenoids are rich in brightly colored orange, red and yellow apricots, broccoli, cantaloupe, carrots, collards, peaches, squash, sweet potatoes and tomatoes. Vitamin C is found in broccoli, citrus fruits, green leafy vegetables, green peppers, strawberries and tomatoes. Vitamin E is abundant in dark green leafy vegetables, liver oil, nuts and seeds, and whole grains. Selenium is plentiful in chicken, eggs, fish and shellfish, garlic, grains and red meat.

Other common phytochemicals are *flavonoids* and *polyphenols*, found in cranberries, pomegranates, purple grapes, red wine, soybeans and tea; *lutein*, found in broccoli, Brussels sprouts, kiwifruit, and dark green leafy vegetables, such as collards, kale and spinach; *lycopene*, found in pink grapefruit, tomato products and watermelon; *lignans*, found in barley, flaxseed, oatmeal and rye; *vitamin-like antioxidants*, such as glutathione and coenzyme Q10 (CoQ10) and *antioxidant enzymes*, including catalase, glutathione peroxidase and superoxide dismutase (SOD), which are all produced by the body.

Research is ongoing as to whether or not antioxidant supplementation is beneficial and, if it is, which antioxidants are helpful and in what amounts. Until research is conclusive, it is prudent to consume whole foods or those with minimal processing to reap the most nature-made antioxidants.

Phytonutrients

Phytonutrients are plant-based chemical compounds. They are sometimes referred to as "phytochemicals." The reason why phytonutrients are of such interest is that they may reduce the risk of certain diseases, such as cardiovascular disease and some cancers. This may be due to their chemical compositions, fibers or some combinations of plant substances.

Plant-based substances have been used to treat disease and maintain health for centuries. For example, during Hippocrates' time (about 460–370 BCE), common aspirin was extracted from willow tree leaves, because willow tree leaves were thought to decrease fever.

Today, phytochemicals from cruciferous vegetables (broccoli, cauliflower, cabbage, kale, Brussels sprouts, and others) are used to treat certain tumors. Selenium, known for its antioxidant quality, is abundant in cruciferous vegetables. In the body, selenium acts as a cofactor in the synthesis of ***glutathione***, an antioxidant that is manufactured in the liver.

322

Lycopene, a phytochemical found in tomato products, has been touted for its protective effects against cardiovascular diseases and cancers of the lungs, prostate and stomach. Studies are mixed and nonconclusive; scientific evidence does not fully support these relationships [78].

Lutein and zeaxanthin, phytonutrients found in eggs and dark green leafy vegetables, may affect eyesight and help prevent age-related macular degeneration (AMD) and cataracts. There is insufficient scientific evidence to fully support these connections. The majority of people in the United States are not consuming enough fruits and vegetables daily to provide ample lutein and zeaxanthin to decrease the risk of age-related macular degeneration and cataracts [79].

The phytonutrients found in spices like cinnamon, cloves, nutmeg and turmeric are thought to have a host of healthy benefits, yet few are thoroughly proven. Turmeric, commonly used in Asian and Mediterranean cooking, reportedly has anti-inflammatory properties, associated with arthritis, Alzheimer's disease and certain cancers. Research is ongoing and nonconclusive.

Phytonutrients can be destroyed by processing and cooking. Vitamin C, a water-soluble vitamin and antioxidant that is found in such foods as citrus fruits, onions and tomatoes, is destroyed by high heat.

Chlorophyll, a green pigment that is found in deep green leafy vegetables, leaches in cooking water, unless it becomes a part of the finished dish. While chlorophyll is not an antioxidant, it is filled with other phytonutrients and magnesium, which is important in protein synthesis, muscular contraction and relaxation, nerve transmission, and teeth and bone mineralization.

Lycopene is actually more concentrated in processed tomato products and better absorbed with some fat. Foods and beverages high in phytonutrients are featured in Table 7-3, with their presumed health-enhancing benefits. The suspected roles of these phytonutrients are provided in Table 7-4.

The preventive effects of fruits and vegetables cannot be explained by just one phytonutrient that is taken out of the context of a healthy diet. Until all research about phytonutrients and disease prevention is confirmed, eating a wide range of fruits and vegetables daily is still the smartest strategy.

TABLE 7-3 Foods High in Phytonutrients

Foods and Beverages	Phytonutrients
Acaí berries	Anthocyanins, dietary fiber, omega-3 and omega-6 fatty acids, phytosterols and polyphenols
Alfalfa	Saponins
Apples	Catechins, flavonols and tartaric acid
Artichoke	Carotenoids
Asparagus	Lignins
Beets	Carotenoids
Bell peppers	Carotenoids and vitamin C
Blackberries and blueberries	Anthocyanins and anthocyanidins, lignans and tannic acid
Black tea	Flavonols
Broccoli (also Brussels sprouts, cabbage, cauliflower and kale)	Allylic sulfides, carotenoids, lignans and vitamin C
Cantaloupe	Carotenoids
Carrots	Carotenoids and lignins
Chili peppers	Capsaicin
Citrus fruits	Carotenoids, flavonols and vitamin C
Citrus peel	Limonoids
Cocoa	Flavonols
Cranberries	Anthocyanins and ellagic acid
Dark chocolate	Catechins
Eggplant	Anthosyanins and anthocyanidins
Flaxseeds and oil seeds	Lignans
Garlic	Limonene, flavonols and allylic sulfides
Goji (wolfberry)	Carotenoids, ellagic acid, vitamin C and selenium
Grapefruit	Flavonols
Grapes	Stilbenes and resveratrol
Green tea	Catechins, flavonols and oxalic acid,
Legumes	Catechins, carotenoids, flavonols, lignans, omega fatty acids and saponins
Mangos	Cryptoxanthin
Mangosteen	Xanthones
Nuts and seeds	Phytic acid, phytosterols and stilbenes (resveratrol)
Oats	Soluble fiber
Okra	Carotenoids
Olive oil	Hydroxytyrosol, oleuropein and oleocanthal
Onions	Flavonols and allylic sulfides
Papaya	Cyptoxanthin
Peanuts	Phytosterols and stilbenes
Pomegranate	Tannins and vitamin C
Pumpkin	Carotenoids and lignans
Purple corn	Anthocyanins
Quinoa	Dietary fiber
Red cabbage	Anthocyanins and anthocyanidins
Red grapes and wine	Catechins, ellagic acid, flavonols and stilbenes (resveratrol)
Red wine	Catechins and stilbenes (resveratrol)
Rice bran	Phytosterols
Sesame	Lignans
Shiitake mushrooms	Lentinan
Soy	Isoflavones, phytic acid, phytosterols and saponins
Spinach	Carotenoids and lignins
Spirulina	Beta-carotene
Squash	Carotenoids
Sweet potatoes	Carotenoids
Tea (green or black)	Catechins
Tomato	Carotenoids and vitamin C
Watercress	Organo or allylic sulfides
Watermelon	Carotenoids
Whole grains	Lignins, organo or allylic sulfides and saponins

Source: [80].

TABLE 7-4 Functions of Phytonutrients

Phytonutrients	Functions
Anthocyanins/Anthocyanidins	Antimicrobial activities, neutralizes free radicals
Carotenoids	Neutralizes free radicals, repairs DNA
Catechins	Neutralizes free radicals
Flavonols	Anticancer activities, neutralizes free radicals
Isoflavones	Anticancer activities, blocks estrogen while produces estrogen-like effects (protects bones, lowers LDL cholesterol)
Lignins	Anticancer activities
Limonoids	Detoxes liver enzymes
Organo or allylic sulfides	Antitumor activities, detoxes liver enzymes, lowers cholesterol
Phytosterols	Reduces tumor growth, lowers cholesterol
Saponins	Anticancer activities, lowers cholesterol
Stilbenes	Anticancer and inflammatory activities, lowers cholesterol

Source: [81,82].

[a]These relationships are conditional; research is ongoing.

Morsel "The value of those wild fruits is not in the mere possession or eating of them, but in the sight and enjoyment of them." —Henry David Thoreau (American environmental scientist, philosopher and poet, 1817–1862)

Functional Foods

Functional foods are described by this name because they have functions in the human body. One can say that most foods are functional because they supply nutrients for the human body to do its work. The term implies that certain foods have functions over and beyond simply nourishing the body: they protect it from foreign invaders, build immunity against future invaders, and help decrease certain disease risk factors.

The term *functional foods* was first coined in Japan in the 1980s. Food for Specified Health Uses (FOSHU) is a special Japanese government approval process for foods that contain ingredients with health functions. The safety of a food and its effectiveness in human health functions; the absence of any safety issues; the use of nutritionally appropriate ingredients; a guarantee of compatibility with product specifications; and established quality control methods and claims must be approved by the Japanese Ministry of Health, Labour and Welfare (MHLW).

In the United States, there is no consensus on an exact definition of a functional food, though the FDA acknowledges that the terms *functional foods* and *nutraceuticals* are "widely used in the marketplace" and that "such foods are regulated by the FDA under the authority of the Federal Food Drug and Cosmetic Act (FFDC) of 1938, even though they are not specifically defined by the law." The FFDC gives the FDA the authority to oversee food, drugs and cosmetics. It covers food colorings, food additives, bottled waters and homeopathic medications, among others [83].

Since 1994, manufacturers in the United States have been permitted to make "structure or function" claims by the FDA, but not health claims. This means that they are able to describe how a product "affects" the human body, but not claim any health "effects." However, in 1997, the FDA approved the first food-specific health claim for foods that contain whole oat sources of soluble fiber (oats, oat bran and oat flour) and the reduced risk of coronary heart disease.

In 1997, the Quaker Oats Company filed a petition with the FDA to permit this claim, based on significant scientific evidence and agreement. The FDA now permits this statement on foods containing 1.7 g per serving of psyllium husk soluble fiber or 0.75 g of oat or barley soluble fiber as beta-glucans ... "*reduced risk of heart disease may result from their regular consumption.*"

While functional foods were originally recommended for specific risk groups, today's processed functional foods may be marketed to the population at large. Some food manufacturers add nutraceuticals to their products, such as extracts, fiber, herbs, pre- or probiotics, vitamins, oils or phytochemicals with presumed health benefits.

Statements, symbols, vignettes and other communications that suggest a relationship between the presence or level of a substance in food and a disease- or health-related condition are considered *implied health claims.* A food is considered misbranded if its labeling is false or misleading in any particular representation or suggestion. The FDA has adopted a case-by-case approach for handling ingredient statements that depends on the overall context of the label. The FDA regulations also provide that certain ingredient statements will be treated as nutrient content claims whenever they appear on labels. This is why label reading by consumers is so complex but imperative [84, 85].

Functional foods are sometimes referred to as *medicinal foods.* They can be fresh or processed foods with reported "medicinal" health-promoting and/or disease-preventing properties that duplicate the attributes of medicine (see "Medicinal herbs").

Functional foods are also sometimes referred to as *nutraceuticals.* Nutraceuticals integrate the features of both nutrition and pharmaceuticals, and imply that some nutrients have a druglike effect. This concept is far from new. The ancient Indian science of Ayurveda is a therapeutic and complementary system of Eastern medicine that stresses moderation and plant-based treatments for therapeutic purposes.

Uncertainty among functional foods, medical foods, and nutraceuticals is common. For example, processed foods that are made from functional food ingredients or fortified with health-promoting ingredients, such as "vitamin-enriched" products, may be considered medicinal foods or nutraceuticals—especially if consumed in quantity. So may fresh foods, such as carrots with beta-carotene or broccoli with sulphorphane, if they are eaten in excess. Fermented foods with live cultures (see "Bite on This: probiotics and prebiotics") are also considered functional foods. Even these foods can disrupt normal gastrointestinal functions if consumed in surplus. Table 7-5 shows other functional foods and their reported benefits.

TABLE 7-5 Functional Foods and Reported Health Benefits

Food Groups	Associations with Health Maintenance and/or Disease Prevention[a]
Dairy products	
Cheese	Improves bone health; reduces osteoporosis risk; maintains desirable body composition and healthy immune function
Ice cream	Improves bone health; reduces osteoporosis risk
Dairy milk	Improves bone health; reduces osteoporosis risk
Yogurt	Improves bone health; reduces osteoporosis risk
	Probiotic; improved gastrointestinal health
Fruits	
Apples	Reduces coronary heart disease and some cancer risks
Bananas	Improves gastrointestinal health
Blueberries	Maintains healthy urinary tract; bolsters antioxidant defense; contributes to brain function maintenance
Cranberries	Maintains urinary tract and heart health; bolsters antioxidant defense; contributes to brain function maintenance
Grapefruit (red)	Maintains prostate health; neutralizes free radicals; contributes to healthy immune function
Grapes and raisins	Contributes to urinary tract and heart health; bolsters antioxidant defenses; contributes to brain function maintenance
Lemons and limes	Antioxidant; neutralizes free radicals
Oranges	Antioxidant; neutralizes free radicals
Plums and prunes	Improves heart health; maintains healthy digestive tract

(Continued)

TABLE 7-5 (Continued)

Food Groups	Associations with Health Maintenance and/or Disease Prevention[a]
Tomatoes	Supports maintenance prostate health
Watermelon	Maintains prostate health
Grains	
Barley	Improves heart health; reduces coronary heart disease risks
Corn	Reduces some cancer risks
Flax	Reduces some cancer risks; maintains heart health and healthy immune function
Oats	Improves heart health; reduces coronary heart disease risks
Psyllium breads/cereals	Improves heart health; reduces coronary heart disease risks
Wheat bran	Reduces some cancer risks; maintains healthy digestive tract
Legumes	
Beans	Improves heart health; maintains healthy digestive tract; reduces some cancer risks
Soy protein	Improves heart health; maintains bone health, healthy brain and immune functions; maintains menopausal health
Meats	
Beef (lean)	Maintains desirable body composition and healthy immune functions
Fatty fish	Improves heart health; maintains mental and visual functions
Nuts and seeds	Improves heart health; maintains mental and visual functions
Vegetables	
Asparagus, broccoli, carrots, collards, corn, kale, spinach	Supports maintenance of eye health
Broccoli, cabbage, cauliflower, kale	Enhances detoxification of undesirable compounds; boosts cellular antioxidant defenses
Carrots, pumpkin, sweet potatoes, spinach, tomatoes	Neutralizes free radicals; boosts cellular antioxidant defenses; converts into vitamin A
Garlic, onions, leeks, scallions	Enhances detoxification of undesirable compounds; supports healthy cardiovascular, immune and digestive systems

Source: [86].

[a]The biologically active components in functional foods may impart health benefits, but these are not definitively clinically demonstrated unless noted.

Bite on This: probiotics and prebiotics

Prebiotics are a category of functional foods. They are nondigestible food ingredients that stimulate the growth and activity of bacteria in the colon to improve colorectal health. Prebiotics are typically carbohydrates, the most common being soluble fibers. Prebiotics act to increase the number and activity of two types of bacteria—***bifidobacteria*** and ***lactic acid bacteria***—which help to improve digestion and mineral absorption, and strengthen the immune system. In the case of soluble fibers, such as oatmeal, consumption of prebiotics may contribute to gastrointestinal health and help prevent colorectal cancer.

Dietary sources of prebiotics include soybeans, inulin (found in Jerusalem artichokes, jicama and chicory), raw oats, and unrefined barley and wheat. Prebiotics may improve colon pH (normal colon pH ranges between 5.5 and 7, which is slightly acidic to neutral), calcium and other mineral absorption, immune system effectiveness, and intestinal regularity. The addition of substantial quantities of prebiotics to the diet may result in a temporary increase in bloating, bowel movements and/or intestinal gas.

Probiotics are dietary supplements that contain live organisms with potentially beneficial bacteria or yeasts. *Lactobacillus* and *bifidobacterium*, are the most widely used probiotic bacteria. *Lactobacillus* converts sugars and other carbohydrates into lactic acid. They provide the characteristic sour taste of fermented dairy products (such as yogurt) and lower the pH in foods so that organisms cannot grow and cause spoilage.

Lactobacillus may impart gastrointestinal benefits by assisting the human body's naturally occurring gut flora to restore itself. Probiotics are recommended after antibiotic use or *candida* (yeast) infection for this purpose. They may also strengthen the immune system.

Bifidobacterium make up the gut flora and reside in the colon. They may aid digestion, help prevent some types of tumor growth, and are associated with a lower incidence of allergies.

Probiotics and prebiotics have become very popular dietary supplements. Like sports and nutritional beverages, they have segued from substances with medical functions to ones with health-enhancing properties. Keep in mind that they still carry calories, nutrients and other substances that may or may not be right in all circumstances. Like many other controversial areas of nutrition, it is easy to consume "too much of a good thing." Before one self-prescribes any of these products, it is best to confer with a health care provider.

Medicinal Herbs

Medicinal herbs are plants that are used for medical purposes, from reducing the severity and longevity of illness to protecting the body from foreign invaders, such as bacteria and viruses. Medicinal herbs have been used throughout history and are still utilized throughout the world. Chinese herbal therapy accounts for the majority of treatments in traditional Chinese medicine (TCM). Over 300 herbs are commonly used today. They include astragalus, cinnamon, coptis, dong quai, ginseng, licorice, peony, rehmannia, rhubarb and wolfberry.

> **Morsel** "Why, then, can one desire too much of a good thing?" —Rosalind in Shakespeare's *As You Like It*, 1600

Traditional Western medicine is more dependent on synthetic chemicals, but many of them have herbal foundations. Some of these are monitored by US or global agencies. The FDA oversees all food and drugs in the United States. Yet, some medical herbs are neither food nor drugs; instead, they fall into the category of dietary or nutritional supplements. Medicinal herbs may only comprise minute quantities in dietary or nutritional supplements. However, these supplements may be consumed in excess and produce druglike or even toxic effects. Furthermore, some people may be sensitive or allergic to certain medicinal herbs and develop allergic-like responses.

The Dietary Supplement Health Education Act (DSHEA) was passed by the US Congress in 1994 and restricts the authority of the FDA over supplements that do not carry a disease claim. This act allows the manufacturer of medicinal supplements to market medicinal herbs without FDA approval.

Medicinal herbs can carry structure and function claims. For example, a product can indicate that it maintains, promotes or supports the human body, but it cannot indicate that it protects the body from disease or reduces a disease state, such as coronary heart disease or diabetes. Products of this nature must also carry a statement that indicates that they have not been reviewed or approved by the FDA.

The US Congress created the National Center for Complementary and Alternative Medicine (NCCAM) in 1998, which is a part of the National Institutes of Health (NIH). Its purpose is to research complementary and alternative medicine. Some of the medicinal herbs that have undergone research include cranberry, echinacea, garlic, ginkgo biloba, hawthorn and saw palmetto.

> **Morsel** "What was paradise, but a garden full of vegetables and herbs, and pleasure? Nothing there but delights." —William Lawson (British author of *The Country Housewife's Garden*, 1553–1635)

Several of the more commonly used medicinal herbs are shown in Table 7-6, along with their reputed health benefits. Many are not fully confirmed in scientific studies. Compare their reputed health benefits with current research for sound advise.

TABLE 7-6 Medicinal Herbs

Herbs	Reputed Health Benefits/Concerns
Artichoke	Reduces cholesterol levels
Basil	Increases antibodies and anthocyanins; destroys intestinal parasites
Black cohosh	Reduces premenstrual symptoms; produces estrogen-like activity
	Problems: Gastrointestinal disorders
Black cumin	Produces analgesic properties, similar to aspirin
Butterbur	Remedies headaches and inflammation
Calendula	Treats acne; reduces inflammation; controls bleeding; soothes irritated tissue
Cayenne pepper (Capsaicin)	Decreases chronic pain from shingles and neuralgia; reduces burning; promotes vasodilation and platelet separation
Cranberry	Aids urinary tract infections
Echinacea (coneflower)	Reduces length, severity of common colds; controls urinary tract infections; speeds wound healing
	Problems: Should not be used by those with HIV, multiple sclerosis or rheumatoid arthritis
Elderberry	Speeds recovery from certain types of influenza
Fennel	Reduces inflammation and recurrent stomach upsets
Feverfew	Remedies migraine headaches, nausea and vomiting
	Problems: Commercial doses too high; acts on blood vessels in brain
Garlic	Combats fungi, parasites and viruses; inhibits blood clots; lowers blood pressure, blood cholesterol and blood sugar
	Problems: Excessive use may cause gastrointestinal problems; should not be taken with anticoagulants
Gawo	Reduces diarrhea, fever and inflammation
German chamomile	Benefits sleep; calms irritable bowel syndrome and other stomach disorders
Ginger	Reduces gastrointestinal problems, including motion sickness and nausea; strengthens cardiac function
	Problems: May cause heartburn, irritate gallstones, and prolong bleeding time
Gingko biloba	Improves short-term memory and concentration
	Problems: May cause allergic skin reactions, headaches and indigestion
Green tea	Inhibits breast cancer cells; helps heal scars
Hibiscus	Acts as antihypertensive, antifungal and antibacterial agent
Honey	Reduces and heals wounds
Lemongrass	Treats common cold, convulsions, cough, digestive tract spasms, exhaustion, fever, high blood pressure, pain, rheumatism, stomachache and vomiting
	Problems: Some toxic side effects after inhaling or swallowing. Unsafe during pregnancy; avoid if breast-feeding
Magnolia	Inhibits bacteria responsible for dental caries and periodontal disease
Milk thistle	Protects liver from toxins; regenerates new liver cells
	Problems: May be harmful in excess
Oregano	Fights drug-resistant bacteria
Pawpaw	Functions as insecticide
Peppermint oil	Aids irritable bowel syndrome
Pokeweed	Treats acne, swollen glands and tonsillitis
Pomegranate	Reduces heart disease risk factors, including LDL oxidation and systolic blood pressure; prevents breast cancer cell production; helps fight dental plaque through antiviral and antibacterial acts
Psyllium	Acts as a laxative; reduces blood cholesterol; reduces colorectal cancer risks
	Problems: May cause gastrointestinal disorders; increases flatulence
Rauvolfia serpentina	Reduces anxiety, high blood pressure and sleeplessness
Salvia	Improves memory
St. John's wort	Decreases mild anxiety and depression
	Problems: Causes sedation; effects increase with sunlight; may mask prostate cancer symptoms
Saw palmetto	Reduces urinary symptoms due to enlarged prostate
	Problems: May mask prostate cancer symptoms

328

(Continued)

TABLE 7-6 (Continued)	
Herbs	**Reputed Health Benefits/Concerns**
Shiitake	Produces antitumor and antiviral properties; provides immunological benefits for allergies and arthritis; inhibits platelet aggregation and thrombosis
Soy	Contains phytoestrogens with estrogen-like activity
Stinging nettle	Prevents inflammation, prostate disorders and osteoarthritis
Tea tree oil	Treats acne
Turmeric	Protects against certain cancers; contains *curcumin* (antioxidant and anti-inflammatory)
Valerian root	Helps insomnia; acts as mild tranquilizer
	Problems: May cause heart function disorders, headache, restlessness and sleeplessness
Vanilla	Increases catecholamines (epinephrine and adrenal); used in essential oils aromatherapy

Source: [87,88].
The biologically active components in medicinal herbs may impart health benefits, but these are not definitively clinically demonstrated unless noted.

Like most nutrient recommendations, if medicinal herbs are used, they should be used under the supervision of a health care provider, in moderation, with respect to the total diet. Herbs such as aconite, belladonna, black cohosh, borage, broom, chaparral, comfrey, ephedra, germander, kava, kombucha, lobelia, pennyroyal, poke root, sassafras, skullcap and wormwood should most likely be avoided due to their potentially harmful effects.

References

[1] Lieberman S, Bruning N. In: The real vitamin & mineral book. New York: Avery Group; 1990.

[2] Rosenfeld L. Vitamine—vitamin. The early years of discovery. Clin Chem 1997;43:680–5.

[3] Funk C. The vitamines, <http://www.mc.vanderbilt.edu/biolib/hc/nutrition/nh3.html/>; [accessed 02.09.08].

[4] Institute of Medicine (IOM). Dietary Reference Intakes (DRIs): estimated average requirements. <http://www.iom.edu/Activities/Nutrition/SummaryDRIs/~/media/Files/Activity%20Files/Nutrition/DRIs/New%20Material/5DRI%20Values%20SummaryTables%2014.pdf/>; [accessed 02.09.08].

[5] Combs GF.. In: The vitamins: fundamental aspects in nutrition and health, 3rd ed. Burlington, MA: Elsevier Academic Press; 2008.

[6] Institute of Medicine, Food and Nutrition Board. In: Dietary reference intakes for calcium and vitamin D. Washington, DC: National Academy Press; 2010.

[7] Office of Dietary Supplements. Vitamin D. <http://ods.od.nih.gov/factsheets/vitamind/>; [accessed 02.09.08].

[8] Office of Dietary Supplements. Vitamin E. <http://ods.od.nih.gov/factsheets/vitamine/>; [accessed 02.09.08].

[9] Oregon State University. Vitamin K. <http://lpi.oregonstate.edu/infocenter/vitamins/vitaminK/>; [accessed 02.09.08].

[10] National Institutes of Health (NIH). Thiamin. <http://www.nlm.nih.gov/medlineplus/ency/article/002401.htm/>; [accessed 02.09.08].

[11] Oregon State University. Riboflavin. <http://lpi.oregonstate.edu/infocenter/vitamins/riboflavin/>; [accessed 02.09.08].

[12] Oregon State University. Niacin. <http://lpi.oregonstate.edu/infocenter/vitamins/niacin/>; [accessed 02.09.08].

[13] Oregon State University. Pantothenic acid. <http://lpi.oregonstate.edu/infocenter/vitamins/pa/>; [accessed 02.09.08].

[14] Staggs CG, Sealey WM, McCabe BJ, et al. Determination of the biotin content of select foods using accurate and sensitive HPLC/avidin binding. J Food Compost Anal 2004;17:767–76.

[15] Office of Dietary Supplements. Vitamin B6. <http://ods.od.nih.gov/factsheets/vitaminb6/>; [accessed 02.09.08].

[16] Oregon State University. Vitamin B6. <http://lpi.oregonstate.edu/infocenter/vitamins/vitaminB6/>; [accessed 02.09.08].

[17] Office of Dietary Supplements. Folate. <http://ods.od.nih.gov/factsheets/Folate-HealthProfessional/>; [accessed 02.09.08].

[18] US Food and Drug Administration (FDA). CFR—code of federal regulations title 21. <http://www.accessdata.fda.gov/scripts/cdrh/cfdocs/cfcfr/CFRSearch.cfm?fr=101.79/>; [accessed 02.09.08].

[19] Office of Dietary Supplements. Vitamin B12. <http://ods.od.nih.gov/factsheets/VitaminB12/>; [accessed 02.09.08].

[20] Tucker KL, Rich S, Rosenberg I, et al. Plasma vitamin B12 concentrations relate to intake source in the Framingham Offspring Study. Am J Clin Nutr 2000;71:514–22.

[21] Oregon State University. Vitamin B12. <http://lpi.oregonstate.edu/infocenter/vitamins/vitaminB12/>; [accessed 02.09.08].

[22] Oregon State University. Vitamin C. <http://lpi.oregonstate.edu/infocenter/vitamins/vitaminC/>; [accessed 02.09.08].

[23] University of Maryland Medical Center. Vitamin C. <http://www.umm.edu/altmed/articles/vitamin-c-000339.htm/>; [accessed 02.09.08].

329

[24] Office of Dietary Supplements. Vitamin C. <http://ods.od.nih.gov/factsheets/VitaminC-HealthProfessional/>; [accessed 02.09.08].

[25] Oregon State University. Calcium. <http://lpi.oregonstate.edu/infocenter/minerals/calcium/>; [accessed 02.09.08].

[26] Oregon State University. Phosphorus. <http://lpi.oregonstate.edu/infocenter/minerals/phosphorus/>; [accessed 02.09.08].

[27] University of Maryland Medical Center. Phosphorus. <http://www.umm.edu/altmed/articles/phosphorus-000319.htm/>; [accessed 02.09.08].

[28] Office of Dietary Supplements. Magnesium. <http://ods.od.nih.gov/factsheets/magnesium/>; [accessed 02.09.08].

[29] Oregon State University. Magnesium. <http://lpi.oregonstate.edu/infocenter/minerals/magnesium/>; [accessed 02.09.08].

[30] United States Department of Agriculture (USDA). Dietary guidelines for Americans, 2010. <http://www.cnpp.usda.gov/DGAs2010-PolicyDocument.htm/>; [accessed 02.09.08].

[31] United States Department of Agriculture (USDA). USDA national nutrient database for standard reference, release 23. <http://www.ars.usda.gov/Services/docs.htm?docid=22115/>; [accessed 02.09.08].

[32] USDA Food and Nutrition Information Center. Sodium and chloride. <http://www.nap.edu/openbook.php?isbn=0309091691/>.

[33] American Heart Association. Sodium (salt or sodium chloride). <http://www.heart.org/HEARTORG/GettingHealthy/NutritionCenter/HealthyDietGoals/Sodium-Salt-or-Sodium-Chloride_UCM_303290_Article.jsp#.Tv-AW9QV2Vo/>; [accessed 05.08.08].

[34] University of Maine. Sodium content of your foods. <http://umaine.edu/publications/4059e/>; [accessed 02.09.08].

[35] United States Department of Agriculture (USDA). USDA national nutrient database for standard reference, release 17. <http://www.nal.usda.gov/fnic/foodcomp/Data/SR17/wtrank/sr17a307.pdf/>; [accessed 02.09.08].

[36] Institute of Medicine. In: A population-based policy and systems change approach to prevent and control hypertension. Washington, DC: National Academies Press; 2010.

[37] Vasan RS, Beiser A, Seshadri S, et al. Residual lifetime risk for developing hypertension in middle-aged women and men: the Framingham heart study. JAMA 2002;287:1003–10.

[38] Palar K, Sturm R. Potential societal savings from reduced sodium consumption in the US adult population. Am J Health Promot 2009;24:49–57.

[39] Bibbins-Domingo K, Chertow GM, Coxson PG, et al. Projected effect of dietary salt reductions on future cardiovascular disease. N Engl J Med 2010;362:590–9.

[40] Strazzullo P, D'Elia L, Kandala NB, et al. Salt intake, stroke, and cardiovascular disease: meta-analysis of prospective studies. BMJ 2009;339:b4567.

[41] Centers for Disease Control and Prevention (CDC) Application of lower sodium intake recommendations to adults—United States, 1999–2006. MMWR Morb Mortal Wkly Rep 2009;58:281–3.

[42] National Institutes of Health (NIH). Chloride in diet. <http://www.nlm.nih.gov/medlineplus/ency/article/002417.htm?debugMode=false/>; [accessed 02.09.08].

[43] Institute of Medicine (IOM). Dietary Reference Intakes: electrolytes and water. <http://www.iom.edu/~/media/Files/Activity%20Files/Nutrition/DRIs/DRI_Electrolytes_Water.pdf/>; [accessed 02.09.08].

[44] http://www.iom.edu/Global/News%20Announcements/~/media/442A08B899F44DF9AAD083D86164C75B.ashx

[45] United States Department of Agriculture (USDA). USDA national nutrient database for standard reference, release 24. <http://www.ars.usda.gov/Services/docs.htm?docid=8964/>; [accessed 02.09.08].

[46] Parcell S. Sulfur in human nutrition and applications in medicine. Altern Med 2002;7:22–44.

[47] Centers for Disease Control and Prevention (CDC). Iron and iron deficiency. <http://www.cdc.gov/nutrition/everyone/basics/vitamins/iron.html/>; [accessed 05.08.08].

[48] National Heart Lung and Blood Institute (NHLBI). What is iron-deficiency anemia? <http://www.nhlbi.nih.gov/health/health-topics/topics/ida/> [accessed 02.09.08].

[49] Office of Dietary Supplement. Iron. <http://dietary-supplements.info.nih.gov/factsheets/iron.asp/>; [accessed 02.09.08].

[50] Office of Dietary Supplement. Zinc. <http://ods.od.nih.gov/factsheets/Zinc-HealthProfessional/>; [accessed 02.09.08].

[51] Oregon State University. Zinc. <http://lpi.oregonstate.edu/infocenter/minerals/zinc/>; [accessed 02.09.08]

[52] Oregon State University. Iodine. <http://lpi.oregonstate.edu/infocenter/minerals/iodine/>; [accessed 02.09.08].

[53] National Institutes of Health (NIH). Iodine in diet. <http://www.nlm.nih.gov/medlineplus/ency/article/002421.htm/>; [accessed 02.09.08].

[54] Office of Dietary Supplement. Iodine. <http://ods.od.nih.gov/factsheets/Iodine-HealthProfessional/>; [accessed 02.09.08].

[55] Office of Dietary Supplement. Selenium. <http://ods.od.nih.gov/factsheets/Selenium-HealthProfessional/>; [accessed 02.09.08].

[56] Oregon State University. Selenium. <http://lpi.oregonstate.edu/infocenter/minerals/selenium/>; [accessed 02.09.08].

[57] Oregon State University. Copper. <http://lpi.oregonstate.edu/infocenter/minerals/copper/>; [accessed 02.09.08].

[58] National Institutes of Health (NIH). Copper in diet. <http://www.nlm.nih.gov/medlineplus/ency/article/002419.htm>; [accessed 02.09.08].

[59] Oregon State University. Manganese. <http://lpi.oregonstate.edu/infocenter/minerals/manganese/>; [accessed 02.09.08].

[60] National Institutes of Health (NIH). Manganese. <http://www.nlm.nih.gov/medlineplus/druginfo/natural/182.html/>; [accessed 02.09.08].

[61] http://www.ars.usda.gov/SP2UserFiles/Place/12354500/Data/SR23/nutrlist/sr23a315.pdf

[62] National Institutes of Health (NIH). Fluoride in diet. <http://www.nlm.nih.gov/medlineplus/ency/article/002420.htm/>; [accessed 02.09.08].

[63] Institute of Medicine. In: Food and Nutrition Board: Dietary Reference Intakes for calcium, phosphorous, magnesium, vitamin D, and fluoride. Washington, DC: National Academy Press; 1997.

[64] Oregon State University. Fluoride. <http://lpi.oregonstate.edu/infocenter/minerals/fluoride/>; [accessed 02.09.08].

[65] Oregon State University. Chromium. <http://lpi.oregonstate.edu/infocenter/minerals/chromium/>; [accessed 02.09.08].

[66] Office of Dietary Supplement. Chromium. <http://ods.od.nih.gov/factsheets/chromium/>; [accessed 02.09.08].

[67] Oregon State University. Molybdenum. <http://lpi.oregonstate.edu/infocenter/minerals/molybdenum/>; [accessed 02.09.08].

[68] Institute of Medicine, Food and Nutrition Board. In: Dietary reference intakes for vitamin A, vitamin K, arsenic, boron, chromium, copper, iodine, iron, manganese, molybdenum, nickel, silicon, vanadium, and zinc. Washington, DC: National Academy Press; 2001.

[69] US Department of Health and Human Services (DHHS). Dietary guidelines for Americans, 2005. <http://www.health.gov/DietaryGuidelines/dga2005/document/default.htm/>; [accessed 02.09.08].

[70] He FJ, Nowson CA, Lucas M, et al. Increased consumption of fruit and vegetables is related to a reduced risk of coronary heart disease: meta-analysis of cohort studies. J Hum Hypertens 2007;21:717–28.

[71] Hung HC, Joshipura KJ, Jiang R, et al. Fruit and vegetable intake and risk of major chronic disease. J Natl Cancer Inst 2004;96:1577–84.

[72] Appel LJ, Moore TJ, Obarzanek E, et al. A clinical trial of the effects of dietary patterns on blood pressure. DASH Collaborative Research Group. N Engl J Med 1997;336:1117–24.

[73] World Cancer Research Fund. Food, nutrition, physical activity, and the prevention of cancer: a global perspective. <http://www.dietandcancerreport.org/>; [accessed 02.09.08].

[74] United States Department of Agriculture (USDA). MyPlate, <http://www.cnpp.usda.gov/MyPlate.htm/>; [accessed 02.09.08].

[75] Bender DA. A dictionary of food and nutrition, 3rd ed. Oxford, UK: Oxford University Press; 2005.

[76] Office of Dietary Supplement. Dietary supplements. <http://ods.od.nih.gov/factsheets/DietarySupplements/>; [accessed 02.09.08].

[77] US Food and Drug Administration (FDA). Guidance for industry: a food labeling guide. <http://www.fda.gov/Food/GuidanceComplianceRegulatoryInformation/GuidanceDocuments/FoodLabelingNutrition/FoodLabelingGuide/ucm064919.htm/>; [accessed 02.09.08].

[78] Cancer Society. Lycopene. http://www.cancer.org/Treatment/TreatmentsandSideEffects/ComplementaryandAlternativeMedicine/DietandNutrition/lycopene/; [accessed 05.08.08].

[79] American Optometric Association. Lutein and zeaxanthin—eye-friendly nutrients. <http://www.aoa.org/x4732.xml/>; [accessed 05.08.08].

[80] Halvorsen BL, Carlsen MH, Phillips KM, Bohn SK, Holte K, Jacobs Jr DR, Blomhoff R. Content of redox-active compounds (i.e., antioxidants) in foods consumed in the United States. Am J Clin Nutr 2006;84:95–135. PMID:16825686. [accessed 12.08.11]

[81] Gollman B, Pierce K. In: The Phytopia cookbook. Dallas, TX: Phytopia Press; 1998.

[82] United States Department of Agriculture (USDA). Phytonutrient FAQs. <http://www.ars.usda.gov/aboutus/docs.htm?docid=4142/>; [accessed 12, 2011].

[83] Ministry of Health, Labour and Welfare. Food for specified health uses (FOSHU). <http://www.mhlw.go.jp/english/topics/foodsafety/fhc/02.html/>; [accessed 02.09.08].

[84] Schneeman BO. Regulatory framework for food labeling related to nutrition. <http://ucanr.org/sites/Zann_test/files/28692.pdf/>; [accessed 02.09.08].

[85] Federal Trade Commission. Enforcement policy statement on food advertising. <http://www.ftc.gov/bcp/policystmt/ad-food.shtm/>; [accessed 05.08.08].

[86] Iowa State University. What you need to know about the health benefits of functional foods. <http://www.extension.iastate.edu/publications/PM1798.pdf/>; [accessed 12.08.11].

[87] MedlinePlus. Herbal medicine. <http://www.nlm.nih.gov/medlineplus/herbalmedicine.html/>; [accessed 12.08.11].

[88] National Technology Program. Medicinal herbs. <http://ntp.niehs.nih.gov/files/herbalfacts06.pdf/>; [accessed 12.08.11].

CHAPTER 8

Fluid Basics: Healthfully Meeting Fluid Needs

Healthy Fluid Choices, Roles and Applications

OBJECTIVES

1. Recognize water sources and functions for normal body activities
2. Identify water sources and roles in cooking and baking
3. Discriminate among the benefits and concerns over alcohol ingestion
4. Incorporate alcohol into recipes and menus for flavor enhancement
5. Compare the pros and cons of caffeine consumption in health and disease
6. Utilize coffee, tea and chocolate in recipe development for flavor and health enhancement

Culinary Nutrition. DOI: http://dx.doi.org/10.1016/B978-0-12-391882-6.00008-X

7. Distinguish the nutritional values among different types of dairy milk and their benefits in health maintenance and disease prevention

8. Describe the advantages and disadvantages of sports drinks for various athletic populations

9. Contrast fortified beverages according to age and nutritional needs

10. Evaluate soft drinks in the human diet

INTRODUCTION: HEALTHFULLY MEETING FLUID NEEDS

The US public has been advised to drink eight glasses of water a day, and more if they live in a hot climate or if they exercise. But is there research that supports this recommendation, or is it just hearsay, like the saying "An apple a day keeps the doctor away"?

Morsel "Eating teaches drinking." —Italian proverb

This chapter examines fluid requirements in humans and how these requirements can be met through an array of fluids, including caffeinated beverages, dairy products, fortified beverages, juices, water and more. It also looks at the effects that substances such as alcohol and caffeine have on fluid balance.

Many foods are high in fluids, including celery, lettuce, tomatoes and watermelon, which break down and release these fluids during digestion and throughout cooking and baking. Informed nutrition and culinary specialists should know how to incorporate these fluids into recipes and meals to maximize their taste, texture and nutrients. Techniques for preserving a variety of fluids in cooking and baking are explored.

Consuming too many fluids can have deleterious effects, as can ingesting too few fluids. By understanding the roles of fluids in human nutrition, one may be more mindful of their use and abuse. Water, an essential nutrient like carbohydrates, proteins, lipids, vitamin and minerals, is critical for health and well-being. Since most of the human body is made up of water, it may be the most quintessential nutrient of all.

MAIN COURSES
Fluid Requirements

The idea that a person should consume eight cups (two liters) of water daily per 2,000 calories can be attributed to the Food and Nutrition Board (FNB) of the Institute of Medicine (IOM) of the National Academies. It established this recommendation for water consumption in the 1940s. This amount was to include all fluids consumed, including those found in solid foods, which could be significant. Foods such as white bread may contain as much as 30 percent water.

Morsel "Water is said to be potable; indeed, some declare it our natural beverage, although even they find it palatable only when suffering from the recurrent disorder known as thirst, for which it is a medicine." —Ambrose Bierce (American writer, 1842–1913)

The concept of water consumption based on daily calories is even more complicated when alcohol and caffeinated beverages are considered. While both of these beverages are fluids, they can act as diuretics in large quantities. *Diuretics* increase urine excretion, which means that they have the potential of decreasing fluids in the body. Normal intake of coffee, soft drinks or tea may cause minimal hydration problems. The same is true about alcohol; average intake of one or two drinks daily should cause little appreciative fluid loss. Normal intake of caffeinated beverages and alcohol, which may account for as much as one-half or more of the daily fluid intake for healthy adults, should be considered when replenishing fluids. Caffeinated beverages and alcohol in excess require greater attention.

What is "normal" intake for one person may not be considered normal for another. This is why parameters have been established to suggest the amounts of fluids that healthy adults should consume daily. Instead of eight cups of water per 2,000 daily calories, four cups of water per 1,000 daily calories, with more water for individual circumstances, may be more achievable and reasonable.

Consuming large amounts of fluids, especially water, does not appear to prevent bladder cancer, kidney stones or urinary tract infections. Nor do copious amounts of water flush the body of toxins. Rather, large amounts of fluids may upset the normal balance of electrolytes in the body, particularly chloride, potassium and sodium, and affect major body systems, including cardiovascular, circulatory and excretory.

Dehydration can also have devastating effects on the body, from back pain and headaches to irregular heartbeats and death. It is commonly thought that once a person is thirsty, the body is already dehydrated and gulping down even a large quantity of fluid may be too late for rehydration.

In reality, the first line of bodily defenses against dehydration is the *antidiuretic hormone (ADH)* and *aldosterone.* When the human body first becomes dehydrated, the blood becomes more concentrated and the watery substance of the blood is reduced. The **antidiuretic hormone** then signals the kidneys to reabsorb more water and return it to the bloodstream. **Aldosterone** is a hormone that is secreted by the adrenal glands. It signals the kidneys to decrease the elimination of sodium in the urine and return this mineral (and electrolyte) to the circulation. Body water seeks this sodium and is conserved.

With normal kidney function, we consume the fluids that we need. If this finely balanced system fails and blood sodium concentrates, the sensation of thirst takes over. If we do not drink enough, then the body's cells, organs and systems may suffer.

Thirst sets in when the blood is concentrated in sodium around 2 percent. Dehydration sets in when the blood is concentrated in sodium about 5 percent. If we listen to our body and consume beverages and high-fluid foods when we are thirsty and hungry, we should be able to maintain **fluid balance**, or **homeostasis**. If we ignore these signals, this is when we can develop fluid-related problems.

A way to understand the importance of fluid balance is to compare it to body weight. After exercising in very hot conditions, a 150-pound person may lose three pounds, which is a 2 percent loss in body weight. At a 4 percent loss of body weight, muscle strength and endurance may suffer. At a 7 to 10 percent loss, severe muscle weakness may result. And at a 20 percent loss of body weight, coma and death may follow. It is recommended that a person weigh himself before and after exercise and replace every 1-pound loss with two 8-ounce cups of water.

Fluid intake should be individualized, like other nutrients. It is a matter of discovering how much fluid helps a person feel best and how much needs to be replaced under extenuating conditions. For the majority of people, a normal intake of fluids with meals, plus more fluids when thirst calls, should be sufficient. Larger, more muscular individuals and those that sweat heavily should probably consume more fluids with meals and between meals.

Certain populations require more attention and response to thirst and hunger signals, such as athletes, children, the elderly and those who live in hot climates. This is why, for example, it is important to tend to the elderly during very hot weather. The elderly, whose kidneys are less able to conserve water when their fluid intake is low, must be reminded to drink, and their diet should have ample foods with fluid, like fruits and vegetables. So should people with gastrointestinal illnesses and children with fever.

From a weight control standpoint, a large quantity of fluid consumed *before* a meal can help a person reach early satiety, or fullness, and eat less. However, since water has no calories, this sensation is just temporary. When it diminishes, hunger will likely return. But if an appreciable amount of fluid is consumed *during* a meal, then satiety may be longer lasting.

The soluble fiber that is found in whole grains and some fruits and vegetables depends on fluids to swell and provide fullness and is indispensible in weight control. Table 8-1 compares the calories and sugar in common beverages. Keep in mind that different types of dairy milk and fortified juices and beverages deliver more nutrients than just sugar calories, but all beverages can have some place in an otherwise healthy diet.

TABLE 8-1 Comparison of Calories and Sugar in Common Beverages

Beverages	Average Calories (calories)	Average Sugar Content (grams)
Juice	90–120 cal	17–28 g
Dairy milk, 2%	120	12.5
Dairy milk, 1%	100	12.5
Dairy milk, skim	85	12.5
Soda	90–100	26–28
Fruit punch/drinks	90–120	25–30
Sports drinks	50–65	14–15
Vitamin water	40–50	8–13
Water	0	0

Morsel "The best wine is the oldest; the best water the newest." —William Blake (English painter, poet and printmaker, 1757–1827)

High-fluid foods and menus that ensure good hydration are presented in this chapter. Special fluids that can be used for targeted groups with increased hydration needs are also discussed [1,2,3].

Water: Functions and Sources

FUNCTIONS OF WATER

Water is an essential nutrient, just like carbohydrates, protein, lipids, vitamins and minerals. Like vitamins and minerals, water does not contain any calories, but it is fundamental in energy production.

Water can be found in practically all cells in the human body, animals and plants. It is also a major component in nearly all of the foods and beverages we consume. Water acts as a medium in cooking and baking to help transfer heat, which directly affects the flavor, stability and texture of foods. Water solutions can be acidic (acid) or alkaline (basic), which can affect the performance of the food molecules that are contained within it. For example, acidic or basic solutions can affect the color of fruits and vegetables and the texture of egg and meat proteins.

Water is a small, simple chemical compound that is composed of hydrogen and oxygen. Its chemical formula is known as H_2O, which means that water contains two hydrogen atoms and one oxygen atom that are bonded together. While the chemical composition of water is simple, its significance cannot be understated. It carries essential oxygen to the cells for energy.

Water provides 60 percent of a person's body weight. In an average 150-pound person, this amount equals about 90 pounds of water. The remaining 60 pounds is divided between body fat and stored protein in muscles, carbohydrates, vitamins and minerals.

Overall, men have proportionally more water in their bodies than women do because they have more muscle mass. Children have proportionally more water than the elderly, whose muscle mass decreases with age. Muscle is about 75 percent water, bone is about 20 percent water, and teeth are about 10 percent water. Raw meat, like human muscle, is about 75 percent water, and many fruits and vegetables can be as much as 95 percent water.

An average of 1,400 to 2,850 milliliters of water is available daily through foods, liquids and the water created by metabolism, called *metabolic water*. Foods provide 700 to 1,000 milliliters, liquids about 550 to 1,500 milliliters, and metabolic water about 200 to 300 milliliters.

336

Generally, daily water output equals daily water intake. A healthy adult excretes about 1½ to 3 quarts of water daily roughly in this manner:

Water Excretion/Losses	Amount (milliliters)
Kidneys excrete	500–1,400 ml
Lungs excrete	350
Fluid losses from the skin	450–900
Fluid losses from feces	100–200
Total output:	1,400–2,850 milliliters = 1.4–2.85 liters or 5.88–11.97 cups

One ounce of fluid equals about 30 milliliters; one liter of fluid equals about 4.2 cups. Consuming about 8 cups of water every day is recommended so water loss equals water intake [4,5].

Water has many vital roles in the body. It is the main component of all of the body fluids both inside and outside of the cells. It serves as a lubricant in the joints and as a shock absorber in the spinal cord and for the fetus in the amniotic sac. Water helps transport nutrients to the cells to be metabolized into energy and carries away waste products. It moistens the mucous membranes and hydrates the hair, nails and skin. Water helps maintain a normal body temperature and participates in numerous chemical reactions throughout the human body.

Water is also a *solvent*, a liquid that dissolves *solutes* in a *solution*. Many substances, including food chemicals, can dissolve in water. This is a very important characteristic for ingredients in cooking and baking. Salt brines and sugar syrups depend on water-based solutions. Water is also essential in *suspensions*, *emulsions*, *gels* and *foams*. Nonfat dairy milk is a milk-protein suspension in water. Cream is an emulsion of butterfat in water, and oil-and-vinegar salad dressing is an emulsion of oil in vinegar. Jellies made with gelatin or pectin are dispersions of water in solid gels, and souffles and beer "heads" are dispersions of gas bubbles in water-based liquids to create lighter textures and/or different mouthfeels.. These applications provide interest and variety to the foods and beverages that we consume.

Water Sources

Water is found in foods with a moist taste and texture, such as lettuce and tomatoes; foods that crunch, such as apples and crackers; and foods that have a fatty taste and texture, such as avocadoes and ground beef. Here are some percentages of water by weight in some common foods [6]:

- Lettuce and tomatoes are about 95 percent.
- One percent dairy milk is about 90 percent.
- Apples with skin are about 86 percent.
- Avocadoes, bananas and white potatoes are about 65 to 79 percent.
- Roasted white meat chicken is about 65 percent.
- Eighty percent of some lean ground meat is about 56 percent.

HARD AND SOFT WATERS

Water in the US food supply varies according to the location and how it is processed. *Hard water* contains minerals from shallow ground, such as calcium, magnesium and sodium. Some hard water may taste a little metallic or salty. It may leave a crystal residue inside tea kettles or coffee pots. Water softeners are sometimes used to make hard water softer.

The minerals in hard water contribute to the total intake of minerals by the human body. The ingestion of hard water may be restricted for some health conditions because of this mineral buildup.

Soft water generally comes from deep within the earth's crust. It tends to have a higher concentration of sodium than hard water. This amount of sodium may need to be taken into account in restricted-sodium diets for hypertension and other conditions. Soft water helps soap to lather better than hard water, but it tends to leaves a ring in the bathtub, sink and toilet. Soft water may dissolve toxic substances from pipes, such as lead, into the water supply.

337

Because water from our food supply is so essential to the human body, water safety is critical. The US Environmental Protection Agency (EPA) is responsible for monitoring the water supply. It sets limits for potential contaminants, including bacteria, lead, mercury, nitrates and silver.

One type of parasite of particular concern in the water supply is *crytosporidium*. It is found in water that contains animal waste or sewage, and it is highly resistant to chlorine (used as a disinfectant). Crytosporidium can cause gastrointestinal or flu-like symptoms and can lead to long-term complications in people with vulnerable immune systems, such as certain cancers and HIV disease.

Lead pipes were banned in US building materials in 1986, but if homes or food service establishments were built earlier than this date, lead-clad pipes could still supply water. Lead-contaminated water may cause kidney, liver and nerve damage, with harmful cardiovascular, gastrointestinal, immunological and/or reproductive effects. Water treatment systems can be used, and/or laboratories can test questionable water for lead content. For precaution, pipes should be "flushed" before use by running cold water, particularly early in the morning.

BOTTLED WATERS

Although the US water supply is considered to be one of the best in the world, the bottled water industry has dramatically grown since the 1990s. Health, safety and contaminant-free water are reasons why some people may choose bottled water over tap water.

Bottled water labels may carry enticing terms and pictures, suggesting that the contents are pure and superior to tap water. To ensure their accuracy, the US Food and Drug Administration (FDA) regulates bottled water products that are in interstate commerce under the Federal Food, Drug and Cosmetic Act (FD&C Act), passed by Congress in 1938 and amended many times.

Under the FD&C Act, bottled water manufacturers are responsible for safe, wholesome and truthfully labeled bottled water products. The FDA has established standards of identity regulations that define different types of bottled water and standards of quality regulations that set maximum levels of contaminants (chemical, microbial, physical and radiological). The International Bottled Water Association (IBWA) is a trade organization that enforces these FDA bottled water regulations.

From a regulatory standpoint, the FDA describes bottled water as "Water that is intended for human consumption and that is sealed in bottles or other containers with no added ingredients, except that it may contain safe and suitable antimicrobial agents. Fluoride may also be added within the limits set by the FDA."

This definition excludes flavored water, seltzer, soda, tonics and water products sold from vending machines. It includes *artesian* and *artesian well water*, *groundwater*, *purified water* (also known as *demineralized*, *distilled*, *deionized*, or *reverse osmosis*), *sparkling bottled*, *well water*, and *community* or *municipality sourced water*, as shown in Table 8-2.

The purity of bottled water is comparable to tap water, since it does not have to meet higher standards. Chlorine levels may be lower than tap water, since bottled water is filtered to remove chemicals that affect taste. Fluoride could be removed in bottling, so some bottled waters may not help to prevent tooth decay or promote oral health. This may be a significant consideration in the type of water that is given to infants and children with emerging teeth.

Chemicals and flavors could be added in bottling—some in significant quantities. The section on fortified beverages in this chapter highlights some of the substances that are used in fortification [7].

WATER BALANCE

Water exists both inside and outside of the cells. *Intracellular water* consists of about two-thirds of the water in the body, while *extracellular water* or *plasma* includes the rest. The balance of intra- and extracellular water is attributed to *electrolytes*, elements or small molecules with electrical charges, such as sodium, potassium, magnesium, chloride and phosphate.

Water volume inside the cell is mostly due to potassium and phosphate ions. Extracellular water is mainly the result of sodium and chloride ions. Changes in concentrations of any of these electrolytes can cause water to

TABLE 8-2 Types and Sources of Waters

Types of Water	Sources of Water
Artesian water	Drawn out of wells from restricted water-bearing rocks or rock formations
Artesian well water	Same as above
Club soda[a]	Artificially carbonated water May contain added salts and minerals; levels vary
Community or municipality water	Source must appear on label, preceding or following brand name
Mineral water	Drawn from underground sources Contains at least 250 parts per million (ppm) total dissolved solids Low mineral content must appear on label If more than 1,500 ppm, high mineral content may appear on label. If 20 milligrams calcium, 0.36 milligrams iron or 5 milligrams sodium, must bear nutritional labeling
Purified water	All minerals removed
Demineralized, distilled, deionized, reverse osmosis	Same as above
Seltzer water[a]	Tap water with artificially added bubbles of carbon dioxide gas
Sparkling water	Contains the same amount of carbon dioxide gas that is naturally present at its source
Spring water	Obtained from underground formation where water naturally flows to surface Mineral content remains same as source Collected at spring or source feeding the spring
Tonic water[a]	Artificially carbonated water Contains added salts and minerals
Well water	Obtained from rock formation through bored or drilled holes, or constructed in ground

Source: [8–11].
[a]Not considered bottled waters by FDA regulations.

shift. If water enters the cells beyond capacity, the cells can burst. If water exits the cells in large amounts, the cells can shrink and die, and the extracellular water can become overladen with minerals. In turn, this could result in *edema*, the accumulation of fluid in the tissues. Water movement throughout the cells is further discussed in Chapters 1 and 7.

Water in the bloodstream is called *plasma*, and the amount of it is called *plasma volume*. Plasma serves to regulate body temperature, among other functions. When muscles give off heat during exercise, the heat is transferred to the plasma, which in turn transfers the heat to the skin. When a person sweats, she gives off this heat which cools the skin and body. If it is humid and the air is filled with moisture, these conditions interfere with normal sweating and make it difficult to cool the body. That is why it is important to drink fluid in humid conditions. If a person does not drink enough fluid, it may be drawn from the muscles and organs and lead to poor attention, cramping, decreased performance and fatigue. These are the early signs of *dehydration*.

Dehydration is the excessive loss of body fluids. Dehydration can be caused by diseases of the gastrointestinal tract, excessive alcohol or caffeine intake, outside temperature and humidity, poor fluid intake, and other factors. Dehydration can be the underlying problem in illnesses and can be severe enough to become life-threatening.

The symptoms of dehydration become increasingly severe with greater water loss. The heart and respiration rates increase to compensate for decreased plasma volume and blood pressure. Body temperature rises from decreased sweating. Still, a healthy adult should be able to successfully rebound.

After age 50, the body's thirst sensation diminishes in effectiveness, which continues with advanced age. Dehydration and *hyperthermia* impose serious risks to seniors, especially in extreme temperatures. Athletes may experience symptoms of decreased endurance, elevated body temperature, flushing, rapid heart rate, rapid onset of fatigue, and reduced performance due to dehydration. Dehydration in the human body progresses as follows:

- *Early symptoms of dehydration (about 2 percent water loss):* decreased blood pressure (orthostatic hypotension), dizziness or fainting when standing, headache, muscle cramps, and visual "snow" or fuzziness
- *Mild dehydration (about 5 to 6 percent water loss):* abnormally dark urine, constipation, decreased urine volume, dry skin, headache, dizziness, dry mouth, insomnia, lack of tears when crying, loss of appetite, thirst, and unexplained tiredness
- *Moderate to severe dehydration (about 10 to 15 percent water loss):* fainting, lethargy or extreme sleepiness, no urine output, seizures, and sunken eyes
- *Untreated dehydration (greater than 15 percent water loss):* delirium, swelling of the tongue, unconsciousness, and death

As dehydration progresses, the heart may have to work harder and beat faster to supply enough oxygen for the working muscles. As the body temperature increases, many organs and systems become stressed to increase output. This may lead to **heat exhaustion** (mild to moderate dehydration), characterized by cool and clammy skin, dry mouth, dizziness, fatigue, headache, muscle cramping, nausea, sweating and/or weak or rapid pulse.

If body temperature remains high, this can lead to **heatstroke** (moderate to severe dehydration). Indicators of heatstroke may include blurred vision, cessation of sweating, confusion, convulsions, delirium, hallucinations, hot and dry skin, increased body temperature of 104 °F or higher, loss of consciousness, and/or death.

Proper hydration is regulated by the **kidneys**. The kidneys filter ions from the blood, including magnesium, phosphate, potassium and sodium, and remove excess liquids from the body through the urine. The kidneys also remove metabolic wastes, such as urea and uric acid, and drugs from the bloodstream. If any of these substances settle out of the urine and crystallize, they can enlarge into a hardened mass, or **kidney stone**. Kidney stones can become lodged in the bladder, causing pain and necessitating their removal.

340

Water intoxication is a condition in which too much water is contained in the bloodstream without enough electrolytes. Water intoxication can occur when a quantity of fluid is consumed in a short amount of time and the kidneys are not able to filter enough water from the bloodstream. This condition dilutes the sodium in the bloodstream and throws off the water balance in the body. As a result, water rushes inside the cells, including the cells of the brain, which may cause confusion, coordination difficulties, coma, dizziness, headache, strange behaviors, or seizures. People with kidney disorders, those who drink large amounts of plain water during heavy exercise, and those who drink copious amounts of water due to psychological or other reasons may risk the consequences of water intoxication.

Recipe: Fruit-Flavored Waters

*These fruit-flavored waters are calorie-free with the essence of fruit flavors and fresh fruit garnishes. Flavored waters are perceived to be tastier, thus encouraging people to consume more of them. These fruit-flavored waters are all variations on the same theme: crisp and clean-tasting water, fresh fruit combinations, and appealing garnishes. Experiment with your own combinations and taste preferences. The recipes for **Fruit-Flavored Waters** can be found in the **Recipe file** which is located within the Culinary Nutrition website at www.culinarynutrition.elsevier.com, and photos are within the centerfold **Photo file** in Plate 8.1.*

WATER IN COOKING AND BAKING

Water is a clear substance that becomes filled with food molecules that bond together during cooking and baking. These chemical bonds are the result of the polar charges that both water and nutrients, such as carbohydrates and proteins, carry. Thanks to these polar charges, water is able to engulf or "swallow" carbohydrates and proteins so they appear to dissolve inside water. Think of a simple sugar solution or pickling brine: the sugar and salt look as if they dissolve into the solution and brine water.

When water is exposed to low temperatures, it crystallizes into solid *ice*. As the temperature increases, ice first melts into liquid water and then it vaporizes into steam. These physical changes are accomplished through reformulating the chemical bonds. Water expands when it freezes into ice. This also happens to food. Plant and animal cell membranes that are filled with water expand and often rupture, which may affect the texture of food. As ice crystals melt and liquid is lost, this may also affect food texture.

Water has high *specific heat*, the amount of energy required to raise its temperature a specific amount. This is because the chemical bonds in water must first be broken down before the molecules can move faster to heat the water. For this reason, water is a good medium for slow heating. Covering a pot or pan will prevent water from turning into steam and will help hold the temperature longer, even after the pot or pan is removed from the heat source.

It also takes a while for water to vaporize into *steam*. Water first needs to absorb a great deal of heat before this transition can occur. This concept can be likened to sweating. Before sweat can dissipate from the skin, it must absorb quite a bit of body heat.

Cooking and baking have utilized this concept for centuries. The hot contents of ancient clay vessels were cooled by the evaporation of moisture that collected on their surfaces. When delicate custards were baked in water baths, the moisture wicked away the heat. Slow oven roasting and simmering gently evaporated the moisture that rose to the surface of food and allowed it to cook gently. The same techniques are used today.

Steam carries a lot of heat. The steam from a bubbling pot of hot liquid can be intense and should be managed with care. Steaming food can be an effective way of cooking without fat. When food is positioned in a steamer basket above boiling water, the steam rises to cook the food; then it circulates back down to cook the food from above. The pot or pan must be covered for this process to occur. Lifting the lid breaks the cycle. Adding a tablespoon of boiling water to a dry saute will slightly steam the contents. Placing a pot of boiling water into a bread oven will cause the loaves to rapidly expand.

Water is a relatively neutral mix of acids and bases; it is neither too acidic nor too alkali. Most foods that we consume are slightly acidic. If they are cooked in water that is also slightly acidic, the food can be affected. It could taste sour, the color could be "off," and the texture could be compromised. In protein foods, this could cause toughening. In fruits and vegetables, this could cause sogginess.

The properties of acids and bases in foods affect almost everything we eat and drink. That is why it is a good idea to familiarize oneself with the pH scale. The *pH scale* has been formulated to indicate the acidity and alkalinity of substances. It runs from 0 to 14, with 7 being neutral. A pH that is lower than 7 indicates that a substance is more acidic, while a pH higher than 7 indicates that a substance is more basic.

Human gastric juice has a pH of 1.3 to 3.0, which is acidic enough to digest animal proteins. Baking soda has a pH of 8.4. Baking soda reacts with acidic ingredients, such as lemon juice or vinegar, which neutralizes the base and acid and releases carbon dioxide (CO_2) gas to help baked goods rise. Adding citrus juice, vinegar or wine to cooking water lowers the pH and increases acidity. Adding baking soda to cooking water increases the pH and may produce a slippery texture.

A common acid in baking is *cream of tartar* (technically potassium hydrogen tartarate), derived from the inside of wine barrels. If cream of tartar is mixed with baking soda, it becomes *single acting baking powder*, which reacts when liquids are added and contributes to rise. *Double acting baking powder* has additional acids that react with heat and add a second rise as recipes bake.

Alcohol: the Good, the Bad and the Ugly

Is alcohol a beverage or a food? Is it a drink or a drug? Is it healthy or harmful? There are many questions and misconceptions about alcohol. Alcohol is included in this chapter because it is a fluid with healthful properties when it is used sensibly. Alcohol also has important roles in cooking, culture and cuisine. Yet, alcohol can have many harmful effects when it is used imprudently as a recreational beverage.

Alcohol is actually a group of organic compounds that include *ethanol (ethyl alcohol)*, *isopropanol (isopropyl alcohol* or *rubbing alcohol)*, and *methanol (methyl alcohol)*. The suffix "-ol" generally means that a substance is a type of alcohol. Most alcoholic beverages that one can drink without harm contain ethanol, a narcotic drug with depressant effects. Contrary to popular opinion, ethanol is not a stimulant because it slows down the central nervous system and decreases motor coordination, reaction time and intellectual function.

Ethanol is produced by the microscopic yeast fermentation of carbohydrates in the absence of oxygen. A number of carbohydrates can be used in this process. These include fruits, grapes, grains, and fruit and grain mixtures.

Humans can metabolize ethanol to produce energy. Ethanol is quite caloric, with 7 calories per gram, compared to 9 calories per gram for lipids and 4 calories per gram for both carbohydrates and protein. But alcohol is not an essential nutrient. It is also not stored by the body. This means that once ethanol is metabolized, it must be removed by the body or it accumulates in the blood and body tissues. For the purpose of this discussion, ethanol will be referred to as alcohol—its familiar name.

ALCOHOL METABOLISM

Once alcohol is consumed, it passes through the esophagus into the stomach, where 10 to 30 percent of the ethanol is absorbed and metabolized into energy. The remaining alcohol proceeds into the small intestine, where about 70 to 90 percent of the alcohol is metabolized and absorbed into the bloodstream.

At this point, the rise in blood alcohol is greater for women than men. This is because women have less body water than men (52 percent for the average woman versus 61 percent for the average man). This means that a man's body is able to dilute alcohol more than a woman's body, even if they weigh the same amount. This explains why men seem to tolerate alcohol better than women, why one drink in a woman has the same effects as two drinks in a man, and why women are more susceptible to alcoholic liver disease, brain damage and cardiac muscle damage.

From the small intestine, alcohol is transported by the bloodstream to the liver, where it is metabolized by the enzyme *alcohol dehydrogenase* into *acetaldehyde* and water. Other enzymes then convert acetaldehyde into *acetate*, and then into carbon dioxide and water for excretion. Some nonmetabolized alcohol can be detected in the urine by urinalysis and by a *Breathalyzer*, a specialized device that estimates blood alcohol content (BAC). Nonmetabolized alcohol is also removed by the body through breast milk, feces, saliva and sweat.

The metabolism of alcohol follows similar pathways as sugars and fats. Alcohol is quickly absorbed, can be filling, and interferes with hunger and satiety. A person may feel "full" after drinking, but the sensation is from alcohol calories, not from food. As a result, chronic alcohol ingestion may lead to malnutrition. It may also lead to weight gain.

Alcohol stimulates insulin production, which speeds up glucose metabolism and can lead to low blood sugar—especially if it is not accompanied by food. This is why diabetics should consume food if they drink alcohol.

Alcohol also dilates the peripheral or secondary blood vessels. It causes heat to transfer from the body's core to the extremities, where it is quickly dispersed. A person who consumes ethanol may initially feel warm, but this may be temporary, and chilling may follow. It is not uncommon to experience a number of body temperature changes, depending on the length of the drinking experience.

Rate of Alcohol Metabolism

There is a limit as to how much alcohol can be metabolized by the body per hour. The rate of alcohol metabolism by the human body is about ½ ounce (15 milliliters) per hour, or about one standard drink every 60 to 90 minutes.

Blood alcohol peaks about 30 to 60 minutes after consumption. If more alcohol is consumed than metabolized, or if alcohol is consumed too fast, blood alcohol can accumulate with increased loss of mental and physical control. A person may lose consciousness or die if he or she continues to drink.

Fatty foods delay the time alcohol spends in the stomach and its passage into the small intestine and bloodstream. The presence of fatty foods, such as chips, nuts, or olives, in the gastrointestinal tract reduces the peak blood level of alcohol to about half that of an unfed person. Fatty foods such as these should accompany alcohol service at taverns and events.

Aspirin and carbon dioxide in carbonated beverages, beer and sparkling wine have the opposite effect: they speed up the passage of alcohol and increase its peak blood level. Food helps moderate this response.

Alcohol absorption is also dependent on the amount of the enzyme alcohol dehydrogenase. Alcohol dehydrogenase is about 40 percent less active in the liver of women, so alcohol may pass undiluted into their bloodstream. Some ethnic groups produce less alcohol dehydrogenase, such as Asians, who develop facial "flushing" from alcohol ingestion. Sensible alcohol consumption in this population is recommended.

Bite on This: alcohol in the bloodstream

The amount of alcohol in the bloodstream is indicated by the **blood alcohol level (BAL)** or **blood alcohol concentration (BAC)**. It is designated in milligrams of alcohol per 100 milliliters of blood. The BAC reflects the amount of alcohol consumed, how fast it is consumed, and the amount of alcohol that is present in the bloodstream after one hour of ingestion. Since the liver can only metabolize about one drink per 60 to 90 minutes, any excess alcohol enters the bloodstream full strength.

A blood alcohol level of 50 to 100 mg/dL may be considered *legal drunkenness*. The lowest known lethal dose of alcohol in humans is about 15 shots for a 220-pound person. Chronic alcohol consumption may cause higher tolerance.

The progressive percentages of BAC, behavior, and mental and physical impairments are shown in Table 8-3.

TABLE 8-3 Progressive Effects of Alcohol on Behavior and Mental and Physical Functions

Percent BAC	Behaviors	Mental and Physical Impairments
0.01–0.029	Normal	Subtle, detected by testing
0.03–0.059	Chatty, comfortable, joyful, outgoing, relaxed, reduced alertness	Awareness, concentration, coordination, reasoning
0.06–0.10	Dulled, extroverted, sexually impaired, unrestrained	Depth perception, distance acuteness, glare recovery, peripheral vision, reasoning, reflex reactions
0.11–0.20	Angry or sad, emotional swings, overly expressive, rowdy	Gross motor control, reaction time, slurred speech, unsteady
0.21–0.29	Bewilderment, failed understanding, impaired sensations	Loss of consciousness, memory blackout, severe motor impairment
0.30–0.39	Severe depression, unconsciousness, possible death	Bladder function, breathing, heart rate
≥0.40	Unconsciousness, death	Breathing, heart rate, pulse

Source: [12,13].

343

EFFECTS OF ALCOHOL ON THE BRAIN

Since alcohol is metabolized quickly, the central nervous system can be affected fairly rapidly. As alcohol reaches the brain, it acts as a narcotic. It stimulates behavior but suppresses higher brain functions and interferes with concentration, memory, muscle coordination, speech, thinking and vision.

The first area of the brain to be affected by alcohol ingestion is the *cerebral cortex*, where judgment and reasoning are controlled. The early signs of intoxication are clumsiness, delayed reflexes and slurred speech.

The next area of the brain to be affected by alcohol ingestion is the *limbic system*, or the sensory area of the brain, which controls behavior, emotions, long-term memory and voluntary muscles. Intoxication to this point can lead to more erratic behavior.

After the limbic system, the *cerebellum* is the next area of the brain that is affected by alcohol ingestion. The *cerebellum* controls the regulation and coordination of balance, movement and posture. Intoxication to this level can lead to staggering. This is why the ability to walk a straight line is factored in a *field sobriety test*, used for DUI arrests.

Then the *hypothalamus* and *pituitary gland*, followed by the *medulla*, or *brainstem*, are affected by alcohol ingestion. This area of the brain is responsible for basic vital life functions, such as blood pressure, heartbeat and respiration. Intoxication that affects this area of the brain can lead to unconsciousness and death.

HANGOVER AND DEHYDRATION

Excessive alcohol consumption may lead to intoxication and a hangover, which may take over when the seemingly euphoric effects of alcohol subside. An alcohol *hangover* resembles a mild case of drug withdrawal with symptoms of dehydration, including a headache. Since alcohol is a central nervous system depressant, heightened sensitivity to activity, light and sound may occur. If a person has a drink to cure a hangover, it only delays recovery. Aspirin or caffeinated products may temporarily alleviate it. Fluids (especially water) are recommended.

This is because alcohol increases urination. It does this by blocking the *antidiuretic hormone (ADH)*, which regulates urine production. In turn, ADH causes the kidneys to conserve fluids. Once ADH is blocked, urination increases, which may lead to dehydration. One ounce of hard liquor or 12 ounces of beer will cause about the same amount of urine loss.

ETHANOL TOXICITY

Ethanol is the only type of alcohol that can be consumed in moderation without serious harm, and only if it is denatured or does not contain toxic impurities. However, even ethanol may be toxic. Chronic alcohol consumption may affect the liver and brain. *Cirrhosis* is a condition that is characterized by the replacement of healthy liver tissue with fibrous scar tissue and nodules, leading to progressive loss of liver function.

Alcohol damages dendrites, the branched ends of nerve cells that carry messages to the cells. Alcohol dilates the channels in the cells that regulate the flow of calcium. This causes excess calcium to flow into the cells and overstimulate their activity. Over time, this may alter their functions. Some forms of cancer, such as oral, esophageal and maybe breast cancer, have been linked to excessive ethanol consumption [14].

ALCOHOL ADDICTION

Ethanol is a potentially addictive substance, with numerous potentially destructive health effects. *Alcoholism*, also known as *alcohol dependence syndrome*, is a disease that is characterized by four main conditions: craving, loss of control, physical dependence and tolerance. Alcoholism is partially genetic and partially environmental. Alcoholic-prone individuals may have different biochemical responses to alcohol than non-alcoholic-prone people.

Alcohol addiction is a compulsive craving for alcohol, coupled with an impaired ability to recognize the negative effects of excessive alcohol consumption. In alcohol addiction, or *alcohol dependency*, the emotional and physical motivations to have a drink overrule the intellectual reasons why not to have a drink. There may also be impaired ability to recognize the negative effects of excessive alcohol consumption.

Continued alcohol consumption builds *tolerance* to the drug, or decreased effectiveness of alcohol in the human body. *Metabolic tolerance* is when alcohol is metabolized at a faster rate than normal and increased amounts of alcohol need to be consumed for comparable effects. This is because a habitual drinker becomes efficient over time in lowering the blood alcohol concentration.

Functional tolerance is an alteration in sensitivity to alcohol. For example, the nerve cells become heightened to counteract the inhibitory effects of alcohol. This is a protective mechanism so that the body can still

344

function despite its drug-induced state. But this heightened nerve activity may also cause convulsions, hallucinations and withdrawal symptoms if alcohol is eliminated, which is often seen in drug withdrawal programs.

There is always a risk of mixing alcohol with other drugs, because the combination may intensify the effects of both substances. Chronic drinking may activate an enzyme that converts over-the-counter pain medications into chemicals that may cause liver damage.

Alcohol can inflame the stomach. Aspirin can also cause inflammation of the stomach lining and lead to bleeding or ulcers. People who take aspirin regularly should probably check with their health care provider about alcohol consumption.

The mixture of alcohol with other drugs may alter sex hormones in both men and women. Men might experience testicular, testosterone or sperm changes, and women might experience altered estrogen levels, which may increase the risk of breast cancer.

Excessive ethanol intake is risky for children, slender people, seniors, and women who have decreased body fluid, which concentrates alcohol. Excessive vomiting, often leading to unconsciousness, is triggered sooner in people with low alcohol tolerance. If someone "passes out," this may prevent alcohol toxicity, unless excessive alcohol is consumed very quickly and the blood alcohol concentration (BAC) is high.

Bite on This: moderate alcohol consumption

The American Heart Association recommends that if a person drinks alcohol, he or she should do so in moderation. Moderate alcohol intake is considered to be an average of one to two drinks per day for men and one drink per day for women. Moderate alcohol consumption may have beneficial or harmful effects, depending on the amount consumed and the age and individual characteristics of the person who consumes the alcohol [15].

One may think that "hard" alcohol contains more alcohol than beer or wine. This is not the case. One glass of wine, a bottle of beer or a shot of whiskey or other distilled spirits contain about equivalent amounts of alcohol. A standard drink is considered to be:

- 1½ ounces 80-proof distilled spirits, straight or in a mixed drink (100 calories)
- 1 ounce 100-proof distilled spirits (80 calories)
- 3 ounces sherry or port (130 calories)
- 5 ounces red or white wine (80 to 100 calories)
- 9¾ ounces malt liquor (135 calories)
- 12 ounces wine, malt or spirit-based cooler (210–230 calories)
- 12-ounce bottle or can of regular beer (150 calories)

Table wines, distilled spirits and malt beverages contain about 14 grams of alcohol per serving. In comparison, regular beer contains about 13 grams of alcohol per serving, and light beer contains about 11 grams of alcohol per serving.

345

ALCOHOL AND DISEASE

Drinking too much alcohol may lead to a variety of conditions that are caused by the alcohol itself or the effects of alcohol on the human body. These include accidents, alcoholism, anemia, bone disorders, brain damage, breast cancer, cirrhosis of the liver, coronary heart disease, fetal alcohol syndrome, gastrointestinal disorders, hypertension, increased blood lipids (especially triglycerides), malnutrition, obesity, pancreatitis, problems with pregnancy and/or lactation, sex hormone disturbances, strokes, suicides, and vitamin and mineral deficiencies. It is not possible to predict which people will be inflicted by these conditions. Some of these conditions have clear connections to alcohol consumption, such as fetal alcohol syndrome. Others are not so obvious, such as sex hormone disturbances.

ACCIDENTS AND INJURIES RELATED TO ALCOHOL

Alcohol consumption is associated with a range of *accidents* and *injuries* due to impaired mental and motor functions. The complex skills required to operate motorized vehicles are susceptible to alcohol intake, which distorts almost every aspect of information that is processed by the human brain.

The brain's voluntary control of eye and hand movements is linked to blood alcohol concentration. Alcohol-impaired drivers tend to require more time to read a street sign and to respond to a traffic signal than nondrinkers. While successful driving requires a series of tasks, alcohol-impaired drivers tend to favor one task over another. For example, alcohol-impaired drivers tend to concentrate more on steering and focus less on overall safety.

ANEMIAS CAUSED BY ALCOHOL

Alcohol may contribute to different *anemias*, lower than normal levels of red blood cells (RBCs). Alcohol blocks the action of folic acid, which is used to create new red blood cells. Chronic alcoholism causes cirrhosis, which slows the passage of blood through the portal vein. This backs up blood into the gastrointestinal tract, which can cause swollen or knotted veins in the esophagus and intestines and lead to hemorrhoids. Hemorrhoids can burst, bleed and further lower the level of red blood cells.

BONE DISORDERS CAUSED BY ALCOHOL

Alcohol intake may affect *bone health* in women. The bone's mechanical properties, such as strength and strain, may be decreased by too much alcohol. This may lead to a loss of bone density and increased susceptibility to osteoporosis.

BRAIN DAMAGE CAUSED BY ALCOHOL

Mild to moderate drinking may adversely affect the *hippocampus*, the learning and memory center of the brain. Alcohol inhibits the systems that store new information, such as long-term memory, and makes it difficult to immediately remember what was recently learned. Mild to moderate drinking may also adversely affect the *prefrontal area* (behind the forehead), which plays an important role in behavior and in forming the adult personality. Anxiety, depression and reckless behavior are common expressions in psychiatric disorders, which may coincide with alcoholism. Long-term, heavy alcohol consumption may potentially have more severe brain consequences.

BREAST CANCER AND ALCOHOL

Moderate alcohol intake may increase the risk of *breast cancer*, especially in postmenopausal women who use hormone therapy. Women with a personal or family history of breast cancer may be at increased risk even with low alcohol intake.

VITAMIN A METABOLISM AND ALCOHOL

Alcoholism affects *vitamin A metabolism*. The enzyme alcohol dehydrogenase is responsible for converting retinol to retinoic acid, a precursor to vitamin A. The availability of alcohol dehydrogenase for this conversion is dependent on its need to metabolize ethanol. With heavy drinking, less alcohol dehydrogenase is available, so less vitamin A may be made. Vitamin A is responsible for healthy hair, skin and tissues; new cell growth; and vision in dim light. Vitamin A deficiency symptoms may appear in alcoholism.

CIRRHOSIS AND ALCOHOL

Morsel "Wine is the most healthful and most hygienic of beverages." —Louis Pasteur (French chemist and microbiologist, 1822–1895)

Cirrhosis is an outcome of chronic liver disease, commonly caused by alcoholism. Alcohol injures the liver by blocking the normal metabolism of carbohydrates, lipids and protein. Cirrhosis, with its fibrous scar tissue and nodules, leads to progressive loss of liver functions. Generally, liver damage cannot be reversed, but treatment may delay progression and reduce complications.

CORONARY HEART DISEASE AND ALCOHOL

While there appears to be a positive association between moderate red wine consumption and *coronary heart disease*, drinking too much alcohol can raise blood pressure, cause irregular heartbeats and heart failure, and increase LDL cholesterol and triglycerides. The fine line between moderation and too much alcohol lies within the USDA guidelines. "Low-risk" drinking is considered no more than 7 drinks per week for women and 14 drinks per week for men, with no more than 4 drinks on any given day for men and 3 drinks on any given day for women [16,17].

FETAL ALCOHOL SYNDROME

Fetal alcohol syndrome (FAS) is a disorder that may cause permanent birth defects in newborn infants as a result of alcohol ingestion during pregnancy. Fetal alcohol syndrome is the leading cause of preventable mental retardation in the Western world.

Alcohol crosses the placental barrier. While the fetus can metabolize alcohol, it does so at a slow rate. Blood alcohol remains high longer in the fetus than in the mother, with more time to accomplish its damaging effects.

The characteristics of fetal alcohol syndrome that are associated with alcohol ingestion during pregnancy include decreased muscle tone and poor coordination; delayed brain development and/or damage to areas of the brain that are involved in movement, social skills, speech and thinking; facial abnormalities; and growth retardation both in the womb and after birth.

The major harm of FAS is permanent damage to the central nervous system, particularly the brain. Alcohol exposure may cause developing brain cells and structures to be underdeveloped or malformed. The risk of brain damage to the fetus exists throughout the entire pregnancy, since the fetal brain develops more each trimester.

Potential central nervous system disorders in the infant include delayed fine and gross motor skills, hyperactivity, impaired language development, learning disorders, memory problems, mental retardation and seizures. These conditions may lead to mental health problems and drug addiction if the infant matures.

While distorted facial features are not as harmful as central nervous system disorders, they are still physically disfiguring. These include flattened cheeks; grooved and thin upper lip; undersized eyes and jaw; short, turned-up nose; and diminutive head circumference.

The US Surgeon General has advised pregnant women to abstain from alcohol use due to the risk of fetal alcohol syndrome. Four or more daily drinks place a woman at greater risk. Even one drink daily may have harmful effects in FAS-prone women. If a woman abstains from consuming alcohol before conception and when she is pregnant, fetal alcohol syndrome may be completely preventable [18].

GASTROINTESTINAL DISORDERS AND ALCOHOL

Alcohol affects the smooth lining of the stomach and may cause inflammation or *gastritis*. Symptoms of gastritis include abdominal pain, belching, diarrhea, fever, hemorrhage, loss of appetite, nausea, ulcers or vomiting. Intestinal enzymes and transport systems may also be affected, which may lead to lethargy, nutritional deficiencies, and/or weight loss.

HYPERTENSION AND ALCOHOL

Hypertension, or high blood pressure, is a risk factor in cardiovascular disease, congestive heart failure, heart attack, kidney failure, and stroke. Numerous studies in diverse populations have shown that alcohol causes hypertension, and this is independent of age, body weight, or cigarette smoking. The exact relationship between the amount of alcohol consumed and the effects of alcohol on hypertension is undetermined at present. Although alcohol influences both systolic and diastolic blood pressure (the level at which the heart is pumping and resting, respectively), its effect on systolic pressure appears to be more significant. Men are more sensitive to the hypertensive effects of alcohol than women.

MALNUTRITION AND ALCOHOL

Excessive alcohol can depress protein synthesis and lead to protein deficiency. Severe thiamine deficiency is common. Folate, vitamin B6 and vitamin B12 absorption may be compromised, which affects red blood cell formation. The liver activates vitamin D less efficiently, which leads to osteoporosis and bone fractures. And the kidneys excrete more calcium, folate, magnesium, potassium and zinc, which cause varying degrees of vitamin and mineral deficiencies.

Since alcohol is caloric at 7 calories per gram, alcohol consumption can result in overweight or obesity. An average serving of alcohol contains 80 to 150 calories. Drinking in excess can add hundreds of calories.

PANCREATITIS AND ALCOHOL

The pancreas undergoes inflammation from excessive alcohol, much like the stomach. Damage can be permanent. *Acute pancreatitis* occurs more often in men than women. It is characterized by fever, nausea, rapid pulse, severe abdominal pain, swollen and tender abdomen, and vomiting. Since the pancreas is responsible for insulin production, critical in glucose metabolism, the excessive alcohol in diabetics can be quite serious.

PREGNANCY AND LACTATION AND ALCOHOL

Alcohol is quickly transferred from the mother's bloodstream to the fetus. Because all of the organs of the fetus are forming during pregnancy, they are vulnerable to toxic substances, such as alcohol, especially during the first three months of pregnancy. The risks of birth defects, growth retardation, mental disorders, and miscarriage increase in direct proportion to the amount of alcohol the mother drinks and the frequency of her drinking. Heavy drinking can gravely affect the fetus.

Abstinence is the safest strategy to ensure the health of the fetus. Of course, the mother's diet, drug use, health, lifestyle, medical history, pollutants, socioeconomic factors, and tobacco use all may have an impact. Even under ideal conditions, women cannot completely control the outcome of pregnancy. A nursing mother should consult with her medical provider about alcohol consumption, as there is conflicting advice. Alcohol is passed to the infant through breast milk.

SEX HORMONES AND ALCOHOL

Alcoholism can modify sex hormones in both men and women. It may cause testicular injury in men and affect sperm production and testosterone synthesis. In women, alcoholism may cause higher blood levels of estrogen than abstainers. This may be because alcohol slows the metabolism of estrogen. Also, there is increased conversion of androgens (male sex hormones) to estrogen with alcohol consumption. Increased estrogen without progesterone could increase a woman's risks of uterine or breast cancer.

> **FOOD BYTE**
>
> *Wine* may have originated in southern Caucasus between Turkey, Armenia and Iran, roughly between 6000 and 4000 BC. The legend of wine's discovery is attributed to a Persian fable. A princess was presumed to have fallen out of the king's favor, so she consumed a jar of what she thought was poison. The king had placed some bad grapes in the jar. Rather than succumb to poison, the princess's behavior became lighthearted. The king celebrated her survival with the "poison," which must have turned into wine.

HEALTH BENEFITS OF ALCOHOL

In moderation, alcohol consumption may have health benefits. These include lower risk of Alzheimer's disease, diabetes, heart attack, and stroke. Alcohol increases "good" HDL cholesterol and decreases "bad" LDL cholesterol, and there are indications that moderate alcohol intake may reduce the risks of blood clots and stroke.

Some research has correlated the protective benefits of moderate alcohol consumption, especially red wine and coronary heart disease. Various studies suggest that French people have a lower rate of heart disease due to their red wine consumption. This is one of the curiosities of the French Paradox. Although the French consume high-fat foods, smoke more than Americans, and exercise less, they have lower mortality from coronary heart disease. The reason might be their red wine consumption with its health-promoting substances.

Flavonoids in red wine and other antioxidants may be beneficial in reducing the risk of coronary heart disease. Some of these substances may be found in other foods, such as grapes or red grape juice. *Resveratrol* is a substance that is found in the skin of grapes. It is thought to act as an antioxidant by inhibiting free radical formation and preventing blood platelets from sticking together. This may reduce blood clot formation and decrease the risk of heart attack or stroke. However, the association between red wine consumption and reduced coronary heart disease may be due to other factors, such as a diet that is high in fruits and vegetables and low in saturated fats and physical activity.

Morsel "The correct order of beverages is starting with the most temperate and ending with the most heady." —Jean-Anthelme Brillat-Savarin (French epicure, gastronome, lawyer and politician, 1755–1826)

Bite on This: types of alcohol for human consumption

Most yeast cannot grow when the concentration of alcohol is higher than about 18 percent by volume. The alcoholic content of beer, sake, and wine generally falls under this limit.

- *Beer* is one of the world's oldest and most consumed alcoholic beverages. It is made by brewing and fermenting starches that are derived from cereals. The most common cereal starch used in beer production is *malted barley*. Corn, rice and wheat are also used, often in combination with barley.

Most beer is flavored with *hops*, a flower from the hops plant. Hops balances the sweetness of malt with bitterness; contributes citrusy, flowery, fruity, or herbal aromas; and acts as a preservative. It favors the activity of brewer's yeast over less beneficial microorganisms. Fruit and herbs are also sometimes added in brewing.

- *Fortified wines* are made by adding brandy or other distilled spirits to reach a higher level of alcohol than by fermentation, such as ginger wine, port, or sherry. Fortified wines have an alcohol content of about 20 percent by volume.
- *Liqueurs* are sweet alcoholic beverages with an alcohol content of 15 to 70 percent by volume. They may be flavored with bark, cream, flowers, fruits, herbs, roots, seeds, or spices that dissolve in the alcohol. Liqueurs are not usually aged for long. They may have resting periods for the flavorings to mingle.
- *Malt liquor* is a North American term for a type of beer with high alcohol content. In the United Kingdom, similarly made beverages are called *super-strength lager*.
- *Sake* is a Japanese alcoholic beverage that is produced by multiple fermentation of polished rice. The starch is converted to sugar by enzymes, and then the sugar is converted to alcohol by yeast. Sake brewing is different from beer brewing. The enzymes come from a mold called *kōji* rather than malt, and the multiple processes of fermentation occur simultaneously, while in beer brewing they occur in a series of steps.

After fermentation, sake is filtered to remove the grain solids, except in *nigori sake*, where it remains clouded. Generally, sake is not aged. It breaks down quickly with air, heat, or light.

- *Spirits*, unsweetened alcoholic beverages with more than 30 percent alcohol by volume, are produced by *distilling* fermented products, concentrating the alcohol and eliminating some by-products. Spirits are sometimes added to wines to create fortified wines. Examples of spirits are whisky, vodka, gin, schnapps, brandy, rum, and tequila.
- *Wine* is made from the fermentation of grape juice. It can ferment without added acids, enzymes, sugars, or other substances due to the natural chemical reactions of the grapes

and yeast. Wine is made by fermenting crushed grapes with various types of yeast. The yeast consumes the sugars in the grapes and converts them into alcohol. The commercial use of the word *wine* is protected by law in many countries, due in part to this highly intricate and classified process.

There are various types of yeast and grapes used in wine production, which give wine its characteristic sensory qualities. Other fruits can be used to make wine, such as apples or berries. They produce wine that is known by its fruit name, such as apple or berry wine.

ALCOHOL IN COOKING

- Alcohol is both an aid and an impediment in cooking. All forms of alcohol—beer, distilled spirits, and wine—can be used in many dishes, from appetizers to desserts. Alcohol lends distinct flavor when it is needed or subtle, background flavor to let other tastes stand out. Alcohol partners with some flavors to create depth and boosts other flavors to heighten flavor and aroma.
- Acidic, bitter, sweet, salty, and savory tastes in foods can all be affected in some way by the presence of alcohol. If alcohol is mismatched with other ingredients in a recipe, or if it is used in high quantity, it can adversely affect a dish or meal.
- Alcohol can be astringent. *Astringency* is not a taste but a quality that can convey unity or harshness. If alcohol is too astringent in a dish, it can have a sharp mouthfeel.

This is also true if too much or the wrong kind of alcohol is used. When it is balanced, the alcohol seems to bring the dish together.

- Alcohol is clear and colorless. Alcohol mixes easily with water and fatty substances. This feature makes alcohol a convenient partner with cream, juice, dairy milk, or soda. Because alcohol mixes with fatty substances, it can permeate cell membranes and extract aromatic and highly colored pigments, such as carotenoids. Add a little alcohol, such as vodka to tomato sauce, and the highly aromatic and colorful compounds in tomato sauce emerge and are amplified.
- Alcohol is more volatile than water. Alcohol has a lower boiling point than water; it quickly comes to a boil and easily evaporates with heat over time. Since alcohol is so flammable, it can be used to flame a dish, such as Crêpes Suzette or Duck a l'Orange, with brandy or rum. The intense heat vaporizes the alcohol, leaving a slightly roasted taste. Some alcohol remains, depending on the type that is used. This also occurs in a long, slow stew. While some alcohol dissipates, some lingers, lending a subtle to robust taste.
- Alcohol has a lower freezing point than water. Alcoholic drinks can be concentrated by freezing. A mixture of alcohol and water is actually lower in density than pure water. This helps explain layered liqueurs. A liqueur floats or sinks, depending on its weight compared to the other liqueurs or liquids. The heaviest liqueurs are creamy, opaque, and thick, like crème de menthe or cacao. Middle-weight liqueurs are more translucent like amaretto, flavored fruit brandies, or triple sec. The lightest liqueurs are lighter in color and sweetness, such as Southern Comfort or peppermint schnapps.
- Most alcohol has some aroma. Some pure grain alcohol has little to no smell or taste. Since alcohol molecules somewhat resemble sugar molecules, they convey subtle to sweet tastes and aromas. At higher concentrations, foods with alcohol can be hot and irritating in both taste and aroma.
- Alcohol easily binds to aromas in foods and beverages. Then aromatic compounds are released into the air. This allows us to experience alcohol food aromas before we experience the taste of alcohol in foods.

ALCOHOL AND THE LAW

Alcoholic beverages are a part of some cultures and cuisines. But because alcohol is a drug, the sale and regulation of ethanol are restricted by many countries. The production of alcoholic beverages may require a license and be taxed. In the United States, the sale of alcoholic beverages is controlled by the counties, local jurisdictions, or states.

The production of distilled beverages is also regulated and taxed. The Bureau of Alcohol, Tobacco, Firearms, and Explosives, and the Alcohol and Tobacco Tax and Trade Bureau enforce federal laws and regulations. All alcoholic product packaging in the United States must contain a health warning from the US Surgeon General reading *"According to the Surgeon General, women should not drink alcoholic beverages during pregnancy because of the risk of birth defects. Consumption of alcoholic beverages impairs your ability to drive a car or operate machinery, and may cause health problems"* [19].

These agencies and services may be helpful for alcohol abuse:

- Alcoholics Anonymous: www.alcoholics-anonymous.org/
- Al-Anon/Alateen: www.alateen.org/
- National Clearinghouse for Alcohol and Drug Information: www.ncadi.samhsa.gov/
- The National Drug and Alcohol Treatment Referral Routing Service: 800-662-HELP (4357)

The Pros and Cons of Caffeinated Beverages

CAFFEINE

Caffeine is a ***methylxanthine alkaloid***, a bitter white crystalline chemical compound, commonly used as a mild stimulant and bronchodilator in asthma. Caffeine is the world's most widely consumed and unregulated psychoactive substance and the most used ergogenic, or energy-producing, aid. In the human body caffeine acts as a mild stimulant and diuretic. It increases the heart rate, raises metabolism, restores alertness, stimulates the central nervous system, and wards off drowsiness. It reaches peak level in the bloodstream between 15 minutes and 2 hours after it is consumed.

Caffeine is found in the beans, fruit, and leaves of over 60 plants. It is most commonly consumed by humans in infusions that are extracted from the beans of the coffee plant, the leaves of the tea bush, and other plants. Caffeine is called *guaranine* when extracted from guarana berries (used for energy drinks); *mateine* when extracted from yerba mate (also used in energy drinks); and *thein* when extracted from tea leaves. Caffeine is also found in the *kola nut*, used to make cola, and the *cacao pod*, used to make chocolate.

Morsel *"Drinking a daily cup of tea will surely starve the apothecary."* —Chinese proverb

351

THEOPHYLLINE AND THEOBROMINE

Theophylline is another member of the methylxanthine family. It has the same psychoactive properties as caffeine. Theophylline is naturally found in trace quantities in tea. Theobromine is a bitter alkaloid of the cacao plant that is found in chocolate. It is also in the methylxanthine class of chemical compounds, like theophylline and caffeine. When the caffeine content of beverages is given, theophylline and theobromine may not be separately listed. The caffeine content of various beverages is shown in Table 8-4.

TABLE 8-4 Caffeine Content in Various Beverages

Types of Beverages	Calories (calories)	Caffeine (milligrams)
8 ounces brewed, drip coffee	2 cal	104 mg
8 ounces instant coffee	5	62
8 ounces decaffeinated brewed or instant coffee	5	3
2 ounces espresso-type coffee	1-2	80
8 ounces brewed black tea	0	67
8 ounces brewed green tea	0	40
12 ounces iced unsweetened black tea	2	47
12 ounces iced sweetened black tea	133	17
12 ounces regular cola with caffeine	136–151	29–99
12 ounces diet cola with caffeine	0	46–70
12 ounces caffeinated noncola beverage (such as Mountain Dew)	165	56
8 ounces cocoa beverage	109	2
8 ounces chocolate milk	200	5–8
8.5 ounces energy-type drink	118	80

> ### Recipe: Peppermint Chai Tea
>
> *Chai tea usually contains deeply brewed black tea, milk, a combination of Indian-type spices, and a sweetener. This recipe for **Peppermint Chai Tea** in the **Recipe file** which is located within the Culinary Nutrition website at www.culinarynutrition.elsevier.com, is filled with two types of tea—pekoe and peppermint—along with black pepper, cardamom, cinnamon, cloves, ginger and nutmeg to spice it up, and low-fat milk and honey to sweeten it. Chai tea is generally served piping hot so its creaminess and spiciness can interplay with cool and sweet desserts. It is also pleasant tasting when chilled, with or without a sprinkling of spices of your choice. The finished beverage is shown within the centerfold **Photo file** in Plate 8.2.*

CAFFEINE AND HEALTH

Caffeine releases fatty acids from fatty tissues in the bloodstream. This gives the illusion that the body has been fed. It also provides fat to exercising muscles for energy, enhances skeletal and heart muscle contractions, and increases mental alertness. It does this by increasing neural activity.

Too much caffeine can cause nervousness, shakiness, and sleep disturbances. Quantities over 600 milligrams are banned by the National Collegiate Athletic Association due to their increased energy and performance capabilities. Pregnant and nursing women, children, seniors, and those with ulcers or drug-dependent medical conditions should restrain their caffeine intake. There may be some association between caffeine consumption and miscarriage and/or low-birth-weight infants, but research has not verified this.

Coffee contains antioxidants, protective against oxidative stress. They combat potentially damaging free radicals, implicated in aging, cancer and coronary heart disease. Medium roasts appear to have the highest quantity of antioxidants.

Several kinds of polyphenols, protective plant chemicals, are also common in green tea and are considered more effective than those in black tea. This feature may have to do with how tea is processed. Green tea consumption may protect against breast, colon, liver, lung, and skin cancers; coronary heart disease; high cholesterol; and hypertension.

Caffeine dependence syndrome is characterized by drug dependency: a need to ingest caffeinated products; an inability to cut them back or out of one's diet; and withdrawal symptoms, including headache and fatigue. Caffeine withdrawal symptoms, including headache, inability to concentrate, irritability and stomachache, may appear soon after the discontinuation of caffeine and last a few days until brain receptors return to normal.

The FDA acknowledges caffeine as a "multiple purpose generally recognized as safe food substance" (GRAS). This assumes that caffeine is not combined with other drugs or by those with medical conditions that may augment its effects.

FOOD BYTE

Coffee was discovered around AD 850. Legend has it that in southern Ethiopia, the Arab goatherd Kaidi observed his goats' friskiness after chewing berries from an evergreen shrub. Arabica coffee grows wild in Ethiopia today and is one of the three main species of coffee consumed worldwide. The Arabic word for coffee is **qahwah**, which means "stimulating drink."

COFFEE

The principle source of caffeine throughout the world is the coffee bean, the seed of the coffee plant, which also contains carbohydrates, protein, lipids, acids, and antioxidants. The roasting process turns these carbohydrates and lipids into aromatic oils, breaks down and builds up acids, and releases coffee's distinctive flavor.

The two most commonly grown coffee species are *arabica* and *robusta*. Arabica is believed to be the first species of coffee to be cultivated. It contains less caffeine than any other commercially cultivated species of coffee. Robusta contains about 40 to 50 percent more caffeine than arabica. It also tends to be bitter. That is why arabica is considered more suitable for consumption and is more cultivated today worldwide.

Coffee beans from different parts of the world have other distinctive characteristics, such as acidity, aroma, body, and flavor. These characteristics are dependent on the growing region, processing, and varietals. Like wine, varietals are known by the region in which they are grown, such as Colombian, Java, or Kona. Most arabica coffee beans originate in eastern Africa, Arabia, Asia, and Latin America. Robusta coffee beans are grown in western and central Africa, throughout southeast Asia, and Brazil.

The caffeine content of coffee varies according to the type of coffee bean and the method of preparation. Lighter-roast coffee tends to have more caffeine than darker-roast coffee because the roasting process reduces the caffeine content (although it lends distinctive flavor).

Bite on This: a comparison of coffee varieties

The standard American roast is medium-light; medium-dark is Viennese roast; dark and full-bodied is French or Italian roast.

- **American (regular) roast:** medium-roasted beans; moderate brew; medium flavor
- **Decaffeinated coffee:** brewed coffee that has undergone chemical solvent or Swiss water process decaffeinating; about 97 percent caffeine-free
- **European roast:** two-thirds heavily roasted beans; one-third regular or medium-roast
- **Freeze-dried coffee:** brewed coffee that has been frozen, then water-evaporated; crystalline form
- **French roast and dark French roast:** heavily roasted beans; strongly colored and flavored
- **Instant coffee:** heat-dried freshly brewed coffee in powdered form
- **Italian roast:** glossy, heavily roasted brown-black beans; strongly flavored
- **Viennese roast:** one-third heavily roasted beans; two-thirds regular or medium-roast

Coffee beans are only 1 to 2 percent caffeine. Coffee also contains trace amounts of theophylline, but not theobromine. A cup of brewed coffee has more caffeine than a cup of brewed tea because a larger weight of coffee is extracted per cup than tea. In general, one serving of coffee ranges from 40 milligrams of caffeine for a single shot of arabica-variety espresso to about 80 to 100 milligrams for an 8-ounce cup of arabica-drip coffee. Good-quality robusta coffee is used in some espresso blends.

Coffee flavoring can be used in cakes, candies, cream pies, ice cream, and with chocolate. If used in meat dishes, it brings out the umami flavor. Instant coffee or *espresso* can be used in baked goods and confections for flavoring. It can also be used full strength in sauces and stews. Coffee-flavored liqueurs can be used in dessert and beverage recipes. They are particularly flavorful with allspice, cinnamon, citrus zest, or nutmeg added.

Coffee is best served around 140°F (60°C). Higher heat accelerates chemical reactions. Volatile molecules may escape, the flavor may noticeably change, and the beverage may become more acidic.

Recipe: Coffee Caribbean

*Coffee trees have flourished in the Caribbean islands for centuries due to the geography of this region with its high altitudes, volcanic soils and warm weather. This recipe for **Coffee Caribbean** in the **Recipe file** which is located within the Culinary Nutrition website at www.culinarynutrition. elsevier.com, relies on the deep and robust coffee flavor along with assertive Caribbean spices. It is particularly flavorsome with foam topping and/or sweetening, which helps to temper the coffee's bitter taste. The finished beverage is shown within the centerfold **Photo file** in Plate 8.2.*

TEA

Tea is another commonly consumed beverage that is available with and without caffeine. Tea is made from the dried and processed leaves of one species of plant called *camellia sinensis*. Herbal teas or infusions are not teas but dried flowers and/or herbs. There are three major tea varietals:

- *Chinese*—small leaves; thrives at higher altitudes
- *Indian (or Assam)*—larger leaves; thrives at lower altitudes
- *Hybrid*—mixture of Chinese and Indian

There are four main methods of processing tea that produce four different types of tea:

- *Black tea*—most consumed; highest in caffeine (30 to 40 milligrams per 8 ounces); antioxidant properties
- *Green tea*—more processing than white; tastes somewhat like fresh leaves or grass; lower in caffeine (10 to 20 milligrams per 8 ounces); higher antioxidant properties
- *Oolong tea*—most difficult to process; hybrid of green and black teas; partially oxidized in processing; lower in caffeine (10 to 20 milligrams per 8 ounces)
- *White tea*—least processed; tastes the most like fresh leaves or grass; lowest caffeine; most antioxidants

Like coffee, the amount of caffeine in tea varies according to the growing location and processing. Tea generally contains about half as much caffeine per serving as coffee, depending on the source of the tea leaves and the strength of the brew. A standard 8-ounce cup of tea can have between 20 and 60 milligrams of caffeine. The color of the tea leaves is not a good indicator of the caffeine content of the tea. Tea also contains a small amount of theobromine and slightly higher levels of theophylline than coffee. Decaffeinated tea is available in most varieties.

Tea should be consumed as soon as it is finished brewing, or it may become harsh. Color and taste may dissipate. If tea is mixed with dairy milk or cream, the taste is less astringent because the acid is buffered by the milk protein. The tannic acid in tea acts as a binder and decreases iron absorption. If tea is brewed slowly for iced tea, less caffeine and *theaflavin*, a polyphenol, are extracted, and the tea remains clear instead of cloudy.

Tea can be used as an aromatic like Jasmine tea; in baked goods like Earl Grey muffins; in desserts like green tea sorbet or ice cream; and in marinades, oils, sauces, spice rubs or tenderizers. Tea leaves can be used for steaming or smoking foods, as in smoked duck. Powdered tea can be used for decoration. Lemon juice boosts the acidity of tea, adds freshness, and lightens the color.

Recipe: Green Tea Shake

*This recipe for **Green Tea Shake** in the **Recipe file** which is located within the Culinary Nutrition website at www.culinarynutrition.elsevier.com, shows how versatile green tea is as an ingredient as well as a beverage. Green is a color that connotes health. This pleasantly colored mint green beverage is as inviting as it is nutritious. It is colored and flavored with green tea with its antioxidants and blended with low-fat yogurt, fat-free dairy milk and fresh fruit with protein, vitamins and minerals for a gustatory and nourishing delight. The finished beverage is shown within the centerfold **Photo file** in Plate 8.3.*

FOOD BYTE

Chocolate was actually discovered by the Olmecs, who cultivated the cacao tree about 3,000 years ago in the Veracruz and Tabasco regions of Mexico. The Mayans name the tree *cacahuaquchtl* (Mayan for "tree"). They thought that the cacao pods were symbols of fertility and life and a gift from God. Christopher Columbus discovered these worshipped pods in the Caribbean in the 1500s and named them *tchocolatl* or *xocolat*.

CHOCOLATE

Chocolate, from the *cacao* pod, contains a small amount of caffeine, theobromine and theophylline. A typical 8-ounce cup of hot chocolate has about 5 milligrams of caffeine, as does 8 ounces of chocolate milk. In comparison, a typical 1.55-ounce milk chocolate bar has about 9 milligrams of caffeine, and 1 ounce of semisweet dark chocolate has about 20 milligrams of caffeine—about one-fourth that of coffee. The amount of caffeine will vary depending on the type of chocolate that is used in beverages, cooking, or baking.

Chocolate has a rich and complex flavor, filled with acidity, astringency, bitterness, and sweetness, depending on the type of chocolate. Some chocolate has salt added to it for "bite" to bring out flavor and create clarity.

Chocolate sauce can be made from chocolate that is high in cocoa solids with a strong chocolate flavor— ideally a dark chocolate with at least 50 percent cocoa solids. Melt the chocolate with water and sugar, and then add cream or butter and flavorings such as extracts or liqueurs. A simpler sauce can be made from cocoa powder and dairy milk or cream. Both can provide the basis for hot or cold chocolate beverages.

Bite on This: types of chocolate

Some of the following types of chocolate can be used in beverages (as noted). Others are better for cooking and baking.

- *Unsweetened chocolate*, also known as *bitter* or *baking chocolate*, contains cocoa solids and cocoa butter. It is typically used in brownies, cakes, and cookies. It has a distinctively chalky taste and texture that become smoother with eggs and butter. It does not contain sweeteners, so it is not suitable for eating out of hand.
- *Sweetened chocolate is similar to semisweet chocolate*. It does not contain milk solids. It has a more pronounced chocolate taste than milk chocolate.
- *Dark chocolate* is chocolate with a high content of cocoa solids and no or very little milk solids (up to 12 percent). It can be unsweetened, bittersweet, semisweet or sweet. If a recipe specifies "dark chocolate," use semisweet.

  Dark chocolate is produced by adding fat and sugar to cacao. With its high cacao content, dark chocolate is a rich source of antioxidants, particularly flavonoids, which are thought to possess protective cardiovascular properties.
- *Semisweet chocolate* is dark chocolate with low sugar content. It is the classic dark baking chocolate in cooking and baking for cakes, cookies and brownies. Semisweet chocolate can be substituted for sweet dark chocolate.
- *Bittersweet chocolate* is chocolate liquor to which cocoa butter, an emulsifier such as lecithin, some sugar, and vanilla are added. It has less sugar and more liquor than semisweet chocolate. Bittersweet chocolate is a chocolate of choice for cooking and baking because of its rich, intense, and bitter flavor. If specified in a recipe, do not substitute semisweet or sweet chocolate.
- *Milk chocolate* is sweet chocolate with milk powder or condensed milk. It contains 10 to 20 percent cocoa solids (cocoa and cocoa butter) and more than 12 percent milk solids. It is seldom used for baking, except for cookies.

- *White chocolate* is a mixture of cocoa butter, milk solids, sugar, and vegetable fat. It does not contain cocoa solids, so it really is not true chocolate. Its rich and creamy texture and sweet and subtle flavor complement other baking ingredients.
- *Hot chocolate*, *hot cocoa*, *drinking chocolate*, *cocoa* or *instant chocolate* is a mixture of chocolate or cocoa powder; cream, dairy milk, or milk powder; and sugar or sugar substitute. It may contain lecithin to help emulsify the mixture. Cocoa powder can be used in frostings and sauces.
- *Dutched* or *alkalized cocoa* is the product of cocoa beans that have been treated with potassium carbonate, an alkaline. It neutralizes the acidity of cocoa or even makes it slightly alkaline, which affects their chemical composition. This changes the taste, making it more alkaline, less roasted and caramel-like, milder, and darker.

Recipe: Mexican Cocoa

One of the indigenous ingredients of Mexico is chocolate. While this recipe for **Mexican Cocoa** *in the* **Recipe file** *which is located within the* Culinary Nutrition *website at www.culinarynutrition.elsevier.com, does not rely on Mexican chocolate, it has a distinctively chocolate taste that enhances this beverage. This nutty, milky, spicy and sugary mix can be stored and mixed with hot water, low- or nonfat dairy milk, or soy milk for a warm, satisfying and nutritious midday snack or after-meal finale. The finished beverage is shown within the centerfold* **Photo file** *in Plate 8.2.*

COLA AND OTHER SOFT DRINKS

Caffeine is a common ingredient in soft drinks such as **cola**, from *kola nuts*. Soft drinks may contain 10 to 50 milligrams of caffeine per serving. The caffeine comes from the ingredients, chemical synthesis, or additives.

Most colas are acidic in nature, with carbonic, citric, or phosphoric acid. A small amount of acid is vibrant to the palate. But if an acidic cola is paired with an equally acidic food, the taste intensifies. That is why colas have so much sugar and other unique flavors—to balance the acid!

Energy drinks may contain more caffeine than colas. The caffeine in energy drinks may range from 80 to 150 milligrams, from natural ingredients plus synthetic chemicals. *Guarana* with caffeine, and theobromine are common ingredients in some energy drinks.

Dairy Beverages and Dairy Substitutes

FLUID FOOD: DAIRY MILK

Dairy milk is an opaque white, watery liquid from mammals. Mammalian breast milk is designed to provide complete nourishment and support growth and development for newborns through infancy. This is until their immature digestive systems are able to digest and absorb dairy milk from another mammal, most often a cow. Formulas designed to replicate human milk are nutritionally similar.

Humans are an exception in the mammalian world for consuming milk past infancy. They may use formulas; the milk of other mammals, such as camel, cow, goat, horse, sheep, yak, or water buffalo; or vegetable-based milks, such as almond, coconut, rice, or soy. The nutrients in milk vary by species.

Lactose Intolerance

Some humans are not able to digest dairy milk past infancy because they are *lactose intolerant*. They lack the enzyme lactase, which reaches the highest level after birth and then declines. Chapters 4 and 9 discuss lactose intolerance and how to cook and bake without lactose to accommodate this disease.

Cow and other mammalian milk, such as goat or sheep, may be processed into food products such as butter, cheese, cream, ice cream, and yogurt, or food additives and industrial food products such as casein, condensed milk, lactose, powdered milk, and whey protein. People with lactose intolerance or milk allergy may not be able to tolerate any of these products because they are lactose-based. Instead, they may use almond, rice, soy, or other grain; legume; and nut-based "milks" like the Strawberry Soy Milk Shake. The use of nondairy milks for lactose intolerance is discussed in Chapters 4 and 9.

TABLE 8-5 Comparison of Milk Nutrients (Per 8 Fluid Ounces)

Type of Milk	Calories (calories)	Total Fat (grams)	Saturated Fat (grams)	Protein (grams)	Carbohydrates (grams)	Calcium (milligrams)
1%	102 cal	2.5 g	1.5 g	8 g	12.18 g	300 mg
2%	121	4.5	3	8	11.71	296
Skim	86	0.5	0.5	8.5	12.15	303
Whole	150	8	5	8	11.71	292
1% chocolate	158	2.5	1.5	8	26.10	287
2% chocolate	179	5	3	8	30.32	284
Whole chocolate	209	8	5	8	25.85	281
Cultured buttermilk	99	2	1.5	8	11.74	285
Goat	168	10	6.5	8.5	10.86	326
Human	171	11	5	2.5	16.95	79

Recipe: Strawberry Soy Milk Shake

*Some soy milk and tofu have distinctive tastes and textures. By blending soy milk and silken tofu with 100 percent fruit preserves or fresh fruit at its peak, these ingredients transform in flavor. Make sure to use reduced-fat soy milk, fresh silken tofu and good-quality fruit preserves or ripe berries to maximize nutrients and flavor. The beauty of this **Strawberry Soy Milk Shake** in the **Recipe file** which is located within the Culinary Nutrition website at www.culinarynutrition.elsevier.com, is that other 100 percent fruit preserves or fresh fruit and flavored soy milk combinations may be easily substituted, depending on availability. The finished beverage is shown within the centerfold **Photo file** in Plate 8.3.*

Dairy Milk Nutrients

Dairy milk is an emulsion filled with globules of butterfat floating around a watery fluid. Phospholipids and protein hold the globules together. Fat-soluble vitamins A, D, E, and K are located in the milk fat component of milk.

Most of the protein in dairy milk is *casein* and *whey*. Both the fat globules and the casein protein, which repels light, create the opaque white color of milk. Skim milk looks slightly blue because the casein protein breaks up short wavelengths of light that appear blue. In some types of dairy milk, the fat globules contain carotenoids, which contribute a creamy color. Riboflavin (vitamin B2) in the whey has a greenish color.

The carbohydrate lactose, or milk sugar, is what gives dairy milk a sweet taste and sugar calories. Lactose is a double sugar that is made of glucose and galactose, two simple sugars. Consuming even a small amount of lactose may cause bloating, cramps, diarrhea, intestinal gas, and/or undigested lactose in those who are lactose intolerant.

Dairy milk delivers a unique combination of essential nutrients and helps to fill important nutrient gaps in many diets. It is abundant in calcium, vitamin D and potassium—identified as shortfall nutrients of public health concern by the *2010 USDA Dietary Guidelines*.

Milk varies according to the type and amount of carbohydrates, protein, lipids, vitamins, minerals, and water it contains. A comparison of milk nutrients is shown in Table 8-5.

One 8-ounce cup of dairy milk contains about 300 milligrams of calcium, about one-third of the daily recommended intake (DRI) of calcium for a healthy adult. The amount of calcium that is absorbed by the human body is disputed. Calcium from dairy products has greater bioavailability than calcium from certain vegetables, such as spinach. Oxalic acid in green leafy vegetables binds calcium and makes it less available to the body.

Dairy milk also contains biotin and pantothenic acid for energy production; iodine for thyroid function; potassium and magnesium for cardiovascular health; selenium for antioxidant value; thiamine for cognitive function; vitamin A for immune function; vitamins B12 and riboflavin for cardiovascular health and energy production; and vitamins D and K for bone health.

357

Dairy Milk and Health and Disease

Studies show a possible link between low-fat dairy milk and the reduced risk of colorectal cancer, coronary heart disease, hypertension, and obesity. Overweight and obese people who consume dairy milk may have decreased insulin resistance and Type II diabetes. One of the health-promoting factors in dairy milk is *conjugated linoleic acid (CLA)*, a fatty acid. CLA is present only in dairy milk and meat from grass-fed cows.

Dairy milk may increase certain health risks. Casein breaks down in the stomach to produce two substances that have been linked with autism. Studies have not confirmed this association. Cow milk allergy (CMA), an adverse allergic reaction to the protein in cow's milk, is unlike lactose intolerance. High dairy milk consumption has also been associated with *Crohn's disease* and other gastrointestinal disorders, and Parkinson's disease and prostate cancer in men. Once again, associations are not proven.

Bovine growth hormone (**BGH**) has been used in cattle to increase milk production. Milking cows naturally produce bovine growth hormone. BGH increases insulin-like growth factor 1 (IGF1) in the liver. Elevated levels of IGF1 in human blood have been linked to increased rates of breast, colon, and prostate cancers.

In the United States, dairy milk is fortified with vitamins A and D. Vitamin A is removed from dairy milk when the fat is reduced, and then low-fat dairy milk is fortified with this vitamin. This practice may cause reduced-fat milk to have higher vitamin A content than whole milk. Milk is also fortified with vitamin D to compensate for reduced sun exposure. This is vital during winter months when sunlight is minimal. Milk sometimes has flavorings added, such as banana, chocolate, or strawberry.

Pasteurization

Pasteurization of cow's milk initially destroys potential pathogens and increases its shelf life. When pasteurized milk spoils, it is unsuitable for consumption; it has an unpleasant odor and taste.

358

FOOD BYTE

Kefir is a fermented milk drink that originated in the Caucasus region, much like wine. It is prepared by adding kefir "grains" to cow, goat, or sheep milk. Kefir grains are a combination of bacteria and yeasts within a lipid, protein and sugar web. This intricate web of microorganisms and nutrients forms grains that look like a head of cauliflower. Traditional kefir was inoculated in bags that were made from animal skins, hung in doorways, and punched as people passed to mix the milk and kefir grains.

Bite on This: types of dairy milk

Dairy milk varies according to cultures, fat content, sweeteners, flavors, pasteurization, processing, and type of mammal, among other factors.

- *Acidophilus milk and a/B milk* are made with bacterial cultures, such as *Lactobacillus acidophilus* and *bifidobacteria*. They are more tolerated by lactose-intolerant individuals than uncultured milk; however, some people still may not be able to digest its partially broken down milk sugar.
- *Buttermilk* was traditionally drained from churned butter. Now cultured buttermilk is made with bacteria cultures to create its tangy flavor and creamy texture. *Lactococcus lactis bacteria* and others are used to ferment the milk sugar lactose. Prolonged fermentation may cause the milk to be too sour for consumption.

In raw milk, lactic acid–producing bacteria ferment the lactose to lactic acid. The acidity of lactic acid prevents or slows the growth of other organisms. During pasteurization most of these lactic acid bacteria are destroyed.

Lactic acid has a low pH that denatures the milk proteins and causes the milk to undergo a variety of different transformations in appearance and texture. Some of these products are buttermilk, cheese, kefir, sour cream, and yogurt.

- **Condensed milk** is evaporated milk with a high proportion of sugar (40 to 45 percent)—thus the alternate name *sweetened condensed milk*. Condensed milk requires less processing than evaporated milk because the added sugar inhibits bacterial growth. It has a thick mouthfeel, with about 8 percent fat.

Condensed milk has a syrupy consistency, glossiness, and ivory color, like evaporated milk. It is used in confections and desserts. Condensed milk can be stored unrefrigerated in well-closed cans for many years, just like canned evaporated milk.

- **Evaporated milk** is also called **dehydrated milk**. It is shelf-stable canned milk with about 60 percent of the water removed by heat. It is available in low-fat and nonfat varieties. Processing develops an ivory color and a caramelized flavor. It has a high proportion of sugar to other calories.

Evaporated milk can be used in thick sauces and puddings to help prevent curdling. If reconstituted with water, evaporated milk can pass as slightly sweetened fresh milk. Evaporated milk has a long shelf life like condensed milk.

- **Half-and-half** is a mixture of cream and milk. It is used in recipes that call for pouring cream. It does not whip.
- **Homogenized milk** has been forced through minuscule holes to disperse its fat globules. This is so they remain suspended in the watery portion of milk. Most milk sold today is homogenized. In fresh, nonhomogenized milk, the cream rises to the surface to be removed and churned into butter.

To prevent spoilage, milk should be kept refrigerated between 35° and 38°F (1.7° to 3.3°C). Most milk is pasteurized by heating and then refrigerated for transport. Milk spoilage can be prevented by using sterilized milk that is heated for a long period of time.

- **Lactose-reduced milk** is low-fat or nonfat milk with the addition of the enzyme lactase. About 70 percent of lactose is converted by lactase into more digestible simple sugars. Lactose-reduced milk is sweeter than normal. It is easier for those who are lactose sensitive to digest, but lactose-free milk is best.
- **Lactose-free milk** comes in low-fat and nonfat varieties. As much as 99 percent of its lactose has been broken down by the addition of lactase. It is beneficial in lactose-intolerant diets.
- **Nonfat milk** contains less than 0.2 percent fat. It is also referred to as skim milk. It has 86 calories and 0.4 grams of fat.
- **1% and 2% milk** refers to the percentage of fat in the milk. One percent milk has 105 calories and 2.4 grams of fat, and 2% milk has 120 calories and 4.7 grams of fat.
- **Powdered milk**, or **dry milk powder**, is the sturdiest form of milk, which is made by removing almost all of the water from milk. The moisture content is usually less than 5 percent. It can be made from nonfat, low-fat, or whole milk. If exposed to light or air, the flavor may deteriorate.

359

Powdered milk can be added in dry form to thicken sauces or soups; in dessert recipes; and in baking to help boost the nutritional value of these recipes. Once reconstituted with water or milk, it can be refrigerated for up to one week.

- **Raw milk** has not been pasteurized, which makes it vulnerable to contamination by bacteria or other foreign substances. People may choose to consume it before pasteurized milk due to processing and health concerns.
- **Ultrapasteurized milk** is heated for a shorter time but at a higher temperature than pasteurized milk. The process increases shelf life, but it might distort flavor.
- **Ultra-heat pasteurized (UHP) milk** undergoes even higher heat processing than ultrapasteurized milk. The purpose of this higher heat is to destroy all microorganisms. It is generally aseptically packaged, which ensures its three-month shelf life.
- **Whole milk** is about 3.5 percent fat, with 150 calories per 8-ounce cup. Nonhomogenized whole milk may have a layer of cream on top.

Cooking with Different Types of Dairy Milk

Dairy milk is used as an ingredient in cooking and baking and as a beverage that accompanies a meal in the United States. This is unlike other areas of the world where populations are lactose intolerant. As an ingredient in cooking and baking, dairy milk supplies body, browning, flavor, liquidity, moisture, protein, sweetness and salts. It is versatile in sauces and soups that require creaminess and in beverages to temper bitterness and add sweetness and creaminess, such as chocolate, coffee and tea.

The proteins in dairy milk may coagulate with heat, which is why it is important to heat dairy milk gently. Coagulated casein and whey protein adheres to calcium and trapped fat. It forms the surface film of scalded milk, sauces and soups. To minimize this film, a saucepan can be covered, the dairy milk can be constantly stirred, or foamed milk can be placed over the surface of the liquid. To reduce scorching on the bottom of a pan or pot, wet it first to prevent the protein from sticking; use moderate heat, or place the milk in a double boiler so that the boiling water heats the milk rather than direct heat.

If the dairy milk solution contains acids from fruits or vegetables, or tannins from coffee and potatoes, these tannins may cause further coagulation. This is particularly important when making a cream soup, such as broccoli; fruit sauce, such as strawberry; or a coffee/caramel recipe. To prevent coagulation, add acidic or tannic ingredients to a milk solution instead of adding a milk solution to one that contains acids or tannins. Also, avoid high temperatures once the milk solution has mixed with the acidic or tannic ingredients.

Evaporated milk can withstand high temperatures without curdling. It can be used whole strength to add creaminess and thickness to sauces and puddings and lend color, crust, flavor, moisture, and tenderness to baked goods. It is an important ingredient in key lime pie. Evaporated milk is useful in slow cooker recipes and as a breading liquid for fish, poultry, meats, and vegetables. If it is very cold, it can whip, but it quickly collapses. Since the milk sugar is concentrated, this sweetness should be accounted for in savory recipes and yeast breads where the sweet taste may compete. One-half cup of evaporated milk plus one-half cup of water is the equivalent of 1 cup of whole milk, unless reduced-fat evaporated milk is used. Evaporated milk can be substituted in equal amounts for cream or half-and-half in most recipes.

Sweetened condensed milk can caramelize or undergo the Maillard browning reaction at low temperatures. Heating sweetened condensed milk in a double boiler or the microwave may help to prevent this reaction. Caramelized condensed milk can be used as a topping for desserts.

Buttermilk is an excellent ingredient in baked goods, cold soups, and salad dressings. It provides a rich, tangy flavor with fewer calories than milk or cream. Its flavor pairs well with sweet fruits, such as cherries, peaches, or pears, like crème fraiche—the European counterpart to sour cream. Its acidity makes buttermilk an effective marinade with protein foods. This acidity balances the discoloration of blueberries and walnuts in baked goods, where it also promotes browning and improves texture. Buttermilk can be used as the liquid for coating foods before breading.

In using **sour cream** or **yogurt** in recipes, there may be some liquid separation. Pour off the liquid, or stir it back into the fermented product. Before adding sour cream or yogurt to hot liquid, bring it to room temperature. It can easily curdle if the temperature is too high. Remove food from heat before stirring in sour cream or yogurt, or add them carefully over a very low simmer. About 1 tablespoon of flour can be added to ½ cup of sour cream to discourage curdling when using it as a thickener. Sour cream or yogurt will separate if frozen and then thawed. This factor should be considered if freezing is called for in a recipe.

Milk can be foamed to add texture and interest to recipes. A *foam* is a light, airy protein structure filled with air bubbles that holds its shape for a period of time. *Meringues* are foams made with egg whites; *whipped cream* is a foam that is made with cream; and the topping on a specialty coffee is a foam that is made with milk.

The protein and the fat in these foams act as stabilizers. Egg proteins easily coagulate, while milk proteins are more resistant. Milk should be slowly heated. Coffee foam prevents a "skin" that forms on the surface of the coffee beverage and helps retain heat. Generally, reduced-fat and skim milk foam well due to their protein fortification. Old milk may curdle when heated.

Recipe: Papaya Yogurt Smoothie

When blenderized, yogurt transforms into a milk-like consistency, as in this recipe for ***Papaya Yogurt Smoothie*** *in the* ***Recipe file***. *which is located within the* Culinary Nutrition *website at www.culinarynutrition.elsevier.com. Once mixed with tropical fruit nectar or juice, like papaya or mango, along with low-fat dairy milk and dry milk powder for protein, this smoothie creates a powerhouse of nutrients with its protein, minerals, vitamins and antioxidants. This smoothie is a healthy beverage for growing teenagers, and it makes a nutritious pairing with a simple salad and soup. The finished beverage in shown within the centerfold* ***Recipe file*** *in Plate 8.3.*

FRUIT AND VEGETABLE JUICES

Fruit and vegetable juices are natural liquids that are extracted from fruit or vegetable tissue. Juice is extracted by mechanical means or by *macerating*, which is softening or breaking foods into pieces with liquid, as opposed to *marinating*, which is soaking foods in a seasoned, often acidic liquid before cooking.

Citrus juice can be extracted from grapefruits, lemons, limes or oranges commercially with electric juicers or by hand. Juices may be filtered to remove fiber or pulp, but this decreases the available fiber. Some high-pulp juices retain the pulp.

Juices may be reduced in acidity for sensitive stomachs. A variety of vitamins, minerals, and health-promoting substances may be added for fortification. Some juices are concentrated and frozen, such as cranapple, grape or orange. They can be used in concentrated forms to enhance sauces and desserts, or reconstituted for drinking. Other processing techniques include canning, evaporating, freeze-drying and pasteurizing.

Common juices include apple, carrot, cranberry, grapefruit, grape, mango, orange, pineapple, pomegranate and tomato. Juice blends, such as cranberry-apple, and pineapple-grapefruit, are increasingly popular for their taste and potential health-enhancing properties. Mild-flavored juice concentrates are used as sweeteners to balance acidity and enhance flavor. For example, white grape juice concentrate is used to enhance and blend the flavors of cranberry and raspberry juices. Apple juice concentrate mellows and smooths the flavor of cherry and apricot juices. And pineapple juice concentrate blends and rounds out tropical juices, like lemon, lime, orange and passion fruit.

The advantage of most vegetable juices is that they do not contain as much sugar as some fruit juices and do not raise insulin levels to the same degree. The exception is some root vegetables with stored carbohydrates, such as beets and carrots. Most vegetable juice is rich in antioxidant vitamins A, C and E; lycopene, which gives tomatoes their red color; calcium; potassium; and magnesium.

FRUIT JUICES AND HEALTH

Beyond hydration, juices are consumed for their health-enhancing benefits. Orange juice is high in antioxidant vitamins A and C and folic acid, which helps prevent neural tube defects during pregnancy. Prune juice is higher in fiber than other juices for digestive health. Cranberry juice helps to keep the urinary tract healthy. Pomegranate juice is a good source of antioxidant polyphenols, pantothenic acid and potassium. A number of tropical juices have been touted for their preventive health benefits. These include açaí, blueberry, goji (wolfberry), guarana, mangosteen, noni and sea-buckthorn.

Juices vary according to their calories and sugar content, as shown in Table 8-6. Some have as much natural sugar as some soft drinks and are higher in calories.

FRUIT JUICES COMPARED TO WHOLE FRUIT

Whole fruit provides the juice, pulp, and sometimes the skin. Unless the entire fruit is pulverized and liquified, these substances and their nutrients might be lower in fruit juice. That is why many fruit juices are fortified.

TABLE 8-6 Comparison of Calories and Sugar in Common Fruit Juices				
Types of Fruit Juices	Calories (calories)	Total Carbs (grams)	Sugar (grams)	Sugar (teaspoons)
12 ounces apple juice	180 cal	48 g	33 g	6.96 tsp
12 ounces cherry juice	210	49.5	37.5	7.9
12 ounces grape juice	192	48	48	10.12
12 ounces orange juice	156	36	36	7.59
In comparison				
12 ounces cola soft drink	145	40	40	8.43

Source: [20].

TABLE 8-7 Orange Juice Compared to a Fresh Orange

8-Ounce Glass Orange Juice	1 Medium-Sized Orange
112 calories	65 calories
0 grams fat	0 grams fat
0 grams saturated fat	0 grams saturated fat
0 milligrams cholesterol	0 milligrams cholesterol
2 milligrams sodium	0 milligrams sodium
26 g carbohydrates	16 g carbohydrates
0 grams fiber	3 grams fiber
21 grams sugar	13 grams sugar
2 grams protein	1 gram protein
10% DV vitamin A	6% DV vitamin A
207% DV vitamin C	106% DV vitamin C
3% DV calcium	6 DV calcium
3% DV iron	1% DV iron

The edible skins of fruit are where the sunlight interacts and forms a variety of colored pigments. These pigments include health-promoting carotenoids and flavonoids. Fruit pulp is a source of fiber and juice that is captured inside the tissues. Fresh fruit juice has active enzymes and reactive and oxygen-sensitive substances, which make them unstable. Apple and pear juice may turn brown, for example, due to these substances.

Orange juice provides a good example of the difference in nutrients between fruit juice and whole fruit, as shown in Table 8-7. A fresh orange is lower in calories, carbohydrates, and sugar, and higher in fiber and calcium than orange juice. Orange juice is slightly higher in protein and in the Daily Values (DVs) of vitamins A and C and iron. Each has a place in a healthy diet.

The pulpy white area of oranges is the primary source of flavonoids. The juicy segments contain most of the vitamin C. When oranges are processed, the pulpy white parts of the oranges are removed, reducing the fiber and the bioavailability of flavonoids. While some commercial products have added pulp, it may not be the same quantity.

JUICE LABELS

"No added sugar" is commonly indicated on fruit juice labels. These products still contain natural fruit sugars. Some juices only contain a small percentage of real fruit juice. The rest may be water and added sweeteners, such as sucrose, or high fructose corn syrup (HFCS). Look for the percentage of juice disclosure on the label. All beverages that contain juice or whose labels picture fruit must include it.

- *Fruit juice* has a standard level of purity in the United States. The term *fruit juice* can only legally be used to describe a beverage that is 100 percent fruit juice.
- *Juice cocktail* or *juice drink* is a blend of fruit juice(s) with other ingredients. The term *juice drink* can be used to describe any drink that includes juice, even if the juice content is just 1 percent of the total volume.
- *Nectar* is a beverage that contains fruit juice or puree and water; it may or may not contain sweeteners.
- *Vegetable juice* is made by extraction of juice from vegetables. They can be freshly made or made by commercial processing. Some commercial brands contain a significant amount of sodium. Typical vegetables may include beets, carrots, celery, cucumbers, dandelion greens, kale, or parsley. Sometimes herbs and fruits may be added, including garlic, ginger, lemon, pumpkin, or tomatoes. Vegetable juices include *aojiru*—a Japanese vegetable juice made from carrot, kale, tomato, turnip, and V8 juices.

SOFT DRINKS

Carbonated soft drinks are commonly known as *soda*. The name "soft drink" infers that the beverage does not contain alcohol, which is considered a "hard drink." Carbonated soft drinks are available in types that are sweetened with sugars or with the sugar substitutes that are described in Chapter 4.

TABLE 8-8 Caffeine Content of Soft Drinks

Soft Drinks	Caffeine (milligrams)
Jolt	71.2 mg
Pepsi One, Mountain Dew, Diet Mountain Dew	55
Tab, Surge, Mellow Yellow, Kick Citrus	46.8–54.0
Diet Coke	45.6
Shasta Cola, Cherry Cola, and Diet Cola	44.4
RC Cola, Diet RC	43
Dr Pepper, Diet Dr Pepper, Diet Sunkist Orange	41
Mr. Pibb, Sugar-Free Mr. Pibb, Red Flash, Sunkist Orange	40
Storm, Big Red, Wild Cherry Pepsi	38
Pepsi Cola, Pepsi Twist, Diet Pepsi Jazz	37.5
Diet Pepsi, Diet Wild Cherry Pepsi, Diet Pepsi Twist, Aspen	36
Coca-Cola Classic, Cherry Coke, Lemon Coke,	34
Vanilla Coke, Diet Cherry Coke, Canada Dry Cola, A&W Crème Soda	29.0–30.0
Canada Dry Diet Cola	1.2
Diet Rite Cola, Sprite, 7-UP, Minute Maid Orange, A&W Root Beer, Slice, Sierra Mist, Fresca	0

Source: [21].

The average sweetened soft drink contains 150 calories per 12 ounces. Most of the calories in soft drinks are in the form of refined cane sugar or corn syrup. High fructose corn syrup (HFCS) is used nearly exclusively in the United States as a sweetener because of its lower cost. Unless soft drinks are fortified, they contain little to no fiber, minerals, protein, vitamins, or other essential nutrients. They may also contain artificial colorings and flavorings. Glucose and fructose, two simple sugars in soft drinks, are fermented by oral bacteria that produce acid, which dissolves tooth enamel during the tooth decay process. Many soft drinks are acidic, and some may have a pH of 3.0 or even lower, which adds to the oral acidity.

363

Some colas contain *phosphoric acid*, a mineral acid that conveys a tangy taste. Phosphoric acid may withdraw calcium from bones, lowering bone density and contributing to osteoporosis. A high-meat diet (which is also high in phosphorus) compounds the situation. It may be that soft drinks replace calcium-containing foods and beverages in the diet, and this is the greater problem at hand.

Many soft drinks contain varying amounts of caffeine. Caffeine is a safe ingredient that has been added to some soft drinks for more than 100 years. Most of the caffeine in cola drinks is added during the formulation process. Caffeine-reduced and caffeine-free soft drinks are also available. The caffeine content of soft drinks is shown in Table 8-8.

Fortified Beverages

The beverage industry comprises a wide range of products, including chocolate beverages, fruit juices and drinks, instant flavored drinks, nectars, meal replacers, milks and milk drinks, supplements, sports drinks and others. Many have been implicated in obesity, diabetes and other degenerative diseases due to their calories and lack of significant nutrients. This may have opened the beverage market to micronutrient-fortified beverages, which may or may not be necessary, depending on one's overall diet.

Micronutrient-fortified beverages, especially those with energy-enhancing ingredients, can be natural and organic or synthetic. Antioxidants, caffeine from guarana and kola nuts, lycopene, omega-3 fatty acids, soy isoflavones, and various forms of protein, such as *taurine* (a type of amino acid), are common ingredients.

Vitamin waters mainly consist of vapor distilled, deionized, and/or reverse osmosis water, with crystalline fructose from corn syrup as a sweetener. They may also contain citric acid, electrolytes, natural flavors, and vitamins, such as vitamins B3, B6, B12, C and E. Some fortified waters are vapor-distilled municipal water with unspecified amounts of electrolytes, such as calcium, magnesium and potassium. Other ingredients may be added, depending on the flavor and intended purpose of the beverage. Vitamin waters may not necessarily be low-sugar drinks. Their sugar content may be comparable to some sweetened soft drinks.

Fruit-based waters may have a light fruit flavor with less crystalline fructose than some fortified beverages. They may not contain any fruit juice.

Energy drinks may contain some similar ingredients as vitamin waters, such as crystalline fructose, electrolytes, natural flavors, and vitamins. They may also contain some form of caffeine and *ribose*, a component of DNA and RNA. Other ingredients may be added for flavor and color.

At the present, a common energy drink is **Red Bull**, a carbonated beverage that is marketed to combat mental and physical fatigue and increase metabolism. Per 8.3 ounces, Red Bull contains about 110 calories; 28 grams of carbohydrates; 26 grams of sugar (sucrose and glucose); *glucuronolactone*, a naturally occurring chemical compound produced by glucose metabolism in the liver; *taurine*, a type of amino acid; niacin; vitamins B6 and B12; pantothenic acid; and about 80 milligrams of caffeine, similar to the amount in an average cup of brewed coffee or twice that of a can of Coke. Sugar-Free Red Bull, sweetened with aspartame and acesulfame potassium, is also available. Red Bull is digested similar to coffee. It does not rehydrate like typical sports drinks.

Sports Drinks

Sports drinks have reached mainstream consumption, but their calories and nutrients are formulated for the sports market—not daily consumption, unless there is regular fluid and electrolyte loss. Sports drinks are designed to help delay the onset of fatigue during exercise and help rehydrate athletes after training or competition by replenishing carbohydrates, electrolytes, protein, and other nutrients. Most sports drinks provide a readily absorbable form of carbohydrates, important to exercising muscles, since carbohydrates are the primary fuel for exercise and are critical to performance.

Overconsumption of plain water can cause **water intoxication** or **hyponatremia**, an electrolyte disturbance in which the sodium concentration in blood plasma is too low. Severe or rapidly progressing hyponatremia can result in swelling of the brain and death. Fluids that supply 60 to 100 calories per 8 ounces help prevent this condition and provide needed carbohydrates, calories, electrolytes, and fluids for continuous performance, especially in extreme conditions over three hours.

The three primary categories of sports drinks are *isotonic*, *hypertonic*, and *hypotonic*. Isotonic sports drinks are said to be in balance with the body's fluids and nutrients; hypertonic sports drinks have more nutrients and other substances than in the blood; and hypotonic sports drinks have fewer nutrients and other substances than in the blood.

- Isotonic sports drinks contain water and other nutrients that are similar in proportion to the fluids and nutrients in the blood. They quickly replace fluids that are lost by sweating and supply absorbable carbohydrates in the form of glucose, the body's preferred energy source. The concentration of glucose in isotonic sports drinks is 6 to 8 percent (13 to 19 grams per 8 ounces). Higher quantities of sugar can delay stomach emptying and increase the risk of cramps.
- Gatorade is a flavored noncarbonated, isotonic sports drink produced by PepsiCo. It is designed for consumption during physically active conditions to rehydrate and replenish carbohydrates, electrolytes and fluids. Per 21.4 ounces, Gatorade supplies 158 calories, 39 grams of carbohydrates, 32 grams of sugar, and 238 milligrams of sodium. POWERade is another isotonic sports drink produced by the Coca-Cola Company.
- Hypertonic sports drinks contain a high level of carbohydrates. They are used to supplement daily carbohydrate intake and are normally consumed after exercise to "top" muscle glycogen stores. Hypertonic drinks may be too high in sugar to be absorbed during exercise. They are sometimes used in ultra-distance events in conjunction with isotonic drinks to replace fluids.
- Hypotonic sports drinks contain a low level of carbohydrates. They can quickly replace fluids that are lost by sweating and provide some energy in the form of sugar calories. They are suitable for athletes who need fluids without a significant boost of carbohydrates.

Taurine, found in energy drinks, often in combination with performance enhancing substances such as *creatine* and *anabolic steroids*, is designed to alleviate muscle fatigue in strenuous workouts and raise exercise capacity. Its safety has been questioned. More information about electrolyte-replacement fluids and exercise can be found in Chapter 10.

SERVE IT FORTH

1a. Many specialty coffee drinks are high in calories, carbohydrates, and fats. Plus, the super-sized cups hold more beverage than one serving; many have as much as three 8-ounce servings!

The local coffee shop wants to offer low-calorie, low-fat, low-sugar coffee drinks but not compromise taste. Design a coffee drink with 100 calories or fewer, 3 grams of fat or fewer, and 5 grams of sugar or fewer

Which ingredients and in what amounts would you use to make this coffee drink? What could you add to bring out the coffee and other flavors without adding more calories, fat or sugar? Support your responses.

2a. Dairy milk consumption has been declining in the United States, and other less nutritious beverages are on the rise. Dairy milk is filled with fluid and nutrients, such as protein; carbohydrates; varying amounts of lipids; vitamins and minerals, especially vitamins A, C, D, and K; calcium; phosphorus; and magnesium—all needed for healthy bones and teeth. A number of drinks try to mimic dairy milk and its nutrients. These are the nutrients in one (8-ounce) serving of reduced-fat (2%) dairy milk:

- 121 calories
- 12 grams of carbohydrates
- 11 grams of sugars
- 0 grams of fiber
- 4.5 grams of total fat
- 3 grams of saturated fat
- 22 milligrams of cholesterol
- 8 grams of protein
- 118 milligrams of sodium
- 296 milligrams of calcium
- 184 IU of vitamin A
- 2 milligrams of vitamin C

List the foods and beverages that supply the same level of nutrients as one 8-ounce serving of dairy milk. (Refer to Chapters 4 to 7.)

With this information, create a marketing message that promotes the nutritional qualities of dairy milk compared to the foods and beverages that provide the same levels of nutrients. Support your comments.

3a. Cocoa beverages are often filled with sugar or sugar substitutes. They may contain too many calories for regular consumption. But cocoa provides flavor, color, antioxidants, and an array of vitamins and minerals like vitamins A, B1, B2, B3, C, E and pantothenic acid, and calcium, copper, iron, magnesium, manganese, potassium and zinc.

The Yummy Company wants to develop a new chocolate beverage for children and teenagers that is lower in sugar and calories than reduced-fat chocolate milk and filled with vitamins and minerals. You have been hired as a food scientist to create its formulation.

Describe the contents of this new chocolate beverage. Analyze its nutrient content by using a nutrition analysis tool, such as the one that can be found at http://nutritiondata.self.com.

How do the nutrients in this new chocolate beverage compare to those in reduced-fat chocolate milk? (This information can be found at http://ndb.nal.usda.gov.) Why would children and teenagers choose this new chocolate beverage rather than reduced-fat chocolate milk? Support your comments.

Three additional activities can be found within the *Culinary Nutrition* website at www.culinarynutrition.elsevier.com.

WHAT'S COOKING?

1. Dissolving rates of solutes
   Objectives
   - To dissolve solutes in fluids and note their dissolving rates
   - To determine why some solutes dissolve faster than others

○ To see if temperature affects the rate that solvents dissipate into solutions
○ To apply this information to cooking and baking

Materials

12 small glasses, measuring cup, ½ cup boiling water, ½ cup ice water, ½ cup room temperature water, powdered juice drink, instant coffee, instant cocoa, instant tea

Procedure

Pour ½ cup ice water into the first glass; ½ cup of room temperature water into the second glass; and ½ cup of boiling water into the third glass. Sprinkle a pinch of the powdered juice drink into each glass and observe the results. Then repeat the process with fresh water—first with the instant coffee, then with the instant cocoa, and finally with the instant tea. With each solute, note the reaction with the ice water, room temperature water, and boiling water. Compare and contrast each solute.

Evaluation

Indicate at which temperature each of the solutes dissolved most easily. What do you think caused this reaction? Does temperature make a difference, and if so, do solutes seem to dissolve easier if they are in hot, cold, or temperate solutions? How does the rate of diffusion differ when a solute has sugar in it (powdered juice drink and instant cocoa) versus one that does not (instant coffee and tea)?

Culinary applications

How can you apply this information to cooking and baking?

2. **Absorption of fluids**

Objectives

○ To observe how water is absorbed by vegetables
○ To see what causes vegetables to wilt
○ To determine the effects of salt in absorption
○ To determine the effects of temperature in absorption
○ To apply this information to cooking and baking

Materials

1 large carrot, 1 large cucumber, 1 large celery stalk, salt, water, vegetable peeler, 6 bowls, measuring spoons, slotted spoon

Procedure

Peel the carrot, cucumber, and celery into strips. Divide each of the vegetable parings into two piles. Put each of the piles into the bowls, filling the first two with the carrot peelings, the second two with the cucumber peelings, and the third two with the celery peelings. Cover the carrot peelings with cold water, the cucumber peelings with room temperature water, and the celery peelings with warm water. Add 1 tablespoon of salt to one of the bowls of carrot peelings, one of the bowls of cucumber peelings, and one of the bowls of celery peelings. Stir each mixture well. Let the mixtures soak for a few hours. They do not have to be refrigerated. About every 30minutes, take one peeling out of each of the bowls and bend it to test for crispness.

Evaluation

Rate which of the carrot, cucumber, and celery peelings are the crispiest: the ones in the salt water or plain water? Which of the peelings absorbed water? Which lost water? Did any of the peelings appear to do neither? How did temperature affect the peelings? Compare and contrast.

The direction in which fluids flow into plants depends on the minerals that are dissolved in the fluids—in the case of this experiment, sodium. If more minerals are inside the plants rather than dissolved in the fluids, the fluids flow into the plants and make them firm. The opposite is true: when there are more minerals dissolved in the fluids than in the plants, the fluids inside the plants flows out, softening or wilting them.

Culinary applications

How can you apply this information to cooking and baking?

3. **Curdled dairy milk**

Objectives

○ To observe how solids can be extracted from liquids
○ To examine the curds (milk protein) and whey (milk liquid) in milk

○ To see the effects that acid and bases have on milk protein
○ To apply this information to cooking and baking

Materials

2 cups skim milk, 6 tablespoons vinegar, nonmetallic or enamel saucepan, ¼ cup water, 1 tablespoon baking soda or borax (a white, crystalline powder that acts as a buffer in solution), strainer or sieve, measuring cups, measuring spoons

Procedure

Slowly heat 2 cups of skim milk and 6 tablespoons of vinegar together in a nonmetallic or enamel saucepan over low heat, stirring constantly. As it begins to curdle or clump together, remove the pan from the heat. Continue stirring the mixture off the heat until the curdling stops. Let the curds settle to the bottom of the saucepan. Strain the curds from the whey through a strainer or sieve until dry. Add ¼ cup of room temperature water and 1 tablespoon of baking soda or borax. Stir gently. The mixture should bubble. In a few minutes, the bubbling should stop, leaving behind a sticky substance.

Evaluation

When the vinegar is added to the skim milk, the milk solids separate from the liquid. How long did this step of the experiment take? Note the texture and any color changes. The solids, or curds, dry to form a hard plastic-like substance called *casein*, which acts as an adhesive, like glue. How long did this step of the experiment take? Note the texture and any color changes. The baking soda or borax neutralizes any acid that remains. How long did this step of the experiment take? Note the texture and any color changes.

Culinary applications

How can you apply these observations to cooking and baking?

OVER EASY

Fluids make up a significant part of the human body. At 60 percent of body weight, water has aptly earned the title as the body's principal chemical component and nutrient. Every cell, organ, and body system requires water to function. A lack of water can lead to the serious complications of dehydration. Mild, moderate, and severe dehydration all take their tolls on the body, from tiredness, headache, dizziness to, at worst, death.

While water is the best fluid to consume for rehydration, in many circumstances, chocolate beverages, coffee, fortified beverages, fruit and vegetables juices, milk, soft drinks, sports drinks, and tea all serve to replace what the body loses through feces, respiration, sweat, and urine. While alcohol contains fluid, it also dehydrates the body. Moderate caffeine consumption may not be as dehydrating as commonly considered.

Alcohol in moderation has some health-promoting features. In addition, it is a useful ingredient in cooking and baking, as are the other highlighted fluids: coffee, chocolate, dairy beverages and milk substitutes, fruit and vegetable juices, tea, and water. They provide aroma, flavor, moisture, texture, and a medium for other ingredients to perform their roles, among other functions.

Specialized beverages with fortification and sports drinks with unique formulations are specifically designed for certain audiences. These include calcium nutrient-fortified fruit juices and soy beverages for those who are lactose intolerant and energy and muscle-building drinks for athletes. Some of their ingredients may not be warranted in nonactive populations.

Controversy stems over the relationship of soft drinks with high fructose corn syrup and overweight and obesity, particularly in children and adolescents. At the current time, direct correlations cannot be made. Other factors, such as increased food intake and inactivity, must be taken into account.

CHECK PLEASE

1. About how much fluid should be consumed daily?
   a. 6 cups per 1,000 calories
   b. 8 cups per 1,000 calories
   c. 6 cups per 2,000 calories

367

   d. 8 cups per 2,000 calories

   e. 2 liters per 1,000 calories

2. Water intoxication is when:

   a. water acts like alcohol in the body

   b. a person is dehydrated

   c. there are too many electrolytes in the blood

   d. there is too much water in the blood

   e. a person needs a drink of water

3. Headache, muscle cramps, decreased blood pressure and/or dizziness or fainting may be symptoms of:

   a. intoxication

   b. dehydration

   c. rehydration

   d. inebriation

   e. exhaustion

Essay Question

1. Coagulation is an important factor when using dairy milk in cooking and baking. Describe what coagulation is, and give five techniques or substitutions that can be used to accommodate for it.

For additional questions, please see the *Culinary Nutrition* website at www.culinarynutrition.elsevier.com.

HUNGRY FOR MORE?

Alcoholics Anonymous   www.alcoholics-anonymous.org

American College of Sports Medicine   http://www.acsm.org

Centers for Disease Control   www.cdc.gov

The Environmental Protection Agency   www.epa.gov

Juice Products Association   http://www.fruitjuicefacts.org

National Coffee Association of USA, Inc.   http://www.ncausa.org

National Confectioners Association/Chocolate USA   http://www.chocolateusa.org/

The National Dairy Council   www.nationaldairycouncil.org

National Clearinghouse for Alcohol and Drug Information   http://ncadi.samhsa.gov

National Organization of Fetal Alcohol Syndrome   http://www.nofas.org

Teas Association of the USA, Inc.   http://www.teausa.com

TAKE AWAY

High Fructose Corn Syrup

High fructose corn syrup (HFCS) is actually a group of corn or potato syrups. They have been processed by enzymes to increase the fructose content; then they are mixed with pure corn syrup (100 percent glucose). HFCS does not contain any artificial or synthetic ingredients or color additives, and it meets the FDA's requirements for the term *natural*. HFCS is relatively inexpensive.

HFCS, table sugar (sucrose), honey, and several fruit juices all contain the same type of simple sugars. Sucrose and HFCS contain nearly the same one-to-one ratio of fructose and glucose. Sucrose is 50 percent fructose and 50 percent glucose; HFCS is 42 to 55 percent fructose, with the remaining sugars from glucose and other sugars. The type of HFCS that is most commonly used in soft drinks is 55 percent fructose and 45 percent glucose (HFCS-55). HFCS-42 is less sweet and is used in many fruit-flavored noncarbonated beverages and in baked goods.

HFCS has the same number of calories per teaspoon as table sugar (4 calories per gram) and is equal in sweetness to table sugar. In addition to its sweetening properties, HFCS helps to keep foods fresh, lowers the freezing point, retains moisture in bran cereals and breakfast bars, enhances fruit and spice flavors, promotes surface browning, and provides fermentability.

The amount of HFCS in fruit juice and soda has been implicated as a contributing factor in obesity and diabetes, but this correlation remains to be proven. Both sucrose and HFCS appear to be metabolized the same way in the body. Pure fructose can stimulate the liver to produce triglycerides and induce insulin resistance, risk factors in diabetes and cardiovascular disease.

Studies that compare HFCS to sucrose conclude that they essentially have the same physiological effects, with little or no evidence that HFCS is different from sucrose in its effects on appetite or the metabolic processes that are involved in fat storage. An expert panel concluded that the current evidence is insufficient to implicate HFCS as a causal factor in overweight and obesity in the United States. Like many other sweeteners and dietary substances, HFCS should be used in moderation along with a well-balanced diet, if at all.

This is another area of nutrition worth watching, as fruit drink and soft drink consumption have dramatically risen since the 1970s, while dairy milk, a more nutritious beverage, has fallen [22,23,24].

Fluid Needs with Exercise

Athleticism requires attention to fluid intake. Inadequate fluid intake can lead to dehydration, heat illness, and reduced performance. The more active a person is, the more fluids he or she requires before, during, and after exercise. These are some simple caveats to keep in mind about fluids and exercise:

- Schedule drinking like eating. Do not wait for thirst, the sensation to drink, because important fluids and electrolytes may already be lost.
- Drink before, during, and after exercise. Fluids fuel the body with liquids and replenish the body when it needs it.
- Drink the right fluids at all times. Carbonation and caffeine have the capacity to bloat and dehydrate the body. Sports drinks have the right balance of fluids, absorbable sugar, and electrolytes to replace what is lost in respiration and perspiration.
- Check hydration after exercise. Urine should be clear or, at best, light-colored.
- Weigh before and after exercise. Have 2 cups of fluid for each pound lost during exercise.

Less active people require eight to ten 8-ounce cups of fluid daily per 2,000 calories. This is about 64 to 80 ounces total daily fluid intake. More active people may need ten to twelve 8-ounce cups of fluid daily, or 80 to 96 ounces. The most active people may need at least 2 cups (16 ounces) of fluid before exercise; ½ to 1 cup (4 to 8 ounces) of fluid every 15 to 20 minutes of exercise; and at least three 8-ounce cups (24 ounces) of fluid after exercise. In very hot and humid climates, fluid needs may increase. Checking hydration and weight are the best strategies.

References

[1] US Department of Agriculture (USDA). USDA national nutrient database for standard reference, release 24. <http://www.ars.usda.gov/Services/docs.htm?docid=8964/>; [accessed 07.02.08]

[2] Harvard School of Public Health. How sweet is it? <http://www.hsph.harvard.edu/nutritionsource/healthy-drinks/how-sweet-is-it/index.html/>; [accessed 07.02.08].

[3] Harvard School of Public Health. Healthy drinks. <http://www.hsph.harvard.edu/nutritionsource/healthy-drinks/>; [accessed 07.02.08].

[4] Brandis K. Fluid physiology: 3.1 water turnover in the body. <http://www.anaesthesiamcq.com/FluidBook/fl3_1.php/>; [accessed 07.02.08].

[5] Mayo Clinic. Functions of water in the body. <http://www.mayoclinic.com/health/medical/IM00594/>; [accessed 07.02.08].

[6] US Department of Agriculture (USDA). USDA national nutrient database for standard reference, release 18. <http://www.ars.usda.gov/Services/docs.htm?docid=9673/>; [accessed 07.02.08].

[7] Centers for Disease Control and Prevention (CDC). Bottled water and fluoride. <http://www.cdc.gov/fluoridation/fact_sheets/bottled_water.htm/>; [accessed 07.02.08].

[8] http://www.cfsan.fda.gov/~lrd/bot-h2o.html/

[9] American Dental Association. Bottled water. <http://www.ada.org/3048.aspx/>; [accessed 07.02.08].

[10] Geological Society of America. Bottled water—where does that water come from? <http://geology.com/articles/bottled-water.shtml/>; [accessed 07.02.08].

[11] Gleick PH. In: Bottled and sold: the story behind our obsession with bottled water. Washington, DC Island Press; 2010.

[12] Virginia Tech. Alcohol's effects. <http://www.alcohol.vt.edu/students/alcoholeffects/index.htm/>; [accessed 07.02.08].

[13]   Centers for Disease Control and Prevention (CDC). Alcohol and public health: frequently asked questions. <http://www.cdc.gov/alcohol/faqs.htm/>; [accessed 07.02.08].

[14]   Cancer.org. Alcohol and cancer. <http://www.cancer.org/acs/groups/content/@healthpromotions/documents/document/acsq-017622.pdf/>; [accessed 07.02.08].

[15]   American Heart Association (AHA). Alcoholic beverages and cardiovascular disease. <http://www.americanheart.org/HEARTORG/GettingHealthy/NutritionCenter/Alcoholic-Beverages-and-Cardiovascular-Disease_UCM_305864_Article.jsp#.Tv9SAtQV2Vo/>; [accessed 07.02.08].

[16]   National Institute for Alcohol Abuse and Alcoholism (NIAAA). Rethinking drinking. <http://rethinkingdrinking.niaaa.nih.gov/>; [accessed 05.03.10].

[17]   National Institute for Alcohol Abuse and Alcoholism (NIAAA). State of the science report on the effects of moderate drinking. <http://pubs.niaaa.nih.gov/publications/ModerateDrinking-03.htm/>; [accessed 05.23.10].

[18]   Office of the Surgeon General. US Surgeon General releases advisory on alcohol use in pregnancy. <http://www.surgeongeneral.gov/pressreleases/sg02222005.html/>; [accessed 07.02.08].

[19]   Alcoholic Beverage Labeling Act (ABLA). United States federal law enacted in 1988, United States Code at title 27, section 213.

[20]   SelfNutritionData. SelfNutritionData: know what you eat. <http://nutritiondata.self.com/>; [accessed 07.02.08].

[21]   Wilstar.com. Caffeine content of popular drinks. <http://www.wilstar.com/caffeine.htm/>; [accessed 15.09.11].

[22]   ScienceDaily. US soft drink consumption grew 135% since 1977, boosting obesity. <http://www.sciencedaily.com/releases/2004/09/040917091452.htm/>; [accessed 07.02.08].

[23]   Barclay L, Vega C. Soft drinks and fruit drinks linked to diabetes risk in African American women. <http://www.medscape.org/viewarticle/578315/>; [accessed 07.02.08].

[24]   Forsee RA, Storey ML, Allison DB, et al. A critical examination of the evidence relating high fructose corn syrup and weight gain. Crit Rev Food Sci Nutr 2007;47:561–82.

CHAPTER 9

Diet and Disease: Healthy Choices for Disease Prevention and Diet Management

Practical Applications for Nutrition, Food Science and Culinary Professionals

OBJECTIVES

1. Identify dietary and culinary strategies to improve blood lipids
2. Plan daily foods and beverages to meet cardiovascular disease goals
3. Identify dietary and culinary strategies to improve blood sugar

Culinary Nutrition. DOI: http://dx.doi.org/10.1016/B978-0-12-391882-6.00009-1

4. Adjust recipes and create meal plans for people with diabetes
5. Identify dietary and culinary strategies for cancer prevention
6. Devise dietary and culinary interventions for cancer prevention and management
7. Identify dietary and culinary strategies to improve hypertension
8. Develop dietary and culinary strategies to reduce hypertension, including the DASH diet
9. Identify dietary and culinary strategies to improve gastrointestinal disease
10. Design dietary strategies and culinary approaches for gastrointestinal disease prevention and management
11. Identify dietary and culinary strategies for food allergy and sensitivity management
12. Experiment with different dietary strategies and culinary approaches for various food allergies and sensitivities

INTRODUCTION: DISEASE PREVENTION AND DIET MANAGEMENT

Many of the degenerative and/or debilitating diseases—allergies, cancer, cardiovascular disease, diabetes, digestive disorders, and hypertension—have diet and nutrition origins. Obesity, as detailed in Chapter 10, is also considered a disease with genetic components and is associated with the development of many other degenerative diseases.

Morsel *"Eat little, sleep sound."*
—Iranian proverb

Eating better does not guarantee freedom from degenerative diseases, but it may offer some preventive advantages. Rather than search for "the fountain of youth" in a pill or potion, diet and nutrition strategies may help to decrease blood pressure, guard against certain cancers, induce weight loss, lower cholesterol and other blood lipids, manage food allergies, normalize blood sugar, and relieve discomforting gastrointestinal tracts. Besides disease interventions, healthy food and nutrition choices may add quality to life.

For example, whole grains from oats and barley may reduce the risk of cardiovascular disease, certain cancers, diabetes and stroke from their fiber and disease-fighting nutrients. Just 5 to 10 grams of soluble fiber daily from fruits, legumes, vegetables and whole grains may reduce LDL cholesterol 3 to 5 percent; 2 grams of plant sterols daily from soy foods may lead to another 5 to 15 percent reduction in LDL cholesterol. This is the equivalent of consuming about two (8-ounce) daily servings of orange juice fortified with plant sterols.

Reducing dietary cholesterol to less than 200 milligrams daily, decreasing dietary saturated fat to less than 7 percent total fat, and losing 10 pounds if one is overweight or obese may bring about an additional 3 to 10 percent reduction of LDL cholesterol. A 10-pound weight loss can be attained in one year by consuming just 100 fewer daily calories. This LDL-lowering potential by food choices is very impressive, since LDL cholesterol is one of the major risk factors in cardiovascular disease [1–3].

Consuming salmon and other fatty fish that are rich in omega-3 fatty acids may help to decrease inflammation in the human body and may lower the risk of cardiovascular diseases and certain cancers, including breast and prostate.

Incorporating legumes into the diet may also be prudent disease prevention. Legumes are low in fat and high in protein and folate. Folate is a B vitamin that may help to lower blood levels of homocysteine, a type of amino acid that has been linked to cardiovascular disease and stroke.

Broccoli and its relatives in the cruciferous family, including Brussels sprouts, cabbage and cauliflower, contain carotenoids and antioxidants with potential cancer protection; folate with reported protective heart defense; and vitamin C with alleged stroke reduction.

Other foods and beverages that contain an array of disease-fighting substances include dairy milk with vitamin D fortification, which may help to lower the risk of certain cancers, diabetes and heart disease; red wine with the antioxidant resveratrol, which may supply anticancer and heart-healthy benefits; berries with the colorful phytonutrient anthocyanin, which may reduce inflammation and offer certain cancer and heart disease protection; and almonds with the antioxidant vitamin E and healthy fats, which may help lower LDL cholesterol.

Nutritional research helps to correlate foods and beverages with diseases; food science helps to translate nutritional research into disease-fighting ingredients and products; and the culinary arts helps to incorporate nutritional research and food science into healthy recipes, meals and menus. This collaboration promotes an integrated approach to disease prevention—much like an integrated approach is used in the treatment of disease. This chapter serves to connect nutrition and disease research with food science translations and culinary applications to illuminate the disease-fighting potential of foods and beverages.

MAIN COURSES
Obesity
OVERVIEW, DIET AND LIFESTYLE MODIFICATIONS

Chapter 10 features overweight and obesity and their impact on health and longevity. The disease of obesity carries a host of risk factors. These risk factors make an obese person more vulnerable to other degenerative diseases, including cardiovascular disease, certain cancers, diabetes and hypertension.

> **Morsel** "More die in the United States of too much food than of too little food." —John Kenneth Galbraith (Economist and author of *The Affluent Society*, 1908–2006)

The roles of nutrition, food science and culinary professionals in obesity, weight loss and weight management cannot be overstated. Well-planned, flavorful and aesthetically pleasing diets are good strategies to address obesity and its side effects. The uses of reduced-calorie, low-calorie and non-calorie ingredients vary. Refer to Chapter 10 for in-depth information about the growing public health issues of obesity, with useful tools for its management.

373

> **FOOD BYTE**
>
> Obesity is more than just eating too much and exercising too little. Obesity requires a multidisciplinary approach in its prevention, treatment and elimination. It is a complicated, multidimensional disease, as the following statement by the National Institutes of Health (NIH) indicates:
>
> *Obesity is a complex, multifactorial chronic disease that develops from an interaction of genotype and the environment. Our understanding of how and why obesity develops is incomplete but involves the integration of social, behavioral, cultural, physiological, metabolic and genetic factors. [4]*

Cardiovascular Disease
OVERVIEW, DIET AND FOOD MODIFICATIONS

> **Morsel** "Don't dig your grave with your own knife and fork." —English proverb

Cardiovascular disease has been one of the major causes of death in the United States for over 50 years. The underlying cause of cardiovascular disease is atherosclerosis. *Atherosclerosis* is a condition that is characterized by *plaque*, fatty deposits in the inner walls of the arteries. These plaques obstruct the flow of blood to the heart and the brain and may lead to heart attack or stroke.

A *heart attack (myocardial infarction)* occurs when one or more regions of the heart muscle undergo severe or prolonged oxygen debt. It happens when a *blood clot* blocks the flow of blood through a *coronary artery*—a blood vessel that feeds blood and nutrients to a section of the heart muscle. A *stroke* occurs when the blood supply to a part of the brain is interrupted or severely reduced, which deprives brain tissue of oxygen and nutrients. Brains cells can begin to die within a few minutes.

Atherosclerosis and hypertension are two conditions that lead to most cardiovascular disease. *Hypertension* is a condition that is characterized by high blood pressure. Blood pressure is a measurement of force against the artery walls as the heart pumps blood throughout the body. Hypertension is a disease with its own set of risk factors that require diet and food modifications.

Plaques are thought to start very early in life. As a person ages, these plaques enlarge and may cause the arteries to narrow, lose their elasticity, and become brittle or harden. This is why atherosclerosis is often referred to as "hardening of the arteries."

Because the blood flow may be impeded, blood pressure may rise, lead to hypertension, and place extra stress on the heart and its associated arteries. Additional plaque may form where there is damage, particularly where the arteries connect. Other blood vessels throughout the body may be affected, including the kidneys, which try to readjust, only to raise blood pressure further.

Some cardiovascular disease risk factors are *fixed*; these include age, gender and genetics (heredity). Other cardiovascular risk factors can be *modified*. These include a high-cholesterol and high–saturated fat diet, abnormal blood fats (particularly high LDL cholesterol and low HDL cholesterol), adult-onset diabetes, cigarette smoking, weight-related hypertension, inactivity, obesity and stress.

FIXED CARDIOVASCULAR RISK FACTORS

- *Age:* As age increases, cardiovascular risks increase. Women over 55 years of age (postmenopause) and men over 45 years of age are at higher risk of cardiovascular disease.
- *Gender:* Women tend to have higher HDL cholesterol before menopause. This is because estrogen is protective against cardiovascular disease and why women are at a greater risk of cardiovascular disease postmenopause.
- *Genetics (heredity):* If a father or brother under 55 years of age or a mother or sister under 65 years of age has cardiovascular disease, then the risk of cardiovascular disease in other family members increases.

More African Americans have hypertension than Caucasians and a higher risk of cardiovascular disease. Cardiovascular disease is also higher among American Indians, native Hawaiians, Mexican Americans and some Asian Americans.

MODIFIABLE CARDIOVASCULAR RISK FACTORS

- *High LDL cholesterol and high–saturated fat diet:* Decrease dietary cholesterol, saturated fats and trans fats and increase omega-3 fatty acids, soluble fiber and soy foods.

  Dietary cholesterol over 200 milligrams daily, without a high-fiber diet to counterbalance this intake, could build up inside the arteries, impede blood flow and increase cardiovascular risks. Consuming less than 200 milligrams of dietary cholesterol daily is prudent. Dietary cholesterol is only available from animal-derived foods and beverages.

  Saturated fats, also from animal-derived foods and beverages and some tropical plant foods, including palm and coconut oils, tend to raise blood cholesterol and increase cardiovascular risks. Trans fats, mostly from processed foods with hydrogenated fats, have similar effects.

  According to the American Heart Association's Nutrition Committee, healthy Americans over the age of 2 should decrease foods and beverages that contain saturated fats to less than 7 percent of total daily calories and limit trans fats to less than 1 percent of total daily calories.

  Switch to mono- and polyunsaturated fatty acids from fish, nuts and nonhydrogenated vegetable oils. Include omega-3 fatty acids from fatty fish and flax; soluble and insoluble fibers from fruits, vegetables and whole grains; and soy foods with soluble fiber, soy protein and other protective factors [5–7].

- *Abnormal blood fats (total cholesterol, high LDL cholesterol and low HDL cholesterol):* Decrease dietary cholesterol, saturated fats and trans fats as described above. To increase protective HDL cholesterol, increase activity and red wine consumption if alcohol is consumed (one drink per day for women and two drinks per day for men).

- *Adult-onset diabetes:* The alterable risk factors of diabetes: high LDL cholesterol and low LDL cholesterol, overweight or obesity, poor blood sugar management, poor fiber intake and inactivity are very similar to the alterable risk factors for cardiovascular disease. Diabetes is a disease that attacks the blood vessels, including the coronary arteries; consequently, cardiovascular risks also multiply.
- *Cigarette smoking:* Quit smoking to eliminate nicotine and carbon monoxide. **Nicotine** is a chemical that increases dopamine, which brings euphoria and relaxation. It constricts the blood vessels, which burdens the heart. **Carbon monoxide** is a chemical that quickly binds with hemoglobin in red blood cells in the lungs. It damages the lining of the blood vessels and decreases the amount of hemoglobin that is available for oxygen transport.
- *Weight-related hypertension:* The risk factors of hypertension include excessive alcohol consumption (more than one drink per day for women and two drinks per day for men), lack of fruits and vegetables, overweight and obesity, and sodium intake. Reducing the risk factors of high blood pressure helps to decrease the risk of hypertension, despite the fixed risk factors of age, gender and genetics.
- *Inactivity:* Aim for at least 30 to 60 minutes of moderately intense physical activity most days of the week for cardiovascular risk reduction. However, shorter amounts of exercise that are performed throughout the day also offer cardiovascular benefits. People who have achieved a moderate fitness level may be less likely to prematurely expire than those with a low fitness level.
- *Obesity:* Obesity by itself increases the risk of cardiovascular disease, even when there are no adverse effects. Just a 10 percent increase in body fat can be stressful and harmful to the heart, as can yo-yo dieting—repeated weight gain and weight loss [8].
- *Stress:* Chronic stress raises **cortisol**, a hormone produced by the adrenal gland in the adrenal cortex. Cortisol is called the "stress hormone," since it increases blood pressure and blood sugar, increases cardiovascular risk factors, and reduces immune responses.

OPTIMAL TOTAL BLOOD CHOLESTEROL AND BLOOD LIPID LEVELS

A blood test known as a **lipoprotein profile**, taken after a 9- to 12-hour fast, shows the levels of total cholesterol; LDL cholesterol (the main source of cholesterol buildup and blockage in the arteries); HDL cholesterol (which helps decrease cholesterol build up in the arteries) and triglycerides (another blood lipid and cardiovascular disease risk factor). Optimal levels for total blood cholesterol and other blood lipids are shown in Table 9-1.

HOMOCYSTEINE

Another indicator of cardiovascular disease is the level of homocysteine. **Homocysteine** is a substance that is produced by the body when protein breaks down. The B vitamins, including folate, vitamin B6 and vitamin B12, help to convert homocysteine into other amino acids. If there are inadequate levels of these B vitamins, the level of homocysteine may rise. This may damage the lining of the arteries, contribute to blood clots and lead to a heart attack or stroke. Folate is abundant in foliage (green leafy vegetables), and vitamins B6 and B12 can be found in protein-rich foods, such as beef, legumes and poultry.

DIETARY STRATEGIES TO IMPROVE BLOOD LIPIDS

The diet-serum lipid connection is well established in cardiovascular disease. Translating the blood cholesterol and lipid guidelines in Table 9-1 into food and beverage choices requires both nutrition and culinary perspectives.

Strategies include decrease total fat; decrease saturated and trans fats; decrease dietary cholesterol; decrease total blood cholesterol; and increase HDL cholesterol and plant sterols in the daily diet.

- *Decrease total fat:* Recommendations by government and health organizations suggest that total dietary fat be limited to 30 percent of daily calories. On a 2,000-calorie-per-day diet, this amounts to about 600 calories or 67 grams of total fat.

  2,000 calories × .30 = 600 calories/9 calories of fat per gram = 67.66 grams of total fat

  For those with higher cardiovascular risks, it is recommended that dietary fat be limited to 20 percent of daily calories. The average US total daily fat intake currently exceeds both amounts.

Culinary Nutrition

TABLE 9-1 Optimal Levels for Total Blood Cholesterol and Blood Lipids

Blood Levels	Interpretations
Total blood cholesterol	
Less than 200 mg/dL	Desirable total blood cholesterol[a]
200 to 239 mg/dL	Borderline high total blood cholesterol
240 mg/dL and above	High total blood cholesterol
Low-density lipoprotein cholesterol	
Less than 100 mg/dL	Optimal
100 to 129 mg/dL	Near optimal[b]
130 to 159 mg/dL	Borderline high[c]
160 to 189 mg/dL	High[d]
190 mg/dL and above	Very high
High-density lipoprotein cholesterol	
Less than 40 mg/dL for men	Major cardiovascular risk factor[e]
Less than 50 mg/dL for women	Major cardiovascular risk factor[e]
60 mg/dL and above	Protective cardiovascular risk factor
Triglycerides[f]	
Less than 150 mg/dL	Normal
150 to 199 mg/dL	Borderline high
200 to 499 mg/dL	High[g]
500 mg/dL and above	Very high

Source: [9].

[a]75–169 mg/dL for those age 20 and younger, and 100–199 mg/dL for those over age 21.

[b]If there is cardiovascular disease or diabetes, then the LDL cholesterol goal is 100 mg/dL or less.

[c]If there is no cardiovascular disease or diabetes, but there are two or more risk factors, then the LDL cholesterol goal is 130 mg/dL or less.

[d]If there is no cardiovascular disease or diabetes and either no or one cardiovascular disease risk factor, then the LDL cholesterol goal is 160 mg/dL or less.

[e]If total blood cholesterol is 200 mg/dL or greater, and if HDL cholesterol is less than 40 mg/dL for men and 50 mg/dL for women, then other blood lipids should be examined, such as LDL cholesterol and triglycerides. Some medical specialists use the ratio of total cholesterol to HDL cholesterol as a cardiovascular risk factor. This ratio is obtained by dividing the HDL cholesterol level by the total cholesterol level. For example, if a person has an HDL cholesterol level of 50 mg/dL and a total blood cholesterol level of 200 mg/dL, then the ratio would be 4:1. The goal is to keep the ratio below 5:1; the optimum ratio is 3.5:1.

[f]Normal triglyceride levels vary by age and gender.

[g]A high triglyceride level with low HDL cholesterol or high LDL cholesterol increases atherosclerosis, though it is unclear how. High triglycerides are often a sign of other conditions that increase cardiovascular disease risks.

- *Decrease saturated and trans fats*: Reduction of saturated and trans fatty acids are two of the most significant dietary changes to reduce total blood cholesterol and LDL cholesterol. Saturated fat should be less than 10 percent of total calories. If there is existing cardiovascular disease or diabetes, saturated fat should be less than 7 percent of total calories. Trans fats should be limited to less than 1 percent of total daily calories. On a 2,000 daily calorie diet, 7 to 10 percent of total calories amounts to about 140 to 200 calories or 16 to 22 grams of saturated fat. One percent of total calories amounts to about 20 calories.

  2,000 calories×.07 = 140 calories/9 calories of fat per gram = 15.5 grams of saturated fat
  or
  2,000 calories×.10 = 200 calories/9 calories of fat per gram = 22.2 grams of saturated fat
  2,000 calories×.01 = 20 calories

- *Decrease dietary cholesterol*: Decreasing dietary cholesterol often goes hand-in-hand with decreasing saturated fat. Government and health organizations recommend that dietary cholesterol be limited to 300 milligrams daily for people without coronary heart disease and 200 milligrams of dietary cholesterol for people with higher cardiovascular risks.

  High-cholesterol foods include egg yolks, fish roe, liver pate, butter, some shellfish, processed meats and dairy products; however, the food industry is developing lower-cholesterol alternatives for many of these items. Plant foods contain no cholesterol.

FOOD BYTE

Long condemned for their high cholesterol content, eggs are reestablishing their place in the US diet. Egg yolks do have a significant amount of cholesterol (about 185 milligrams of cholesterol per yolk), and they may affect blood cholesterol levels. But eggs also contain nutrients that may help lower the risk for cardiovascular disease, which include folate, riboflavin, vitamins B12 and D, and protein. For most people, cholesterol in food has less effect on total blood cholesterol and harmful LDL cholesterol than the *ratio* of fats in the blood. Moderate egg consumption—up to one a day— does not appear to increase cardiovascular disease risk in healthy individuals without coronary heart disease [10,11].

- *Decrease total blood cholesterol*: Inclusion of plant-based phytonutrients might help to lower total blood cholesterol and preserve artery elasticity. Phytonutrients such as these include allyl sulfide, found in the allium family, which includes chives, garlic, leeks, onions, scallions and shallots; soluble and insoluble fibers, found in foods such as oatmeal and oat bran; phytosterols, found in almonds and walnuts, among other nuts; and lignans, found in foods like rye, soybeans, flax and sesame seeds.
- *Increase HDL cholesterol*: Consuming fish with omega-3 fatty acids and foods with soluble fibers, found in apples, barley, kidney beans, oats, pears, prunes and soy foods may help to lower LDL cholesterol, *which may boost the amount of HDL cholesterol*. (This is because as one type of cholesterol decreases, another may increase.) Moderate alcohol consumption also raises HDL cholesterol.

  Additionally, fish with omega-3 fatty acids may help to reduce blood pressure and the risk of developing blood clots. In people who have already had heart attacks, fish with omega-3 fatty acids may reduce the risk of sudden death. Soluble fibers may reduce cholesterol absorption in the bloodstream. Five to 10 grams or more of soluble fiber daily may decrease total and LDL cholesterol. Soy foods may slightly reduce LDL cholesterol, but they probably do not significantly lower total cholesterol.

- *Increase dietary plant sterols*: **Phytosterols**, which are plant sterols, mimic the action of steroid hormones, such as estrogen, in the body. They have the ability to block cholesterol absorption and reduce total blood cholesterol when they are consumed with a low-fat diet. Phytosterols do not appear to affect LDL cholesterol or triglycerides.

  Phytosterols are found in some margarines, orange juice, soy foods and yogurt drinks. A 10 percent or greater reduction in LDL cholesterol may be attained by consuming at least 2 grams of phytosterols daily—the equivalent of about two 8-ounce servings of phytosterol-fortified orange juice. Margarines that contain phytosterols may carry a cholesterol-lowering claim that is monitored by the FDA [12,13].

LIFESTYLE GOALS AND STRATEGIES TO REDUCE CARDIOVASCULAR DISEASE

In 2006, the American Heart Association formulated diet and lifestyle recommendations for cardiovascular disease risk reduction in the general population. These lifestyle goals and practical tips still serve the test of time:

1. **Use as many calories as you consume**. It is easy to underestimate the amount of food consumed and overestimate the amount of activity performed. Refer to Chapter 10 to determine daily caloric requirements and the foods and beverages that meet these requirements. Become familiar with how many calories are expended daily in various activities. Several online activity calculators and applications for mobile devices are available. A pedometer can be used to compute distance walked throughout the day. Then compare calories consumed versus calories used. This eye-opening approach to caloric balance may curtail excessive overeating and underexercising and impress their importance for cardiovascular health [14].
2. **Eat a variety of nutritious foods from all the food groups**. Replacing solid fats with heart-healthy oils is a prudent strategy, but all food groups should be taken into consideration when planning a heart-healthy diet and recipes. Include fiber-rich whole-grain foods to help lower blood cholesterol and provide satiety for weight management. Most fruits and vegetables are high in fiber, minerals and vitamins and low in calories, which help to manage weight and control blood pressure. Oily fish such as salmon,

sardines and trout, while higher in fat and calories than cod, halibut or scrod, provide heart-healthy omega-3 fatty acids.

3. **Eat fewer nutrient-poor foods**. Limit foods and beverages that are high in fats, sugars and calories but low in nutrients, such as alcohol, candy and other confections, chocolate, soft drinks and fruit-flavored beverages. Alcohol increases insulin sensitivity, which predisposes carbohydrates that are ingested with alcohol to be converted to fat. Plus alcohol intake is correlated with hypertension—one of the risk factors in cardiovascular disease.

4. **Follow these food guidelines:**

Choose fewer . . .

- Oversized beverages and foods with added sugars, such as some specialty coffees, teas, juice drinks and breakfast cereals.
- Foods with partially or fully hydrogenated fats and oils and shortening, such as some commercial frostings, margarines, microwave popcorn, crackers and salad dressings.
- Foods that are high in dietary cholesterol and/or saturated fat, such as some egg yolks, fatty meats, poultry skin, tropical vegetable oils like palm and coconut, and full-fat dairy products.
- Fried foods with nonspecified polyunsaturated oils, such as "vegetable oil."
- Alcoholic beverages if consumed. Practice moderation, which is considered to be one drink daily for women and two drinks daily for men.

Choose more . . .

- Antioxidant-rich fruits and vegetables—five or more daily, *including carrots (beta-carotene), ruby-red grapefruit (lycopene), tomatoes (vitamins A and C) and spinach (lutein).*
- Herbs and spices with phytonutrients, *including cumin, ginger, garlic, pepper and turmeric.*
- Fat-free, 1% fat and low-fat dairy products, *including cheese, frozen desserts, dairy milk and yogurt.*
- Legumes, *including black beans, garbanzo beans, kidney beans, soybeans and peanuts (if nonallergic).*
- Whole grains—at least three (3-ounce) servings daily, *including barley, brown rice, millet, oats, quinoa and rye.*
- Monounsaturated fatty acids, *including canola, olive and peanut oils, avocadoes, nuts, olives and seeds.*
- Fish with omega-3 fatty acids, lean meats and skinless poultry, prepared with little to no fats and oils, *including salmon, mackerel and trout; flank, shank, rump or round cuts and boneless, skinless poultry*

Choose and prepare . . .

- Foods with little to no extra salt—limit to less than 1 teaspoon of salt or 2,300 milligrams of sodium daily, as described in Chapter 7.
- Foods with lower-fat cooking methods, such as baking, broiling, grilling, stir-frying, or steaming, as discussed in Chapter 6.
- Foods and beverages with sensible portion sizes, as reviewed in Chapter 1 [15,16].

CULINARY STRATEGIES TO REDUCE CARDIOVASCULAR DISEASE

Translating dietary recommendations into culinary strategies challenges nutrition, food science and culinary professionals alike. It can be accomplished through innovative ingredients and food products, realistic and appealing recipe adaptations, and consumer-friendly heart-healthy meals and menus. The following are some culinary strategies to consider for heart-healthy cooking:

- Reduce the frequency of recipes that call for fried foods [17,18]. Frying should be used only occasionally if at all, since it adds so many calories and fat. Compare the following:
  - A *fried* chicken breast contains about 193 calories, 7 grams of total fat, and 1.62 grams of saturated fat.
  - A *roasted* chicken breast contains about 130 calories, 3 grams of total fat, and 0.92 grams of saturated fat.
  - A *sauteed skinless* chicken breast contains about 120 calories, 2 grams of total fat, and 0.5 gram of saturated fat.
  - A large order of *fast-food french fries* contains about 539 total calories, 28.8 grams of total fat, and 6.7 grams of saturated fat.
  - A 5-ounce serving of *oven-roasted french fries* contains about 110 calories, 9 grams of total fat, and 1.5 grams of saturated fat.

- Use mostly lean meats (beef flank; round, rump or shank; pork center loin; loin roast; rib chop; sirloin, tenderloin, or top loin) with the least amount of visible fat or skin. These cuts require moist-heat cooking methods as described in Chapter 3. Use very small amounts of higher-fat meats (beef blade, rib eye, or porterhouse; pork belly, shoulder, or bacon) as flavorsome ingredients in some recipes. They can provide the "missing" flavor in ordinary recipes. Compare the following:
  - One ounce of beef blade contains about 62 calories, 4 grams of total fat, and 1 gram of saturated fat.
  - One slice of pork bacon contains about 41 calories, 3 grams of total fat, and 1 gram of saturated fat. Consider the following:
    - Smoky tea, which imparts a sweet, bacon-like smoky flavor when used as a rub, contains no calories or fat.
- Experiment with reduced-fat ingredients. Reduced-fat ingredients work better in recipes where they are not the focal ingredients or exposed to heat. For example, reduced-fat cheese has a better consistency inside a lasagna or casserole where it blends with moist ingredients rather than on the top of pizza or in a cheese fondue. Compare the following:
  - One ounce of reduced-fat provolone cheese contains about 77 calories, 5 grams of total fat, and 3 grams of saturated fat.
  - One ounce of whole-milk provolone cheese contains about 98 calories, 7 grams of total fat, and 5 grams of saturated fat.
- A white sauce that is made from reduced-fat or skim dairy milk is thinner with less mouthfeel than a white sauce that is made with whole dairy milk or cream. Pureed vegetables, such as cauliflower or potatoes, can give the sauce more body, and a touch of monounsaturated oil, such as canola, can round out the taste and texture. Compare the following:
  - One cup of thick white sauce contains about 465 calories, 35 grams of total fat, and 9 grams of saturated fat.
  - One cup of thin white sauce contains about 262 calories, 17 grams of total fat, and 5 grams of saturated fat.
- Lean meats can be succulent when braised or stewed by using low heat. While searing improves appearance and flavor in lean meats, it does not necessarily lock in flavor. As meat is heated, muscle fibers contract and force out moisture—especially from cut surfaces.
- Use nuts and nut butters where they make a sensible addition or replacement. Chopped or crushed nuts can top salads and vegetables to add taste and texture. They can also extend the amount of salad dressing, butter or margarine that is used in some recipes. Almond, cashew or hazelnut "butters" can enrich some sauces, soups and desserts. Besides adding multidimensional taste and texture, nuts and nut butters add protein, minerals, vitamins and healthy fats. Compare the following:
  - One tablespoon of butter contains about 102 calories, 11.5 grams of total fat, 7.3 grams of saturated fat, and 0.12 gram of protein.
  - One tablespoon of almond butter contains about 101 calories, 9.5 grams of total fat, 0.9 gram of saturated fat, and 2.4 grams of protein.
  - One tablespoon of peanut butter contains about 94 calories, 8 grams of total fat, 1.6 grams of saturated fat, and 4 grams of protein.
- Reduce butter and oil in recipes by one-quarter where suitable; some recipes may be able to withstand a greater reduction. First, check the amount of fat or oil in a recipe. Then, look at their function(s) in the recipe to decide if they can be reduced and the integrity of the recipe maintained. Compare the following:
  - One-fourth cup of vegetable oil for sauteing contains about 482 calories, 55 grams of total fat, and 4 grams of saturated fat.
  - One tablespoon of vegetable oil for sauteing contains about 124 calories, 14 grams of total fat, and 1 gram of saturated fat.
  - One ounce of traditional vinaigrette-style salad dressing (three parts oil to one part vinegar) contains about 82 calories, 8 grams of total fat, and 1 gram of saturated fat.
  - One ounces of modified, lower-fat vinaigrette (one part very flavorful oil, like walnut or extra-virgin olive oil, two parts stock or low-calorie liquid thickened with arrowroot, and one part vinegar or other acid) contains about 33 calories and 3 grams of total fat, with negligible saturated fat.
- Replace a portion of the meat in recipes with lower-fat, nutrient-dense ingredients, such as cooked whole grains. Some processed meats average 80 to 90 percent fat; regular ground beef, cooked bacon and chicken

379

wings average 60 to 79 percent fat; fried chicken and corned beef average 40 to 59 percent fat; and roasted poultry with skin averages 20 to 39 percent fat. Compare the following:

- ○ One pound of regular ground beef (80 percent lean) contains about 291 calories, 18 grams of total fat, and 6 grams of saturated fat.
- ○ One-half cup of cooked soybeans contains about 173 calories, 9 grams of total fat, and 1 gram of saturated fat.
- ○ One-half cup of cooked bulgur wheat contains about 83 calories, 0 grams of total fat, and 0 grams of saturated fat.
- ○ Either cooked soybeans or bulgur wheat can replace about 4 ounces of the ground beef to decrease calories, total fat and saturated fat. They also add fiber and phytonutrients to dishes.

- Use less salad dressings, sauces and toppings. These flavorful additions enhance simple foods, often with too many calories and fats. Use one-quarter to one-half the amount; lightly dress vegetables, proteins and grains to bring out the natural flavors of foods without smothering them. Modifications such as these retain the delicious flavors—just less. Compare the following:

- ○ One-quarter of a cup of ranch salad dressing contains about 284 calories, 32 grams of total fat, and 4 grams of saturated fat.
- ○ One tablespoon (one-quarter of the amount above) contains about 71 calories, 8 grams of total fat, and 2 grams of saturated fat, *for a savings of about 213 calories, 24 grams of total fat, and 2 grams of saturated fat.*
- ○ Two tablespoons of classic butter sauce contain about 400 calories, 46 grams of total fat, and 28 grams of saturated fat.
- ○ One tablespoon (one-half of the amount above) contains about half this amount: about 200 calories, 23 grams of total fat, and 14 grams of saturated fat, *for a savings of about 100 calories, 23 grams of total fat, and 14 grams of saturated fat.*

Recipe: Frisee, Grapefruit, Avocado and Cranberry Salad with Cranberry Vinaigrette

Like an olive, an avocado is a fruit that contains heart-healthy monounsaturated fats. A little avocado is all that is needed to balance the bitter frisee salad greens, tart grapefruit, tangy cranberries and vinaigrette in this **Frisse, Grapefruit, Avocado and Cranberry Salad with Cranberry Vinaigrette** *in the* **Recipe file** *which is located within the Culinary Nutrition website at www.culinarynutrition.elsevier.com. When a higher-fat ingredient such as avocado is used sparingly in a recipe, it tricks the palate into thinking there is more to come. Plus, a little fat helps the absorption of phytonutrients, healthful plant compounds in the other ingredients. The finished dish is shown within the centerfold* **Photo file** *in Plate 9.1.*

- Replace solid fats with softened fats or liquid oils wherever possible. There are logical places for using solid fats, softened fats and liquid oils in recipes, such as in a pie crust (solid fat), bread spread (softened fat) or sauteing (liquid oil). Substituting one for another does not always work. For example, oil is not meant to be on toast, while butter is not intended to be on salad greens. But when they can be swapped, calories; total fat; and saturated, monounsaturated and polyunsaturated fatty acids may improve. Compare the following:

- ○ One cup of vegetable shortening contains about 1,812 calories, 205 grams of total fat, 51 grams of saturated fat, 91 grams of monounsaturated fat, and 54 grams of polyunsaturated fat.
- ○ One cup of butter contains about 1,628 calories, 184 grams of total fat, 117 grams of saturated fat, 48 grams of monounsaturated fat, and 7 grams of polyunsaturated fat.
- ○ Three-quarter cup of vegetable oil contains about 1,445 calories, 164 grams of total fat, 12 grams of saturated fat, 103 grams of monounsaturated fat, and 46 grams of polyunsaturated fat.

- Use fat for flavor rather than as a central ingredient in recipes. Classic Caesar salad dressing has a pronounced umami taste and creamy texture. It relies on anchovies, egg yolk, oil and Parmesan cheese—very flavorful and higher-fat ingredients that are difficult to replicate. To retain the salad's character, cut back, not out of, these highly flavorful salad ingredients. Instead of pouring high-fat Caesar salad dressing over low-to-no calorie salad greens, use it sparingly from the bottom up. Place a set amount of dressing in the bottom of a salad bowl, and then mix the salad ingredients very well to disperse the salad dressing and unite the flavors.

- Loaded baked potatoes contain more calories and fats than the baked potato itself. Use less butter that is brightened with lemon juice to let the potato flavor star. Add Parmesan cheese for a low-fat umami finish [19,20]. Compare the following:

  ○ One classic entree Caesar salad contains about 500 calories, 45 grams of total fat, and 11 grams of saturated fat.
  ○ One reduced-calorie and -fat Caesar salad contains about 140 calories, 8 grams of total fat, and 2 grams of saturated fat.
  ○ One medium baked potato with 1 tablespoon of butter, 1 tablespoon of sour cream and 1 tablespoon of cheddar cheese contains about 286 calories, 14 grams of total fat, and 9 grams of saturated fat.
  ○ One medium baked potato with 1 pat of butter and 1 teaspoon of lemon juice contains about 191 calories, 4 grams of total fat, and 2 grams of saturated fat.
  ○ One tablespoon of Parmesan cheese contains about 22 calories, 1 gram of total fat, and 1 gram of saturated fat.

Bite on This: cooking and baking with eggs, egg whites and egg substitutes

Eggs are one of the most versatile ingredients in both cooking and baking. Among their many functions, eggs are needed for binding, clarifying, delaying crystallization, emulsifying, leavening, moistening and thickening. As important as eggs are to the consistency of foods and beverages, some people need to eliminate or reduce egg yolks in their diet due to their cholesterol content (one large whole egg contains 185 milligrams of dietary cholesterol) or because they are allergic to egg whites. Eliminating whole eggs or egg yolks in recipes requires creative use of egg whites in cooking and baking.

If eggs are the main liquid ingredient in a recipe, it is probably safe to assume that the main function of the eggs is to add moisture. If eggs are the only leavening agent in a recipe, it is probably safe to assume that the main function of the eggs is for leavening. If there is one egg in a recipe and there is also a considerable amount of baking powder or baking soda, then it is probably safe to assume that the main function of the egg is to act as a binder because the baking powder and baking soda may be responsible for leavening.

Do not replace more than two whole eggs in a recipe to ensure its consistency. The fewer eggs in a recipe, the easier it is to substitute without losing too much taste or texture. For each one whole egg in a recipe, use two egg whites. Sometimes one-half yolk is added for color, taste and/or texture. Too many egg whites will make a cake tough and rubbery. If a recipe calls for 100 mL (0.4 cup) of liquid egg whites, this is equal to about 3 egg whites. To extend egg whites, add 1 teaspoon of cold water to each 2 egg whites. This equals about 3 egg whites. For food safety, only use reconstituted powdered egg whites or pasteurized egg whites that are sold in the dairy section of supermarkets.

Most egg substitutes contain 99 percent egg whites. The other 1 percent is made of natural colorings, flavorings, salt, spices and gums, such as guar gum or xanthan gum for consistency. Many do not contain fat or cholesterol; some contain vegetable oil.

Egg substitutes that are made from egg whites can be used in breads, cakes, cookies, muffins and puddings, but not in cream puffs or popovers, which require some fat for emulsification. One-fourth cup of liquid egg substitute equals about 1 large fresh egg. For recipes that call for egg yolks, use about 3 tablespoons of egg substitute per yolk.

Choose an egg substitute according to baking needs. Eggs mostly act as leaveners in cakes to make them light and fluffy. In cookies and muffins, eggs mostly add moisture and bind ingredients.

Cookies and pancakes do not necessarily need eggs for leavening, since they are flat, so whole eggs may be able to be omitted from some recipes. If eggs are omitted, add 1 to 2 tablespoons of additional fruit juice, dairy milk, oil or water to restore the moisture that eggs would have contributed. Baking powder, baking soda, egg whites or yeast can be used in some cookie or pancake recipes instead of whole eggs.

Egg whites can be used in whipped toppings as a substitute for whipped cream. Mascarpone or ricotta cheese can be incorporated for volume and texture and a small amount of gelatin can be added to bind the ingredients.

Commercial egg replacers, made from potato flour and leaveners, are available in some supermarkets, specialty stores and online. They are relatively flavorless and are best used for cakes, cookies and muffins; they can also be used for binding ingredients in cooking. To replace 1 whole egg, use about 1 teaspoon of egg replacer plus 2 tablespoons water (products may vary). A little more water or other liquid may have to be added to some recipes.

- The following egg substitute recipe is quick and easy and may be useful in breads, cakes, cookies, muffins, puddings or whipped toppings. Like other egg substitutes, it requires experimentation for best results. Other egg substitute ideas can be found in Chapter 5.

Quick and Easy Egg Substitute
1 tablespoon nonfat dry milk powder 2 egg whites from large eggs dash of annatto*, saffron or yellow food coloring (optional)

1. Sprinkle nonfat dry milk powder over egg whites.
2. Beat until smooth.
3. Add annatto, saffron or yellow food coloring, if desired.
4. Beat until well blended.
5. Use immediately, or place in a tightly sealed container and refrigerate up to 4 days.
   Yield = ¼ cup or 1 large egg

* Annatto is a natural plant extract used as a food coloring.

Bite on This: a closer look at butter and butter substitutes

There is no denying the distinctive taste of butter in cooking and baking. Besides its delicious flavor, butter provides color, crispness and tenderness, among its other attributes. But some people need to reduce or eliminate butter from their diet due to its total fat, saturated fat and cholesterol content, or because of a food allergy to the milk protein in butter.

Many recipes require a certain amount of fat to be successful. While this fat does not have to be butter, some fat substitutes may not work as well as butter. It is important to compare and contrast the taste and functionality of fat substitutes in recipes with the fats that they replace. It is also important to compare and contrast their nutrients, because using some fat substitutes may not save calories or total fat.

Oil that is extracted from seeds or nuts, such as corn kernels, flaxseeds, peanuts, rapeseeds (used for canola oil), safflower seeds, soybean seeds and/or sunflower seeds, is often processed into margarines or spreads. *Margarine* is an emulsion of these oils and water, along with other emulsifiers; antispattering agents; colors; vitamins A, D and sometimes E; and preservatives. *Regular margarine* contains at least 80 percent oil. This standard is mandated by the FDA. *Reduced-fat* or *reduced-calorie/diet margarine* contains no more than 60 percent oil. It contains 25 percent less fat and calories than regular margarine. *Light/lower-fat margarine* contains no more than 40 percent oil. It contains at least 50 percent less fat and calories than regular margarine. *Fat-free margarine* contains less than ½ gram of fat per serving, with gelatin, lactose, rice starch and other ingredients that are not calorie-free. The average nutrients in 1 tablespoon of salted butter, regular margarine, light margarine and fat-free margarine are shown in Table 9-2 for comparison.

TABLE 9-2 Comparison Between Different Fats

Salted Butter 1 Tablespoon (14 grams)	Regular (Solid) Margarine 1 Tablespoon (14 grams)
102 calories	102 calories
0 grams carbohydrates	0 grams carbohydrates
0.1 gram protein	0 grams protein
11.5 grams total fat	11.4 grams total fat
7.3 grams saturated fat	1.8 grams saturated fat
3.0 grams monounsaturated fat	6.6 grams monounsaturated fat
0.4 gram polyunsaturated fat	1.8 grams polyunsaturated fat
31 milligrams cholesterol	0 milligrams cholesterol
82 milligrams sodium	132 milligrams sodium

Reduced-Fat Margarine 1 Tablespoon (14 grams)	Light Margarine 1 Tablespoon (14 grams)
87 calories	50 calories
0 grams of carbohydrates	0 grams of carbohydrates
0 grams of protein	0 grams of protein
10 grams of total fat	5 grams of total fat
1.9 grams of saturated fat	1 gram of saturated fat
4.7 grams of monounsaturated fat	1.5 grams of monounsaturated fat
2.8 grams of polyunsaturated fat	1.5 grams of polyunsaturated fat
0 milligrams of cholesterol	0 milligrams of cholesterol
98 milligrams of sodium	80 milligrams of sodium

Vegetable oil *spreads* are products that contain less than 80 percent of the oil that is mandated by the FDA for regular margarine. Spreads tend to be mild in flavor and can be heated to higher temperatures than butter because they have higher smoke points.

One tablespoon (14 grams) of a typical vegetable oil spread contains about:

77 calories
0.1 gram of carbohydrates
0 grams of protein
8.6 grams of total fat
1.6 grams of saturated fat
4.2 grams of monounsaturated fat
2.4 grams of polyunsaturated fat
0 milligrams of cholesterol
112 milligrams of sodium

Some vegetable oil spreads, with just 32 percent fat, act as *functional foods* to reduce dietary cholesterol. They contain *plant stanol esters*, shown to lower cholesterol levels and reduce the risk of coronary heart disease. Some anticancer benefits of these plant stanol esters have also been demonstrated. The FDA has allowed vegetable oil spreads such as these to carry "qualified health claims" for reducing the risk of coronary heart disease.

The main source of fat in some of these spreads is rapeseed (canola) oil, which contains a proportionally high amount of unsaturated fatty acids and only 7 percent saturated fatty acid. This is one of the lowest amounts of saturated fatty acids among vegetable oils.

One tablespoon (14 grams) of a typical cholesterol-lowering spread contains about:

70 calories
0 grams of carbohydrates
0 grams of protein
8 grams of total fat
1 gram of saturated fat
4.5 grams of monounsaturated fat

2 grams of polyunsaturated fat
0 milligrams of cholesterol
110 milligrams of sodium

Cholesterol-lowering spreads are best used for spreading on breadstuffs and as a topping on vegetables and other side dishes. Some of these spreads are used for cooking and baking, but oils and other ingredients vary, which may affect a recipe's outcome. Like other fat substitutes, it is best to experiment [19,21–23].

Cooking with Margarines and Vegetable Oil Spreads

An ever-changing multitude of margarines and vegetable oil spreads are available for use. They can be used in the following ways:

- Products that are *at least 80 percent oil* can be used in most recipes where hardened margarine or butter is specified.
- Products that are *60 percent or more oil* can be used in almost any recipe where hardened butter or margarine is specified. Modified margarines (such as reduced-fat, light, etc.) or vegetable oil spreads should not be used for baked goods that require precise amounts of fat and moisture, such as pastries. Exceptions do occur.
- Products that are *50 to 59 percent oil* can be used in many cooking applications, including sauteing, as well as for spreading or topping foods. They may not work in baking applications that require precise amounts of specified fats.
- Products that are *49 percent or less oil* should *only* be used for spreading or topping foods and for adding flavor to recipes that do not depend on fat or oil for moisture (such as macaroni and cheese). These products *should not* be used for baking or frying.

In general, the higher the oil content of a margarine or vegetable oil spread, the more total fat it contains. Substituting either margarine or vegetable oil spread for butter *will not necessarily save calories*. The opposite is also true: the lower the oil content of a margarine or spread, the less fat it contains. Like butter, oil contributes browning, flavor and texture. This is important when considering a butter substitute for sauteing or baking, since products with less fat or oil may affect the flavor, moisture, texture and other qualities in the finished product.

Perhaps the wisest advice when choosing a fat substitute for butter is to use less butter if calories and cholesterol permit; use a margarine or vegetable oil spread with the highest percentage of oil for taste and performance if cholesterol is a concern; or use a combination of butter and oil, as in the following recipe:

Butter-Oil Blend
½ teaspoon fine-grained kosher or sea salt
2 tablespoons room-temperature water
1 cup canola or light olive oil
1 cup softened unsalted butter
2 tablespoons nonfat dry milk powder
¼ teaspoon liquid lecithin
Dash annatto, saffron or yellow food coloring (optional)

1. Dissolve salt in water in small bowl; reserve.
2. Place oil, butter, nonfat dry milk powder and annatto, saffron or yellow food coloring (if using) into food processor or blender.
3. Add salt water; blend until smooth.
4. Use immediately, or refrigerate.

Yield = about 2½ cups

Nutrients per recipe: About 3,608 total calories, 6.6 grams of carbohydrates, 6.4 grams of protein, 395 grams of total fat, 132.9 grams of saturated fat, 185.7 grams of monounsaturated fat, 68.7 grams of polyunsaturated fat, 490.5 milligrams of cholesterol, and 255 milligrams of sodium.

Nutrients per 1 tablespoon: 90.2 total calories, 0.16 gram of carbohydrates, 0.16 gram of protein, 9.87 grams of total fat, 3.3 grams of saturated fat, 4.64 grams of monounsaturated fat, 1.71 grams of polyunsaturated fat, 12.26 milligrams of cholesterol, and 6.37 milligrams of sodium.

Diabetes

OVERVIEW, DIET AND FOOD MODIFICATIONS

Whereas cardiovascular disease is mostly concerned with *dietary fat* management, diabetes is mostly concerned with *blood sugar* management. In *diabetes*, the response to blood sugar in the bloodstream by the hormone insulin is either slow or ineffective. As a result, sugar cannot move inside the cells effectively to provide energy, and it lingers in the bloodstream for a long period of time. This is why this disease is referred to as *hyperglycemia* (high blood sugar). One of the devastating effects of diabetes is vascular (vessel) damage due to this abnormal condition.

> **Morsel** "He who does not mind his belly will hardly mind anything else."
> —Samuel Johnson (English biographer, editor, essayist, lexicographer, literary critic, moralist, novelist, and poet, 1709–1784)

The human body goes through some adaptations to accommodate high blood sugar in the bloodstream. For one, the kidneys transfer some of the glucose into the urine for excretion. This may cause increased urination, thirst and problems with concentration, speech and vision, since there may be less available glucose for brain functions. Urine test strips are used to test for this condition.

Diabetics may feel hungry if they do not eat regularly scheduled and balanced meals. Diabetics should have some protein, carbohydrates and healthy fats at each scheduled meal or snack. Both protein and carbohydrates help to regulate blood sugar, and healthy fats provide satiety, so a combination of all three nutrients is ideal.

Normal blood glucose levels after fasting should be between 70 to 100 mg/dL; prediabetic blood glucose levels are between 100 and 125 mg/dL, and diabetes is characterized by a blood sugar level after fasting at 126 mg/dL or above after two consecutive blood tests [24].

TYPE I AND TYPE II DIABETES

As described in Chapter 4, the two main types of diabetes are *Type I* (previously known as juvenile diabetes) and *Type II* (previously known as adult-onset diabetes). Type I diabetes generally strikes children under 12 years of age. It is the result of very little or no insulin production by the pancreas. Type I diabetes requires injected insulin to properly manage blood sugar.

There is speculation but not consensus about the cause(s) of Type I diabetes. It may be the result of an allergic reaction or virus that affects the insulin-producing cells in the pancreas. It also has a strong genetic component.

Type I diabetes can emerge suddenly. Clinical signs include insatiable thirst, rapid weight loss and frequent urination. Immediate medical care is required, including insulin administration. If insulin is not immediately provided, glucose will not be available for the brain and other vital organs. This condition may cause hypoglycemia, or low blood sugar. Undetected and untreated hypoglycemia may lead to confusion, dizziness, fatigue, headache, irritability, nervousness, sweating, unconsciousness, weakness or even death.

The more common type of diabetes is Type II diabetes, which usually affects adults over the age of 45 years old, although more children are now faced with this disease. The risk factors of Type II diabetes include genetic predisposition, family history and central-type obesity (too much fat around the abdomen and visceral organs). People with Type II diabetes may not be able to produce enough insulin, or there may be insulin resistance at the cellular level. Overweight or obesity may interfere with proper insulin function. An increase in diabetes may parallel the epidemic of global obesity.

Type II diabetes drives body fatness because more fat is stored than burned for energy. The liver removes excess sugar in the bloodstream that is converted into fat and sent to the cells for metabolism into energy or storage. In Type II diabetes, this fat has a difficult time entering the cells to be metabolized into energy, so more fat ends up in storage fat cells.

The cells requiring energy send messages to the hypothalamus (the hunger control center of the brain) that they need to "be fed." If a person responds by overeating, then the cycle continues and more fat is stored than metabolized into energy. The storage fat cells may become larger and more resistant unless this cycle is broken. Losing weight on a calorie-, fat- and carbohydrate-controlled diet is a sensible strategy. Exercise is an equally important approach.

Type II diabetes now affects an increasing number of children and teenagers due to childhood and adolescent obesity. While Type II diabetes is controllable, Type I diabetes is a lifelong disability.

KETOSIS

When glucose is not available for energy, the human body may turn to an intermediary state for its energy needs. This state is called *ketosis*, in which the body produces *ketones*, which are by-products that form when the body burns stored fat for energy (see Chapter 6).

Some high-protein/low-carbohydrate diets rely on ketosis for weight and fat loss. However, this is not an advantageous or healthy state, especially for diabetics, because it may cause too much weight loss and make the blood too acidic. This condition is called *acidosis*, which may result in coma or death.

The treatments for Types I and II diabetes differ. Type I diabetes is mainly treated by injected insulin, a healthy and well-balanced diet, exercise, and weight loss (if required). Type II diabetes is mainly treated by weight loss (if required), a healthy and well-balanced diet, and exercise. Oral medications to help control blood glucose and boost insulin effectiveness, and occasionally injected insulin are used if blood sugar is poorly managed.

Since the treatments for both Types I and II diabetes require a healthy and well-balanced diet coupled with weight loss, this is where nutrition and culinary specialists can be effective.

DIETARY STRATEGIES TO IMPROVE BLOOD SUGAR MANAGEMENT

A major goal in diabetes prevention and control is blood sugar management. Normal blood pressure and cholesterol are also essential. Many of these strategies will improve all three risk factors of diabetes:

1. **Eat enough calories for optimal weight.** Eat fewer calories to lose weight and the right amount of calories to maintain weight. Specific guidelines for determining ideal body weight and healthy weight loss can be found in Chapter 10. Here are some guidelines:
   - Choose foods that are naturally lower in calories, such as some fruits, lean meats, legumes, low-fat dairy products, vegetables and whole grains, *and* control the portion sizes of these foods.
   - Replace higher-calorie side dishes, such as french fries, with lower-calorie vegetables, such as side salads. As recommended by the USDA MyPlate Guidelines, fill half the plate with vegetables and fruits. The extra fiber is not only filling, but it also helps to stabilize to blood sugar.
   - Increase water consumption because soluble fiber depends on it, and water assists in fat metabolism. But *decrease* other sweetened liquid calories, including fruit drinks, soft drinks, and coffee and tea beverages. Even pure fruit juice should be consumed in moderation.
2. **Eat regularly spaced meals.** The exact number of meals and the precise timing of these meals are not as critical as once thought. Consistency, meal size and composition are essential in blood sugar management. Here are some guidelines:
   - Try to consume meals and snacks no more than three to four hours apart. Three well-balanced healthful meals, plus one or two proportional snacks may help to normalize and maintain blood sugar.
   - Ideally, each meal and snack should contain some lean protein, whole-grain carbohydrates and healthy fats as described in the "Food choices to improve blood sugar management" section that follows.
3. **Eat a consistent amount of healthy carbohydrates throughout the day.** The carbohydrates in processed fruit drinks and refined starches tend to raise blood sugar quicker than those in whole fruits, vegetables and grains. The *glycemic index* or *GI* addresses this difference in carbohydrates by ranking them according to their effects on blood sugar levels (see Chapter 4). Here are some guidelines:
   - A good rule of thumb is to consume three to five servings (45 to 60 grams) of carbohydrates at each meal and one or two servings (15 to 30 grams) of carbohydrates at each snack.
   - Avoid consuming refined carbohydrates, such as soft drinks or alcoholic beverages, on their own. Have some foods with a little protein or fat, such as cheese, nuts, or peanut butter and crackers, to buffer rapid spikes in blood sugar that these refined beverages may induce.

○ Follow a food pattern similar to the one that is shown in "Food choices to improve blood sugar management." It should be individually designed for specific needs as determined by a diabetes specialist.

4. **Eat just enough fat and the right kind of fat.** A higher total fat intake–even healthy monounsaturated fatty acids—is associated with insulin resistance. Here are some guidelines:

○ Another good rule of thumb is to limit "added fats" such as butter or salad dressing, to three or four servings daily. One serving is equal to about 1 teaspoon of butter, margarine, oil or mayonnaise; 1 tablespoon of reduced-fat butter, margarine or mayonnaise; 1 tablespoon of regular salad dressing; or 2 tablespoons of reduced-fat salad dressing.

○ Substitute monounsaturated fats (avocado, canola oil, nuts and nut oils, olives and olive oil, and peanuts and peanut oil) for saturated fats (butter, cheese and lard).

○ Replace higher-fat dairy products (butter, coffee cream and whipping cream) with lower-fat dairy products (light butter, half-and-half and light cream).

○ Look for labels that read "no trans fat." Since 2006, all packaged foods, including dietary supplements, must list the amount of trans fat on the Nutrition Facts label. But unless there is at least 0.5 gram or more of trans fat in a food, the label can claim 0 grams. Like saturated fat, trans fat tends to increase blood cholesterol levels [25].

○ Limit deep and shallow frying of meat, poultry, fish and vegetables to reduce excess oil. Even sauteing may add too much oil, so limit the quantity.

○ Use herbs and spices to expand the flavor of butter, margarine or cream sauces so that less can be used. Cut back but not necessarily eliminate these flavorsome additions.

5. **Keep a food log.** A food log helps to improve self-awareness and it encourages a person to modify his or her food intake to improve blood glucose levels. Food logs can track portion sizes, the timing of meals and snacks, and their satisfaction.

6. **Read food labels.** Labels that read "low-fat" and "sugar-free" may still contain unwanted calories and other substances. For example, a low-fat food might be higher in sugars and a sugar-free food might be higher in fats. Review favorite foods and beverages to find the best-tasting products with the least fat, calories and other ingredients that fit diabetic diet requirements.

387

DIABETES INDIVIDUALIZED MEAL AND LIFESTYLE PLAN

The **American Diabetes Association (ADA)** recommends an individualized meal and lifestyle plan for managing diabetes and body weight. The ADA also supports balancing food intake with daily physical activity. For a more specialized meal plan, the ADA recommends that individuals with diabetes consult a registered dietitian (RD) or certified diabetes educator (CDE). Some of these clinicians work with culinary specialists to design and create diets for people with diabetes. A sample approach to blood sugar management follows.

FOOD CHOICES TO IMPROVE BLOOD SUGAR MANAGEMENT

It is important to space healthy carbohydrates throughout the day to help manage blood sugar between meals and snacks. This sample meal and snack pattern is designed for a person who consumes about 2,200 calories a day—the standard amount of calories that is used as a reference for the USDA Daily Values (DV). A diabetes specialist can adjust the number of calories and number of carbohydrate servings, depending on individual needs.

Starches: 6 to 11 Servings Daily

2 servings at breakfast
1 serving at morning snack
3 servings at lunch
3 servings at dinner

Starches That Equal 1 Serving (15 grams of Carbohydrate)

1 slice whole-grain bread
½ bagel or English muffin
¾ cup unsweetened, ready-to-eat high-fiber cereal

3 cups cooked pasta, rice,
½ cup cooked legumes, lentils or peas

Fruit: 2 to 4 Servings Daily

1 serving of fruit at breakfast
1 serving of fruit at morning snack
1 serving of fruit at afternoon snack
1 serving of fruit at evening snack

Fruits That Equal 1 Serving (15 grams of Carbohydrates)

1 fresh small-sized fruit
½ cup cooked fruit
½ cup fruit juice
⅓ to ½ cup fresh fruit juice (depends on sugar content)
¾ cup to 1¼ cups berries or melon (varies by size)
2 tablespoons dried fruit

Low-fat Dairy Products: 2 to 3 Servings Daily

1 serving of low-fat dairy products at breakfast
1 serving of low-fat dairy products at afternoon snack
1 serving of low-fat dairy products at dinner

Low-Fat Dairy Products That Equal 1 Serving (12 grams of Carbohydrates)

1 cup fat-free (skim) or low-fat (1%) dairy milk
1 cup fat-free or low-fat plain yogurt
1 cup reduced-fat kefir or buttermilk

Nonstarchy Vegetables: 3 to 5 Servings Daily

At least 1 serving at lunch
At least 2 servings at dinner
1 or more servings at afternoon snack

Nonstarchy Vegetables That Equal 1 Serving (5 grams of Carbohydrates)

½ cup cooked vegetables
1 cup raw vegetables
(Salad greens are considered "free foods" with <5 grams carbohydrates per serving.)

Sweets, Desserts, Other Carbohydrates: 1 to 2 Servings Daily (Calories and Blood Sugar Permitting)

1 serving of sweets with lunch
1 serving of sweets with dinner

Sweets, Desserts and Other Carbohydrates That Contain 1 Serving (15 grams of Carbohydrates)

3 gingersnaps
5 vanilla wafer cookies
1 tablespoon honey or 100 percent fruit spread
1 (100%) frozen fruit juice bar
½ cup sugar-free/fat-free pudding and some frozen yogurt and ice cream*
*Read food labels on frozen yogurt and ice cream to ensure grams of carbohydrates per serving.

Total Carbohydrate Per Meal or Snack

60 grams of carbohydrates at breakfast (2 starches, 1 fruit, 1 low-fat dairy)
30 grams of carbohydrates at midmorning snack (1 starch, 1 fruit)
65 grams of carbohydrates at lunch (3 starches, 1 nonstarchy vegetable, 1 sweet)
35 grams of carbohydrates at midafternoon snack (1 fruit, 1 low-fat diary, 1 nonstarchy vegetable)
85 grams of carbohydrates at dinner (3 starches, 1 low-fat dairy, 2 nonstarchy vegetables, 1 sweet)
15 grams of carbohydrates at evening snack (1 fruit)

Total daily carbohydrates = 290 grams or 1,160 calories (290 grams × 4 calories per gram = 1,160 calories)

On a 2,200-daily calorie diet, 1,160 calories from carbohydrates equal about 52 percent of total calories. This allows for about 30 percent or fewer calories from fat and 20 percent or more calories from protein. The ratio of 50:30:20 (50 percent carbohydrates, 30 percent fat and 20 percent protein) can be applied to other calorie levels for blood sugar management. This ration is also heart-healthy and sensible for weight control.

FOODS AND BEVERAGES THAT MEET THE 50:30:20 GOALS

A day's worth of foods and beverages that approximate 2,200 calories and meet these 50:30:20 goals might resemble this plan:

Breakfast

2 starch servings (1 slice whole-grain bread *plus* ¾ cup ready-to-eat high-fiber cereal)
1 fruit serving (1 small peach)
1 low-fat dairy serving (1 cup skim dairy milk)

Midmorning Snack

1 starch serving (½ bagel)
1 fruit serving (1 small apple)

Lunch

3 starch servings (2 slices whole-grain bread *plus* ½ cup lentil soup)
1 nonstarchy vegetable serving (1 cup fresh mixed bell pepper slices)
1 free food (lettuce for sandwich)
1 sweet serving (5 vanilla wafer cookies)

plus

3 ounces turkey breast
2 tablespoons reduced-fat butter, margarine or mayonnaise for sandwich

Midafternoon Snack

1 fruit serving (½ cup fruit juice)
1 low-fat dairy serving (1 cup fat-free plain yogurt)
1 nonstarchy vegetable serving (1 cup fresh carrot strips)

plus

2 tablespoons reduced-fat ranch-style dressing for carrots

Dinner

4 starch servings (1 cup cooked brown rice *plus* 1 small whole-grain dinner roll)
1 low-fat dairy serving (1 cup skim dairy milk)
2 nonstarchy vegetable servings (1 cup steamed broccoli)
1 free food (1 cup salad greens)
1 (100%) frozen fruit juice bar

plus

  5 ounces broiled ground round
  2 tablespoons reduced-fat butter, margarine or mayonnaise for roll, rice and broccoli

Evening Snack

  1 fruit serving (1 cup fresh berries)

TOOLS FOR CREATING HEALTHY RECIPES AND MENUS FOR DIABETES

Three reliable tools can be used to create healthy and appealing diabetic diets. These are *exchange lists,* *carbohydrate counting* and *nutritional analysis.*

Exchange Lists

Exchange lists provide detailed information about the nutrients in many foods and beverages. They are designed to help manage diabetes, weight management, cardiovascular risk reduction and general healthy eating. When used knowledgeably, exchange lists help to ensure balance and moderation. There are three main groups of foods and beverages in the exchange lists: carbohydrates, proteins (meats and meat substitutes) and fats. Within these groups, there is nutrient information about carbohydrates (dairy products, fruits, starches and starchy vegetables, nonstarchy vegetables, sweets, desserts and other carbohydrates); proteins (meats and meat substitutes); and fats. There are also exchange lists for "free foods" with few calories, combination foods, fast foods and alcohol.

Each of the exchange groups contains a list of foods and beverages that equal about the same number of calories, carbohydrates, proteins and fats. Foods and beverages can be "exchanged" or "traded" within an exchange group because they are similar in nutrients.

390

Exchange lists for diabetes and meal planning are created and updated by the Academy of Nutrition and Dietetics[1] and the American Diabetes Association. They are the basis for the "Foods and beverages that meet the 50:30:20 goals" section [26,27].

Carbohydrate Counting

Counting carbohydrates provides a total amount of daily carbohydrates and helps clarify how each type of carbohydrate (starches, dairy products, starchy and nonstarchy vegetables, sweets, desserts and other carbohydrates) affects blood glucose. The amounts and types of each of these carbohydrates can be adjusted at each meal and snack as needed.

In carbohydrate counting, carbohydrates are first calculated as a percentage of total calories and then in calories and grams. About one-half (50 percent) of total calories should come from carbohydrates. On a 2,200-calorie diet, 50 percent of total calories equals about 1,100 calories (2,200 calories × .50 = 1,100 calories). Since there are 4 calories per gram of carbohydrate, this amounts to 275 grams (1,100 calories/4 = 275 grams). This is the total amount of daily carbohydrates. One could then divide this amount into three meals (275 grams/3 = 92 grams of carbohydrates/meal) or five meals and snacks (275 grams/5 = 55 grams of carbohydrates/meal or snack). A diabetes specialist can help to translate these carbohydrate counts into food and beverage servings.

Carbohydrate counting was used to determine the amounts and balance of carbohydrates in the meals and snacks in the "Food choices to improve blood sugar management" section. It is widely recognized and used in diabetic meal planning. Information about carbohydrate counting can be found at http://www.diabetes.ca/Section_Professionals/ng_carbcounting.asp.

---

[1]The American Dietetic Association (ADA), the world's largest organization of food and nutrition professionals, officially changed its name to the Academy of Nutrition and Dietetics (AND) in 2012.

Nutritional Analysis

Many print and online recipes now incorporate the nutritional analysis of recipes, much like the nutrient breakdowns that follow the recipes in this text. Nutritional analysis makes it easy to look at the carbohydrate content of a recipe and determine if it will fit into a diabetic meal plan or if the recipe needs to be adjusted.

Several nutrition analysis programs are available online for free or for a fee. Make sure they are based on the USDA Nutrient Database for Standard Reference at http://www.nal.usda.gov/fnic/foodcomp/search/, and that the programs are regularly updated.

Follow these steps when considering a recipe for a diabetic meal plan:

1. Look up each ingredient in the recipe for the calories, carbohydrates and other nutrients.
2. Add the total calories and grams of carbohydrates of all of the ingredients in the recipe.
3. Divide the total number of calories and grams of carbohydrates in the recipe by the number of servings of the recipe.
4. The answer is the total number of calories and grams of carbohydrates per serving of food.

A person can determine if a serving of this recipe fits into the calories and carbohydrates that are allotted for a meal, snack and in the daily meal plan, as shown in this example:

Tapioca Pudding

Ingredients	Calories	Grams of Carbohydrates
⅓ cup sugar	258 cal	67 g
3 tablespoons tapioca	102	25
2¾ cups dairy skim milk	228	33
1 egg, well beaten	71	0.6
1 teaspoon vanilla	12	0.3
Totals:	671 calories	125.9 grams

Yield: 6 (½-cup) servings
Total calories: 671 calories
Total grams of carbohydrates: 125.9 grams
Grams of carbohydrates per serving: 125.9 total grams carbohydrates/6 servings =
   20.98 grams of carbohydrates per (½-cup) serving

A (½-cup) serving of this tapioca pudding (20.98 grams of carbohydrates) could be consumed along with one small piece of fresh fruit (15 grams of carbohydrates) at the midafternoon snack, for a total of about 35 grams of carbohydrates. By using nutritional analysis in this manner, other recipes can be included in diabetic meal plans.

FOOD BYTE

A common misconception is that sugar causes diabetes because blood sugar is uncontrolled. People with diabetes do need to watch their dietary sugar and total carbohydrate consumption to properly manage their blood sugar, but sugar is only one part of the carbohydrate picture. Nutritional researchers have reported that there is no definitive connection between sugar intake and the risk of developing Type II diabetes. A diet high in calories of all kinds, being overweight or obese, and an inactive lifestyle are the main risk factors. This does not mean that a person can eat sugar-laden foods without guilt. They are still high in calories, and calories count [28].

ADJUSTING RECIPES AND MEALS FOR PEOPLE WITH DIABETES

Like cooking and baking for people with cardiovascular disease, adapting favorite recipes for diabetics requires scrutinizing ingredients and techniques and experimenting with different products and cooking methods. In some cases, taste and texture will hardly be affected. In other instances, changes to the original recipes may be significant. Sugar and fat substitutes do not taste the same or react the same way to the ingredients they mimic. Using real ingredients but less of them, just like heart-healthy cooking, is also a good strategy for diabetic cooking.

Portion size is critical because it reduces calories, and fewer calories may help blood sugar management. However, smaller portions may look insignificant on a plate. That is where the use of fresh and cooked vegetables with only 5 grams of carbohydrates per serving comes in. Free foods (such as salad greens) with virtually no calories come in handy.

Draw an imaginary line through the center of the lunch or dinner plate and then another line that dissects one-half of the plate into two sections. One of these sections (about one-fourth of the plate) should be filled with whole grains, such as cooked brown rice or quinoa, or starchy vegetables, such as corn, peas or root vegetables. The other section (also about one-fourth of the plate) should be filled with lean protein foods, such as lean meats, seafood, skinless poultry or tofu.

The other one-half of the plate should be filled with nonstarchy vegetables, such as broccoli, carrots, cauliflower, mushrooms or tomatoes, fresh fruit and/or free foods that are low in carbohydrates, such as cabbage, cucumbers and salad greens. One cup of dairy skim milk and a small whole-grain roll or a small piece of fruit (if calories and carbohydrates permit) round out this imaginary plate [29]. Figure 9-1 shows a healthy diabetic plate that is also the composition of MyPlate, recommended by the ADA as a guide for building a healthy plate.

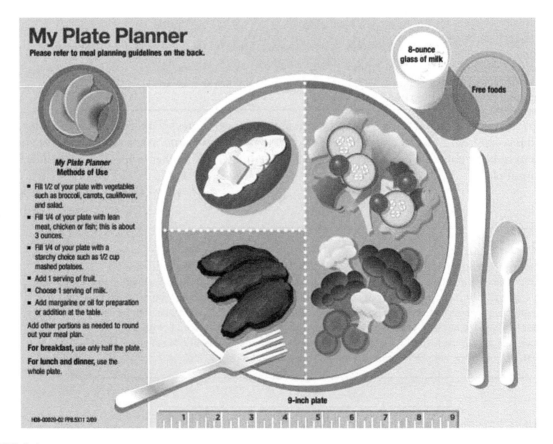

FIGURE 9-1
The healthy diabetic plate. **Source:** [30]. OptumRx. MyPlate planner.

Bite on This: sugar substitutes in cooking and baking

Under normal conditions, sugar is recommended before the use of sugar substitutes in cooking and baking. This is because sugar has many essential functions. Sugar provides color, sweetness, tenderness and texture, to name a few.

Under exceptional conditions, such as diabetes, sugar may need to be reduced or eliminated in recipes. In some recipes, sugar can be reduced by one-fourth to one-third without altering the taste or texture. Fruit juices and frozen fruit juice concentrates may be used for natural sweetening. But even natural sweeteners may be too high in carbohydrates for some diabetics, depending on their daily carbohydrate requirements.

That is why sugar substitutes and sugar-free products provide options. They contain zero grams to a few grams of carbohydrates and some have little to no calories with little effect on blood sugar. Sugar substitutes and sugar-free products can be useful tools in both carbohydrate and calorie management—essential for both people with diabetes and people who are overweight or obese.

The safety of sugar substitutes has been questioned throughout the years. To date, six artificial sweeteners have been approved by the FDA. These include aspartame, acesulfame-K, neotame, saccharin, sucralose and tagatose. They have not been indisputably shown to initiate or promote disease. Rebaudioside A (Reb-A) is a highly purified form of stevia that was approved by the FDA for use in 2008.

Regardless, no artificial sweetener should play a major role in a diabetic diet or weight-loss diet. Sugar substitutes contribute very little to a diet and then tend to replace more nutritious foods if used excessively. It is best to check the labels or contact the manufacturers for any questions about their use.

The following are the most common sugar substitutes (and their brand names) used in product development, cooking and baking.

Acesulfame K or Ace K (Sweet One or Sunett)

Description: *Acesulfame K* ("K" is for potassium) is a calorie-free artificial sweetener that was discovered in 1967. It is 180 to 200 times sweeter than sucrose.

Cooking and baking applications: Unlike aspartame, acesulfame K is stable with heat, even in moderately acidic or basic conditions. It can be used in baking and in products that require a long shelf life.

Limitations: Acesulfame K is often blended with other sweeteners, such as aspartame or sucralose, to offset its slightly bitter aftertaste.

Equivalents: 1 packet of Sweet One = 4 calories; 1 packet of Sweet One = 2 teaspoons of sugar (30 calories or 7.5 grams of carbohydrates); 12 packets of Sweet One (48 calories) = 1 cup of sugar (774 calories or 193.5 grams of carbohydrates)

Aspartame (Equal)

Description: Equal is a calorie-free artificial sweetener that contains aspartame, dextrose and maltodextrin. These ingredients break down into amino acids in the body. Equal is about 200 times as sweet as sucrose. It was first sold in the United States in 1982.

Cooking and baking applications: Equal can be used in hot or cold beverages and in recipes where sugar is primarily used to sweeten. Equal loses sweetness when it is used at high temperatures for long periods of time. It can be incorporated into a recipe at the end of cooking.

Limitations: People who have *phenylketonuria (PKU)*, a rare genetic condition in which the body cannot metabolize *phenylalanine* (an amino acid and component of aspartame), should not use this sweetener.

Equivalents: 1 packet of Equal = 4 calories; 1 packet of Equal = 2 teaspoons of sucrose (30 calories or 7.5 grams of carbohydrates); 24 packets of Equal (96 calories) = 1 cup of sucrose (774 calories or 193.5 grams of carbohydrates)

Saccharin (Sweet 'N Low)

Description: Saccharin is 300 to 500 times sweeter than sucrose. It was first synthesized in 1879 from hydrocarbon derivatives.

Cooking and baking applications: Saccharin is used to improve the taste of many diet foods and beverages. It is often blended with other noncaloric sweeteners to minimize its bitter aftertaste. Sweet 'N Low can be used in cooking and baking applications without losing much of its sweetness because it is heat-stable. A baking version, a liquid, and a brown sugar blend are available.

Limitations: The bitter aftertaste may be eliminated in prepared foods by combining saccharin with another sweetener (or a little sucrose in recipes).

Equivalents: 1 packet of Sweet 'N Low = 4 calories; 1 packet of Sweet 'N Low = 2 teaspoons of sucrose (30 calories or 7.5 grams of carbohydrates); 12 packets of Sweet 'N low (48 calories) = 1 cup of sucrose (774 calories or 193.5 grams of carbohydrates).

Brown Sweet 'N Low contains 20 calories per 1 teaspoon. One teaspoon of Brown Sweet 'N Low = ¼ cup of brown sugar; 4 teaspoons of Brown Sweet 'N Low = 1 cup of brown sugar

Stevia rebaudioside A or Reb-A (Truvia, PureVia, SweetLeaf)

Description: *Stevia rebaudioside A* is extracted from the leaves of a South American plant. Only the highly purified form of stevia (Reb-A) is approved safe by the FDA. Stevia is 250 to 300 times sweeter than sucrose. It is found in baked goods, candy, chewing gum, desserts and as a tabletop sweetener.

Use in cooking and baking: The Reb-A form of stevia is heat stable and can be substituted for sucrose in baking.

Limitations: Reb-A has less of an aftertaste than the sweetener that is derived from the whole leaf, which leaves a licorice taste.

Equivalents: 24 packets of stevia Reb-A = 1 cup of sucrose; each stevia brand recommends its own sugar-to-stevia ratio. Some brands sell stevia in liquid or bulk form.

Sucralose (Splenda)

Description: *Sucralose* is a chlorinated sugar that is 600 times sweeter than sucrose. It is used in beverages, frozen desserts, chewing gum and baked goods, among other applications.

Cooking and baking applications: Unlike other artificial sweeteners, sucralose is stable when heated and can be used in baked and fried recipes. For every 1 cup of Splenda used in cakes, add ½ cup of sifted nonfat dry milk powder and ½ teaspoon baking soda to the dry ingredients. For every 1 cup of Splenda used in muffins and quick breads, add ½ teaspoon of baking soda and 1 to 2 tablespoons of honey or molasses for flavor and moistness. A Splenda-sugar blend is available that helps to create moistness, sweetness and volume. It acts more like 100 percent sugar because it helps products brown, rise and spread.

Limitations: Splenda may not work well in certain cake recipes that rely on sugar for structure. Finished recipes that contain Splenda may require refrigeration.

Equivalents: 1 packet of Splenda = 3 calories; 1 teaspoon of Splenda = 1 teaspoon of sucrose (30 calories or 7.5 grams of carbohydrates); 1 cup Splenda = 1 cup of sucrose (774 calories or 193.5 grams of carbohydrates). If the half-sugar blend or half–brown sugar blend is used, replace 1 cup of sucrose with one-half cup of the blend.

*The FDA allows the designation of "calorie-free" if there are 5 calories or fewer per serving [31,32]: The caloric value of a product containing less than 5 calories may be expressed as zero or to the nearest 5 calorie increment (i.e., zero or 5 depending on the level). Foods with less than 5 calories meet the definition of "calorie-free" and any differences are dietarily insignificant. (US FDA Regulation # 21 CFR 101.9 (c) (1))

Cancer

OVERVIEW, DIET AND FOOD MODIFICATIONS

Cancer is not a new disease. It was described in early medical records that dated about 2500 BC. Breast cancer and its treatments were recorded about 1600 BC. Theories about cancer have been proposed since the 1700s.

Among its many descriptions, cancer has been labeled "black bile," "lymph abnormality" and "hard growing mass." Considering that the first statistics about cancer were published in the 1800s and radiation and chemotherapy treatments for cancer began in the 1900s, research has come far in identifying what cancer really is and what it actually does to the human body.

Cancer is not a singular disease but rather a group of diseases that are characterized by *unrestrained* cell division and growth. This condition may disrupt the normal functioning of organs by transforming or mutating cells, causing tumor development and metastasizing or spreading beyond the tissues where it began. Dietary factors may account for significant cancer deaths. The process of cancer progression comes in stages.

Cancer Progression and Diet Strategies

In *Stage I* of cancer progression, cancer *initiators* or *carcinogens*, including alcohol, cigarette smoke, dietary factors, environmental chemicals, hormone replacement therapy (HRT), oxygen-free radicals, x-rays and ultraviolet (UV) radiation and viruses transform or *mutate* the *DNA* within cells.

In a healthy person, damaged genes are repaired or replaced, and tumors do not necessarily develop. In *Stage II* of cancer progression, *promoters*, such as alcohol, estrogen and fat, may initiate tumor development. Tumors may disrupt normal cell function. In some cases, tumors can be surgically removed. If they are not detected and removed, then in *Stage III*, cancer *metastasizes* to local tissues. In *Stage IV*, cancer spreads beyond the tissues where it began into organs and/or throughout the body. During each of these stages, a healthy diet and lifestyle might be protective and restorative.

In the initiation phase of Stage I, antioxidants such as green tea with polyphenols and tomatoes with lycopene may help to neutralize oxygen-free radicals and protect against DNA damage. Also in Stage I, most cancer-causing initiators enter the body as precarcinogens that must be broken down in the human body by liver enzymes. If these initiators are not broken down, they may turn into full carcinogens that are capable of damaging DNA. Garlic, onions, shallots and leeks with allyl sulfide may limit this process.

Still in Stage I, if these precarcinogens are broken down by the liver, liver enzymes can carry away their remains. Cruciferous vegetables, such as broccoli and cauliflower with sulforaphane, help to increase the production of these enzymes by the liver.

If the body's defenses in the initiation phase of Stage I cancer progression fail and cells undergo DNA mutations during the promotion phase of Stage II cancer progression, then the next dietary approach to arrest cancer progression includes fatty fish, flaxseed and a common weed called purslane—all with omega-3 fatty acids. Omega-3 fatty acids in fatty fish actually come from plant substances in plankton and algae that fatty fish, such as salmon and trout, feed upon. Omega-3 fatty acids tend to crowd out other fats from the cells and help to prevent tumor growth. Foods with corn and soy oil that contain omega-6 fatty acids tend to promote cancer cell division and growth. This is partially the reason why eating too many fried foods is discouraged.

Reproductive tissue divides rapidly when it is triggered by sex hormones, such as estrogen or testosterone. This may cause increased cancer growth in the breasts, cervix and uterus. Soy foods with isoflavones may act as weak plant estrogens and block stronger cancer-causing estrogens during the promotion phase of Stage II. The relationship between soyfoods and cancers is controversial, especially when there is a genetic predisposition to breast cancer.

In Stage III, cancers are locally advanced. Cancerous tumors invade the local (surrounding tissues) because they need blood. The tumors release a growth factor in order to develop new blood cells. This process is

> **Morsel** "Everything I eat has been proven by some doctor or other to be a deadly poison, and everything I don't eat has been proven to be indispensable for life. But I go marching on." —George Bernard Shaw (Playwright, 1856–1950)

called angiogenesis. COX-2 inhibitors in red wine, grapes, grape juice, peanuts with resveratrol, and turmeric suppress this growth factor and act as anti-inflammatory and analgesic agents, much like common aspirin.

In Stage IV, cancers have often metastasized, or spread to organs and/or throughout the body. Nutritional challenges increase. Foods and beverages should be viewed in conjunction with medical treatments to help to boost the immune system and energy. A nutritional care plan should be developed by a registered dietitian in collaboration with a health care provider.

If appetite is poor or if underweight, then small meals and/or nutritional beverages should be consumed throughout the day to meet needed calories and nutrients. Precise nutritional guidance before, during and after treatments is available from qualified providers.

RISK FACTORS AND INTERVENTIONS FOR VARIOUS FORMS OF CANCER

Some types of cancers have unique risk factors, while others share similar risk factors. Likewise, some dietary interventions are targeted to specific types of cancer, while others may be targeted to many cancer types, such as breast, colon and rectal, esophageal, and prostate cancer, among others.

Breast Cancer

Only heart disease claims more American women's lives than cancer. Dietary risk factors that are associated with female cancers include alcohol consumption, body fat in postmenopausal women, elevated blood fats and dietary fats, excessive weight, inactivity, poor fiber intake and reduced intake of fruits and vegetables. The connection between soy foods and female cancers is speculated, but conflicted.

Nondietary risk factors include age, atypical hyperplasia (irregular cells in noncancerous breast tissue), early age of first menstrual period, education, family history, first live birth at late age, never given birth, inactivity, late menopause, oral contraceptives, pesticides, postmenopausal estrogen (HRT), smoking and socioeconomic status.

396

Colon and Rectal Cancer

Next to lung cancer, colon and rectal cancer are the most deadly types of cancer. To date, the ten-year life expectancy for people with colon and rectal cancer is not very promising. But there is better evidence about the causes and effects of colon and rectal cancer than other cancers.

Dietary and lifestyle strategies include avoiding excess weight around waist; eating more fruits, legumes, vegetables and whole grains; getting sufficient calcium; increasing selenium (a trace mineral in plants that is deficient in some geographic locations); increasing physical activity; and limiting red meat and saturated fat.

Recipe: Curried Garbanzos with Fruited Basmati Rice

*This recipe for **Curried Garbanzos with Fruited Basmati Rice** in the **Recipe file** which is located within the Culinary Nutrition website at www.culinarynutrition.elsevier.com, incorporates garbanzo beans (also called ceci beans or chickpeas) with soluble and insoluble fiber for healthy digestive tracts. Adding fruit to rice also raises the fiber content and adds visual appeal. Curries often contain spices such as coriander, cumin, fenugreek, red pepper and turmeric, which are minuscule cancer fighters. Fiery hot chili peppers that frequently accompany curries are filled with antioxidants vitamins A and C for added cancer protection.*

Esophageal Cancer

The incidence of esophageal cancer has risen more rapidly than any other cancer in the United States since the 1970s. It usually strikes men who are of above-average weight and those who consume caffeine, drink alcohol, eat high-fat foods and smoke cigarettes. Esophageal cancer may be partially due to acid reflux (heartburn). A plant-based diet tends to lower the risks of esophageal cancer, especially those with high vitamin C from citrus fruits, berries, melons, bell peppers, broccoli and tomatoes.

> **FOOD BYTE**
>
> Does coffee cause cancer? Speculations about the association between coffee consumption and the risk of certain cancers have been popularized and denied. In the late 1900s, the World Cancer Research Fund and the American Institute for Cancer Research concluded, "Most evidence on coffee suggests that coffee drinking has no relationship with cancer risk." There is little indisputable scientific evidence that moderate coffee consumption increases the risk of developing cancer at any site in the body. In fact, there is an inverse relationship between coffee consumption and certain cancers (oral, esophageal and pharyngeal, prostate and skin), and coffee has reported antioxidant benefits. But excessive coffee consumption might be a marker for other indulgent lifestyle habits, such as overeating, undue alcohol consumption, and/or smoking, which are associated with some types of cancer [33].

Prostate Cancer

Overweight men are more likely to die from prostate cancer than normal-weight men because body fat stimulates prostate cancer growth. Men should keep their weight stable from their 20s through the rest of their lives. Dietary strategies include decreased saturated fat and red meat. Red meat induces higher testosterone levels that seem to promote the development of prostate cancer.

At one time it was thought that selenium and vitamin E might be effective dietary measures to help prevent prostate cancer. Selenium-rich foods include Brazil nuts, codfish, oats, and turkey, and vitamin E–rich foods include nuts, seeds and oils. Lycopene, a phytochemical in bright orange, red and yellow fruits and vegetables such as guava, pink grapefruit, tomatoes and watermelon, was also thought to be a preventative.

Much of the research on the association of these nutrients and prostate cancer is changing. Until definitive, it is best to use selenium, vitamin E and lycopene-containing foods and supplements in moderation—like the other dietary approaches to cancer prevention that follow [34].

397

DIETARY STRATEGIES FOR CANCER PREVENTION

Following certain dietary strategies may help to prevent certain cancers, but they are not guaranteed. Dietary strategies may also curtail the progression of certain cancers, but they are not ensured. By incorporating the following dietary strategies, other nutrition-related diseases, such as cardiovascular disease and diabetes, may also benefit:

- **Decrease grilled foods, such as blackened meats**. Broiled or grilled, "muscle meats" have been linked with the production of *heterocyclic amines (HCAs)*. HCAs have caused tumors in animals and possibly increase the risk of breast, colon, prostate and stomach cancers in humans. When animal fat drips onto hot coals or stones, *polycyclic aromatic hydrocarbons (PAH)* may form. PAHs are carried upward and back onto food through smoke and by flare-ups. The US Environmental Protection Agency classified seven PAH compounds as possible human carcinogens [35].

Safe grilling tips include control drippings and flare-ups, cook at lower temperatures, cover grill, flip food frequently, keep portion sizes small, marinate meats to break down muscles, minimize grilling time, precook meats, remove charred portions, trim fat and use tongs (do not pierce meats).

- **Decrease salt-cured, smoked and nitrite-cured foods, such as sausages and hot dogs**. In countries where people consume a significant amount of salt-cured, smoked and nitrite-cured foods, there is a higher rate of esophageal and stomach cancers. Examples of these foods include bacon, ham, hot dogs and salt-cured fish, common in Japan and Iceland diets [36].
- **Decrease total fat, saturated fat and cholesterol**. Dietary fat does not necessarily initiate cancer, but it may promote cancer. Monounsaturated fatty acids from avocados, olives and peanuts and their oils and omega-3 fatty acids from fatty fish, flaxseed and purslane may be protective against certain types of cancer, while polyunsaturated fatty acids with omega-6 fatty acids from corn and soy oil may be certain cancer promoters. This is because excessive intake of omega-6 fatty acids may cause an imbalance with omega-3 fatty acids. This condition may cause cell membranes to be unstable and tumors to thrive.

Saturated fats, found in animal fats and coconut and palm oil, have an *indirect* relationship to cancer. Saturated fats may cause excessive body weight, which may trigger certain cancers. Whether or not saturated fatty acids independently *cause* cancer is controversial. Trans fats, made from physically and chemically manipulated vegetable oils, may increase some cancer as well as cardiovascular risks [37].

- **Include an abundance of fruits and vegetables (especially cruciferous) with phytochemicals and antioxidants (beta-carotene, vitamins C and E).** Phytochemicals are minute, cancer-fighting plant compounds that help supply watermelon's red color, broccoli's strong smell and wine's full body. Examples of cancer-fighting phytochemicals include allyl sulfides in garlic and onions; carotenoids in carrots, sweet potatoes and tomatoes; fiber in fruits, vegetables and whole grains; flavonoids in wine and tea (especially green tea); indoles in cruciferous vegetables; isoflavones in soy products; lignin in berries, flaxseed and whole grains; lutein in spinach and collard greens; lycopene, in ruby-red grapefruit, watermelon and tomato products; phenols found in almost all fruits, vegetables and whole grains; phytoestrogen in soy foods; prebiotics in barley, oats and soybeans; sulforaphane in broccoli, cauliflower, cabbage and kale; resveratrol in wine and grapes; and zeaxanthin in corn and eggs.

Antioxidants are chemical magnets and cancer fighters. They are able to unite and disable oxygen-free radicals so they cannot oxidize cell membranes and mutate DNA. Beta-carotene, which converts to vitamin A in the liver, vitamins C and E, and selenium are common antioxidants for cancer prevention. Some of the top foods that contain phytochemicals and their suspected cancer prevention roles are shown in Table 9-3.

Recipe: Brussels Sprouts with Caramelized Onions

Brussels Sprouts with Caramelized Onions may turn these cruciferous vegetables into favorites. A little bit of fat and umami help to balance the bitterness of cruciferous vegetables. In this recipe, the caramelized onions have both: by sauteing the onions in a little oil until they are caramelized, their flavor deepens. Brussels sprouts are rich in vitamins and minerals and the photonutrient sulforaphane and may offer some cancer protection. The recipe for *Brussels Sprouts with Caramelized Onions* can be found in the **Recipe file** which is located within the Culinary Nutrition website at www.culinarynutrition.elsevier.com. The finished dish is shown within the centerfold *Photo file* in Plate 9.2.

- **Incorporate high-fiber foods (especially whole grains).** Dietary fiber increases the rate that food passes through the gastrointestinal tract. It also binds with bile acids, retains water, reduces the conversion of organisms in the colon to cancer-causing substances, and softens the stool. Singularly and combined, these activities protect against the development of colorectal cancer.

AMERICAN CANCER SOCIETY NUTRITION AND PHYSICAL ACTIVITY GUIDELINES FOR CANCER PREVENTION

The American Cancer Society (ACS) recommends that for cancer prevention, individuals should adopt a physically active lifestyle, eat a healthy diet, and maintain a healthy body weight.

Adults should engage in at least 30 minutes of moderate to vigorous physical activity, beyond their usual activities, on five or more days per week; 45 to 60 minutes are preferable. Children and adolescents should engage in at least 60 minutes per day of moderate to vigorous physical activity at least five days per week [41].

A healthy diet means choosing foods and beverages in amounts that help to achieve and maintain a healthy weight. Choose most of the foods consumed from plant sources, including legumes and whole grains. Eat five or more daily servings of a variety of fruits and vegetables. Choose whole grains over processed (refined) grains. Limit processed and high-fat red meats.

Salt consumption should be limited. Studies in other countries link diets with foods that are preserved by salting and pickling with increased risk of nasopharyngeal, stomach and throat cancers. No evidence confirms that moderate levels of salt in cooking or flavoring foods affect cancer risks.

TABLE 9-3 Foods, Phytochemicals and Cancer Prevention Roles

Foods	Phytochemicals	Suspected Cancer Prevention Roles
Almonds	Saponins	Strengthen immune system; interfere with DNA replication
Apples	Flavonoids, fiber, antioxidants	Deactivate carcinogens; inhibit cancer development
Black beans	Saponins	Strengthen immune system; interfere with DNA replication
Blueberries, blackberries	Flavonoids, antioxidants	Deactivate carcinogens; inhibit cancer development
Broccoli	Isothiocyanates	Stimulate protective enzymes that detoxify carcinogens
Brussels sprouts	Isothiocyanates	Stimulate protective enzymes that detoxify carcinogens
Cantaloupe	Carotenoids, antioxidants	Strengthen immune system; contribute anticancer properties
Carrots	Carotenoids, phenols	Strengthen immune system
Chocolate	Flavonoids, antioxidants	Deactivate carcinogens; inhibit cancer development
Cranberries	Flavonoids	Deactivate carcinogens; inhibit cancer development
Eggplant	Flavonoids; antioxidants	Deactivate carcinogens; inhibit cancer development
Flaxseed	Flavonoids; lignans	Antioxidant properties
Garlic	Organosulfur compounds	Strong antibacterial activity
Ginger	Gingerols	Block carcinogens
Grapefruit	Monoterpenes, antioxidants	Help dispose of carcinogens
Green tea	Phenolic compounds	Scavenge free radicals; interrupt cancer development
Hot peppers	Capsaicin, antioxidants	Cancer defense
Jerusalem artichokes	Flavonoids, prebiotic	Restore colon bacteria
Kale	Lutein and zeaxanthin	Neutralize free radicals
Oats	Beta glucan	Prevent carcinogen formation
Onions	Organosulfur compounds	Block cancer-causing chemicals
Orange peel	Monoterpenes, antioxidants	Help dispose carcinogens
Parsley	Flavones, antioxidant beta-carotene	Cellular defense
Pomegranates	Favonoids, fiber, antioxidants	Deactivate carcinogen; inhibit cancer development
Red grapes/wine	Flavonoids, antioxidants	Inhibit enzymes that activate carcinogens
Rosehips	Lycopene	Inhibit cancer cell proliferation
Rosemary	Antioxidant	Cellular defense
Sesame seeds	Phytosterols	Anticancer activities
Soybeans	Isoflavones, saponins, fiber	Block hormones, strengthen immune system, interfere with DNA replication
Spinach	Lutein and zeaxanthin	Neutralize free radicals
Sweet potatoes	Antioxidant beta-carotene	Strengthen immune system
Tomatoes	Antioxidant beta-carotene, vitamin C	Anticancer immunity protection
Walnuts	Phytosterols, saponins	Strengthen immune system; interfere with DNA replication

Source: *[38–40].*

Reduce cured and smoked food intake. Some studies have linked large amounts of processed meat to increased risk of colorectal and stomach cancers. This association may (or may not) be due to nitrites, which are added to ham, hot dogs and luncheon meats to maintain color and prevent bacterial growth. Processed meats and meats that are preserved by smoke or salt increase human exposure to potential cancer-causing agents and should be reduced.

If you drink alcoholic beverages, limit your intake. Drink no more than one drink per day for women or two per day for men.

Maintaining a healthy weight throughout life means balancing calories consumed with physical activities, avoiding excessive weight gain, and maintaining a healthy weight if currently overweight or obese.

GENERAL GUIDELINES FOR COOKING FOR CANCER PREVENTION
Visualize Color

To convert the American Cancer Society recommendations into foods and beverages, start by visualizing very colorful recipes and meals. Normally, the more colorful a dish or meal is, the greater the array of cancer-fighting fruits, vegetables, whole grains and other proactive substances.

- **Breakfast choices** could include bright orange cantaloupe melon (beta-carotene), dark brown whole-grain cereal (fiber), crystal-white yogurt (probiotics) and lemon-yellow pineapple juice (vitamin C).
- **Lunch choices** could include a bright green salad (flavonoids), vivid red tomatoes (beta-carotene and vitamin C), burgundy kidney beans (fiber and isoflavones), brilliant green bell peppers (phenols and vitamins A and C), and blueberries and blackberries (carotenoids and flavonols).
- **Dinner choices** could include crimson wild salmon (omega-3 fatty acids), deep green broccoli (sulphorophane), slate black beans or kelly green peas (fiber and isoflavones), caramel-colored whole-grain pasta (lignans), ruby-red wine or grape juice (resveratrol), bright yellow and orange tropical fruit (beta-carotene and vitamin C), and dark brown bitter chocolate (flavonoids and polyphenols).

> ### Recipe: Linguini and Peas with Roasted Garlic Wine Sauce
> *Linguini and Peas with Roasted Garlic Wine Sauce is a full-bodied dish that can serve as a side dish or entree. The roasted garlic wine sauce is filled with allyl sulfide from the garlic and resveratrol from the wine sauce, two potential cancer-fighting phytochemicals. Broccoli, with its antioxidant vitamins A and C and sulforaphane, can be added for additional disease-prevention abilities. The recipe for **Linguini and Peas with Roasted Garlic Wine Sauce** can be found in the **Recipe file** which is located within the* Culinary Nutrition *website at www.culinarynutrition.elsevier.com. The finished dish is shown within the centerfold **Photo file** in Plate 9.3.*

400

Choose Antioxidant and Photochemical-Rich Foods and Beverages

Round out each meal and menu with high-antioxidant and phytochemical-rich foods and beverages. Use the list in Table 9-3. For example, the following foods can be added to the breakfast, lunch and dinner choices above:

- **Breakfast:** Add walnuts to cereal (phytosterols and saponins) and green tea (phenolic compounds).
- **Lunch:** Add almonds (saponins) and fresh spinach (lutein and zeaxanthin) to salads.
- **Dinner:** Add garlic (organosulfur compounds) and ginger (gingerols) to salmon and grated orange zest (monoterpenes and antioxidants) to broccoli.

Lose Weight and Maintain Weight Loss

Like the *2010 USDA Dietary Guidelines*, the American Cancer Society guidelines also recommend balancing calories consumed with exercise and emphasize the prevention of obesity and achieving and maintaining a healthy body weight. Refer to the recommendations for weight management in Chapter 10—particularly for establishing an ideal body weight and calorie level.

The same dietary goals for cardiovascular disease and diabetes prevention—50 percent carbohydrate, 30 percent fat and 20 percent protein—can be applied to cancer prevention. Attention to calories and the proportion of carbohydrates, fat and protein should help to keep excess nutrients under control.

Table 9-4 shows a daily menu for cancer prevention that is high in antioxidants and phytonutrients. It approximates the 2,200-calorie, 50:30:20 pattern that is recommended for diabetes, cardiovascular disease, weight management and general health.

TABLE 9-4 High Antioxidant and Phytonutrient, Reduced-Calorie and Fat Menu for Cancer Prevention

Breakfast	Lunch	Dinner
1 cup whole-grain, high-fiber cereal 1 cup nonfat dairy milk or soy milk 1 cup blueberries 1 slice whole-grain toast with 1 teaspoon nut butter 1 cup orange juice	Spinach salad: 　1 cup spinach 　2 tablespoons each chopped carrots, cauliflower and tomatoes 　½ cup black beans 　3 tablespoons olive oil and lemon juice dressing 　4 whole-grain crackers 　1 cup minestrone soup 　1 cranberry and walnut oatmeal cookie 　1 slice watermelon 　1 cup nonfat dairy milk or soy milk	Salmon and vegetable fajitas: 　1 whole-grain tortilla 　4 ounces grilled salmon 　¼ cup each stir-fried sweet red peppers and onions 　¼ cup salsa 　½ cup brown rice with black beans 　½ cup plain nonfat yogurt 　¼ cup raspberries 　1 tablespoon chocolate syrup

Nutrition Facts:
2,277 calories
31% calories from fat
52% carbohydrates
17% protein
37 grams dietary fiber

Hypertension

OVERVIEW, DIET AND FOOD MODIFICATIONS

Hypertension, or high blood pressure, is a singular disease, as well as a contributor to other diseases, such as cardiovascular disease and diabetes. Similarly, cardiovascular disease, diabetes and obesity may contribute to hypertension. Hypertension is often confused with anxiety, mental tension and stress. While chronic anxiety is sometimes associated with the complications of hypertension, it does not cause it.

Hypertension is a medical condition in which the pressure of the blood is chronically elevated. It is identified as either *essential (primary hypertension)* or *secondary hypertension*. The most common type of hypertension is essential. The following risk factors contribute to essential hypertension:

- Age (blood pressure rises with age in the United States)
- Buildup of plaque in the arteries accompanied by inelasticity
- Excessive alcohol consumption
- Family history of high blood pressure
- Inactivity
- Overweight or obesity
- Race (African Americans and Hispanics are the most vulnerable)
- Stress
- Tobacco use
- Too much sodium and too little potassium and vitamin D in the diet

Secondary hypertension is a result of another (or secondary) condition, such as an endocrine defect, kidney disease or tumors. If corrected, blood pressure could return to normal values.

DIAGNOSING HYPERTENSION

Hypertension is diagnosed by gauging blood pressure. A cuff with a stethoscope is tightened around the upper arm to listen to heartbeats. Two readings are taken: the *systolic*, or "upper" level, which is the force exerted by the heart as it *contracts* to pump blood throughout the body, and the *diastolic*, or "lower" level, which is the pressure that the blood exerts on the artery walls *between* heart beats. Hypertension is diagnosed when both the systolic and diastolic levels are elevated; otherwise the diagnosis is *prehypertension*, or increased risk of hypertension.

- Optimal blood pressure is blood pressure less than 120/80 mm Hg.
- Prehypertension is blood pressure from 120/80 mm Hg to 139/89 mm Hg. Prehypertension is not true hypertension but rather a classification that identifies people who are at increased risk of developing hypertension.
- Hypertension is blood pressure greater than 140/90 mm Hg.

Hypertension usually is asymptomatic, which means that many people do not realize they have this condition. Some people may experience blurred vision, dizziness, fatigue, flushing, headaches, insomnia or difficulty sleeping and/or *tinnitus* (ringing in the ears).

Chronic hypertension is a risk factor in an *aneurysm* (a weakness in a cerebral artery or vein), chronic renal failure, heart attacks, heart failure and stroke. Even the moderate elevation of arterial blood pressure may contribute to shortened life expectancy.

DIETARY STRATEGIES TO IMPROVE HYPERTENSION

Some hypertension risk factors, such as age, ethnicity and family history, are fixed. Dietary risk factors that are associated with hypertension are changeable. These include body fat and body weight, alcohol and sodium consumption, and dietary fats and cholesterol intake. Fruits and vegetables (especially with potassium), low-fat dairy products (with minerals such as calcium, magnesium and potassium) and whole grains (with vitamins, minerals and iron) seem to be protective against hypertension.

Overweight and obesity

Achieving and maintaining an ideal body weight are important for minimizing the risks of hypertension, as well as other diseases. Even a small weight loss has the capability to reduce or prevent high blood pressure. As much as one-half of US adults with elevated blood pressure are also overweight, so calorie reduction is a good overall strategy to normalize blood pressure [42].

Sodium

Sodium reduction is a preventive approach for reducing the risk of hypertension and a necessary approach for reducing existing hypertension. The *2010 US Dietary Guidelines* recommend consuming less than 2,300 milligrams of sodium daily and 1,500 milligrams of sodium daily for people 51 years of age or older, African Americans, or those who already have hypertension, diabetes or chronic kidney disease.

The goal of 2,300 milligrams of sodium daily is equivalent to about 1 teaspoon of table salt (sodium chloride). Sodium chloride is about 40 percent sodium and 60 percent chloride. The Adequate Intake (AI) for sodium for adults, as established by the US National Academy of Sciences, Institute of Medicine, Food and Nutrition Board is 1,500 milligrams per day. In comparison, humans require only 180 to 500 milligrams of sodium daily.

It is possible to obtain the sodium that is needed daily through dietary sources. These include high-protein foods, such as meat and dairy milk, and vegetables, such as some leafy greens, celery and tomatoes. To reduce sodium in the diet, avoid salty condiments, do not add salt at the table, limit processed and prepared foods, and eliminate or reduce salt from recipes when possible. Other suggestions can be found in the "General guidelines for cooking for people with hypertension" section [43,44].

Alcohol

There is a direct relationship between alcohol and hypertension. People who consume alcohol on a daily basis have a greater risk of developing hypertension than those who abstain. Ethanol activates the sympathetic nervous system, which constricts blood vessels and increases the force in which the heart contracts. It also affects several substances that play important roles in cardiac function, including calcium and magnesium.

Consuming more than three drinks at one time may increase blood pressure. Repeated binge drinking may lead to sustained increase in blood pressure. Heavy drinking that is moderated may help to lower systolic blood pressure by 2 to 4 mm Hg and diastolic blood pressure by 1 to 2 mm Hg [45–47].

Dietary fats and cholesterol

Reducing dietary cholesterol, saturated fats and trans fats may lower blood pressure and reduce hypertension. In addition, reducing dietary fats and cholesterol lowers the risks of cardiovascular disease and obesity, which are intricately liked with hypertension. Cholesterol is only found in animal foods. Saturated fats are mostly found in animal products and tropical oils, such as palm and coconut. Trans fats were used in hydrogenated vegetable oils, but are transitioning out of the US food supply. The DASH diet (see below) helps to reduce dietary fats and cholesterol and increase fruits, vegetables and whole grains.

Potassium

Dietary potassium is associated with blood pressure. This is because potassium works together with sodium and other electrolytes to help regulate the body's water balance. When sodium is too high and potassium and other electrolytes are too low, it can lead to high blood pressure. The adult AI for potassium as established by the US National Academy of Sciences, Institute of Medicine, Food and Nutrition Board is 4,700 milligrams [48].

Fruits and vegetables are particularly rich sources of potassium. These and other potassium-rich foods include 1 baked potato (844 mg), 1 cup of plain yogurt (529 mg), 1 cup of orange juice (496 mg), 1 medium banana (422), ½ cup of cooked spinach (419 mg), 1 cup of dairy skim milk (407 mg), ½ cup of cooked pinto beans (400 mg), 3 ounces of cooked salmon (425 mg), 4 ounces of cooked pork (398 mg), and 4 ounces of cooked hamburger (297 mg).

In total, these common foods and beverages equal about 4,736 milligrams of potassium—fulfilling the AI level for potassium. These fruits and vegetables alone provide about 2,581 milligrams of potassium—over 50 percent of the AI level.

Calcium and Low-Fat Dairy Products

A recent area of interest in the prevention and control of hypertension is the relationship between calcium and hypertension. This is because people who have low calcium and vitamin D intake appear to be at higher risk for hypertension. The Dietary Reference Intake (DRI) for adults up to age 50 is 1,000 milligrams of calcium daily, which is the equivalent of about three (8-ounce) cups of dairy skim milk, plain nonfat yogurt or calcium-fortified orange juice. Women aged 51 years and older should aim for 1,200 milligrams of calcium daily. Men require this amount at 70 years of age and older. More information about calcium sources can be found in Chapter 7 [49].

Fruits, Vegetables and Whole Grains

Besides potassium and calcium, fruits, vegetables and whole grains that are rich in magnesium and fiber may be helpful in lowering blood pressure. Broccoli and spinach are good sources of magnesium, as are almonds, black beans, spinach and tofu.

Whole grains increase fiber intake and contribute several B vitamins (thiamine, riboflavin, niacin and folate) and minerals (iron, magnesium and selenium) that may collectively be effective with fiber in lowering blood pressure.

THE DIETARY APPROACHES TO STOP HYPERTENSION DIET

The *Dietary Approaches to Stop Hypertension (DASH)* diet started in 1993 as a research study funded by the National Heart, Lung and Blood Institute (NHLBI) to determine if a specific diet could lower blood pressure and reduce its complications. The DASH diet study, which lasted four years, examined the effects of three dietary patterns on a group of healthy Caucasian and African American and other minority men and women with an average age of 46 years and average blood pressure of less than 160/80–95 mm Hg. African Americans and other minorities were to comprise about two-thirds of the study sample, and about 50 percent of the sample were to be female. The three diets included a typical American diet, a typical American diet plus additional fruits and vegetables, and the DASH diet (see Tables 9-5 and Table 9-6) [54].

All three groups consumed about 3,000 milligrams of salt daily, which was slightly less than the average US daily intake at the time of 3,600 to 4,000 milligrams. Caloric intake was similar for the three test groups. Alcohol was limited in all the groups to one to two drinks a week.

TABLE 9-5 The DASH Diet

Food Groups	Daily Servings and Serving Sizes	Nutrients
Grains and grain products	6 to 8 servings: 1 slice bread, 1 ounce dry cereal, ½ cup cooked rice, pasta or cereal	Carbohydrates, fiber
Vegetables	4 to 5 servings: 1 cup raw leafy green vegetable, ½ cup cut-up raw or cooked vegetable, ½ cup vegetable juice	Calcium, potassium, magnesium, fiber
Fruits	4 to 5 servings: 1 medium fruit, ¼ cup dried fruit, ½ cup fresh, frozen or canned fruit, ½ cup fruit juice	Calcium, potassium, magnesium, fiber
Legumes, nuts, seeds	4 to 5 servings per week: ⅓ cup or ½ ounce nuts, 2 tablespoons peanut butter, 2 tablespoons (½ ounce) seeds, ½ cup cooked legumes (dry beans), lentils, peas	Protein, calcium, potassium, magnesium, fiber
Fat-free or low-fat dairy products	2 to 3 servings: 1 cup dairy milk or yogurt, 1½ ounces cheese	Protein, calcium, potassium, magnesium
Lean Meats, poultry, fish	Serving of 6 ounces or less: 1 ounce cooked lean meats, poultry or fish, 1 egg	Protein, magnesium
Fats and oils	2 to 3 servings: 1 teaspoon soft margarine, 1 teaspoon vegetable oil, 1 tablespoon mayonnaise, 2 tablespoons salad dressing	Mono- and polyunsaturated fats

Source: [50,52–54].

404

The participants who added more fruits and vegetables to their diet and those who followed the DASH diet lowered their blood pressure the most. Those who exclusively followed the DASH diet had the greatest reduction in blood pressure, especially if they had hypertension before the study. The results also indicated that reducing sodium intake lowered blood pressure in both the typical American diet and the DASH diet groups.

The more sodium was reduced, the greater the fall in blood pressure. The biggest reduction was found in the group that followed the DASH diet at 1,500 milligrams of sodium daily. Blood pressure decreased as much or more by dietary sodium restriction than any antihypertensive medication. The researchers also concluded that the DASH diet may be more effective for African Americans than for Caucasians because they have a greater genetic disposition toward developing hypertension [50,51].

It should be noted that the original DASH diet did not require stringent sodium restriction or weight loss—two traditional dietary tools that may effectively control blood pressure. Combining the original DASH diet with sodium restriction appears to be more effective than just dietary manipulation.

The DASH diet plan is low in total fat, saturated fats and cholesterol. It features whole grains, vegetables, fruits and legumes, nuts and seeds, and low-fat dairy products. Meats, poultry and fish are minimized. Sweets, added sugars and sugar-containing beverages are lower compared to the typical American diet. The diet is rich in calcium, magnesium, potassium, fiber, and other minerals and vitamins, and it supplies about 2,000 calories. It can be adapted according to individualized needs. The DASH diet daily meal plan in Table 9-6 is based on the DASH diet servings in Table 9-5.

DIETARY STRATEGIES FOR PEOPLE WITH HYPERTENSION

The Nutrition Facts Panel on food labels carries essential information about the sodium content of foods and beverages. An array of terms describes the type and amount of sodium. By learning how to decipher this information, a person can choose lower-sodium foods and beverages that comply with sodium-reduced diets.

TABLE 9-6 A Typical DASH Diet Daily Meal Plan

Breakfast	Lunch	Dinner	Snack
2 slices whole grain bread 1 tablespoon unsalted peanut butter 1 tablespoon all-fruit preserves 1 cup dairy skim milk ½ medium grapefruit	**Salad** 3 cups fresh spinach leaves 1 medium tomato ½ cup reduced low-sodium garbanzo beans **Salad dressing** 1 tablespoon olive oil ½ to 1 tablespoon lemon juice 12 unsalted whole-grain crackers 1 medium orange 1 cup dairy skim milk	3 ounces baked halibut 1 cup cooked brown rice ½ cup steamed broccoli 1 whole-grain roll 1 tablespoon reduced-fat butter 1 cup fresh berries	1 cup plain low-fat yogurt 3 gingersnaps ½ cup pineapple in own juice

DASH Diet Components	DASH Diet Servings
Grains and grain products	9 (2 slices whole-grain bread, 12 whole-grain crackers, 1 cup cooked brown rice, 1 whole-grain roll, 3 gingersnaps)
Vegetables	5 (3 cups fresh spinach, 1 medium tomato, ½ cup steamed broccoli)
Fruits	5 (½ medium grapefruit, 1 medium orange, ½ cup pineapple in own juice, 1½ cups fresh berries)
Dairy foods (low-fat or fat-free)	3 (2 cups dairy skim milk, 1 cup plain low-fat yogurt)
Meats, poultry, and fish	1 (4 ounces baked halibut)
Legumes, nuts, and seeds	2 (1 tablespoon peanut butter, ½ cup garbanzos)
Fats and oils	2 (1 tablespoons olive oil, 1 tablespoon reduced-fat butter)
Sweets	0 servings

Nutrition Facts:

1,947 total calories, 52% carbohydrates, 17% protein, 30% fat, 7% saturated fat, 5% polyunsaturated fat, 16% monounsaturated fat, 30.4 grams fiber, 94.8 milligrams cholesterol, 4,308 milligrams potassium, 2,054.1 milligrams sodium

Source: [50,52–54].

The Nutrition Facts Panel shows the percentage of sodium that is provided by *one serving* of a food or beverage in comparison to the DV for sodium (2,400 milligrams). If more than one serving of a food or beverage is consumed, this percentage should *reflect the number of servings*. For example, a 1-ounce serving of pretzels supplies about 15 percent of the DV for sodium (2,400 milligrams $\times$ .15 = 260 milligrams). If two (1-ounce) servings of pretzels are consumed, this amounts to 30 percent of the DV for sodium (15% DV $\times$ 2 = 30% DV) or 520 milligrams, which is about one-fifth of the DV for sodium in just two servings of pretzels. Try not to exceed 100 percent of the DV for sodium in one day.

Sodium terminology that appears on US food labels is established and regulated by the FDA. It provides valuable information about the quantity of sodium in foods and beverages. Some of these terms include the following:

- **Sodium-free:** less than 5 milligrams (mg) of sodium per serving
- **Very low-sodium:** 35 milligrams (mg) or less of sodium per serving
- **Low-sodium:** 140 milligrams (mg) or less of sodium per serving
- **Light-in-sodium:** at least 50 percent less of sodium per serving than an average amount of the same food that does not have sodium reduction
- **Lightly salted:** at least 50 percent less of sodium per serving than an average amount of the same food that does not have sodium reduction

- **Reduced or less-sodium:** at least 25 percent less of sodium per serving than an average amount of the same food that does not have sodium reduction
- **Salt-free:** sodium-free
- **Unsalted, without added salt, no salt added:** no salt added during processing [55]

Follow the portion sizes that are provided on the Nutrition Facts Panel. These portion sizes are often smaller than expected. Additionally, they are usually for one serving in a larger can or bottle, and it is easy to consume everything at once. For example, ½ cup (4 fluid ounces) of vegetable juice contains just 25 calories and 310 milligrams of sodium. One 12-ounce can of vegetable juice contains three times this amount, or 930 milligrams of sodium (about 40 percent of the DV for sodium). In comparison, ½ cup of low-sodium vegetable juice contains about 70 milligrams of sodium or 210 milligrams of sodium for one 12-ounce can or bottle.

GENERAL GUIDELINES FOR COOKING FOR PEOPLE WITH HYPERTENSION

The guidelines for cooking for people with hypertension are comparable to the guidelines for cooking for people who have cardiovascular disease, diabetes or need to lose weight. The attention to and reduction of high-sodium foods and beverages is what differentiates these guidelines.

BALANCE the amount of sodium in recipes, meals and daily menus. If a high-sodium ingredient is used in a recipe, balance it with ingredients that are lower in sodium in the recipe or meal. For example, 2 tablespoons of commercial vinaigrette salad dressing contain about 240 milligrams of sodium. If 2 tablespoons of extra-virgin olive oil and balsamic vinegar are substituted and topped with 2 large chopped olives (80 milligrams sodium), then 160 milligrams of sodium can be saved. This combination will still convey a salty note.

LIMIT the amount of sodium in some foods and ingredients. These include additives and preservatives and substances in beverages, canned foods, ethnic foods, ready-to-use ingredients, luncheon meats and cured poultry and fish, packaged and prepared foods, entrees, and processed cheese and cheese products.

One may see the following additives and preservatives on the food label (look for the word *sodium*):

- Disodium phosphate (stabilizes and buffers quick-cooking cereals and processed cheese)
- Monosodium glutamate or MSG (enhances the flavor in meats and vegetables)
- Sodium alginate (gels chocolate milk, ice cream and jams)
- Sodium benzoate (preserves condiments, including relishes, salad dressings and sauces, fruit juices and soft drinks)
- Sodium caseinate (emulsifies coffee creamers, ice cream and milkshakes; binds processed meats)
- Sodium citrate (buffers, emulsifies and flavors gelatin desserts, ice cream, jams and yogurts)
- Sodium hydroxide (softens and loosens fruit and vegetable skins such as olives)
- Sodium nitrite (cures meats and sausages)
- Sodium propionate (inhibits mold in breads, cakes and pasteurized cheese)
- Sodium saccharin (sweetens beverages and candies)
- Sodium sulfite (bleaches fruits prior to coloring, such as maraschino cherries; preserves dried fruits, such as prunes)

Beverages are also sources of high sodium. The average amount of sodium in 12 ounces of regular soda is 126 milligrams, and 12 ounces of sugar-free soda contain 41 milligrams. Some soda contains potassium, which helps to neutralize some of the acidic flavor of drinks that are made with soda water.

Other beverages, including dairy milk, contain a wide range of sodium as follows. Specific brands vary, so compare the Nutrition Facts Panels.

- 1 cup tomato juice contains 650 mg sodium
- 1 cup homemade cocoa contains 150 mg sodium
- 1 cup skim dairy milk contains 103 mg sodium
- 1 cup carrot juice contains 55 mg sodium
- 1 cup unsweetened fruit juice contains 5 to 10 mg sodium

Canned foods, including legumes, olives, pickles, pickled vegetables, vegetable juices, vegetables with seasoned sauces, soups, and sauerkraut, may be high in sodium per serving. Most vegetables contain sodium as a preservative. Some reduced- and low-sodium varieties are available. Drain and rinse canned foods where possible before adding to recipes to reduce the sodium content. Draining and rinsing some canned vegetables can reduce the sodium content as much as 25 percent [56].

Ethnic foods and ingredients are often higher in sodium. It may be that their original cuisines primarily used salt as a preservative or that they developed in locations where the climate is hot and salt replaced what was lost in perspiration. Ethnic cuisines still rely on higher-sodium ingredients for their pronounced flavors. These include Chinese and Japanese foods made with teriyaki or soy sauce; East Indian, Thai and Vietnamese foods with curries and fish sauce; Italian foods and sauces made with canned and bottled tomato products; and Mexican foods and sauces made with canned chilies, taco and/or enchilada sauce.

Reduced- and low-sodium products are available in specialty stores for some of these cuisines. However, there are no global labeling standards. Some imported products may not carry sodium information on their labels because imported foods tend to follow the labeling regulations of the country in which they are sold.

Common ingredients like baking soda and baking powder (found in many baked goods); condiments and dressings, such as catsup, mayonnaise, mustard, pickle relish and salad dressings; seasoned salts, such as celery, garlic and onion; meat tenderizers; sauces, such as barbecue, chili, cocktail, pasta, smoke-flavored, soy, steak, teriyaki, tomato and Worcestershire; and bouillon; gravies and marinades often contain significant amounts of sodium. Some foods contain multiple high-sodium ingredients, so a dribble or dash may be all that is needed for a salty taste.

Luncheon meats and cured meats, such as bacon, bologna, Canadian bacon, chicken, corned beef, dried fish or dried meats, frankfurters, ham, liverwurst, pastrami, salami, sausages and turkey products; canned poultry and fish, such as chicken, salmon, tuna and shellfish, including crab, clams, lobster, oysters, scallops and shrimp; and soy protein products, including miso and marinated tofu contain both naturally occurring sodium and have additional sodium from processing. Like higher-sodium ingredients, use processed meats, poultry, fish and shellfish as salty accents rather than the focus of a dish.

Packaged foods and beverages, including baked goods, cold and instant hot cereals, Dutch process cocoa and instant cocoa mixes, rice or noodles with seasonings and sauces (such as instant au gratin or scalloped potatoes, rice pilaf and Ramen noodles), snack foods (such as chips, crackers, popcorn and pretzels), soups and soup mixes, and stuffing mixes that contain 200 milligrams or more of sodium per serving should only be used with discretion, if at all. Some reduced- and low-sodium options are emerging as the food industry seeks lower-sodium ingredients for processing.

Prepared entrees, including canned and frozen dinners and entrees, such as chili, hash and stews; entrees with sauce and seasoning mixes, such as macaroni and cheese; and TV-type dinners that contain 200 milligrams or more of sodium per serving should also only be used with discretion, if at all. Entrees that are designed for popular diet programs are frequently reduced in sodium. Compare and contrast the Nutrition Facts Panels for sodium and other nutrients. Sometimes sodium-reduced entrees are higher in some fats and other nutrients.

Processed cheese and cheese products, including American and some Swiss cheese; higher-sodium cheese, such as blue cheese, cottage cheese, feta, Parmesan and Roquefort; and dairy milk–based drinks, such as buttermilk and yogurt beverages, may be higher in sodium than similar dairy products. Either use less of these dairy beverages and food, or select reduced-sodium varieties.

USE low-, reduced- or no-sodium alternatives. In some instances it may be necessary to reduce extra sodium in the diet to a minimum. *Select foods and ingredients that provide 5 percent or less sodium per serving as shown on the Nutrition Facts Panel.* Very low-sodium ingredients and foods may have to be enhanced with citrus juices, flavorful vinegars, fresh fruits and vegetables, and herbs and spices to boost their flavor. More suggestions for reducing sodium in the diet can be found in Chapter 7.

COMPARE, contrast and save. It cannot be emphasized enough: salt is an integral ingredient in cooking and baking, and its absence can cause a recipe to fail and customer or consumer disloyalty. Instead of eliminating

TABLE 9-7 Sodium Comparisons and Savings

Higher Sodium Foods and Beverages	Lower Sodium Foods and Beverages	Sodium Savings (Milligrams of Sodium)[a]
Apple pie (⅓ pie)	Apple (1 medium)	481 mg
Breaded fish fillet (3 ounces)	Grilled fish fillet (3 ounces)	388
Canned biscuit (1)	Homemade biscuit (1)	95
Canned corn (1 cup)	Fresh ear of corn (1)	399
Cheese soup (1 cup)	Cheddar cheese (1 ounce)	845
Chicken pot pie (1)	Baked chicken (3 ounces)	777
Club soda (12 ounces)	Flavored water (12 ounces)	86
Cooking wine (1 ounce)	Drinking wine (3½ ounces	660
Seasoned breadcrumbs (¼ cup)	Uncooked oatmeal (¼ cup)	469
Prebasted turkey (½ breast)	Fresh turkey (½ breast)	3,271
Potato chips (10)	Baked potato (1 ounce)	195
Saltwater fish (3 ounces as sea bass)	Freshwater fish, as trout (3 ounces)	16
Margarine (1 tablespoon)	Unsalted butter (1 tablespoon)	148
Peanut butter cookies (3)	Unsalted peanuts (1 ounce)	186
Sauerkraut (1 cup)	Cabbage (1 cup)	1,738
Self-rising flour (1 cup)	All-purpose flour (1 cup)	1,585
Spaghetti sauce (1 cup)	Tomato paste (1 cup)	1,940
Salt (1 teaspoon)	Juice of 1 fresh lemon	2,297
Tuna noodle casserole (1 cup)	Tuna in water (3 ounces)	343
Tomato sauce (1 cup)	Tomato (1 medium)	1,296

Source: [18].
[a]Milligrams of sodium "savings" approximate.

salt or using salt substitutes, compare and contrast higher- and lower-sodium foods and beverages options as shown in Table 9-7. Many milligrams of sodium can be saved with this simple approach.

FRESH is usually best. Many of the substitutes in Table 9-7 emphasize "fresh." While there is natural sodium in many foods and ingredients, there is no "added sodium." Fresh citrus juice, unseasoned vinegar or drinking-quality wine can be substituted in some recipes for condiments, gravies or sauces with a sodium savings. For example, 1 tablespoon of soy sauce contains 1,029 milligrams of sodium and 1 tablespoon of catsup contains 156 milligrams of sodium, compared to the juice of one fresh lemon, which contains only 1 milligram of sodium.

Similarly, fresh pureed tomatoes (one medium tomato contains about 6 milligrams of sodium) can be substituted for tomato products in some recipes with a sodium savings. These include tomato juice (1 cup of tomato juice contains about 878 milligrams of sodium); tomato soup (1 cup of tomato soup contains about 932 milligrams of sodium); or tomato sauce (1 cup of tomato sauce contains about 1,498 milligrams of sodium).

Bite on This: salt substitutes in cooking and baking

Salt substitutes may be helpful for some people to help reduce and regulate their sodium intake. Some salt substitutes that are labeled "lite" or "low sodium" likely contain some sodium. The amounts vary, so make sure to read the labels.

Some salt substitutes contain potassium that replaces all or part of the sodium. Too much potassium can offset the balance of sodium and potassium in the body. People who are under medical supervision for kidney problems or those who take blood pressure medications should check with their health care provider before using potassium chloride salt substitutes. Look for potassium chloride salt substitutes that are labeled "sodium-free," since some of these products may contain a mixture of sodium chloride and potassium chloride.

Salt substitutes may have an "off" or metallic taste, especially when they interact with other ingredients. Ideally, the best "salt substitute" is the natural sodium in foods and beverages that can be tasted once salt and salt-containing condiments are removed. A sodium-restricted diet must take this natural sodium in foods and beverages into account. When purchasing reduced-sodium foods and beverages, it is wise to look for 140 milligrams of sodium or less per serving, which is considered a "low-sodium food."

Some salt substitutes are mixtures of spices and herbs and do not contain any sodium or potassium. These salt substitutes, as well as homemade seasoning blends without salt, can be used fairly liberally to flavor foods. Check the recommendations for cooking with herbs and spices in Chapter 7 and/or try one of the following no-salt herb and spice blends. These herb and spice blends should be used during cooking to maximize their flavors. They can also be used as dry rubs for fish, meats, poultry, seafood or vegetables. Herbs and spices are dried unless noted. Store these blends in clean containers away from light and heat.

- *All-purpose herb and spice blend:*
  - 1 teaspoon *each* dried basil leaves, coarsely ground black pepper, ground cloves, ground mace, dried marjoram leaves, dried oregano leaves, dried parsley leaves, ground savory and dried thyme leaves, *plus* ¼ teaspoon *each* ground cayenne pepper and ground nutmeg
- *Herbal spice blend 1:*
  - 2 tablespoons *each* dried basil leaves and granulated onion; 1 teaspoon *each* dried oregano leaves and celery seeds, *plus* ¼ teaspoon dried lemon peel and ⅛ teaspoon coarsely ground black pepper
- *Herbal spice blend 2:*
  - 1 tablespoon *each* onion powder, garlic powder and dried parsley leaves, *plus* 2 teaspoons dried basil leaves, *plus* 1 teaspoon *each* dried thyme leaves, dried marjoram leaves and coarsely ground black pepper, *plus* ½ teaspoon *each* ground sage, dried grated orange peel and ground paprika
- *Lemon spice blend:*
  - 2 teaspoons dried parsley leaves, *plus* ½ teaspoon *each* dried basil leaves, granulated garlic, dried lemon peel and dried marjoram leaves, *plus* ¼ teaspoon *each* ground allspice and coarsely ground black pepper
- *Spicy blend 1:*
  - 2 tablespoons ground savory, *plus* 2½ teaspoons granulated onion, *plus* 1 tablespoon mustard powder, *plus* 1½ teaspoon curry powder, *plus* 1¼ teaspoons *each* *ground* cumin and ground white pepper, *plus* ½ teaspoon granulated garlic
- *Spicy blend 2:*
  - 2 tablespoons *each* ground mustard and onion powder, *plus* 1 tablespoon each garlic powder, ground paprika, dried basil leaves and ground thyme, *plus* 1 teaspoon curry powder, *plus* ½ teaspoon ground white pepper

---

FOOD BYTE

Since the 1930s, treatment for hypertension has been peppered by controversies, heroics, misconceptions and myths by both health care providers and patients. Health care providers have attempted to lower blood pressure by administering medications—sometimes with severe side effects; injecting typhoid bacteria; and performing extensive surgery. Patients have been subjected to these treatments in addition to rigid low-sodium diets. Many of these misconceptions and missteps have now been clarified and corrected by long-term clinical trials. It appears that the *degree to which blood pressure is lowered* may be more important than the specific treatments. Lowering blood pressure requires a multitude of efforts; reducing sodium intake is just one approach [57].

Digestive Disorders
OVERVIEW, DIET AND FOOD MODIFICATIONS

Digestive diseases cover a whole range of disorders, from a simple stomachache to colorectal, gastric and pancreatic cancers. Digestive diseases include acid reflux, cirrhosis of the liver, celiac disease, colitis,

Crohn's disease, diverticulosis and diverticulitis, gallstones, gastritis, hepatitis, inflammatory bowel disease, irritable bowel syndrome, liver failure, pancreatitis, peptic ulcers and ulcerative colitis, among other disorders. While some of these conditions have genetic roots, many are diet related. The symptoms vary widely, as do the treatments.

The digestive system is a series of hollow organs that are connected together through a long and twisted tube. The digestive system extends from the mouth to the anus and includes the esophagus, stomach and small and large intestines, as well as accessory organs, including the gallbladder, liver and pancreas. With such a large and complex multi-organ system, it is not uncommon for some of the organs to malfunction. In general, if a person has heartburn that is not relieved by antacids; changes in bowel habits, such as frequent constipation or diarrhea that are not relieved by over-the-counter medications; or ongoing nausea, severe abdominal pain or unintentional weight loss, then they should seek professional health care.

The typical US diet contributes to digestive system disorders with too many calories and fats and too few vegetables, fruits and whole grains with fiber. Poor eating habits, such as eating too quickly, skipping meals and/or late-night eating may also contribute to some digestive system disorders. Sometimes digestive system disorders may lead to significant nutrient malabsorption. *Atrophic gastritis* may lead to the malabsorption of vitamin B12. *Cirrhosis* of the liver may result in the reduced ability to store vitamins A and B12. The fat-soluble vitamins A, D, E and K; calcium; magnesium; and zinc may be more adversely affected than other nutrients.

A well-balanced diet is usually sufficient to provide and maintain the right amounts of vitamins and minerals in the body. Sometimes dietary supplements are necessary. An examination of the major food-related digestive system disorders reveals each of their nutrient needs.

MAJOR FOOD-RELATED DIGESTIVE SYSTEM DISORDERS

The major food-related digestive disorders are bacteria and foodborne illness, celiac disease, colon polyps, diverticulosis and diverticulitis, gastritis, irritable bowel syndrome, lactose intolerance and ulcers.

Bacteria and Foodborne Illness

410

Foodborne illness is usually caused by consuming foods or beverages that are contaminated with bacteria, parasites or viruses. Symptoms may include abdominal discomfort, dehydration, diarrhea, fever and/or vomiting. In most instances, foodborne illness is mild. People of any age may become infected. Those most vulnerable to foodborne illness include people with compromised immune systems, pregnant women, older adults and young children.

Harmful bacteria in raw or undercooked foods and beverages are the most common cause of foodborne illness. Infection by *Escherichia coli (E. coli)* bacteria may cause diarrhea, urinary tract infections, respiratory illness and pneumonia. Some *E. coli* bacteria make a toxin called "shiga." These bacteria, called *shiga toxin-producing E. coli, or STEC*, may cause hemolytic uremic syndrome (HUS), where the kidneys and other organs shut down. Very young children and the elderly are more susceptible to developing HUS or other severe illnesses, which may lead to permanent disabilities or death. *E. coli* outbreaks have included beef, cheese, cookie dough, lettuce, processed meats, spinach, strawberries and other foods.

Proper food handling can prevent most cases of foodborne illness. These include cooking food long enough and at a high enough temperature to kill bacteria; defrosting food in the refrigerator, under cool running water, or in the microwave—never on the kitchen counter; refrigerating prepared food within two hours before bacteria multiply; washing all raw fruits and vegetables under cool running water before using; and washing hands, surfaces, and utensils with hot soapy water before and after food preparation.

Celiac Disease

Celiac disease is a condition that damages the lining of the small intestine and prevents it from absorbing certain foods and beverages. The exact cause of celiac disease is unknown. The damage to the small intestine is due to a reaction by the body's immune system to gluten. *Gluten* is a protein that is mostly found in barley, rye and wheat.

Once the body's immune system overreacts to this common protein and the lining of the small intestine is damaged, the body cannot obtain certain nutrients. Anemia, brittle bones and infertility could develop over time. Untreated, people with celiac disease have increased risk of osteoporosis and intestinal cancers.

People may not feel sick from celiac disease, or they may confuse the symptoms of diarrhea, gas, itchy skin, lethargy, mood changes, stomach pain and weight loss with other causes. These symptoms may occur simultaneously while gluten damages the intestines. The only real "test" of celiac disease is a gluten-free diet to determine if the symptoms diminish. By following a gluten-free diet, the damage to the intestinal lining may heal from a few months in children to a few years in adults.

Celiac disease has a genetic component. If a family member is stricken with celiac disease, it may indicate to a relative that his or her symptoms are disease-related. Celiac disease is frequently associated with other genetic and autoimmune conditions, including Type I diabetes and rheumatoid arthritis, lactose intolerance and thyroid disease. The disorder is most common in women, Caucasians and persons of European ancestry. The treatment for celiac disease is a gluten-free diet, which is described in the following section on cooking for people with gastrointestinal disorders and in Chapter 4.

Colon Polyps

Colon polyps are small clumps of extra tissue that grow inside the colon in the large intestine. Most are noncancerous (or benign), but some larger ones can become cancerous—particularly with neglect. People who are over 50 years of age with a family history of polyps or colon cancer, overweight or obese, and inactive, consume fatty foods on a regular basis, drink alcohol, and/or smoke cigarettes have increased risk of colon polyps.

Mostly colon polyps are asymptomatic, which means that they can form without symptoms. Once formed, colon polyps may cause bleeding, constipation or diarrhea. Colon polyps can be removed during a minor procedure called a *colonoscopy*. Dietary prevention includes alcohol reduction or elimination and a reduced-fat and higher-fiber diet.

Diverticulosis and Diverticulitis

Diverticulosis is a condition that is caused by *diverticula*—small, bulging pouches *(diverticula)* in the lining of the colon, which is located at the end of the small intestine. If these pouches become blocked with waste, allowing bacteria to build up and cause infection, this condition is called *diverticulitis.*

411

Diverticulosis is common as people age. The predominance of diverticulosis occurs over 80 years of age, but it can start much younger. Most people with diverticulosis do not have discomfort. Some may have bloating, constipation, cramps or distress in the lower abdomen or pain.

Diverticulitis may cause severe abdominal pain, change in bowel habits, chills, cramps, nausea, tenderness in the lower left side of the abdomen, or vomiting. It may also lead to bleeding, blockage, or infections or tearing and require immediate health care.

If the infection worsens, an abscess can form in the wall of the colon, which can leak and form a larger abscess in the abdominal cavity. This state is called *peritonitis*, which is often accompanied by fever, nausea and severe abdominal tenderness. Without quick medical attention, peritonitis can be fatal. If the peritonitis causes scarring, it may lead to partial or total intestinal blockage. This condition is called *intestinal obstruction*. The colon is unable to move its contents and emergency surgery may be necessary.

A low-fiber diet is thought to contribute to diverticular disease, which is most common in developed or industrialized countries, but rare in Asia and Africa, where the diet is higher in fiber. Inactivity is also implicated.

Women should try to eat at least 21 to 25 grams of fiber a day, while men should aim for at least 30 to 38 grams of fiber daily. High-fiber foods include fruits (without tiny seeds); vegetables, such as asparagus, broccoli, cabbage, carrots, celery, spinach and squash; legumes; and whole-grain breads, cereals and cooked whole grains. Avoidance of nuts, popcorn and seeds is not warranted. It was once thought that these foods may enter, block or irritate the diverticula; however, no scientific data supports this measure. A high-fiber diet is recommended. See http://digestive.niddk.nih.gov/ddiseases/pubs/diverticulosis/.

Gastritis

Gastritis is a set of conditions that inflame the stomach lining. Gastritis can be caused by drinking too much alcohol, prolonged use of nonsteroid anti-inflammatory drugs (NSAID) such as aspirin or ibuprofen, or bacterial infection, such as *Helicobacter pylori (H. pylori).*

Gastritis can develop from autoimmune disorders (such as AIDS), bile reflux, burns, injury, major surgery, pernicious anemia (from vitamin B12 deficiency), severe infection or trauma. The most common symptoms of gastritis include abdominal bloating, pain or upset, belching, bloody stool, burning in the upper abdomen, fullness, nausea and/or vomiting.

Reducing stomach acid, which irritates the inflamed tissues, helps to relieve the symptoms of gastritis and promotes healing. Avoidance of troublesome beverages, foods and medicines is also recommended.

Irritable Bowel Syndrome

Irritable bowel syndrome (IBS) is a condition whereby the large bowel does not function properly. IBS is called a "syndrome," not a disease, because it is really a group of symptoms, which may include abdominal pain or discomfort, bloating, chronic constipation or diarrhea and mucous in the stool.

There is no specific medical test for IBS—just the identification of symptoms. Women may be more symptomatic during their menstrual periods. There is also no cure for IBS, but nutritional strategies include avoiding foods that trigger symptoms, such as carbonated beverages, dairy products and fatty foods; eating smaller, more frequent meals and snacks; and increasing fiber through fruits, vegetables and whole grains.

Lactose Intolerance

Lactose intolerance is the inability to digest foods and beverages that contain the milk sugar lactose. Lactose intolerance may cause bloating, cramping, diarrhea, gas or general ill-feeling. Lactose is in the majority of dairy foods and daily products, but in varying amounts, and in ingredients such as curds, whey, dried milk, dried milk solids, milk by-products and powdered milk. Lactose may also be added to prepared foods such as breads, cereals, frozen entrees, luncheon meats, dry mixes for baked goods and salad dressings.

Some people may be able to consume a small amount of foods or beverages with lactose—especially where the milk sugar is partially broken down, as in yogurt, cottage cheese and Swiss cheese. This is very individualized and may require self-testing. Lactose-reduced and lactose-free products are available, as are lactase enzyme caplets or drops that are taken before meals.

Adequate calcium and vitamin D are concerns for people with lactose intolerance when dairy milk and milk products are limited. Many foods can provide calcium, vitamin D and other nutrients found in dairy products, including fish with small bones, leafy green vegetables and fortified soy foods and fruit juices. More information about lactose intolerance can be found in Chapter 4 and in the following section on cooking for people with gastrointestinal diseases.

Ulcers

Peptic ulcers are sores or wounds that form in the stomach. If they form in the upper part of the small intestine, they are called *duodenal ulcers*. Peptic ulcers are very common. They develop as a result of uncontrolled acid production in the stomach and changes in a person's immune system. Most peptic ulcers are caused by a bacterial infection, certain medications or smoking. In 1982, physicians Barry Marshall and Robin Warren discovered that *Helicobacter pylori (H. pylori)* bacteria caused an infection, which, in turn, caused peptic ulcers. They won a Nobel Prize for their discovery.

Peptic ulcers may be caused by the combination of *H. pylori* infection and the level of stomach acid. Bacteria weaken the protective coating of the stomach and upper small intestine, and stomach acid then permeates the sensitive tissues that line the digestive system; bacteria and acid directly irritate this lining, which results in sores or ulcers.

Ulcers can also be caused by nonsteroidal anti-inflammatory drugs (NSAIDs) that are taken to treat long-term, painful conditions such as arthritis; pain relievers, such as aspirin or ibuprofen, that are used to treat inflammation; smoking, which causes the stomach to produce more acid; alcohol, which wears down the lining of the stomach and intestines; and, in certain instances, severe emotional or physical stress.

The most common symptom of an ulcer is stomach pain between the breastbone and the crest of the stomach, which may occur a few hours after eating. Pain can also be sensed when the stomach is empty, such

TABLE 9-8 Dietary Approaches to Manage Gastrointestinal Diseases

Gastrointestinal Diseases	Dietary Approaches
Bacteria and foodborne illness	Proper food handling
Celiac disease	Gluten-free diet (no barley, rye or wheat)
Colon polyps	Decreased alcohol and fat; increased fiber
Diverticulosis and diverticulitis	Increased fiber from fruits, vegetables and whole grains
Gastritis	Decreased alcohol; proper food handling
Irritable bowel syndrome	Decreased carbonated beverages, dairy products and fat; increased fiber; small meals
Lactose intolerance	Decreased or no dairy products
Ulcers	Decreased acid and alcohol; proper food handling

as during the night or early in the morning. Pain may be alleviated by consuming foods or beverages or by taking antacids.

Other symptoms of an ulcer may include a bloody or blackish bowel movement, frequent burping or hiccupping, loss of appetite, nausea, vomiting and/or weight loss. Untreated ulcers may cause a fissure or crack in the digestive system and chronic bleeding, which can lead to anemia and, if there is serious internal bleeding, death.

H. pylori bacteria are transmitted from person to person through feces, food, saliva, vomit or water. The best advice for ulcer prevention is hand washing, cleaning and washing food, and ensuring that water is safe to drink.

DIETARY STRATEGIES TO MANAGE GASTROINTESTINAL DISEASES

A combination of the right diet and a healthy gastrointestinal tract delivers nutrients to the cells, prevents nutritional deficiencies, maintains normal intestinal function, repairs and restores damage to the gastrointestinal tract, and establishes intestinal bacteria and immune functions.

413

The amount of food, frequency of eating and composition of the diet all may impact gastrointestinal health. The right diet can also affect the management and recovery from chronic gastrointestinal diseases. The converse is also true: the wrong diet may cause or aggravate gastrointestinal diseases. The best dietary approaches to help manage gastrointestinal diseases are summarized in Table 9-8.

DIETARY GUIDELINES FOR PEOPLE WITH GASTROINTESTINAL DISORDERS

These general dietary guidelines provide a collective approach for the management of gastrointestinal diseases and their broad spectrum of disorders.

Avoid:

- Alcohol and caffeine, which affect the nerve endings of the gastrointestinal tract.
- Fructose (fruit sugar) and sorbitol (sugar alcohol), particularly if they are both used in the same recipe. Fructose can be found in soda and many fruit juice drinks; sorbitol can be found in chewing gum, candy, diet products, popsicles and some medications.
- Foods with guar gum or cellulose gum, if they cause sensitivity. Guar gum is used to thicken and stabilize dressings and sauces and improve the moisture retention in baked goods. Cellulose gum is used in instant beverages, where it provides texture; in baked goods, where it prevents staling; and in ice-cream.
- Spicy foods, until symptoms are resolved.

Consume with care:

- Jerusalem artichokes, leeks, legumes, lentils, onions, peas and potatoes, since they may have a laxative-like effect.
- Refined starches, such as rice and pasta, since they may be constipating.
- Bell peppers, broccoli and cabbage, since they may be gas-forming and cause pain.

Consume:

- Five or six small meals daily with adequate water, which may be better tolerated than three larger meals.
- Fiber in gradual amounts to allow the gut time to adjust without nerve sensitivity and to prevent a laxative-like effect.

Minimize:

- High-fat foods, particularly those with saturated fat from high-fat meats and dairy products.

Consider:

- Over-the-counter enzyme products before meals to help rectify some gastrointestinal discomfort. Make sure to first discuss this consideration with a health care provider.

GUIDELINES FOR COOKING FOR PEOPLE WITH GASTROINTESTINAL DISORDERS

These general guidelines are designed for cooking for people with gastrointestinal diseases and their broad spectrum of disorders.

If a person is restricted to a liquid diet:

- Prepare only clear liquids, such as nourishing broth or stock; fruit, meat or vegetable-flavored gelatin; ices; or strained juices.
- Prepare five to six liquid "minimeals" such as these to prevent dehydration.

If a person is restricted to a soft diet:

- Explore methods to make soft-textured foods more appetizing.
- Make each meal visually appealing to compensate for lack of texture.

If a person is restricted to a regular bland diet:

- Serve food warm, rather than too hot or too cold.
- Remove pits, seeds and skins.

Regular bland diets are often recommended after stomach or intestinal surgery. They allow the digestive tract time to heal before reintroducing more difficult-to-digest foods.

If a person is restricted to a strict bland diet:

- Divide main meals into five to six small minimeals.
- Use only tender protein foods.
- Do not serve fruit juice alone between meals.

Strict bland diets often limit breaded, fibrous, fried, heavily seasoned and/or processed protein foods and favor softer protein foods, such as eggs, smooth peanut butter and/or tofu.

If a person has undergone gastrointestinal surgery:

- Restrict highly seasoned and fried foods.
- Limit fluids; avoid alcoholic beverages.
- Keep high-fiber foods at a minimum until recovery.

If a person needs more roughage (fiber):

- Gradually add fruits, legumes, vegetables and whole grains.
- Progressively add more fluids.

In general, cooking for people with gastrointestinal disorders should be highly individualized. Nutrition and culinary specialists should integrate the range of nutritional needs with food and beverage preferences for maximum effectiveness.

FOOD BYTE

Some folk remedies suggest that a warm cup of dairy milk and honey consumed before bedtime soothes stomach ailments. While other folk remedies have stood the test of time (such as the medicinal use of certain herbs and spices), this rumored gastrointestinal pain reliever may do more harm than good. Dairy milk can actually *cause* acid reflux during sleep. But the real root of nightly gastrointestinal disturbances may be grounded in overconsuming dinner. Eating too much at dinner may cause the stomach to produce more acid. While drinking milk (especially higher-fat varieties) may seem like a quick fix, milk has rebound action that may cause more stomach acid to be secreted, in addition to acid reflux. Though nighttime eating is generally discouraged, a smaller dinner and a simple after-dinner snack might be easier on the gastrointestinal tract than milk alone [58].

Allergies and Intolerances

OVERVIEW, DIET AND FOOD MODIFICATIONS

An *allergy* is an immune system disorder. An *allergic reaction* occurs when a substance in the environment, known as an *allergen*, causes a reaction by the body. Common allergic reactions include asthma, eczema, food allergies, hay fever, hives and the venom of stinging insects, such as bees and wasps.

An allergic reaction is characterized by the excessive activation of white blood cells, or *mast cells*, by an antibody known as *immunoglobulin E (IgE)*. IgE is a type of protein that circulates through the blood and causes an extreme inflammatory response. Mast cells are specific cells that occur in all body tissues but especially in areas of the body where allergic reactions occur, including the nose and throat, lungs, gastrointestinal tract and skin.

A *food allergy*, or *hypersensitivity*, is a reaction to a substance in a food or beverage. The ability of a person to form IgE against the allergens in foods or beverages is often inherited. There are eight confirmed food allergens: eggs, fish, dairy milk, peanuts, shellfish, soy, tree nuts and wheat. Certain fruits, vegetables and seeds also act as food allergens to some people.

Children with food allergies to eggs, dairy milk, soy and wheat may outgrow these allergies. Allergies to fish, peanuts and tree nuts often endure throughout life. A shellfish allergy may develop during later childhood or adulthood. An allergy to shellfish is the most common food allergy among adults. The most severe and often fatal food allergies are from peanuts and tree nuts.

Before an allergic reaction to a food or beverage occurs, a person first has to be exposed to the allergen in the food or beverage. Because this food or beverage is digested, it triggers the production of IgE in large amounts, which attaches to the surfaces of the mast cells. The next time a person consumes the same food or beverage, it interacts with IgE and triggers the cells to release certain chemicals, including histamine.

Histamine and other chemicals dilate blood vessels and make the vessel walls abnormally permeable. If histamine is released in the ears, nose or throat, then breathing, itching and swallowing problems may occur. If it is released in the gastrointestinal tract, then abdominal pain or diarrhea may occur. If it is released in the skin, then eczema or hives may occur.

It is very important for people to identify potential food allergies because they can cause serious illness and, in some cases, death. If there is no family history and no knowledge of food allergies, then early reactions can be hazardous. If there is family history, the best advice is avoidance of suspected allergens through careful label reading and inquiry. To help this effort, the Food Allergen Labeling and Consumer Protection Act (FALCPA), established in January 2006, requires that food manufacturers disclose in plain language the top eight food allergens in food products.

A *food intolerance* is nonallergic food or beverage hypersensitivity. It is different from a food allergy. A food intolerance does not cause an abnormal response to protein in foods and beverages, though some of the symptoms may be similar. Symptoms of food intolerance may include bloating, cramping, diarrhea, headaches, heartburn, irritability, nausea, nervousness, stomach pain and/or vomiting.

Food intolerances are more common than food allergies. Nearly everyone has had an unpleasant reaction to something they ate at one time or another. Lactose intolerance is the most common food intolerance.

A person may have a lactose or wheat intolerance and experience uncomfortable gastrointestinal symptoms, but the symptoms may not be abnormal like a food allergy and they may not be triggered by the immune system. Furthermore, the symptoms may not be life-threatening. This is not to dismiss their importance or sometimes lifelong discomfort.

DIETARY STRATEGIES AND GUIDELINES FOR COOKING FOR PEOPLE WITH FOOD ALLERGIES

There are a number of steps that nutrition and culinary specialists can take to eliminate food allergens in cooking and baking and reduce food sensitivities, including the following:

- **Know what food allergens must be avoided.** If cooking for friends, it is easy to ask about food restrictions. If cooking for guests, inquire about any food allergies or sensitivities in advance. If cooking for customers, instruct the waitstaff to inquire about food allergies and sensitivities in advance of food orders. In each circumstance, have descriptions of recipes and ingredients handy.
- **Be aware of allergen cross-contamination.** *Cross-contamination* occurs when a food allergen is transferred to a food or beverage that does not originally contain this substance. It may cause neighboring foods and/or beverages to be dangerous to consume.

Cross-contamination may occur during food manufacturing if production and packaging equipment are common; during retail sales if presentation and storage space is common; during food service and home use through handling, equipment and utensils—especially, if common, when there is poor food sanitation.

- **Do not serve food "family style."** When preparing and serving allergen-free food, make sure guests or customers do not share or trade containers, dishes, food, or utensils and that they are free of residue. Minute allergen particles may adhere and cause allergic reactions.

There is also a chance that these particles adhere to hands or clothing and are unconsciously transferred to allergic guests or customers. Frequent hand washing is required while working with food allergens and before and after one eats. While disposable food preparation gloves are an option, these, too can become contaminated and must be changed after each use.

- **Keep all surfaces clean and, if possible, restricted for certain foods.** Surfaces that are used for the preparation and service of meals must be properly cleaned and sanitized. In preparation areas, the work surface, all utensils, and pots and pans must be washed with hot soapy water. Soap deactivates proteins that cause allergies.

Work surfaces, counters and cutting surfaces must be thoroughly cleaned between uses. A color-coded cutting board system can minimize cross-contamination risks. Use a separate food slicer for meats and cheeses. Wash trays after each use, since oils and minute particles can seep through liners and cross-contaminate food.

- **Read product labels carefully.** Be aware that there are many terms for food allergens, including dairy milk (whey), wheat (semolina) and egg (albumin), as shown in Table 9-9. While some are common, others

TABLE 9-9 Food Allergen Labeling

Common and Other Terms for Food Allergens

Dairy	
Common	butter, buttermilk, condensed milk, cottage cheese, cream, cheese, custard, dry milk powder and solids, evaporated milk, ghee, goat milk and cheese, half-and-half, malted milk, nougat, paneer (Indian cheese), pudding, sour cream, sweetened condensed milk, whipped cream, yogurt
Other	acidophilus, calcium caseinate, casein, curds, delactosed whey, demineralized whey, hydrolyzed milk protein, iron caseinate, lactalbumin phosphate, lactalbumin, lactoferrin, lactoglobulin, lactose sodium caseinate, lactulose, magnesium caseinate, milk solids, potassium caseinate, rennet casein, whey and whey protein concentrate

Eggs	
Common	albumin, cholesterol-free egg substitute, dried egg and egg solids, mayonnaise, meringue and meringue powder, powdered eggs, egg whites, egg yolks, egg wash, eggnog, fat substitutes, globulin
Other	apovitellin livetin, lysozyme, ovalbumin, ovoglobulin, ovomucoid, ovomucin, ovotransferrin, ovovitelia, ovovitellin, silici albuminate, simplesse®, vitellin

(Continued)

TABLE 9-9 (Continued)

Common and Other Terms for Food Allergens

Fish

Common	anchovies, caviar and roe, Caesar salad dressing, deli meats and hot dogs (with gelatin), steak sauce, gelatin, marinara sauce (anchovies), marshmallows, omega-3 supplements, salad dressings, sushi, Worcestershire sauce
Other	bouillabaisse (fish soup or stew), caponata (eggplant and anchovy relish), ceviche (acid-marinated fish), cioppino (fish soup or stew), fumet (fish stock), kamaboko (fish cakes), nam pla and nuoc mâm (fish sauce), pissaladière (tart with anchovies), surimi (ground reformed fish), taramasalata (fish roe spread)

Peanuts

Common	Asian prepared foods, beer nuts, cold-pressed peanut oil, eggs rolls, glazes and marinades, goober peas, ground nuts, mandelonas (peanuts soaked in almond flavoring), Mexican prepared foods, meat substitutes, mixed nuts, monkey nuts, nutmeat and nut pieces, peanut butter, peanut butter chips, peanut butter morsels, peanut flour, peanut paste, peanut syrup, potato pancakes, sauces (chili sauce, gravy, hot sauce, mole, pesto), salad dressings, sweets (cookies, hot chocolate, puddings), Spanish and Virginia peanuts
Other	arachis (peanut) oil, hydrolyzed plant and vegetable proteins, hypogaeic acid

Shellfish

Common	abalone, clams (cherrystone, littleneck, pismo, quahog), cockles (periwinkle, sea urchin), crab, crawfish (crayfish, ecrevisse), lobster (langouste, langousine, scampi, coral, tomalley), mollusks, mussels, octopus, oysters, prawns, shrimp (crevette), snails (escargot), squid (calamari)
Other	Bouillabaisse, fish stock, seafood flavorings (such as crab, clam extract), surimi

Soy

Common	edamame (soybeans in pods), hydrolyzed soy protein, lecithin, miso (fermented soybean paste), soy and soybeans (albumin, soy butter, soy curd, soy concentrate, soy fiber, soy flour, soy formula, soy grain, soy grits, soy milk, soy nuts, soy oil, soy paste, soy sauce, soy sprouts), soy protein isolate, soya flour, tamari, tempeh, teriyaki sauce, texturized soy flour, texturized soy protein, texturized vegetable protein (TVP), tofu
Other	kinako (roasted soybean flour), kyodofu (freeze-dried tofu), natto (fermented soybeans), okara (soy pulp), shoyu (soy sauce), supro (soy protein isolate), yakidofu (grilled tofu), yuba (bean curd)

Tree nuts

Common	almond, beechnut, Brazil nut, bush nut, butternut, cashew, chestnut, coconut, filbert, ginko nut, hazelnut, hickory nut, lichee nut, macadamia nut, nangai nut, pecan, pine nut, pistachio, shea nut, walnut
Other	almond paste, anacardiam nuts, artificial nuts, barbecue sauce, breading, caponata, chinquapin, gianduja, honey, Indian nut, karite (shea nut), mandelonas (peanuts soaked in almond flavoring), marzipan, mashuga nuts, natural and artificial flavoring, natural nut extract (e.g., almond or vanilla extract), nougat, Nu-Nuts®, nut butters (e.g., almond or cashew butter), mortadella (may contain pistachios), nut meal, Nutella®, nutmeat, nut oil (e.g., almond or walnut oil), nut paste, nut pieces, pancakes, pasta, pesto, pie crusts, pili nut, pine nut variations (Indian, pigndi, pigñolia, pignon, pinon, piñon, pinyon), salads and salad dressings, vegetarian "burgers", walnut variations (English, Persian, black, Japanese, California)

Wheat

Common	bran, bread (made with wheat flours), bread crumbs, bulgur, cereal extract, couscous, crackers, cracked wheat, cracker meal, farina, flour (also all-purpose [AP], bread flour, cake flour, durum flour, enriched flour, graham flour, high-gluten flour, high-protein flour, instant flour, pastry flour, plain flour, self-rising flour, soft wheat flour, steel ground flour, stone ground flour, unbleached flour, wheat flour, white flour, whole wheat flour, germ), gluten, malt and malt extract, matzo (also matzoh, matzah, matza, matsa, matso), matzo meal (also matzoh meal, matzah meal, matza meal, matsa meal, matso meal, matsah meal and matsoh meal), noodles, pasta, semolina, wheat, wheat berries, wheat bran, wheat germ, wheat gluten, wheat grass, wheat malt, wheat starch, wheat sprouts, whole wheat, whole wheat berries
Other	ancient grains (spelt, einkorn, triticale, emmer), bromated flour, phosphated flour, fu (wheat gluten), kamut (related to durum), seitan (wheat gluten), tabbouleh (wheat salad). Amaranth, quinoa, buckwheat, millet and teff are ancient grains, but gluten-free.

417

are less familiar. If an ingredient list shows that a product "may contain" a particular allergen, it is best to avoid it. If an ingredient is not recognizable, then check it out with a health care provider, the Food Allergy and Anaphylaxis Network at http://www.foodallergy.org, or the Kids with Food Allergies Foundation at http://www.kidswithfoodallergies.org before using.

Manufacturers may occasionally change their recipes and use different ingredients in order to create distinctive varieties of the same brand. Also, products may carry different labeling or precautionary warnings in different languages for foreign distribution. Be especially careful to review these labels for potential allergens.

- **Find safe ingredients**. Locating allergy-free ingredients for allergen-free recipes may be challenging. The Food Allergy and Anaphylaxis Network is a reliable starting point. Specialty diet food manufacturers have developed worldwide to meet the food and nutrition needs of allergic people. It is best to scrutinize their websites (if available) and food labels and ask questions through their consumer hotlines before use.
- **Adapt favorite recipes for food allergies, intolerances and sensitivities**. Become acquainted with "safe" ingredients that can be incorporated into allergy-free recipes. These substitutes have the best chance of producing allergy-free dishes that taste and look like the originals. If the recipes do not perform well after using these ingredients, then it is probably best to try different recipes altogether.

Allergy-free cooking requires a very creative approach and openness to new ingredients and foods with new applications. Allergens can be omitted while the essence of the food or recipe is preserved. For instance, pureed cauliflower can substitute for cheese sauce; flaxseeds can substitute for ground nuts or peanuts; coarse bread crumbs can substitute for pine nuts in pesto; and soy or rice "milk" can substitute for dairy milk.

- **Determine the role of food allergens in recipes**. Among the eight confirmed food allergens—eggs, fish, dairy milk, peanuts, shellfish, soy, tree nuts and wheat—the food allergens that are essential to cooking and baking are eggs, dairy milk and wheat.

While it is possible to prepare acceptable allergen-free versions of some recipes, meringues without eggs, ice cream without dairy cream, and bread without wheat flour may produce different aroma, taste and texture—and unsure acceptance.

It is safer to select recipes where eggs, dairy milk and wheat are the secondary ingredients and can be substituted without sacrificing a recipe's success. Then it is a matter of trial and error until the right amounts of allergy-free ingredients create the best results.

For example, in recipes that call for batter, flour is typically used to coat fish, meat or vegetables. A little egg, buttermilk or reduced-fat milk with herbs and seasonings may provide just enough coating.

In recipes that require sauce, flour is frequently used for thickening. Pureed plain-tasting vegetables may provide the right amount of thickness without sacrificing taste.

- **Consider the nutrients in the ingredients that are substituted or omitted**. Egg whites are mostly protein and water, much like dairy milk or tofu, and wheat flour is mostly protein and starch. These nutrients are required for the success of recipes—not the ingredients themselves.

If egg whites or wheat flour is eliminated from a recipe, consider which ingredients can be substituted for the protein, water and starch that they contribute. Substituting fruit puree for egg whites or soy flour for wheat flour may not take their nutrient functions into account. Some gluten-free flour blends approximate all-purpose flour, but not all gluten-free baking powders and baking sodas are effective.

- **Have an emergency plan handy for allergic guests and customers, including staff training**. Severe and fatal allergies often emerge very suddenly and require immediate attention. With food allergies on the rise, particularly in children, it is essential that food service operations have an emergency plan for handling allergic customers and that customers have an awareness of the severity and progression of allergic reactions.

The National Restaurant Association at http://www.restaurant.org is an important resource for staff training. The US Food and Drug Administration provides resources on food allergens at http://www.fda.gov/Food/ResourcesForYou/Consumers/SelectedHealthTopics/ucm119075.htm.

FOOD BYTE

As the incidence of food-related allergies and sensitivities increases in the United States, explanations have been sought. The "hygiene hypothesis" suggests that we live in an ultra-clean society where our immune system no longer has to defend the body against childhood infections. According to this hypothesis, the immune system is acting in "allergic readiness" state instead of one that is "infection fighting." The majority of US children no longer grow up on farms around livestock and plants and are given multiple antibiotics and immunizations. As a result, they have less exposure to environmental allergens. This may be just one of the complex reasons why the immune system has shifted from managing life-threatening infections to handling allergy-alertness and why allergies are on the rise [59].

SERVE IT FORTH

Table 9-10 shows a typical weekly menu that one might find at cafes and roadside diners where people eat around-the-clock. There is an adjacent lounge where alcohol is available at dinner and early evening. Use this menu to address the nutrition and disease issues that are raised in the following three scenarios.

1a. The American Heart Association has decided to target the menus of roadside diners throughout the United States to help make them more heart healthy. Travelers who stop at these diners often seek quick

TABLE 9-10 Cafe or Diner Menu

	Breakfast	Lunch	Dinner	Snacks
Monday	Canned fruit cup Mini sweet rolls Coffee or tea	Chicken salad Potato chips Fruit drink	Fried fish French fries Mixed vegetables Beer	Chocolate bar Soft drink
Tuesday	Applesauce Coffee cake Coffee or tea	Macaroni and cheese Tossed salad Apple juice	Chicken Parmesan Pasta marinara Bread sticks Red wine	Fruit cup Brownie Sparkling water
Wednesday	Orange segments Sausage and egg sandwich Hot chocolate	Turkey pot pie Biscuit Sweetened ice tea	Blackened catfish Dirty rice Green beans Soft drink	Hot dog on bun with condiments Coleslaw Milkshake
Thursday	Banana Chocolate chip waffles Orange juice	Chef's salad Ranch dressing Grape drink	Grilled minute steak Baked potato Creamed corn Mixed drink	Taco Corn chips with salsa Lemonade

Friday	Grapes
	Ham and cheese
	  omelet
	Tomato juice
		BLT
		Sweet potato fries
		
		Soft drink
			Smothered chicken
			Baked beans
			Canned corn
			Fruit punch
				Cheese and
				  crackers
				Beer

Saturday	Grapefruit Egg and cheese muffin Specialty coffee	Fish sticks Potato nuggets Yogurt drink	Shrimp scampi Linguine Garlic bread White wine	Chips and dip Mixed drink
Sunday	Berries Pancakes and bacon Smoothie	Pork chop suey Fried rice Almond cookies Tea	Hamburger Steak fries Tomato and lettuce Beer	Energy bar Sports drink

and filling meals. You have been hired as a nutrition and culinary specialist to improve the menu in Table 9-10 by following the AHA diet and lifestyle recommendations that are summarized below.

- ○ What would you advise to improve the diner menu? Support your comments.
- ○ Address each of the AHA recommendations and incorporate specific foods and beverages in your responses.

AMERICAN HEART ASSOCIATION DIET AND LIFESTYLE RECOMMENDATIONS

- Use up at least as many calories as are taken in.
- Eat a variety of nutritious foods from all the food groups.
- Choose foods like vegetables, fruits, whole-grain products and fat-free or low-fat dairy products most often.
- Eat fish at least twice a week.
- Eat less nutrient-poor foods.
- Choose lean meats and poultry without skin; prepare without added saturated and trans fats.
- Select fat-free, 1% fat and low-fat dairy products.
- Cut back on foods containing partially hydrogenated vegetable oils to reduce trans fats.
- Cut back on foods and beverages that are high in cholesterol; consume less than 300 milligrams of dietary cholesterol daily.
- Cut back on beverages and foods with added sugars.
- Choose and prepare foods with little or no salt; aim to consume less than 1,500 milligrams of sodium daily.
- If you drink alcohol, drink in moderation: one drink daily for women and two drinks daily for men.
- Follow the American Heart Association recommendations when eating out and watch portion sizes [60].

2a. The American Diabetes Association wants to target cafes to help control the rise of diabetes in the United States. Some of these cafes are owned or operated by major food service corporations to help control costs. In additional to providing healthy menus, the ADA wants to offer economical food choices.

You have been hired as a nutrition and culinary specialist to improve the menu in Table 9-10 by following the ADA tips for making healthy food choices that are summarized below. You are also contracted to recommend economical food choices.

- ○ What would you advise to improve the cafe menus? Support your comments.
- ○ Address each of the ADA tips for making healthy food choices and incorporate specific foods and beverages in your responses.
- ○ What would you recommend for economical food choices?

AMERICAN DIABETES ASSOCIATION TIPS FOR MAKING HEALTHY FOOD CHOICES

- Eat lots of vegetables and fruits; pick from the rainbow of colors available to maximize variety.
- Eat non-starchy vegetables, such as spinach, carrots, broccoli or green beans.
- Choose whole grain foods over processed grain products.
- Include dried beans (like kidney or pinto beans) and lentils in meals.
- Include fish in meals 2-3 times weekly.
- Choose lean meats, like cuts that end in "loin," such as pork loin and sirloin. Remove poultry skin.
- Choose non-fat dairy products, such as skim dairy milk, non-fat yogurt and non-fat cheese.
- Choose water and calorie-free "diet" drinks instead of regular soda, fruit punch, sweet tea and other sugar-sweetened drinks.
- Choose liquid oils for cooking instead of solid fats that can be high in saturated and *trans* fats.
- Cut back on high-calorie snack foods and desserts.
- Watch your portion sizes; eating too much of even healthful foods can lead to weight gain [61].

3a. The American Cancer Society wants to try to reduce the incidence of cancer in the civil service organizations throughout the US (city governments, police and fire departments, etc.). The ACS has initiated smoking cessation programs, but now it wants to tackle dietary factors. Many of these civil service organizations are located by cafeterias.

420

The ACS has hired you to revise the menu shown in Table 9-10 to one that is more cancer protective for these cafeterias. The ACS would also like you to generate a cancer-protective grocery list that is based on this revised menu. You are to use the ACS Guidelines on Nutrition and Physical Activity for Cancer Prevention that are summarized below.

○ What would you advise to improve the cafeteria menus? Support your comments.
○ Address each of the ACS guidelines and incorporate specific foods and beverages in your responses.
○ What would you include on a cancer-protective grocery list?

AMERICAN CANCER SOCIETY GUIDELINES ON NUTRITION AND PHYSICAL ACTIVITY FOR CANCER PREVENTION

- Maintain a healthy weight throughout life.
  —Balance calorie intake with physical activity.
  —Avoid excessive weight gain throughout life.
  —Achieve and maintain a healthy weight if currently overweight or obese.
- Eat a healthy diet, with an emphasis on plant sources.
  —Choose foods and drinks in amounts that help achieve and maintain a healthy weight.
  —Eat five or more servings of a variety of vegetables and fruits daily.
  —Choose whole grains over processed (refined) grains.
  —Limit intake of processed and red meats.
- If you drink alcoholic beverages, limit your intake.
  —Drink no more than one drink per day for women or two drinks per day for men[62].

Also:
- Adopt a physically active lifestyle.

  —Adults: Engage in at least 30 minutes of moderate to vigorous physical activity, above usual activities, on five or more days of the week; 45 to 60 minutes of intentional physical activity are preferable.
  —Children and adolescents: Engage in at least 60 minutes per day of moderate to vigorous physical activity at least five days per week.

Three additional activities can be found within the *Culinary Nutrition* website at www.culinarynutrition.elsevier.com.

WHAT'S COOKING?

1. Exploring protein in different flours and gluten development
   Objectives
   ○ To discover the "skeleton" protein that supports baked goods
   ○ To compare and contrast different flours and gluten development
   ○ To apply this information to gluten-free baking
   Equipment
   3 medium bowls, 1 small sauté pan, 1 (12-cup) nonstick muffin tin, 1 large spoon, 1 spatula, measuring cups, measuring spoons, flour sifter, waxed paper, electric or hand mixer, oven
   Procedure
   Part 1: Prepare the following muffin recipe:
   Muffins Prepared with All-purpose and Cake Flour
   Nonfat cooking spray
   1 cup all-purpose flour
   1 cup cake flour (not self-rising)
   3 tablespoons sugar
   3 teaspoons baking powder
   1½ teaspoons salt
   3 tablespoons butter
   1 cup dairy milk
   3 eggs

1. Preheat oven to 350°F.
2. Prepare nonstick muffin tin with nonfat cooking spray.
3. Sift 1 cup all-purpose flour onto waxed paper.
4. Resift into medium bowl with 1 tablespoon sugar, 1 teaspoon baking powder and ½ teaspoon salt.
5. Repeat same process with cake flour.
6. Melt 1 tablespoon butter in saute pan; cool.
7. Beat ⅓ cup milk with 1 egg in medium bowl; add butter.
8. Mix milk-egg-butter mixture with all-purpose flour mixture just until moist.
9. Beat with electric or hand mixer until smooth.
10. Repeat same process with cake flour.
11. Put all-purpose flour batter into 4 muffin cups on one side of muffin tin.
12. Put cake-flour batter into 4 muffin cups on opposite side of muffin tin; leave empty muffin cups down the center. (Remember on which side you placed each batter.)
13. Bake about 15 minutes, or until muffin tops are lightly browned.
14. Remove from oven; place on wire rack to cool slightly (5–10 minutes); remove from muffin tin.
    Yield = 8 muffins (½ from all-purpose flour and ½ from cake flour).

Evaluation

Cut in half one muffin that was made from all-purpose flour muffin and one muffin that was made from cake flour. Compare their aroma, crumb, grain, taste, tenderness, tunnels and any other similarities and/or differences. What can you conclude? Use the following Data Sheet.

Data Sheet

Muffin type	Aroma	Crumb	Grain	Taste	Tenderness	Tunnels	Other
All-purpose flour							
Cake flour							

Some flour does not contain any gluten, while other flour contains a lot of gluten. Wheat flour does not truly contain gluten but contains two substances that convert into gluten under the right circumstances. All-purpose wheat flour has more gluten than cake flour; that is why the muffins have different structure and texture.

A gluten-free flour, such as soy flour, cannot be substituted in the same proportion to wheat flour in a recipe with the expectation that it reproduces the structure and texture of wheat flour. This is why a combination of gluten-free flour and starch is needed to build the support that wheat flour alone supplies. The following flour blend is an all-purpose mixture of gluten-free flours and starches that is good for cookies, cornbread, piecrust, pizza crust, sandwich bread and scones.

Gluten-Free Rice Flour Blend

1 cup brown rice flour
1 cup arrowroot starch/flour or cornstarch
⅔ cup sorghum flour
⅓ cup corn flour (not cornmeal)

Part 2: Repeat the muffin recipe above by using 1 cup of this **Gluten-Free Rice Flour Blend** in place of 1 cup of wheat flour. Compare and contrast the aroma, crumb, grain, taste, tenderness and tunnels and other characteristics of these muffins to those that are made with all-purpose flour and cake flour. What can be concluded about products that are made with gluten-free baking blends as opposed to all-purpose flour or cake flour that contains gluten?

Culinary applications

How can this information be applied to gluten-free diets? Food product and recipe development?"

2. **Cooking vegetables for sensitive stomachs**
   Objectives
   ○ To become aware of cellulose, a fibrous structure in plants
   ○ To observe the different states that cause cellulose to soften
   ○ To apply this information to cooking for gastrointestinal disorders

Equipment

Acorn or butternut squash, water, 1 teaspoon vinegar, ½ teaspoon baking soda, vegetable parer, sharp paring knife, chef's knife, cutting board, measuring spoons, teaspoon, fork, slotted spoon, 3 saucepans, stove top

Procedure

1. Cut squash in half on cutting board with chef's knife.
2. Peel squash with vegetable parer and/or paring knife on cutting board.
3. Remove squash seeds with teaspoon.
4. Cut squash into uniform 1-inch cubes with chef's knife.
5. Divide squash among three saucepans; cover squash with water.
6. Place 1 teaspoon of vinegar in the first saucepan, ½ teaspoon of baking soda in the second saucepan, and do not put anything in the third saucepan.
7. Heat each saucepan to the same temperature, and bring each saucepan to a boil at the same time.
8. Continue boiling until the squash softens in each of the saucepans (it will likely be at different times).
9. Record these times and note your observations on the Data Sheet as shown:

Data Sheet

Squash samples	Boiling time to soften (10, 15, 20 minutes, etc.)	Observations
Squash #1 *plus 1 teaspoon vinegar*		
Squash #2 *plus ½ teaspoon baking soda*		
Squash #3 *without any addition*		

Evaluation

1. Remove one piece of squash from each of the saucepans about every 10 to 15 minutes to test for softness. Use the back of a fork to try to mash these pieces.
2. Record your observations.
3. Rate the order in which the pieces of squash become tender.
4. Does the vinegar (an acid) speed up or slow down the softening rate?
5. Does the baking soda (a base) speed up or slow down the softening rate?
6. What is the effect of cooking the squash in plain water?
7. What do you think would happen if the squash was cooked in salted water?

The length of cooking time for vegetables depends on the amount of cellulose that a plant contains. Foods with more cellulose generally will take a longer time to cook.

Some gastrointestinal diseases first require a "soft" diet and then might switch to a higher-fiber diet. Based on this experiment, if you were to create a soft diet for someone with a sensitive gastrointestinal tract, would you choose spinach or celery, and why? How would you cook these vegetables, and why? Which vegetables would you choose for a higher-fiber diet? How would you cook these vegetables, and why?

Culinary applications

How can this information be applied to food product and recipe development?

3. **One cake two ways: baking with egg substitutes**

Objectives

○ To determine if a cake can be made with or without eggs
○ To observe a cake's quality by using different rising agents
○ To apply this information for people who cannot eat eggs

Equipment

Measuring cups, measuring spoons, 13 × 9 × 2-inch baking pan, large and medium bowls, medium saucepan, flour sifter, electric or hand mixer, large spoon or spatula, stove top, oven, toothpicks

Plus Clean set of ingredients for egg substitute recipe (see below)

Procedure

Part 1: Prepare the following **Golden Raisin Spice Cake** recipe; note volume and texture of the final product.

423

Golden Raisin Spice Cake

1 cup golden raisins
2 cups water
½ cup butter or vegetable shortening, *plus* additional to prepare baking pan
1 egg
1 teaspoon each allspice, cinnamon and cloves
1 teaspoon baking powder
¼ teaspoon salt
2 cups all-purpose flour, *plus* additional to prepare baking pan

1. Preheat oven to 350°F.
2. Prepare a 13×9×2-inch baking pan with butter and flour.
3. Simmer raisins in water in medium saucepan until water reduces to about 1 cup (about 10 to 15 minutes).
4. Sift allspice, cinnamon, cloves, baking powder, salt and flour together into large bowl; reserve.
5. Beat butter and egg with electric or hand mixer in medium bowl until creamy; reserve.
6. Alternately combine flour mixture and butter-egg mixture in large bowl.
7. Add raisins and raisin water; stir to blend.
8. Bake in prepared baking pan 25 to 30 minutes, or until toothpick in center comes out clean.

Part 2: Remake the cake using one or more of the following egg substitutes; note the volume and texture of the final product and any other differences.

When eggs are used as a binder (typically one egg per recipe), substitute:

○ 1 tablespoon ground flaxseed *plus* 3 tablespoons warm water
○ 1 tablespoon unflavored, unsweetened gelatin *plus* 3 tablespoons warm water
○ ¼ cup pureed soft tofu
○ 3 tablespoons pureed fruit (such as bananas, applesauce or prunes)

When used as a leavener (typically 2 to 3 eggs or more per recipe), substitute one of the following for *each egg* called for in the recipe:

○ 1 heaping tablespoon Ener-G-Food Egg Replacer* *plus* 2 tablespoons warm water
○ 1 heaping tablespoon baking powder *plus* 1 tablespoon vegetable oil *plus* 1 tablespoon warm water
○ 1 heaping tablespoon baking powder *plus* 1 tablespoon apple cider vinegar *plus* 1 tablespoon warm water

Evaluation

Some people need to reduce the number of whole eggs they consume because of their cholesterol content. Others need to eliminate eggs because of an egg allergy. Nevertheless, eggs are important in cooking and baking; it is difficult to eliminate them. Eggs provide color, richness and tenderness in recipes. Beaten egg whites provide volume and air. Eggs also act as binding and leavening agents. Eggs add protein and fat-soluble vitamins, among other nutrients.

When this **Golden Raisin Spice Cake** is made according to the original recipe, it contains both 1 whole egg plus 1 teaspoon of baking power for leavening. It should have normal rise and texture. By removing and substituting the egg, both the binding and leavening ability of the cake batter may be affected. Both functions should be taken into consideration when choosing an egg substitute.

Baking with egg substitutes is often a matter of trial and error to determine exactly which egg substitute can be used and in what quantity. This is why there is no one specific answer as to the best egg substitute for this recipe—or other recipes. If the combination that you chose did not work to your liking, a different combination might be more acceptable. Baking (and cooking) for allergies are matters of trial and error.

Culinary applications

How can this information be applied to food product and recipe development?

OVER EASY

The relationship among food, diet and disease is complicated and far from definitive. Though certain nutrients are associated with cardiovascular disease, diabetes, cancer, hypertension, digestive disorders and allergies, other nutrients are related to their cure.

* Presently, Ener-G-Food Egg Replacer can be obtained in some specialty food stores or at www.ener-g.com.

For example, higher-fat diets are linked to cardiovascular disease, while dietary fibers are used in its prevention. The dietary strategies for cardiovascular disease prevention have swung from high-carbohydrate diets to higher-protein diets. Dietary cholesterol, once thought to be highly contributory to cardiovascular disease, has yielded to saturated and trans fats.

The backlash is public skepticism about the relationship between food and health. But ignoring the precursors of disease may lead to early development, complications, and, in some instances, death. A case in point is diabetes. Obesity, poor blood sugar management, high dietary fats, inactivity and a host of other factors have contributed to the surge in adult-onset diabetes. The US public, however, is yet to be proactive to help curb this growing public health crisis.

Food and nutrition research dispels old beliefs and presents new possibilities. This research drives US government and association guidelines. The guidelines that the United States Department of Agriculture, the American Heart Association, the American Diabetes Association, and the American Cancer Society have developed over the years provide the best possible road maps for disease prevention.

Some food and nutrition guidelines are common to each of the diseases in this chapter. They may help people eat better, feel better, lose weight, ward off disease and maybe live longer. Here are some food and nutrition commonalities:

- Almonds and other nuts with monounsaturated fatty acids lower LDL cholesterol.
- Berries with colorful anthocyanin phytonutrients reduce inflammation and offer heart disease and cancer protection.
- Broccoli and other dark leafy green vegetables with antioxidants defend against certain cancers and protect the heart and brain.
- Legumes, peas and lentils with soluble fiber, plant proteins and B vitamins scavenge and eliminate cholesterol and lower homocysteine linked to heart disease and stroke.
- Dairy milk or lactose-free dairy milk with calcium and vitamin D lowers the risk of heart disease, diabetes and certain cancers and strengthens bone density.
- Red wine with phytonutrient resveratrol protects against heart disease and certain cancers and strengthens the immune system.
- Whole grains with insoluble and soluble fibers reduce the risks of diabetes, heart disease, stroke and certain cancers.
- Salmon and other fatty fish with omega-3 fatty acids decrease inflammation, lower heart disease risk, and lower the risk of certain cancers.
- Spices with phytochemicals keep the brain healthy, protect the heart, and control blood sugar.
- Decreased portion sizes control calories, overweight and obesity.

425

Incorporating these nutrient-rich health-promoting foods into products, recipes, meals and menus requires some paradigm shifts. It is true that some of these are higher in calories, such as salmon, or in carbohydrates, like legumes. Think "nutrient-rich foods" instead of labeling foods "good foods" or "bad foods." Focus on the big picture—the whole diet, not any one food or ingredient. When the basic diet is a good one, balanced in nutrients and moderate in calories, then occasional splurges are tolerated and add deliciousness and interest to meals. Perhaps the best advice about diet and disease is to lighten up. Less may be best for long-term disease prevention and health.

CHECK PLEASE

1. Atherosclerosis is characterized by:
- **a.** pain
- **b.** heart attack
- **c.** plaque
- **d.** old age
- **e.** genetics

2. Alterable risk factors of atherosclerosis include:
a. genetics
b. diet
c. activity
d. b and c
e. a, b and c

3. Phytosterols, which have the ability to reduce total blood cholesterol when consumed with a low-fat diet, can be found in:
a. beef
b. margarine
c. butter
d. fish
e. dairy milk

Essay Question

1. Describe three gastrointestinal disorders and five general guidelines for cooking for people with gastrointestinal disorders.

For additional questions, please see the *Culinary Nutrition* website at www.culinarynutrition.elsevier.com.

HUNGRY FOR MORE?

Allergies

The American Academy of Allergy, Asthma and Immunology   www.aaaai.org
The Food Allergy and Anaphylaxis Network   www.foodallergy.org
National Institute of Allergy and Infectious Diseases   www.niaid.nih.gov

Cancer

American Cancer Society   www.cancer.org
Gollman B, Pierce K. *The Phytopia Cookbook: A World of Plant-Centered Cuisine.* Dallas, TX: Phytopia, Inc. 1999.
Weihofen D, Marino C. *The Cancer Survival Cookbook: 200 Quick & Easy Recipes with Healthful Eating Tips.* Minneapolis, MN: Chronimed Publishing, 1998.

Diabetes

American Diabetes Association   www.diabetes.org
Diabetes Public Health Resource   www.cdc.gov/diabetes

Gastrointestinal Diseases

Celiac Disease Foundation   www.celiac.org
Gluten Intolerance Group of North America (GIG)   www.gluten.net
National Digestive Diseases Information Clearinghouse (NDDIC)   http://digestive.niddk.nih.gov

Heart Disease and Hypertension

American Heart Association   www.heart.org
The Cleveland Clinic—Heart & Vascular   http://my.clevelandclinic.org/heart
National Heart, Lung and Blood Institute (NHLBI)   www.nhlbi.nih.gov

Obesity

International Association for the Study of Obesity   www.iaso.org
The Obesity Society   www.obesity.org
Calorie Count (Online diet program)   www.calorie-count.com
FitDay (Diet and Weight Loss Journal)   http://www.fitday.com

TAKE AWAY
Traditional Chinese Medicine

Traditional Chinese medicine (TCM) is an assortment of traditional medical practices that originated in China thousands of years ago. While TCM is considered as the preferred primary medical treatment in Asia, it is mostly considered as complementary or alternative medicine in the Western world.

TCM treats the human body as a whole that is subdivided into several "systems of function," which are named after the anatomical organs. The Chinese term for these systems of function is *zang fu*. *Zang* is roughly translated as *solid organs* (the heart, liver, lung, kidney, pericardium and spleen), and *fu* is roughly translated as *hollow organs* (the gallbladder, large intestine and small intestine, stomach, urinary tract and bladder). Diseases are treated by manipulating these imbalanced systems through heat, herbs, needles, pressure, and so forth on or by sensitive body parts. The manipulation is to restore balance.

In TCM, health is considered a balance between yin and yang. *Yin* is cold, dark, feminine, negative, passive and wet, while *yang* is active, bright, dry, hot, masculine and positive. According to TCM, the interactions and balance between yin and yang in people and nature affect both their behavior and fate. These are the main components of TCM:

- *Acupuncture* regulates the free flow of blood, which is yin, and *qi*, or "vital energy," which is yang. Reportedly, acupuncture tones the body where there is deficiency, drains the body where there is excess, and promotes free flow where there is inactivity.

In acupuncture, a specialist inserts fine needles into specific points on the body that correspond with meridians through which the qi and blood flow. The most common points are considered 12 primary channels, or *mai*, which correspond to the bladder, gallbladder, heart, kidneys, large intestine, liver, lungs, pericardium (the lining of the heart), spleen, stomach and small intestine.

- *Diet therapy* includes dietary recommendations that are based upon a person's individual needs in relation to TCM theories. A balanced TCM diet incorporates foods of various energies, flavors and organic actions.
- *Herbal medicine* utilizes herbal mixtures that are tailored for patients and their yin/yang disorders. Unlike Western medications that are used to treat illness, in TCM the balance and interaction of herbal mixtures are considered more important than the effects of specific drugs.
- *Qi gong* is a 4,000-year-old technique that involves preventative and therapeutic health care, physical training and philosophy. There are nearly 5,000 styles of qi gong; *taiji* is one of the most widely recognized.

There are six paths that a person might follow through taiji and other styles of qi gong. These include self-reliance and empowerment, self-healing, the healer's path, the path of supreme strength and conflict resolution, the supernatural path, and the path of transcendence and immortality.

- Qi gong is frequently practiced with *tai ji (chi)*, an internal Chinese martial arts technique. Tai ji (chi) is thought to improve functional and health status—particularly in older people—to promote longevity.
- *Tui na* massage is similar to acupressure. *Shiatsu* massage uses the fingers and palms to apply pressure to specific areas of the body to correct imbalances, heal specific illnesses, and maintain and promote health.

Today, TCM has been modernized by transforming some of the herbal remedies into soluble granules and tablets. There are both plant and nonplant sources used. Some TCM ingredients have been formulated into Western-style drugs.

Acupuncture has become more common throughout Westernized countries, as have different types of massage, tai chi and TCM diet therapies. Some health practitioners combine both Eastern and Western medical remedies in treating patients. Some patients are becoming more proactive and self-reliant about their health, as qi gong advocates.

As modern and traditional societies continue to globalize, many different approaches to diet, health and longevity may result, including some of the components of TCM. Dual training in both Western and Eastern medicines provides a multifaceted approach to disease, health and wellness.

Recipe: Stir-fried Asian Vegetables

This recipe for Stir-fried Asian Vegetables abounds with plenty of cancer-fighting foods and substances: cruciferous vegetables, including bok choy (Chinese mustard greens), broccoli and Napa cabbage; garlic, onions and scallions from the protective allium family and ginger and red chili, little powerhouses of defense. Stir-frying is quick and preserves nutrients so that these vegetables can be consumed at their peak for a taste of Asian cuisine. The recipe for **Stir-fried Asian Vegetables** *can be found in the* **Recipe file** *which is located within the* Culinary Nutrition *website at www.culinarynutrition.elsevier.com. The finished dish is shown within the centerfold* **Photo file** *in Plate 9.4.*

Living Healthfully to 100 Years and Beyond

The challenge to live to be 100 years old is a dream of some people and a reality of others. A look at societies where living longer is common helps to identify their health-enhancing lifestyles and acquire diet and health advice.

On the Japanese island of Okinawa, out of a population of around 1 million people, about 900 are centenarians. This may not sound like a high number, but it is about four times higher than the average number of centenarians in either the United States or Great Britain. What is even more astonishing is that this number is about equal in gender: almost the same number of men live to be 100 years or over as women do.

It may be that Okinawans age slower than normal. Scientists have discovered a hormone called dehydroepiandrosterone (DHEA) that is produced by the adrenal glands and is a precursor to the female and male hormones estrogen and testosterone. DHEA decreases after 30 years of age. It also decreases with AIDS, adrenal insufficiency, anorexia, end-stage kidney disease and Type II diabetes and by drugs such as corticosteroids, insulin and opiates.

The level of DHEA declines at a much slower rate among centenarians in Okinawa. This may be attributed to the Okinawan diet. People in Okinawa eat tofu and soy products, and they consume a considerable array of antioxidant-rich fruits and vegetables.

428

Okinawans also practice calorie restriction and only eat until they are about 80 percent full—not stuffed. This practice is called *hara hachi bu*. Feeling a little hunger may signal the appetite control center of the brain to protect itself by hoarding calories, since famine might be forthcoming. A typical day's worth of calories in an Okinawan diet is about 1,200. This level is considered dieting to some people in Westernized countries. It is difficult to meet nutrient needs when diets are any lower than 1,200 calories a day.

In Sardinia, the second-largest island in the Mediterranean Sea south of Italy, calories and tofu, hallmarks of the Okinawan diet, are not as important as meat. The population in Sardinia is smaller than in Okinawa, but there are still an equal number of men and women who live to be over 100 years old. What makes Sardinians unique is that they marry their relatives. While there is an increased probability of genetic disorders in Sardinians, there is also a remarkable increase in longevity.

A limited pool of genes is associated with centenarians in Sardinia. One particular gene on the X chromosome may be defective and fail to produce an enzyme known as G6PD. This enzyme can have a negative or positive impact upon health. In the case of these centenarian Sardinians, it appears to be positive.

In Loma Linda, California, living to be 100 years old very much has to do with lifestyle. The city is primarily composed of Seventh-Day Adventists, who abstain from alcohol and nicotine. Many also follow a vegetarian diet. On the average, Seventh-Day Adventists have a long life expectancy, which may also be explained by their spiritual life. Longevity and lifestyle of Seventh-Day Adventists have been studied for years. Part of their healthfulness may be due to lower levels of stress hormones as a result of their religiosity.

In Ecuador, the Vilcabambans live in the Valley of Longevity. A combination of a good year-round climate, plus lots of fresh fruits and vegetables may contribute to these healthy and longer-living people. The Vilcabambans remain healthy throughout their life due to their diet, high activity level, leanness and low cholesterol. Besides fresh fruits and vegetables, they consume almost no animal products or processed foods. They hike and cultivate their own food. By and large, the Vilcabambans take their lives easy and treat their aging with admiration and respect.

What can we learn by studying these centenarians? First, to live longer, inherit healthy genes. Next, live among people who practice healthy habits. Also, do not eat too much or too little; eat plenty of fruits and vegetables and little meat if at all. Be sure to exercise and practice some type of stress reduction and spirituality. It does not hurt to live in a temperate climate that is conducive to healthy lifestyles either. Living to 100 years of age may be more a matter of genetics, but practicing prudent lifestyle approaches such as these might bring more quality of years, if not more quantity.

References

[1] National Heart, Lung and Blood Institute (NHLBI). Your guide to lowering cholesterol with TLC, <www.nhlbi.nih.gov/health/public/heart/chol/chol_tlc.pdf>; [accessed 21.08.08].

[2] US Food and Drug Administration (FDA) Health claims: oats and coronary heart disease—final rule. Fed Regist 1997;62:3583–601.

[3] Rosamond W, Flegal K, Furie K, et al. Heart disease and stroke statistics—2008 update. Circulation 2008;117:e25–e146.

[4] National Heart, Lung and Blood Institute (NHLBI). Clinical guidelines on the identification, evaluation, and treatment of overweight and obesity in adults, <http://www.nhlbi.nih.gov/guidelines/obesity/ob_gdlns.htm>; [accessed 2.09.08].

[5] <http://www.ncbi.nlm.nih.gov/pubmed/12949380>

[6] American Heart Association (AHA). Know your fats, <http://www.heart.org/HEARTORG/Conditions/Cholesterol/PreventionTreatmentofHighCholesterol/Know-Your-Fats_UCM_305628_Article.jsp>; [accessed 2.09.08].

[7] Messina M. Soyfoods and coronary heart disease: beyond cholesterol reduction, <http://www.soyconnection.com/newsletters/soy-connection/health-nutrition/article.php/Soyfoods + and + Coronary + Heart+Disease%3A + Beyond+Cholesterol + Reduction?id = 221>; [accessed 2.09.08].

[8] American Heart Association (AHA). Obesity information, <http://www.heart.org/HEARTORG/GettingHealthy/WeightManagement/Obesity/Obesity-Information_UCM_307908_Article.jsp>; [accessed 2.09.08].

[9] National Heart, Lung and Blood Institute (NHLBI). High blood cholesterol: what you need to know, <http://www.nhlbi.nih.gov/health/public/heart/chol/wyntk.htm>; [accessed 2.09.08].

[10] Fernandez ML. Dietary cholesterol provided by eggs and plasma lipoproteins in healthy populations. Curr Opin Clin Nutr Metab Care 2006;9:8–12.

[11] Djoussé L, Gaziano JM. Egg consumption and risk of heart failure in the Physicians' Health Study. Circulation 2008;117:512–6.

[12] Mayo Clinic. Cholesterol: top 5 foods to lower your numbers, <http://www.mayoclinic.com/health/cholesterol/CL00002/NSECTIONGROUP=2>; [accessed 2.09.08].

[13] American Heart Association (AHA). Meet the fats, <http://www.heart.org/HEARTORG/GettingHealthy/FatsAndOils/Fats-Oils_UCM_001084_SubHomePage.jsp>; [accessed 2.09.08].

[14] Calorie Control Council. Lighten up and get moving! <http://www.caloriecontrol.org/healthy-weight-tool-kit/lighten-up-and-get-moving>; [accessed 2.09.08].

[15] <http://circ.ahajournals.org/content/114/1/82.full>

[16] <http://circ.ahajournals.org/content/114/1/82/T3.expansion.html>

[17] SelfNutritionData. Nutrient search, <http://nutritiondata.self.com>; [accessed 2.09.08].

[18] US Department of Agriculture (USDA). Search the USDA National Nutrient Database for standard reference, <http://www.nal.usda.gov/fnic/foodcomp/search/>; [accessed 2.09.08].

[19] FatSecret. My FatSecret, <www.fatsecret.com>; [accessed 2.09.08].

[20] Good Housekeeping Magazine. Healthy makeover: Caesar salad, <http://www.goodhousekeeping.com/recipefinder/caesar-salad-healthy-ghk>; [accessed 2.09.08].

[21] Katan MB, Grundy SM, Jones P, et al. Efficacy and safety of plant stanols and sterols in the management of blood cholesterol levels. Mayo Clin Proc 2003;78:965–78.

[22] International Food Information Council Foundation. Functional foods fact sheet: plant stanols and sterols, <http://www.foodinsight.org/Resources/Detail.aspx?topic = Functional_Foods_Fact_Sheet_Plant_Stanols_and_Sterols>; [accessed 8.04.08].

[23] Margarine Awareness Resource Group. Margarine makes for healthier meals, <http://www.cookingwithmargarine.com/guidelines.html>; [accessed 2.09.08].

[24] Virginia Mason Medical Center. What are normal blood glucose levels?, <https://www.virginiamason.org/service.cfm?id = 511>; [accessed 2.09.08].

[25] Harvard School of Public Health. Shining the spotlight on trans fat, <http://www.hsph.harvard.edu/nutritionsource/nutrition-news/transfats/>; [accessed 2.09.08].

[26] Academy of Nutrition and Dietetics (AND), <http://www.eatright.com>; [accessed 2.09.08].

[27] American Diabetes Association (ADA), <http://www.diabetes.org>; [accessed 2.09.08].

[28] Janket SJ, Manson JE, Sesso H, Buring JE, Liu S. A prospective study of sugar intake and risk of Type 2 diabetes in women. Diabetes Care 2003;26:1008–15.

[29] US Department of Agriculture (USDA), ChooseMyPlate.gov <http://www.choosemyplate.gov/>; [accessed 2.09.08].

[30] OptumRx. MyPlate planner, <http://www.dlife.com/diabetes/information/inspiration_expert_advice/expert_columns/PrescriptionSolutionsPlatePlannerEnglish_LetterSize_3-09.pdf>; [accessed 14.03.12].

[31] Pollard JM, Bielamowicz MK. Sugar substitutes—weight loss, diabetes, safety, nutrition?, <http://fcs.tamu.edu/health/healthhints/2010/may/index.php>; [accessed 2.09.08].

[32] About.com. Cooking with sugar substitutes. <http://homecooking.about.com/library/weekly/bl010598b.htm>; [accessed 2.09.08].

[33] Glade MJ. World cancer research fund. Food, nutrition, and the prevention of cancer: a global perspective, 1997. Nutrition 1999;15:523–6.

[34] American Cancer Society (ACS). ACS diet and physical activity factors that affect risks for select cancers, <http://www.cancer.org/Healthy/EatHealthyGetActive/ACSGuidelinesonNutritionPhysicalActivityforCancerPrevention/acs-guidelines-on-nutrition-and-physical-activity-for-cancer-prevention-diet-activity-cancer-risk>[accessed 2.09.08].

[35] Luch A. In: The carcinogenic effects of polycyclic aromatic hydrocarbons. London: Imperial College Press; 2005.

[36] Haytowitz DB. Effect of draining and rinsing on the sodium and water-soluble vitamin content of canned vegetables, <http://www.ars.usda.gov/SP2UserFiles/Place/12354500/Articles/EB11_DrainedVeg.pdf>; [accessed 2.09.08].

[37] Milton S. Pennsylvania State Hershey Medical Center. Diet and cancer, <http://printer-friendly.adam.com/content.aspx?productId = 117&pid = 1&gid = 002096&c_custid = 758>; [accessed 2.09.08].

[38] Breastcancer.org. Trans fats linked to breast cancer risk in study, <http://www.breastcancer.org/tips/nutrition/new_research/20080411b.jsp>; [accessed 2.09.08].

[39] Liu RH. Potential synergy of phytochemicals in cancer prevention: mechanism of action. J Nutr 2004;134:3479S–3485S.

[40] Wilson T. Foods and phytonutrients: Table of potential benefits for health and weight loss, <http://www.dietivity.com/foods-and-phytonutrients-table-of-potential-benefits-for-health-and-weight-loss/>; [accessed 19.09.08].

[41] Johnson I, Williamson G. In: Phytochemical functional foods. Cambridge, UK: Woodhead Ltd; 2003.

[42] American Cancer Society (ACS). Common questions about diet and cancer, <http://www.cancer.org/Healthy/EatHealthyGetActive/ACSGuidelinesonNutritionPhysicalActivityforCancerPrevention/acs-guidelines-on-nutrition-and-physical-activity-for-cancer-prevention-diet-cancer-questions>; [accessed 2.09.08].

[43] American Heart Association (AHA). High blood pressure may be due to excess weight in half of overweight adults, <http://www.sciencedaily.com/releases/2007/09/070928180348.htm>; [accessed 22.09.08].

[44] Mayo Clinic. Healthy diet: end the guesswork with these nutrition guidelines, <http://www.mayoclinic.com/health/healthy-diet/NU00200>; [accessed 2.09.08].

[45] Center for Disease Control and Prevention (CDC). Americans consume too much sodium (salt), <http://www.cdc.gov/features/dsSodium/>; [accessed 2.09.08].

[46] National Heart, Lung and Blood Institute (NHLBI). Limit alcohol intake, <http://www.nhlbi.nih.gov/hbp/prevent/l_alcohol/l_alcohol.htm>; [accessed 2.09.08].

[47] National Heart, Lung and Blood Institute (NHLBI). Reduce salt and sodium in your diet, <http://www.nhlbi.nih.gov/hbp/prevent/sodium/sodium.htm>; [accessed 2.09.08].

[48] Stewart SH, Latham PK, Miller PM, Randall P, Anton RF. Blood pressure reduction during treatment for alcohol dependence: results from the COMBINE study. Addiction 2008;103:1622–8.

[49] Food and Nutrition Board, Institute of Medicine. Potassium. In: Spears E, editor. Dietary reference intakes for water, potassium, sodium, chloride, and sulfate, 186–268. Washington, DC: National Academies Press; 2005.

[50] Institute of Medicine (IOM). Dietary reference intakes tables and applications, <http://www.iom.edu/Activities/Nutrition/SummaryDRIs/~/media/Files/Activity%20Files/Nutrition/DRIs/5_Summary%20Table%20Tables%201-4.pdf>; [accessed 2.09.08].

[51] Anderson J, Prior S, Braithwaite D, et al. DASHing to lower blood pressure, <www.ext.colostate.edu/PUBS/FOODNUT/09374.html>; [accessed 2.09.08].

[52] National Heart, Lung and Blood Institute (NHLBI). Dietary approaches to stop hypertension—sodium study, <https://biolincc.nhlbi.nih.gov/studies/dashsodium/>. [accessed 2.09.08].

[53] Appel LJ, Moore TJ, Obarzanek E, et al. A clinical trial of the effects of dietary patterns on blood pressure. N Engl J Med 1997;336:1117–24.

[54] US Department of Health and Human Services (DHHS). Your guide to lowering your blood pressure with DASH, <http://www.nhlbi.nih.gov/health/public/heart/hbp/dash/new_dash.pdf>; [accessed 2.09.08].

[55] National Heart, Lung and Blood Institute (NHLBI). Food exchange lists, <http://www.nhlbi.nih.gov/health/public/heart/obesity/lose_wt/fd_exch.htm>; [accessed 2.09.08].

[56] US Food and Drug Administration (FDA). The new food label: scouting for sodium and other nutrients important to blood pressure, <http://www.foodinsight.org/Hot-Topics/Healthy-Eating-Active-Living/Food/Sodium/tabid/1418/Default.aspx>; [accessed 13.03.11].

[57] Moser M. Lowering blood pressure: do specific levels or medications affect outcomes? myths, misconceptions, and heroics in the management of hypertension. Am J Hypertens 2003;16:267A–8A. doi:S0895-7061(03)00806-9

[58] MedlinePlus. Heartburn, <http://www.nlm.nih.gov/medlineplus/heartburn.html>; [accessed 19.09.08].

[59] Hopp RJ. Genetics and epidemiology of allergic disease. In: Naguwa SM, Gershwin ME, editors. Allergy and immunology secrets (1st ed.). Philadelphia: Penn: Hanley and Belfus; 2001.

[60] American Heart Association (AHA). Diet and lifestyle recommendations, <http://www.heart.org/HEARTORG/GettingHealthy/Diet-and-Lifestyle-Recommendations_UCM_305855_Article.jsp>; [accessed 2.09.08].

[61] American Diabetes Association (ADA). Making healthy food choices, <http://www.diabetes.org/food-and-fitness/food/what-can-i-eat/making-healthy-food-choices.html>; [accessed 2.09.08].

[62] American Cancer Society (ACS). American Cancer Society guidelines on nutrition and physical activity for cancer prevention, <http://www.cancer.org/Healthy/EatHealthyGetActive/ACSGuidelinesonNutritionPhysicalActivityforCancerPrevention/acs-guidelines-on-nutrition-and-physical-activity-for-cancer-prevention-intro>. [accessed 2.09.08].

Weight Management: Finding the Healthy Balance
Practical Applications for Nutrition, Food Science and Culinary Professionals

431

OBJECTIVES

1. Identify the risks of overweight and obesity
2. Compute ideal body weight and desirable body weight
3. Describe body composition, total body fat and body fat distribution in relationship to ideal body weight (IBW)
4. Apply body fat measurements and the body mass index (BMI) to determine IBW
5. Explain metabolism and basal metabolic rate (BMR) in the context of body weight

Culinary Nutrition. DOI: http://dx.doi.org/10.1016/B978-0-12-391882-6.00010-8

6. Describe the relationship among calories, caloric balance and calorie expenditure in weight gain and weight loss
7. Monitor and scrutinize current diets, dieting and diet aids, and distinguish among commercial weight-loss programs
8. Evaluate medical treatments for obesity
9. Identify the techniques of eating right when eating out
10. Recognize behavior modification techniques for weight management

> **Morsel** Be moderate in order to taste the joys of life in abundance. —Epicurus (ancient Greek philosopher, 341 BC–270 BC)

INTRODUCTION: FINDING THE HEALTHY BALANCE

The human body was designed for consuming foods and beverages when they were accessible and withstanding periods of time when they were not. It intuitively and physically struck a balance between calories consumed and calories expended. Our ancient ancestors were hunter-gatherers who sustained such periods of feast and famine. Walking was their means of transportation, and daily tasks were the antithesis of life today with all of its labor-saving devices.

People did not farm until around 12,000 years ago, when a climate change made the world hotter and drier. The global population increased and life could not be sustained by fishing, hunting or gathering alone. As society became agrarian (farm-based) and grains, fruits and vegetables entered the food supply, the diet was essentially based on whole grains, fruits, vegetables and lean protein. People were of average weight. They perished from contagious diseases from living in close proximity, rather than degenerative diseases of overconsumption.

Then animals became domesticated. Transportation moved crops and people around; cities spread and people enjoyed the "fat of the land." New technologies in rapidly expanding countries helped to make life easier, much as it has done exponentially today.

Fast forward to the twenty-first century, with its innumerable factors that contribute to overweight and obesity. Genetics, the environment, food accessibility, and inactivity and urban spread are big contributors. The concept of finding the balance between "calories in" versus "calories out" is more difficult than it was during antiquity, because people have so much weight to lose and they do not have to hunt or gather their food, or toil at daily tasks.

Instead of increased activity, the tendency today is to go on very restrictive diets, only to rebound and gain even more weight. The people who do exercise and/or monitor their diet may not be the ones who need to exercise and diet the most.

Understanding the fundamentals of weight management is the first step in discriminating among the multitude of diet and weight control approaches. Integrating exercise into a sensible diet program that is based on healthy foods and beverages is the next step in a reasonable approach to weight control. Incorporating behavior modification with tried-and-true behavioral strategies is the third step toward successful and permanent dietary and exercise changes. Finally, learning the principles of reduced-calorie cooking and baking is the all-encompassing step toward permanent lifestyle changes. This chapter addresses each of these steps to help people lose weight intelligently and keep it off sensibly.

MAIN COURSES
Weight Management
THE HISTORY OF DIETING

Dieting is not a new strategy for a modern problem. In fact, dieting in its broadest sense is far from new. The world's oldest surviving medical document, the Ebers Papyrus, originated about 1550 BC. It reportedly contained a recipe for an antidiabetic diet of wheat germ and okra. This whole grain and vegetable approach to diabetes is not much different from the dietary approach for this ever-growing disease today.

Modern dieting, as we consider it today, has been attributed to the New Jersey preacher Sylvester Graham and his vegetarian and whole grain advice. In the early 1800s, Graham likened gluttony to sinfulness and correlated dietary difficulties, such as indigestion and constipation, with overeating. Graham developed a pure food, brown bread diet to help settle gastrointestinal disorders. Little did Graham realize that this "brown bread" was the whole-grain bread still praised today for its nutritional and health benefits.

By the late nineteenth century, health concerns about excessive overweight paralleled Victorian moral prudishness and vanity. Victorian society did not value sloth; it promoted skinniness to a fault. Victorian women wore restrictive corsets to make their waists look artificially tiny, while emphasizing their hips and buttocks. The first depiction of the eating disorder anorexia nervosa captured daughters of the very wealthy.

But fashions sway according to the times, and so do acceptable body types. Suffocating corsets became passé, and buxom bodies again became vogue. Robust people depicted prosperous life in the early 1900s—until the world wars dictated food restrictions. Then body sizes diminished and fashions became somber.

After World Wars I and II, body types again became bigger than life, mirroring the booming US economy. In the 1950s, life insurance tables (called actuarial tables) based their premiums on healthy body weight compared to frame size. These weight tables were some of the earliest published statistics in the United States that correlated increased weight and decreased longevity, which resulted in higher insurance premiums.

Weight tables do not necessarily take issues such as race or body composition into account. These are important considerations as the United States is rapidly becoming more racially diverse. Some of the highest rates of obesity exist in African Americans and Latinos. The body mass index (BMI) is a more accurate reflection of body fat, which is what is implicated in degenerative diseases—more so than total body weight. However, the BMI also has its faults, since it is not a good measure for people with dramatic body composition differences, such as body builders or seniors with decreased muscle mass.

433

While the methodology for measuring body fatness is more sophisticated than thousands of years ago, and the treatments for diabetes and other degenerative diseases defy the medical approaches of former times, widespread obesity and lack of physical activity characterize the world in the twenty-first century—unlike any other times.

A svelte, model-like shape still exists as an unrealistic "ideal" body, attained through gastric reductions, plastic surgery, radical diets and more. Still, about one-half of the US population is obese, and the number is growing. This chapter examines the growing dilemma of weight management and provides practical and sensible approaches for food and culinary professionals to help tackle this major public health issue [1–3].

Morsel "The biggest seller is cookbooks and the second is diet books—how not to eat what you've just learned how to cook." —Andy Rooney (Television commentator, 1919–2011)

THE MODERN AGE OF DIETING

The "ideal diet" in the United States in the 1950s was like the economy: gradual. It was a time of rebirth after World War II, characterized by the Four Basic Food Groups: meat, milk, breads and cereals, and fruits and vegetables. The US public was advised to eat the 2-2-4-4 way: 2 servings of meats, 2 servings of dairy foods, 4 servings of fruits and vegetables, and 4 servings of breads and cereals. A number of diet potions, including thyroid and herbal extracts, sold by door-to-door salesmen, promised sensational cures. But for the most part, diet was viewed as balanced and sensible, and it provided a road map for family nutrition.

In the 1960s, fruit, meat and pastry consumption were high. One of the earliest food guide pyramids was conceived in the 1960s out of a growing concern over the increased incidence of coronary heart disease [4, 5]. In the 1970s, the association between the overconsumption of foods high in total fat, saturated fat, cholesterol and sodium and increased risks of cardiovascular disease and diabetes was established. The concept that this association between food and disease should drive US dietary recommendations was recognized. Prior to this time, dietary recommendations were based mostly on weight.

The late 1980s saw the development of the first food guide pyramids, which emphasized grains and other plant foods. The growth of the diet industry in the mid-1900s focused on pills to speed metabolism and garments to "melt away" pounds.

A number of diets paralleled the heightened interest in diets and dieting. These include, but are not limited to, dietary supplements, food combining, high fiber/whole foods, high protein/ high fat, low carbohydrate/ high protein, low fat, rigid calorie control, and raw foods—many with celebrity endorsement. While some of these programs and dietary aids caused initial weight loss, weight often crept back unless long-term weight management strategies were incorporated.

The 2000s brought a diet backlash and a return to comfort foods, contributing to the expanding US waistline. What is the best twenty-first-century approach for losing and maintaining weight? There is no magic cure for overweight or obesity, nor is there just one approach that guarantees weight loss and weight maintenance. This is because weight management is complex and multifactorial.

Overweight and obesity now present monumental health risks, with momentous strain on health care systems. While medical approaches are sought, nutrition, food science and culinary professionals can help by creating healthy products, recipes, meals and diets that are reduced in calories from added sugars and fats and high in nutrients and flavor. To begin this challenging undertaking, a solid understanding of the complexities of overweight and obesity is essential.

OVERWEIGHT AND OBESITY

The terms *overweight* and *obesity* both designate weight ranges that are greater than what is considered healthy for a given height. They are used synonymously, but technically they are distinctively different. ***Overweight*** is defined as 10 to 20 percent above the desirable weight for height, or a body mass index (BMI) of 25.0 to 29.9. It is important to note that some people may be categorized as overweight, but they may not be overly fat due to their body composition. For example, weight lifters may be labeled as overweight according to their weight in pounds, but muscle mass is dense and weighs more than fat. ***Obesity*** is defined as 20 percent or greater above the desirable weight for height, or a body mass index (BMI) of 30 or greater.

REASONS FOR OVERWEIGHT AND OBESITY

The body is like a cashier that needs to balance the amount of money that is taken in by the money that is paid out. By day's end, a person should balance the amount of calories that he consumes with the amount of calories he expends. Sometimes, even in the best-case scenarios, this formula just does not work: we simply eat too much and are too tired to exercise. People claim to eat less and exercise more, and yet the number on the scale keeps rising. Why? The reason is because many factors affect this balance of calories: eating behavior, environment, enzymes, fat cells, genetics, leptin, set point, and thermogenesis.

People should eat when they are hungry and stop eating when they are ***satiated***, or satisfied. This assumes that they "listen" to their internal cues of when they are hungry and when they are full. But where do these cues come from and what interferes with the ability to recognize these internal cues and respond accordingly? A look at hunger and appetite offers some explanations.

Hunger is a physiological need to eat. It is that gnawing feeling in the stomach and the feeling of being weak and in need of food or beverages. The opposite of hunger is ***appetite***, which is the psychological need to eat. In some people, just the appearance or aroma of food may trigger the desire to eat. Other people seem to be less dictated by the sensory qualities of food and rely more on their hunger signals. Learning to recognize these differences is challenging. Plus, the media and other environmental factors may affect appetite and overrule hunger.

It has been speculated that the brain sends neurological signals to the stomach and the stomach sends them back to the brain, and this circuit is responsible for monitoring and responding to food in the environment. In the brainstem, the ***hypothalamus*** senses hunger and satiety. It monitors nutrient levels and conditions in the blood, such as glucose, lipids, protein, sodium, and temperature. Then it sends messages to organs and systems through hormones and nerves to raise or lower levels of these substances in the blood.

In rare instances, the hypothalamus does not operate properly, and individuals may have metabolic and other disorders. Mostly people confuse hunger with appetite. They are triggered to eat by the sights, sounds, aromas, textures and tastes of food in the environment and other emotional, genetic and physical factors, including the following:

- *Environment:* There is some speculation that overweight and obese people are persuaded to eat by **external cues**, such as buffets, food commercials on television, grocery shopping, pictures of food in magazines, and so on. These external cues may override the body's internal regulatory system of hunger and satiety. **Behavior modification** enables overweight and obese people to employ alternative strategies. Its strategies are described in the "Take away" section at the end of this chapter.
- *Enzymes:* It has been speculated that overweight and obese people might produce more of the enzyme **lipoprotein lipase (LPL),** which determines the rate at which adipose (fat) cells store fat. Larger cells produce more LPL, which causes cells to take in more triglycerides for storage. Unfortunately, when weight is lost, and particularly if it is rapidly lost, these cells are quick to pull in more triglycerides, which is partially the reason why weight rebounds so easily.
- *Fat cells:* It is thought that people are born with a certain number of fat cells and that there are a few times in life when these fat cells increase in number: infancy and childhood, adolescence, maybe pregnancy, and perhaps during gross obesity.

  Extra fat cells may sabotage dieting. When overweight and obese people diet and their fat levels decrease, extra fat cells may send additional signals to the brain to refuel more than normal. Despite loss of fat, their bodies may seek more calories. The only way that these fat cells can decrease in number is by **liposuction**—a medical procedure for "sucking out" fat cells by the use of a saline (salt) solution.

- *Genetics:* Heredity may determine who is programmed to be overweight or obese and who is predestined to be thin. The study of genetics can show the relationship between overweight and obese parents and grandparents and the likelihood of overweight and obesity in their children and grandchildren. The notion that environmental factors can override this genetic predisposition for overfatness has not been proven to date.
- *Leptin:* A gene named *ob* (for obese) has been identified that likely produces a hormone called leptin. **Leptin,** from the Greek word that means "slender," exists in fat cells, and when it is released, it signals the body to stop eating.

  It seems when fat increases inside cells, leptin also increases. When a person is fed and satiated, leptin signals her to stop eating. The opposite also appears to be the case: when fat cells are depleted, leptin levels decrease, which stimulates hunger and decreases energy expenditure. In normal-weight people, this regulatory process works efficiently. The leptin gene may be unresponsive or defective in overweight and obese people.

- *Set point:* The **set point** theory suggests that people are programmed to be at a certain weight despite over- or underfeeding. This set point may be established by genetics. Some speculation has been given to the body's ability to reset its set-point—either to lower it by calorie restriction and regular exercise or to increase it by repeated episodes of yo-yo dieting. **Yo-yo dieting** is also known as **weight cycling,** the repeated loss and gain of weight. At this time, neither hypothesis is conclusive.
- *Thermogenesis:* It is possible that overweight and obese people have inherited a regulatory mechanism that limits the rate of fat metabolism and **thermogenesis**, or heat production. This means that the release of energy and the breakdown of carbohydrates, protein, and lipids may be slower when people are overfat. Exercise programs designed for overweight and obese individuals help target body fat. With less body fat, people may be able to use calories more efficiently. [6–8]

Morsel Don't dig your grave with your own knife and fork." —English proverb

RISKS OF OVERWEIGHT AND OBESITY

The risks of overweight and obesity outweigh the advantages.
Overfat people may sustain fewer serious injuries in accidents because of their protective fat, and they are more insulated for cold weather than thinner people. Otherwise, the risks are mighty:

- *Coronary heart disease:* The chances for coronary heart disease and heart attack increase as body mass increases. Obesity also can lead to **congestive heart failure,** a condition in which the heart cannot pump enough blood to meet the body's needs.

435

- *Hypertension (high blood pressure):* There is greater risk of hypertension when overweight or obese. This is because there is more resistance to the force of the blood pushing against the walls of the arteries.
- *Gallbladder disease:* People who are overweight or obese have greater chances of developing gallstones. Too much fat may cause the gallbladder to enlarge and become dysfunctional.
- *Lipidemia:* Overweight or obese individuals have a greater chance of abnormal blood fat levels, which are risk factors for coronary heart disease. These include elevated low-density lipoproteins (LDL), triglycerides, and total cholesterol, and decreased high-density lipoproteins (HDL)
- *Metabolic syndrome:* Overweight and obesity increase the risks of **metabolic syndrome,** a condition that occurs when a person has at least three of the following risk factors:
  - Large waistline
  - Abnormal blood fat levels
  - High triglycerides and low HDL cholesterol
  - Elevated blood pressure
  - Elevated fasting blood sugar

Metabolic syndrome increases the risks of coronary heart disease, diabetes and stroke.

- *Osteoarthritis:* **Osteoarthritis** is a common joint problem of the hips, lower back, and knees. It occurs when protective joint tissues wear away. Extra weight may cause pain, pressure and wear.
- *Sleep apnea* and *respiratory problems:* Overweight and obese people may have more fat stored behind their neck, which can cause the airways to become smaller and make breathing more difficult.
- *Some cancers:* Overweight and obesity may increase the risks of breast, colon, endometrial and gallbladder cancers.
- *Some gynecological problems:* Overweight and obese women may experience menstrual irregularities and infertility.
- *Stroke:* The risk of having a stroke rises as body mass increases. Being overweight or obese may cause a buildup of fatty deposits in the brain. This condition may cause blood clots that can impede the flow of blood and oxygen and cause a stroke or cerebral hemorrhage.
- *Type II diabetes:* Diabetes is a leading cause of blindness, heart disease, kidney disease, premature death, and stroke. A significant percentage of people with Type II diabetes are overweight or obese.

IDEAL BODY WEIGHT AND DESIRABLE BODY WEIGHT

While people may want to weigh a certain amount, there is not one definitive number that is the right weight. A weight range is more likely, and there are a number of methods to determine this range. This is a simple method for estimating **desirable body weight:**

- Women: 100 pounds for the first 5 feet of height, plus 5 pounds for each additional inch
- Men: 106 pounds of body weight for the first 5 feet of height, plus 6 pounds for each additional inch
- Small body frame: subtract 10 percent from this figure
- Large body frame: add 10 percent to this figure

A common weight scale can be used to compare actual body weight to desirable body weight, but it does not show the amount of lean muscle mass compared to fat weight. **Ideal body weight (IBW)** often incorporates more variables. It identifies the weight that people should weigh based on age, gender, height, and muscular development. It factors body composition more into consideration. Sometimes a number of these and other approaches are used and then averaged to determine a weight goal.

BODY COMPOSITION

Some nutritional scientists believe that **body composition** may be more important than total body weight in determining health disease risks such as coronary heart disease and diabetes. The body consists of **lean body mass** (body water, bones, cells, muscles, and organs that provide both structure and function), and **total body fat.** According to antiquated **height-weight tables**, a person can be "overweight" but not "overfat." For example, a male bodybuilder can weigh 260 pounds and be considered overweight, but he may have only 3 percent body fat.

TOTAL BODY FAT

Total body fat includes *essential fat*, found in some cell membranes, bones, and nerve tissues; *subcutaneous fat*, located right under the skin within subcutaneous tissue; and *visceral fat*, fat that is deeply situated in the abdomen. Subcutaneous fat maintains body temperature and cushions the body from accidents. Visceral fat is called organ fat because it clothes the organs.

Adipose cells are found in these adipose or fat tissues. They specialize in storing fat. The two types of adipose tissue are white adipose tissue (WAT) and brown adipose tissue (BAT), known as white fat and brown fat. White fat cells are particularly skillful at storing triglycerides, the storage form of fatty acids. They are very responsive to the level of fatty acids in the blood. When fatty acids are abundant after a high-fat meal, they are moved from the blood into white fat cells for storage. When fatty acids are low from dieting, fasting, or starvation, then white fat cells release fatty acids into the blood for energy. It is theorized that a person creates new white fat cells during periods of growth, including extreme obesity. Methods to reduce white fat cells include liposuction and surgery.

Brown fat, also known as brown adipose tissue, is engorged with blood. Its color is richer than other adipose tissue, which is typically white. BAT generates heat because it is metabolically active like lean body mass, as opposed to white adipose tissue that only stores fat. People have more BAT between their shoulder blades, and babies have more BAT in their abdomens, which is why these areas feel so warm to the touch.

Brown fat distribution tends to be genetically determined. It may prove to have an important role in energy metabolism. Newborns tend to have more brown fat that dissipates with age. Bears that hibernate during the winter are known to have a sizable amount of brown fat to stay warm and still have enough calories to live throughout cold months. They demonstrate the importance of the ratio of lean body mass and adipose tissue in regulating metabolism and body weight.

Cellulite is not fat. It is a collection of substances that push against the connective tissue under the skin, which causes the surface of the skin to dimple, pucker and look lumpy. Aerobic exercise that burns fat and muscular activities that build muscle are probably the best defense against cellulite.

437

BODY FAT DISTRIBUTION

Men tend to carry more visceral fat in their upper torso. This fat distribution, called ***upper-body obesity***, is characterized by an "apple" shape and correlates with a higher risk of health-related diseases, such as coronary heart disease and diabetes. It may be that visceral fat crowds the organs and releases more fatty acids into the portal vein that leads to the liver. This burdens the liver's ability to produce lipoproteins for fat transport and disposal. As a result, free fatty acids circulate though the blood, interfere with normal glucose metabolism, and elevate blood cholesterol.

Women tend to store fat in their hips, buttock and thighs for reproductive purposes. This fat distribution, called ***lower-body obesity***, tends to make people look "pear shaped." It may cause stress on the bones and joints of the ankles, hips, and knees. Lower-body obesity is not associated with coronary heart disease or diabetes [9].

BODY MASS INDEX

The ***body mass index (BMI)*** is a number that is calculated from a person's weight and height. It provides a reliable indicator of body fatness for most people. BMI is used to screen and classify weight categories that may present health problems. By using the BMI, people can compare their weight to the weights of the general population and assess their health risks. BMI is both age-and sex-specific for children and teenagers, because the amount of body fat changes with age and differs between girls and boys.

The following formula is used to calculate the BMI. The BMI for various heights and weights can be found at http://www.nhlbi.nih.gov/guidelines/obesity/bmi_tbl.htm.

$$weight\ (lbs) \div height\ (in)^2 \times 703 = BMI$$

Calculate the BMI by dividing weight in pounds (lbs) by height in inches (in) squared (i.e., height × height); then multiplying this figure by a conversion factor of 703.

Example 1: Female – Weight = 160 lbs; height = 5'5" (65")
Calculation: $160/(65)^2$ [4,225] × 703 = 26.62 BMI—*overweight*
Example 2: Male – Weight = 220 lbs; height = 5'10" (70")
Calculation: $220/(70)^2$ [4,900] × 703 = 31.56 BMI—*obese*

An adult with a BMI between 25 and 29.9 is considered overweight, as shown in Example #1. An adult with a BMI of 40 or higher is considered extremely obese, and 30 or higher is considered obese, as shown in Example #2. A BMI of 18.5 to 24.9 in adults is considered a healthy weight. A BMI below 18.5 in adults is considered underweight.

BODY FATNESS

Although BMI correlates with body fat, BMI does not directly measure body fat. Some very muscular people, especially athletes, may have a BMI that identifies them as overweight even though they do not have excess body fat. This is because the BMI overestimates body fat in athletes. This is also the case with the elderly: the BMI may underestimate body fat in people over 65 years of age.

A more direct measurement uses the ***percentage of body fat***, which is the percentage of fat in the body versus muscle and water. The percentages of body fat in healthy, overweight, obese, and extremely obese adult men and women as determined by the American Council on Exercise are shown in Table 10-1. These percentages of body fat can be used to plan a realistic loss of body fat and preserve lean body mass.

For example, if a woman weighs 140 pounds, and she has 32 percent body fat, this means that she has 44.8 pounds of body fat and 95.2 pounds of lean body mass (bone, blood, muscle, organs, tissue, etc.). Here is the plan for her fat loss:

Current body fat: 140 pounds × .32 fat = 44.8 pounds of body fat
Current lean body mass: 140 pounds – 44.8 pounds of body fat = 95.2 pounds of lean body mass
Desirable body fat: 23% body fat or 32.2 pounds of body fat (140 pounds × .23 fat)
Desirable lean body mass: 140 pounds – 32.2 pounds body fat = 107.8 pounds lean body mass
Fat loss: 44.8 pounds (current body fat) – 32.2 pounds (desirable body fat)=12.6 pounds of body fat to lose

On a reduced-calorie diet with exercise, at a rate of one to two pounds of fat loss per week, fat loss should take about six weeks. Exceptions may be due to a variety of factors, including degree of overweight or obesity.

BODY FAT MEASUREMENT

Methods of measuring body fat and body fat distribution include bioelectrical impedance (BI), computed tomography (CT), magnetic resonance imaging (MRI), skinfold thickness, ultrasound, underwater weighing, waist circumference, waist-to-hip circumference ratios (WHR), and x-ray absorptiometry (DXA). Skinfold thickness using a simple hand caliper or pincer, waist circumference, and waist-to-hip circumference ratios are the easiest and most convenient. The other methods are used more in research, such as in specialized weight loss and sports nutrition laboratories.

- *Bioelectrical impedance (BI):* This method conducts a weak electrical current through the body. Body fat resists the electrical current because it contains less water and electrolytes than lean muscle mass. The measure of body fat is accurate, assuming hydration is normal. Dehydration from exercise, excessive sweating, or premenstrual water retention may distort the measurement.

438

TABLE 10-1 Percentages of Body Fat in Adult Women and Men

Classifications	Body Fat in Women (%)	Body Fat in Men (%)
Healthy	23 to 31%	13 to 21%
Overweight	32 to 37	22 to 25
Obese	38 to 42	26 to 31
Extremely obese	43 *plus*	32 *plus*

Source: *[10].*

- *Computed tomography (CT):* This medical imaging method supplements x-rays and ultrasounds. It is also used for preventive medicine and screening for disease.
- *Magnetic resonance imaging (MRI):* This medical imaging technique is commonly used to visualize the structure and function of the body. It provides detailed images of body fat in any plane.
- *Skinfold thickness:* This simple method is manually taken with a skinfold caliper. Body fat is pinched at multiple sites and then the results are compared to a mathematical formula. The caliper will not show a small amount of body fat lost over a short amount of time. Plus, if someone is overfat or overmuscular, the results can be skewed.
- *Ultrasound:* This method measures the distance between skin, fat, and muscle layers, and allows the measurement of fat and muscle at various body sites. It has research significance, but it is neither economical nor practical for the general public.
- *Underwater (hydrostatic) weighing:* This process submerges a person underwater and then measures his or her weight. Body fat weighs less than lean muscle mass, which is denser than water. Someone who is overfat will weigh less under water. Special, expensive equipment is required, so this method is not entirely practical.
- *Waist circumference:* A simple way to determine body fat distribution is to use a measuring tape to measure waist circumference. The tape should be placed around the waist, parallel to the floor and at the top of the upper hip bones for the hip measurement—not at the narrowest point. Upper-body obesity is considered a waist circumference measurement that is greater than 35 inches in women and 40 inches in men.
- *Waist-to-hip circumference ratios (WHR):* This is a ratio of the waist circumference measurement to the hip circumference measurement. It is determined by measuring the waist circumference just above the upper hip bone, divided by the hip circumference at its widest part (waist circumference/hip circumference). Having more abdominal fat than hip fat places individuals at higher risks of diseases such as heart disease and diabetes.
- *X-ray absorptiometry (DXA):* This procedure uses low-energy x-rays to scan the body; then it displays a total image of all body structures, including fat deposits. While accurate, the equipment is expensive and impractical for general use, much like bioelectrical impedance, computed tomography, magnetic resonance imaging, and ultrasound equipment.

METABOLISM

While the role of body composition in weight management cannot be overemphasized, the role of metabolism is also fundamental. *Metabolism* is the set of chemical reactions that maintain life in living organisms. These chemical reactions help organisms to grow, maintain their structures, reproduce, and react to their environments.

Metabolism is actually two sets of chemical reactions: catabolism and anabolism. **Catabolism** breaks down large molecules, such as food, into energy. **Anabolism** uses energy to construct cell components, such as carbohydrates, proteins, and lipids into cells, organs, and body systems.

Several factors affect a person's metabolism, which in turn can affect a person's body weight, including the following:

- *Age:* After 30 years of age, there is usually a gradual decline in lean body mass and an increase in stored fat in both men and women. This decline in lean body mass lowers metabolism because lean body mass is more active in burning calories than stored fat.
- *Body temperature:* Metabolism is affected by fever and cold because energy must be expended to either cool or warm the body.
- *Climate:* Hot or cold climates can affect metabolism. Shivering contracts and relaxes muscle cells to produce heat energy to warm the body. Sweating requires a complex system of reactions to cool the body.
- *Diet:* A small amount of energy is used for digesting and absorbing nutrients. This process is called *thermogenesis*. It contributes to about 5 to 10 percent of daily total calorie expenditure (see "The thermic effect of food" that follows). This is why small, frequent meals are said to increase metabolism and burn calories. Thermogenesis is greater when protein is a part of a meal, rather than just carbohydrates or lipids.
- *Drugs:* Pharmaceutical drugs may influence metabolism. Caffeine and nicotine can affect metabolism, but in modest amounts, depending on a number of variables.

- *Fasting and starvation:* Both fasting and starvation may slow metabolism because the body tries to hold onto its calories. Vital organs and systems are nourished at the expense of lean body mass and fat stores.
- *Gender:* Men have a higher percentage of lean muscle mass than women, which means they have the potential to burn more calories. This difference in lean muscle mass and body composition is mainly due to male sex hormones. Sports training can change the proportion of lean muscle mass in women, but only to a certain extent without steroids.
- *Growth:* During periods of growth, such as pregnancy, lactation, infancy, childhood, and adolescence, metabolism increases to meet all of the body's demands.
- *Height:* Taller people have a higher metabolism than shorter people because they have more surface area that needs to be heated or cooled, which requires energy.
- *Heredity:* We inherit the predisposition for fast or slow metabolism from our ancestors. Genes may also affect the production of certain enzymes that assist fat uptake and use. This is why family members may come in all sizes and shapes and why losing weight for one family member may be harder for the other.
- *Hormones:* Because hormones control many of the body's chemical processes, they can slow or speed up metabolism. If hormones increase lean muscle mass and change body composition, this could raise metabolism, and the opposite is also true. **Thyroid hormone** is responsible for regulating normal metabolism. **Hypothyroidism** may be caused by too little thyroid hormone and contribute to weight gain. **Hyperthyroidism** may be cause by too much thyroid hormone and contribute to weight loss. Medical attention is needed for both disorders.
- *Lifestyle:* A decline in our metabolism can be attributed to lifestyle changes, such as more sedentary living. This is a factor that is in our control. Regular exercise throughout adulthood will slow the rate at which lean body mass is lost and help maintain metabolism to prevent weight gain.
- *Sleep:* Metabolism is still operative during sleep; it just slows down. That is why one might feel cold in the morning before the voluntary muscles are called into action.
- *Stress and anxiety:* Specialized hormones are secreted under stress or anxiety. They send messages to the cells to speed up metabolism for heightened needs. Fidgeting also increases metabolism, but the contribution is small.

440

BASAL METABOLISM RATE AND WEIGHT

The **basal metabolic rate (BMR)** is the amount of energy that is expended at rest in a neutral environment after the digestive system has been inactive for about 12 hours. It is the rate of one's metabolism when waking in the morning after "fasting" during sleep.

The BMR is enough energy for the brain and central nervous system, heart, kidneys, liver, lungs, muscles, sex organs, and skin to function properly. People who are overweight or obese do not necessarily have a slow BMR. In fact, their BMR is usually faster to accommodate for extra fat and for their body to work harder to perform normal body functions. Building lean muscle mass can increase BMR, but there is a limit for both men and women as to how much lean muscle mass can be built. Some supplements may increase BMR, but also only to a limit, and they may have serious side effects (see "Diet aids").

Expending extra calories through increased physical activity is the most sensible way to increase metabolism. When a person diets, BMR slows down to conserve energy and protect vital organs. A regimen of reasonable dieting with increased exercise maintains or increases BMR and promotes weight loss and weight maintenance. It all depends on calories and caloric balance.

CALORIES

A **calorie** (from the Latin *calor*, meaning "heat") is a unit of energy. It was first called a "kilogram-calorie" by Nicolas Clément, a French physicist and chemist, in 1824 [11]. Today, the term *calorie* has two meanings: the small calorie (cal) and the large calorie, kilocalorie (kcal). The calorie (cal) is the amount of heat or energy that is required to raise the temperature of 1 gram of water by 1°C. The kilocalorie (kcal) is the amount of heat or energy that is needed to increase the temperature of 1 kilogram of water by 1°C. This is the name that is commonly used to describe food energy. For example, 1 gram of carbohydrate or protein has 4 kilocalories, 1 gram of alcohol has 7 kilocalories, and 1 gram of fat has 9 kilocalories. Common usage has dropped the prefix "kilo," but this is the accurate designation.

CALORIE BALANCE

It takes roughly 3,500 kilocalories over and beyond the body's needs to gain 1 pound of body fat, and 3,500 calories less than the body requires to lose 1 pound of body fat. These calories can be all consumed or expended at the same time or over the course of time. Unfortunately calorie balance is not as easy as it seems. This is because calories are not equal. As discussed in Chapter 1, carbohydrates, protein, lipids and alcohol all contain different amounts. And caloric expenditure is highly individualized. By learning how to determine the number of calories expended daily, one can create a healthy weight-loss diet to lose body fat.

CALORIC EXPENDITURE

The three factors that contribute to the amount of calories that a person expends daily are *basal metabolism, physical activity,* and the *thermic effect of food (thermogenesis)*:

- *Basal metabolism (60 to 65 percent of total energy expenditure):* The body expends most of its calories digesting food, maintaining the heartbeat and respiration, and normal brain functioning. The amount of calories needed for basal metabolism is about 1,200 to 1,300 calories daily, based on a 2,000-calorie diet.
- *Physical activity (25 to 35 percent of total energy expenditure):* Physical activity is the total amount of activity that a person carries out daily, from walking in a mall to playing pickup basketball. While basal metabolism is a fairly fixed energy expenditure, physical activity is highly individualized. The more active a person is, the more calories a person may burn.

  People with different body compositions may burn calories differently during physical activity. The amount of muscle mass and total body weight factor into the number of calories expended. Fitness level, intensity, and time are also considerations. Energy is required to move the skeletal muscles, raise the heartbeat, and increase breathing. The more body mass, conceivably the more calories are burned.

  > **Morsel** "To lengthen your life, shorten your meals." —Proverb

- *Thermic effect of food (5 to 10 percent of total energy expenditure):* Thermic means "heat." The thermic effect of food (or thermogenesis) is the creation of heat. It is the amount of calories that it takes to digest, absorb, and process foods and beverages to create energy. If one consumes small meals throughout the day, the thermic effect of food will help to active the metabolism to produce energy after each meal or snack.

441

DETERMINING DAILY ENERGY NEEDS

This is a simple method to use for determining daily energy needs. It accounts for basal metabolism, physical activity, and the thermic effect of food. Computerized methods can be found on the Internet. Check out "Hungry for more?" later in this chapter.

1. Multiply weight in pounds by 10.9 if male or 9.8 if female. These values have been established based on BMR factors. _____
2. Select level of physical activity: _____
   Very light—mostly seated or standing
   Light—mostly moving about
   Moderate—mostly physical work; exercise 1 *or more* hours at least every other day
   Heavy—mostly manual labor; longer and/or more frequent exercise
3. Choose activity factor: _____
   Very light (men and women)—1.3
   Light (men)—1.6
   Moderate (men)—1.5
   Moderate (women)—1.7
   Heavy (men)—2.1
   Heavy (women)—1.9
4. Multiply activity factor in #3 by basal metabolic needs in #1:
   _____ activity factor ×_____ basal metabolic needs=_____ kilocalories

5. Multiply kilocalories in #4 by 5 to 10% to account for the thermal effect of food. _____ kilocalories

6. Add the number of kilocalories needed daily in #4 with the kilocalories that account for the thermic effect of food in #5. _____

This is the total number of kilocalories that are required daily.

> **Example:** A 170-pound man who participated in heavy activity
> **Basal metabolism:** 1,853 kilocalories
> **Physical activity:** factor 2.1
> 1,853 kilocalories (BM) × 2.1 (activity factor) = 3,891.3 kilocalories
> **Thermic effect of food:** 7.5% (.075)
> 3,891.3 kilocalories (BM *plus* physical activity) × .075 (thermic effect of food) = 291.9 kilocalories
> **Total number of kilocalories needed daily:** 3,891.3 (BM *plus* physical activity) *plus* 291.9 (thermic effect of food) = 4,183.2 kilocalories required daily

In order for this man to maintain his body weight, he needs to consume 4,183.2 kilocalories daily. Just 100 additional calories daily will cause him to consume 36,500 extra calories by year's end. Without additional exercise to expend these 100 calories, he can expect to gain 10.4 pounds (36,500 kilocalories/3,500 kilocalories in one pound = about 10.4 pounds!). This is the reason why every calorie counts—both as calories consumed and calories expended [12–14].

Bite on This: 100-calorie foods and beverages

Consuming 100 calories over and beyond what is required each day is easy, so be careful! These calorie-dense foods and alcoholic beverages can be reduced without too much effort. Portion sizes are averaged.

¼ cup potato salad
½ ice cream sandwich
½ croissant
1 can light beer
1 tablespoon butter or margarine
1 tablespoon mayonnaise and salad dressing
1⅓ ounces whole egg caviar
1½ tablespoons pate de foie gras
2 tablespoons chocolate syrup
2 tablespoons cream cheese
2 creme-filled chocolate sandwich cookies
2 slices crisp-fried bacon
2 chocolate graham crackers
2 slices salami
3½ tablespoons French onion dip
4 chocolate kisses
4 ounces extra-dry champagne
4 small Tootsie Rolls
6 ounces Chablis wine
8 potato chips

Need to gain weight? The following 100-calorie portions are nutrient dense versus calorie dense. Once again, the portion sizes are approximate:

½ cup low-fat cottage cheese
½ pound Chinese pea pods
1 cup dairy skim milk
1 medium apple, banana, grapefruit, or orange
1 medium baked potato
1 cup plain, nonfat yogurt
1 large shredded wheat-type biscuit

2 cups fresh strawberries

2 cups tomato juice

2 ounces cooked skinless chicken

3 ounces turkey breast

2 stalks fresh broccoli

3 graham crackers

4 tablespoons low-fat ricotta cheese

4 tablespoons Parmesan cheese

4⅓ cups popped popcorn without butter

12 medium almonds

5 large prunes

6 clams on the half-shell

15 walnuts halves

Source: *[15]*.

WEIGHT GAIN AND WEIGHT LOSS

FOOD BYTE

Starch has important roles in cooking and baking as well as weight management. Starch is responsible for *gelatinization,* when grains and legumes absorb cooking water. It is also responsible for *retrogradation*, when the starch molecules reform and firm up. **Retrograded starch** is good for the body. It resists digestive enzymes, so it is less digestible; therefore, it slows the rise of blood sugar following a meal and prolongs satiety. There is retrograded starch in converted rice and breakfast cereals. Leftover grains, such as risotto, can be reformulated into risotto cakes or balls. This may be why these foods seem so satisfying.

443

WEIGHT GAIN

The body stores excess carbohydrate, protein and fat calories. It metabolizes these calories for energy or stores them as fat, and eliminates their by-products. When digesting and metabolizing carbohydrates, those that are not broken down into glucose for energy may be stored in the muscles and liver as glycogen. Carbohydrates in excess of what is metabolized or stored may be converted into fat.

Protein foods and beverages are broken down into amino acids for growth, maintenance, and repair. Amino acids over and beyond what is necessary for these functions are converted into fat, and the nitrogen portion is excreted in the urine. Lipid-containing foods are metabolized into fatty acids for energy and other lipid-dependent functions. Unused lipids are stored in adipose tissues and adipose cells.

Protein cannot be reformed into protein if it is needed by the body unless all the essential amino acids are present. But new carbohydrates can be formed when the body needs energy. In extraordinary situations the body can break down its protein stores in the muscles to be converted into energy. This is a survival mechanism that the body uses during times of famine or highly restrictive calories.

WEIGHT LOSS

During periods of calorie deprivation, as in dieting, fasting, and illness, the body stores of carbohydrates, protein and lipids are activated. Liver glycogen stores are used in about 4 to 6 hours between meals or about 12 to 14 hours during an overnight fast.

If the absence of food exceeds this amount of time, liver glycogen breaks down into glucose to fuel the brain and the central nervous system. Muscle glycogen is spared for muscular work, and the body strives to keep itself alive by "feeding" the brain.

The body cannot convert fat into glucose for energy, but it does convert protein in the muscle cells into glucose if carbohydrates are not available. This protein is used up twice as fast as fat because protein contains 4 calories per gram and fat contains 9 calories per gram. The muscles may shrink from the loss of protein and water, because with each pound of protein that is used for energy, 3 to 4 pounds of water are freed and excreted. This is why early weight loss is mostly water.

An unrestrained fast of this nature would eventually cause the body to consume its muscles for energy. The heart is a muscle; its stored protein would also be converted into glucose to stay alive. Once the heart is compromised in this manner, death may follow in about 10 days.

Before this happens, the body undergoes further efforts to stay alive by using its fat stores for energy. This condition is called *ketosis*, and the substances that the body lives on are called *ketone bodies* or *ketones.* Ketosis may extend a fasting person's life about 6 to 8 weeks.

Ketones first fuel the central nervous system to keep the brain alive. The body can use about one-half of the remaining ketones for energy. This places a reduced demand on the muscles to release protein for energy, so the muscles are "spared." The concept of "protein-sparing diets" originated in the mid-1800s and then became popular in the mid-1950s. They are still used with and without medical supervision today.

The downside of ketosis is that it can affect the acid-base balance in the bloodstream, making it more acidic. Also, some muscle cells will still continue to break down, and metabolism will slow down, since there are fewer muscle cells. Plus, it is not uncommon for weight loss to plateau or stop from fluid imbalance. People may "rebound" and rapidly regain most or all of the weight that they have lost unless they carefully reintroduce calories and learn behavior modification techniques [16–21].

DIETS AND DIETING

Ketosis compromises the body and is not healthy long term. A well-planned diet can healthfully induce weight loss and preserve muscle mass. A *diet* is the sum of all the food and beverages that are consumed by an organism. *Dieting* is the purposeful choice of foods and beverages to control body weight and/or nutrient intake. The words *diet* and *dieting* are often used interchangeably.

A well-chosen diet meets all nutrient and energy needs. A weight loss of 1 to 2 pounds per week is generally recommended for healthy adults. This amounts to a 3,500- to 7,000-calorie deficit from less food, more exercise, or a combination of the two approaches.

A daily 2,000-calorie diet is used for the US Daily Values, which have been calculated according to what nutritional experts consider to be a healthful diet for adults. This is about the amount of calories that is recommended for most moderately active women, teenage girls and sedentary men. A nutritionally sound weight-loss diet has no fewer than 1,200 calories daily.

Different types of dietary approaches include a very low-calorie diet, a low-calorie diet, a low-carbohydrate/ high-protein diet, a high-carbohydrate/moderate-protein diet, a moderate-carbohydrate/moderate-protein diet, a quick-fix diet, a meal replacement diet, and diet aids, among others.

Different dietary approaches have different percentages of carbohydrates, protein, and fats. Each dietary approach has advantages and disadvantages. No one diet is best for anyone.

- *Very low-calorie diets* are generally less than 800 daily calories of prescribed foods and beverages under medical supervision. Nutritional supplements are often used, many of which are high-protein-based. These diets are generally designed for people with a BMI over 30 or over 27 with other risk factors besides obesity. Sometimes very low-calorie diets are used without medical supervision. **When food and beverage intake is less than 1,200 daily calories, the risks of nutrient deficiencies increase.**
- *Very low- to low-fat/high-carbohydrate diets* range from 60 to 65 percent carbohydrates, 10 to 20 percent or more protein, and less than 10 to 19 percent fat. These diets were popularized in the late 1980s when they were idealized as the diets that healthy societies followed. These diets are typically very low in lean protein and healthy fats and very high in complex carbohydrates and fiber. **Some versions of these diets are still popular today and are effective if portion sizes and calories are controlled.**
- *Moderate-fat/high-protein/moderate-carbohydrate diets* tend to be based on current dietary recommendations, about 50 to 55 percent carbohydrates, 15 to 20 percent protein, and 20 to 30 percent fat, with about

1,200 to 1,800 calories daily. This would create a calorie deficit of about 200 to 800 calories daily. **Weight loss is slow but steady**.

- *High-fat/high-protein, low-carbohydrate diets* typically have less than 20 percent carbohydrate, 25 to 40 percent protein, and 55 to 65 percent or more fat. Carbohydrates are limited to less than 100 to 125 grams per day to ensure ketosis. These very popular diets promote quick weight loss that is mostly water weight. Because they tend to depress appetite and increase energy with ketosis, they are easier to follow than diets where hunger and lethargy may be issues. **These diets may be high in saturated fats and cholesterol and low in fiber, minerals, and vitamins. They may not promote long-term compliance**.

- *Moderate-fat/moderate-protein, moderate-carbohydrate, moderate-calorie diets* contain 40 to 50 percent carbohydrates, 25 to 40 percent protein and 30 to 40 percent fat. This amount of carbohydrates is usually enough to prevent ketosis. Carbohydrates feature whole grains for fiber, minerals, and vitamins; protein is lean; and fats are essential and healthy. These diets were developed as an alternative to *high-fat/high-protein, low-carbohydrate diets*. **They may successfully improve blood fats and blood sugar levels, and induce weight loss** [22,23].

WEIGHT-GAIN DIETS

Certain people need to gain weight. These include some athletes, people with eating disorders such as anorexia, and those who have undergone serious weight loss due to illness or medical treatments, such as chemotherapy.

> **Morsel** "If I can't have too many truffles, I'll do without." —Colette (French novelist and performer, 1873–1954)

Weight gain requires an *increase* of 3,500 calories to gain 1 pound. An easy way to accomplish this is by eating lots of high-calorie, fatty and sugary foods. A more nutritious approach is a balance of carbohydrates, protein, and fat, much like the moderate-fat/high-protein/moderate-carbohydrate diet described above.

It is challenging for some to consume enough food to gain weight, even when presented with a healthy and flavorsome diet. This is where nutritional supplements may have their place. The best nutritional supplements are balanced in nutrients in a highly digestible liquid form. One to two of these liquid nutritional supplements daily can provide 350 to 700 calories in addition to a moderate-fat/high-protein/moderate-carbohydrate diet.

Other ways to add healthy calories include the use of nut butters as spreads instead of pure fat. One tablespoon of peanut butter provides about 90 calories, 4 grams of protein, and 6 grams of fat, compared to 108 calories and 12 grams of fat per tablespoon of butter. Sprinkle nuts or seeds on grains, salads, vegetables, and desserts such as custard, fruit, ice cream, and pudding. Add a few slices of avocado or olives to salads and sandwiches, and use salad dressings with canola, olive, or walnut oil to add healthy fats. Shred squash into sauces, scrape corn kernels into pasta, and mix legumes into meatloaf. Add milk or milk powder to beverages, sauces and soups. Thicken creamy sauces and soups with silken tofu; each slice adds 4 grams of lean protein. Snack on dried fruits and higher-calorie vegetables, such as carrots and edible pea pods with dips. Eat several small meals daily rather than larger meals, so as not to overwhelm the body.

Recipe: Chocolate Pudding

A diet that contains some sweets may be effective for those who struggle with more restrictive diets. If chocolate is incorporated into a diet in a portion-controlled manner, it satisfies cravings for taste and texture. This **Chocolate Pudding** *is mindful of both nutrients and flavor. Dutch process cocoa powder, nonfat milk, some sugar, and cornstarch to thicken create a delicious and nutritious dessert or snack. The recipe can be found in the* **Recipe file** *which is located within the Culinary Nutrition website at www.culinarynutrition.elsevier.com, and the finished dish is shown within the centerfold* **Photo file** *in Plate 10.1.*

COMMERCIAL WEIGHT-LOSS PROGRAMS

A number of commercial weight-loss programs offer a variety of weight-loss diets, with or without individual or group counseling. Typically these diets range between 1,000 to 1,500 calories, but some are

445

very low-calorie. Some programs require daily weigh-ins; others incorporate exercise. Many require foods or supplements that are unique to their program.

The most successful programs offer some combination of behavior modification, convenience, cooking and menu planning, lifestyle management, motivation, nutrition advice, daily exercise plans, slow and steady weight loss, strong support, and weight maintenance. Some employ nutrition and culinary specialists for diet, meal, menu, and recipe creations.

The following questions should be asked when evaluating commercial weight loss programs:

- Are there specific meal plans?
- Do you have to keep food records?
- Can you make changes based on your food preferences?
- Is the program sensitive to your lifestyle and cultural needs?
- What is the rate of weight loss?
- What is the long-term success rate of keeping the weight off?
- What are the credentials of the program leaders?
- Are there short- and long-term health risks?
- Is there ongoing support from a health care professional?
- Is there personalized counseling?
- Is there an exercise component?
- Are there special foods and supplements?
- What are the membership costs?
- Are there weekly fees?
- Is there a follow-up program?

Bite on This: Lena's story

Lena S. is a healthy 30-something normal-weight mother and wife, but she claims that she was not always this way. She was raised in a European country where the notion was that a fat child was a happy child. So Lena's grandmother (who was her primary care provider) overfed her by mixing cereal into milk and preparing rich and starchy foods.

As a child, Lena was overweight, though active. She had a body type much like her mother's, who dieted to control her weight. Lena's mother was her role model. This admiration triggered Lena's lifetime of dieting, except that she did not have the right foods to diet healthfully. She admits to practicing starvation, which continued throughout high school. Then Lena developed a digestive problem that continued through adulthood.

Lena used a diet aid to lose weight fast—about 15 to 20 pounds in one month. She then turned to acupuncture and aggressive exercise. In her early twenties, Lena traveled to the United States, married, became pregnant, and gained a normal amount of weight with her pregnancy. But she developed gallbladder disease during her pregnancy and went back to Europe for surgery. For nine months, Lena could only eat toast and tea, and she lost a considerable amount of weight.

When she recovered, Lena traveled back to the United States and resumed a normal life. She cooked for her husband and son the way she was taught to do in Europe. The weight returned. So Lena used the diet aid again and ate nothing at all every other day to lose weight. And then she regained the weight that she had lost.

About four years ago, Lena joined a popular commercial weight-control program in the United States. She gradually lost about 25 pounds, but she exercised about two hours daily to help achieve this loss. Due to a change in her lifestyle, Lena regained this weight once again.

During the past four months, Lena returned to the commercial weight-control program, relost the 25 pounds, and exercises for enjoyment. She does not feel deprived, and she does not miss any foods. She knows that food is an addiction for her and that she must watch her weight and exercise forever. The commercial weight-loss program is considered the finest in the industry. So Lena is now eating a balanced nutritional diet and incorporating exercise into her busy life in a sensible and healthful way.

The constant battle of losing and gaining weight has taken a toll on Lena's body. But now Lena's weight has stabilized—hopefully forever. She attributes her poor eating habits to her early feeding. Providing a healthy start for children is essential in preventing the potential devastating effects of overweight and obesity like the ones Lena experienced during her young life.

DIET AIDS

Losing weight and keeping it off is difficult because it takes a conscious daily effort to monitor calories and activities. The temptation to use dietary aids is alluring. Turning to pills and potions to take the weight off fast is a lot easier than dieting and exercising, no matter what the cost. But are they safe, and what are the long-term effects?

Herbal and dietary supplements are common weight loss aids. In the United States, the Dietary Supplement and Health Education Act of 1994 (DSHEA) allows manufacturers to classify herbal products and nutritional supplements as foods. But it also allows manufacturers to bypass some strict regulations of the FDA. As a result, weight-loss aids are not subject to the same rigorous standards as prescription drugs or over-the-counter medications. Some can be marketed with limited proof of effectiveness or safety. Manufacturers may make health claims based on their own review and interpretation of studies without FDA authorization. However, the FDA can take a product off the market if it is proven to be dangerous. This is especially important with the number of products that are now available through the Internet. The US Federal Trade Commission (FTC) helps to monitor trafficking. Some of these diet aids are shown in Table 10-2 [24–27]. Because there is no assurance that these products are safe or effective, like other alternative approaches to diet and health, let the buyer beware. Some potential long-term effects can be quite dangerous.

A number of prescription and over-the-counter drugs are available to combat the growing health problem of obesity. They act by inhibiting the enzyme lipase that is needed for fat digestion; numbing the taste buds; raising the brain chemical norepinephrine, which signals satiety; suppressing appetite; and other means.

Potential side effects include decreased absorption of fat-soluble vitamins, gastrointestinal disorders, and increased blood pressure and heart rate. Even "Dieter's Tea," readily available at some supermarkets, may cause severe extreme dehydration, gastrointestinal problems, and sometimes even death.

MEDICAL TREATMENTS FOR OBESITY

There are circumstances when diet and exercise may not be enough for major weight loss. This is when more drastic measures may be taken to reduce weight. *Bariatric medicine* specializes in treating obesity. *Bariatric surgery* is an effective means for severely obese people (those with a BMI greater than or equal to 40 or with a BMI over 35 with serious health problems) to lose a significant amount of weight, reduce blood lipids and blood pressure, and improve health status. But bariatric surgery also has disadvantages.

The three most common types of medical treatments involve *gastric banding, gastric bypass,* and *gastroplasty (stomach stapling),* which reduce the stomach's capacity to hold about 1 ounce of food (the stomach's capacity is about 1 quart in an adult). More than 50 percent of excess weight can be lost long term with these techniques.

Gastric banding uses a silicone band around the upper section of the stomach that limits food intake and causes early satiety. *Gastroplasy* staples the stomach to decrease its volume. The most common surgical intervention is *gastric bypass,* which first decreases the size of the stomach with a band or staples and then creates a pouch that bypasses the lower stomach. Instead, the food moves to the upper part of the small intestine.

Side effects of these techniques may include diarrhea, heartburn, nausea, pain, vomiting, and band or staple slippage or engorgement. The stomach pouch may stretch to 2 to 3 ounces from overeating.

447

TABLE 10-2 Diet Aids, Uses, Effects, and Long-Term Outcomes

Diet Aids	Uses	Effects	Long-Term Outcomes
Bitter orange	Ephedra substitute	Increases calories burned	Not known
Chaso	FenPhen substitute (*also* Fenfluramine)	Appetite suppressant	Heart disease
Chitosan	Safe; may be ineffective	Blocks fat absorption	Not known
Chromium	Unlikely weight loss	Reduces body fat, decreases appetite, builds muscle	Gastrointestinal (GI) problems
Clenbuterol	Similar to ephedrine	Increases metabolism	Impaired heart, lung function
Conjugated linoleic acid (CLA)	May decrease body fat, increase muscle	Decreases appetite; possible reduction body fat, increased muscle	GI problems; may *not* reduce body weight
Ephedra[a]	Banned for safety issues; sold online	Decreases appetite	High blood pressure, irregular heartbeat, heart attacks, seizures, strokes, death
Green tea extract	Caffeine generated	Increases calorie and fat metabolism; decreases appetite	GI problems
Guar gum[b]	Decreases calorie intake from fullness	Blocks fat absorption	GI problems
Heartleaf (*also* country mallow)	Contains ephedra	Decreases appetite, increases calorie expenditure	Not known
Hoodia	No conclusive support	Decreases appetite	Not for children; should not be used during pregnancy
Methylcellulose	Fullness	Appetite suppressant	GI problems with misuse
Phenylpropanolamine (PPA) (*also* Dexatrim)	Diuretic	Appetite suppressant	Increased blood pressure, stroke
Spirulina	No conclusive benefits	Suppresses hunger	Rare cases of side-effects
Starch blockers[c]	Banned	Inhibit starch digestion	GI problems

Source: [28,29].
[a]Ephedra is derived from the herb Ephedra sinica, also known as Chinese Ma Huang.
[b]Guar gum is a type of carbohydrate that swells with liquids. It is used as an emulsifier, stabilizer, and thickener in cooking and baking.
[c]Starch blockers are concentrated raw legumes. They inhibit the starch-digesting ability of the enzyme alpha amylase. Unabsorbed starch then moves to the bowel for elimination.

Liposuction, surgery that uses a vacuum-like procedure to remove fat cells from specific areas of the body, is considered *cosmetic surgery.* Body fat may shift back into the treated areas unless calorie and fat reductions are maintained. Liposuction may also cause body water to redistribute, which may potentially disrupt normal fluid balance and increase the risk of stroke or heart attack.

FASTING

Fasting is the process of consciously refraining from food and drink for a period of time. It may be total or partial, extended or intermittent. Fasting for religious and spiritual reasons has been practiced for millennia. It has biblical roots in the Old and New Testaments and other religious texts, including the Muslim Qur'an, the Indian Mahabharata, and the Hindu Upanishads [30].

Fasting also refers to the condition of the body after a meal is digested. For example, the body fasts between dinner and breakfast. Most people are asked to fast before their annual medical appointment. This is because fasting is used to detect hypo- and hyperglycemia and to measure blood lipids. Fasting is also used in preparation for surgery or anesthetic-based procedures. In naturopathic medicine, fasting cleanses the body of toxins and old or diseased tissues, and gives the gastrointestinal system opportunity to rest.

Some fasts use juices, water or limited amounts of food. Fasts of this nature should be preceded and followed by a healthy diet and should be supervised by knowledgeable health care professionals. A considerable amount of water weight can be lost at the start of a fast, but lean body mass may also be lost as in other very low-calorie diets. Sometimes fasting is used to "jump-start" other diets. The transition to more calories and fluids should be carefully planned to avoid major shifts in body fluids.

There is some interest in fasting to help prolong the life span and reduce the diseases that are associated with aging, inflammation, and oxidative stress. Reducing portion sizes, overhauling recipes to make them healthier, and consuming foods and beverages in their natural states may accomplish similar ends.

> **Morsel** "Life itself is the proper binge." —Julia Child (American author, chef and television personality, 1912–2004)

Disordered Eating

DIET AND EATING DISORDERS

The polar opposites of the disorders of overweight and obesity are *anorexia nervosa* and *bulimia nervosa*. *Anorexia nervosa* is a complex bodily condition that involves neurobiological, psychological, and sociological components. It is characterized by low body weight and distorted body image, with an obsessive fear of gaining weight. People with anorexia nervosa may display behaviors that include the ingestion of diet pills and diuretics, excessive exercise, purging, starvation, vomiting, or other extreme measures. Anorexia nervosa primarily affects female adolescents. About 10 percent of those diagnosed with anorexia nervosa are male.

While medical diagnosis confirms anorexia nervosa, physical symptoms may include the following:

- Abnormal mineral and electrolyte levels
- Amenorrhea (lack of menstrual periods)
- Anemias
- Body mass index less than 17.5 in adults and 85 percent of expected weight in children
- Bradycardia (slow heart rate)
- Brittle fingernails
- Bruising
- Constant coldness
- Constipation
- Creaking joints and bones
- Difficulty moving feet
- Dry skin and lips
- Decreased libido
- Endocrine disorders
- Extreme weight loss
- Fainting
- Fluid in ankles and around eyes
- Fragile appearance
- Frail body image
- Headaches
- Hypotension (low blood pressure)
- Hypothermia (low body temperature)
- Lanugo (fine body hair that insulates skin from lack of fat)
- Male impotence
- Nerve deterioration
- Pale complexion
- Poor circulation ("'pins and needles")
- Purple extremities
- Reduced immune system function
- Reduced metabolism

449

- Reduced white blood cell count
- Stunted growth
- Sunken eyes
- Thin hair
- Tooth decay
- Zinc deficiency

The behavioral, emotional, interpersonal, psychological, and social symptoms of anorexia nervosa may include the following:

- Aggressive when forced to eat
- Chronic moodiness
- Clinical depression
- Denial of basic bodily needs
- Deterioration in family relationships
- Distorted body image
- Excessive exercise
- Excessive food restriction
- Intense fear of overweight
- Low self-esteem and self-efficacy
- Mood swings
- Obsessive compulsive disorder (OCD)
- Perfectionism
- Poor insight
- Preoccupation/obsession about food/weight
- Secretive about eating/exercise behaviors
- Self-evaluation based on body shape/weight
- Belief that control over food/body equals control over life
- Refusal to accept healthy weight concepts
- Refusal to accept reality of dangerously low weight
- Self-mutilation and self-harm
- Sensitive to remarks about body weight
- Substance abuse
- Suicide attempts
- Withdrawal from friendships, other relationships

Bulimia nervosa is a condition that is characterized by incidents of *bingeing*, or overeating, and restrictive eating, much like anorexia nervosa. Like anorexia nervosa, this condition affects more females than males. Some elements of this disorder are the abuse of enemas, diuretics, and laxatives; fasting; overexercising; and self-induced vomiting. Bulimia nervosa may first present itself during adolescence and continue through adulthood. Relapse is common. Bulimia nervosa is more difficult to detect than anorexia nervosa because in general bulimics tend to look healthy and they have few immediate nutrition or health issues.

The two main types of bulimia nervosa are *purging bulimia* and *nonpurging bulimia*. **Purging bulimia** is common. It involves purging through self-induced vomiting to rapidly eliminate food from the body before it is digested. *Nonpurging bulimia* occurs in only approximately 6 to 8 percent of diagnosed cases. It involves excessive exercise or fasting after bingeing to counterbalance the calories consumed.

While medical diagnosis may not confirm bulimia nervosa, the following behavioral, emotional, interpersonal, nutritional, physical, psychological, and social symptoms may lead to its diagnosis:

- Altered heartbeat
- Anorexia nervosa
- Blood chemistry abnormalities
- Dental problems
- Eating in fixed time

- Esophageal bleeding
- Excessive exercise beyond fitness
- Excessive food consumption per episode
- Fasting
- Feeling loss of control
- Hand sores
- Inappropriate behavior to prevent weight gain
- Misused diuretics and/or laxatives
- Recurrent bingeing episodes
- Self-induced vomiting
- Sense of self measured by body image
- Swelling of salivary glands

BINGE-EATING, NIGHT EATING, AND NOCTURNAL SLEEP-RELATED EATING DISORDERS

There is some debate about whether *binge-eating disorder, night eating syndrome,* and *nocturnal sleep-related eating disorder* fall into the same realm of eating disorders such as anorexia nervosa or bulimia nervosa. People who display these behaviors often have histories of alcoholism, drug abuse, or sleep disorders, which may have genetic roots. Episodes may go unnoticed, since most peculiar eating is done alone to conceal the circumstances. Emotional connections are common. Some of these behaviors may lead to anorexia nervosa or bulimia nervosa unless medical, nutritional, and psychological interventions occur.

Binge-eating disorder is a condition that involves food and/or beverage binges without episodes of purging. People with serious binge-eating disorders consume unusually large amounts of foods and beverages and may or may not believe their eating is out of control.

The signs and symptoms of binge-eating disorder may include eating alone to avoid embarrassment; eating large amounts of food when not hungry; eating quickly until uncomfortably full; feeling disgusted, depressed, or guilty after overeating; and feeling ashamed about the amount of food consumed.

Binge-eating disorder is common. It affects about 3 percent of all adults in the United States. It is most common in people aged 46 to 55 years, in women more than men, and in people who are severely obese.

The signs and symptoms of *night eating syndrome* include anxiety over late-night eating; arousal during sleep to eat; consumption of excessive carbohydrate-rich foods and beverages after dinner; depression or stress over night eating; and little appetite for breakfast. Depression, sleep disorders, and stress are suspected triggers. It is estimated that only 1 to 2 percent of US adults have night eating disorder. Others may not seek treatment.

Nocturnal sleep-related eating disorder appears to be more of a sleep-related disorder than an eating disorder. In this disorder, people eat while they seemingly are sound asleep. These eating episodes may be related to sleep-walking; they occur in a state somewhere between wakefulness and sleep. The foods and beverages consumed tend to be high in fat and sugar—foods that may be denied while awake. Hunger and chronic dieting, sleep apnea, stress, and anxiety are speculated to blame. One to 3 percent of US adults may be subject to this disorder. Restrictive dieting during the day may leave people hungry and vulnerable to nocturnal eating at rest [31–37].

Spa Cuisine

SPA APPROACHES TO WEIGHT MANAGEMENT

The term *spa* may have originated from the town of Spa, Belgium, as early as the fourteenth century, where iron deficiency was treated by drinking "iron-bearing" spring water. But the practice of traveling to a hot or cold spring to cure an ailment may even date back to prehistoric times. People were thought to "take the waters" for their cleansing properties, much like a water fast.

Today, two commonly visited spas are *medical* and *destination spas*. **Medical spas** are facilities with comprehensive health care services by licensed health care professionals. While some medical spas focus on cosmetic procedures, others cater to individuals who are overweight or obese.

Medical spas with therapeutic residential weight management programs help participants achieve better health through weight loss, physical conditioning, and improved self-care. Comprehensive programs last one to four weeks or longer. They help empower participants to take charge of their body weight with behavioral strategies, educational programs, food and nutrition strategies, on-site counseling, and ongoing support for long-term changes.

The composition of weight loss in a typical medical spa program is shown in Table 10-3. Note how much water is lost the first week and how little fat. Notice that water loss subsides by the third week and that fat loss is significant.

Destination spas are facilities that offer spa services and guidance toward lifestyle transformations. Comprehensive programs may include cooking demonstrations, healthful cuisine, health and wellness programming, physical fitness activities, and a quick weight-loss diet. The average stay at a destination spa is about 5 to7 days.

Destination spas typically offer portion-controlled, reduced-calorie, flavorful meals and snacks, around 1,500 calories per day for women and 1,800 calories per day for men. The diets are usually nutritionally balanced to initiate slow, safe, and permanent weight loss. Sample higher-protein diets are depicted in Table 10-4. Menus are mostly vegetarian, supplemented by fish, lean poultry, and low-calorie dairy products to make plants, rather than animals, the center of a meal. Higher-complex carbohydrates (fresh fruits, legumes, vegetables, and whole grains) are featured, and fats and sodium are minimized. Emphasis is placed on sensory-satisfying meals that are rich in flavor, texture, and presentational appeal. A day's worth of foods and beverages at approximately 1,500 calories, typical of a destination spa, is shown in Table 10-5.

TABLE 10-3 Composition of Weight Loss in a Typical Medical Spa Program

Food Restriction (Number of Days)	Daily Weight Loss (Pounds)	Composition of Weight Loss (% Nutrients)
1–3 days	1.8 lbs	70% water; 5% protein; 25% fat
11–13	0.5	19% water; 12% protein; 69% fat
21–24	0.4	0% water; 15% protein; 85% fat

TABLE 10-4 Higher-Protein 1,500- and 1,800-Calorie Diets

Higher-Protein Diet	1,500-Calorie Diet Equivalent	1,800-Calorie Diet Equivalent
27 to 37% carbohydrate	480 calories carbohydrates	576 calories carbohydrates
34 to 40% protein	555 calories protein	666 calories protein
29 to 33% fat	465 calories fat	558 calories fat

TABLE 10-5 Typical Destination Spa Daily Menu (approximately 1,500 calories)

Meal or Snack	Calories
Breakfast	
1 cup fresh orange slices with toasted almonds	100 cal
2 small corn muffins	100
½ cup reduced-fat cottage cheese	90
1 cup caffeine-free tea	0
Lunch	
6 ounces Grilled Scallops with Herbed Feta Sauce	360
1 cup broccoli with cauliflower "cream" sauce	100
1 cup herbed brown rice	100
1 cup pineapple ice	90
12 ounces sparkling water with lemon	0

(Continued)

TABLE 10-5 (Continued)

Meal or Snack	Calories
Dinner	
1½ cups Garlic and Almond Soup	80 cal
1 cup mixed bean salad with vegetables	200
1 cup frozen strawberry mousse	100
Snack	
1 cup apricot nectar	120
5 graham cracker squares	110
Total calories	1,550

Exercise and Sports Nutrition

EXERCISE FOR WEIGHT MANAGEMENT AND HEALTH

At the other end of the weight control spectrum from diet is exercise. Too much food and not enough exercise, and people will gain weight over time. The opposite is also true: too much activity and not enough food, and people will lose weight over time. Finding the right balance between healthy food intake and exercise is the solution. But it is easier said than done, since exercise is hard work—the way life was before today's convenient lifestyles.

> **Morsel** "The sovereign invigorator of the body is exercise, and of all the exercises walking is the best." —Thomas Jefferson (US founding father and president, 1743–1826)

Exercise is the performance of physical activities to achieve ideal body weight, physical fitness, and health. It boosts the immune system, builds muscles and bone density, develops athletic skills, helps prevent disease, improves mental health and prevents depression, maintains joint mobility, reduces surgical risks, and supports weight loss or weight maintenance. Frequent and regular aerobic exercise may prevent or support the treatment of coronary heart disease, diabetes, hypertension, obesity and Type II diabetes. But exercise is only part of the bigger issue, which is physical activity.

PHYSICAL ACTIVITIES AND FITNESS

Physical activities are bodily movements that use the skeletal muscles. These muscles apply force to the bones and joints by contraction. The skeletal muscles mostly contract voluntarily. This means that a person consciously sends messages through nerve impulses to the *voluntary muscles* to work, like walk or run. *Involuntary muscles*, like the heart and the muscles that line the gastrointestinal tract, mostly work unconsciously.

The energy that fuels the involuntary muscles is reflected in basal metabolism (see "Determining energy needs"). The energy that fuels voluntary muscles is in addition to basal metabolic needs. The more physically active that a person is, the more calories expended. Regular exercise not only helps people to lose weight, but it also helps them to achieve physical fitness: the ability to participate in moderate to vigorous activities without becoming too fatigued.

TYPES OF PHYSICAL FITNESS

The four types of *physical fitness* are *general*, *cardiovascular*, *muscular*, and *flexibility*. They are all important for achieving and maintaining healthy weight.

General fitness is the ability to engage in moderate-intensity activity on most days. The benefits of being generally fit include improved overall health; the reduction of risk factors in chronic disease; and the achievement, management, and sustainability of ideal body weight throughout adulthood. Some examples of general fitness activities are walking or "active play," such as pickup basketball or recreational bicycling. These moderate-intensity activities should be performed at least 150 minutes per week; 30–60 minutes five days per week; or 20–60 minutes of vigorous-intensity exercise (such as running, swimming laps or playing basketball) three days per week. Longer periods of time, such as 60 to 90 minutes per session, may bring about a calorie deficit and weight loss, assuming that caloric intake does not exceed daily requirements [6].

453

Cardiovascular fitness is the efficiency of the heart, lungs and vascular system in delivering oxygen to the working muscles. It is affected by cardiac output, heart rate, maximal oxygen consumption, and stroke volume. Cardiovascular fitness helps lower blood pressure and cholesterol, and it reduces the risks of cardiovascular disease, certain types of cancer, diabetes, and obesity. Some examples of cardiovascular activities are biking, jogging, swimming, and walking at a 4- to 5-mile-per-hour pace. The activities should be performed at a sustained level at least 20 minutes three to five times weekly. Longer duration or increased frequency may lead to accelerated weight loss, assuming caloric intake does not exceed daily requirements.

Endurance is the ability to perform an effort over time. The two types of endurance are *cardiovascular* and *muscular*. *Cardiovascular endurance* is being able to perform sustained cardiovascular activities. This means keeping a tennis ball in play rather than running for it. Cardiovascular activities should be sustained for at least 20 minutes. To be most effective, cardiovascular endurance should be performed within a person's *target heart rate (THR)*.

TARGET HEART RATE

Target heart rate (THR), or *training heart rate*, is a desirable heart rate range during aerobic exercise. It enables a person's heart and lungs to receive the cardiovascular benefits from a workout. There are two steps for determining one's target heart rate:

1. First, determine the *maximum heart rate (MHR)* for a person's age. The MHR is the highest number of time that the heart can contract in one minute, or the highest heart rate that is achievable during maximal physical exertion.
2. Subtract your age from 220 beats per minute (BPM)
   Example for 18-year old person: 220−18 = 202 BPM

Therefore, 202 BPM is the maximum number of beats per minute that this person's heart should undergo. This theoretical rate may vary, based on age, physical condition, and prior training:

1. Multiple the maximum heart rate (MHR) by 60 to 65 percent for the low end, and 80 to 85 percent for the high end of this range. Unfit individuals should be conservative in their estimates—say, 60 to 80 percent of their MHR; more fit individuals may be able to aim for a higher range—say, 65 to 85 percent of their MHR.
   Example for same 18-year old person: 202 BPM × .65 = 131.3 BPM
   202 BPM × .85 = 171.7 BPM

This person's target heart rate is 131.3 to 171.7 BPM.

2. Count your pulse for 10 seconds, then multiply this figure by 6 for a minute count. This is taken on the radial artery of the wrist or the carotid artery on the side of the neck with the index and middle fingers, not the thumb, which has a pulse of its own.
   Example: 10 beats per second × 6 = 60 BPM

This number, in beats per minute, should correspond to your target heart rate. If it is too low, you should increase the intensity of the activity. If it is too high, you should decrease the intensity of the activity. In the preceding example, 60 BPM is less than the low end of the target heat rate at 131.3; therefore, this person needs to exercise harder. This method allows one to monitor the target heart rate throughout cardiovascular activities to ensure that one is exercising at a safe and effective level for cardiovascular fitness and endurance.

Muscular fitness includes both muscular strength and muscular endurance. *Muscular strength* helps to maintain muscle mass and strength, promote strong bones, reduce arthritis risk, and improve glucose tolerance. These benefits help to reduce the risks of injury, obesity, and osteoporosis.

Some examples of muscular activities include push-ups, sit-ups, and weight lifting. The activities should be performed 20 to 45 minutes per session, two to three days a week on alternating days. The benefits of muscular fitness include *larger muscle mass* over time, which helps to increase metabolism and burn calories, even at rest.

Muscular fitness also helps to build *strength*, which is the ability of muscles to work against resistance. Strong muscles are more efficient at burning calories and preventing injuries. Strong muscles also provide healthy resistance for bones, which protects against osteoporosis. Strength can and should be maintained throughout aging.

Muscular endurance is the ability for a muscle to contract repeatedly over a time period without exhaustion, about 20 minutes. A goal for muscular endurance is one to three sets of exercises, with 10 to15 repetitions of eight or more exercises

Flexibility helps reduce the risks of injury and falls by restoring, maintaining, and increasing muscular and joint elasticity. Some examples of flexibility activities include ballet, stretching, and yoga. The activities should be done almost every day, both before and after cardiovascular and muscular activities. While flexibility does not necessarily help weight loss, because it helps to keep muscles and joints flexible, it allows overweight and obese individuals to participate in more calorie-burning activities.

One should stretch before cardiovascular or muscular workouts to prepare the body for exercise. Stretch after workouts to promote better range of joint motion in the joints and to help remove lactic acid (see "Aerobic and anaerobic metabolism" following). Aim for 5 to 10 minutes of gentle, full-body stretching; breathing freely, without tension.

THE F.I.T. PRINCIPLE

A handy way to incorporate each of these fitness regimens into a weight-loss/weight-maintenance or wellness program is the *F.I.T. principle*, which stands for *frequency, intensity,* and *time. Frequency* is the number of times an activity is performed; intensity is how hard it is performed; and time is duration of the activity. It is recommended that individuals exercise at least three times weekly, at least 30 minutes per session, within their target heart rate for cardiovascular fitness and overall health. For weight loss, it is recommended that individuals exercise five times weekly, at least 30 minutes per session, also within their target heart rate. Recommended schedules for cardiovascular fitness and weight loss follow.

Overall Health: Monday—Wednesday—Friday

Cardiovascular fitness: 30 minutes of brisk walking, jogging, and so on, within the target heart rate range
Muscular fitness: 20 minutes of weight lifting
Flexibility: 5 to 10 minutes of stretching before/after cardiovascular and muscular workouts

Weight Loss: Monday—Wednesday—Friday—Saturday or Sunday (Increase Frequency)

Cardiovascular fitness: 30 to 45 minutes at increased intensity (increase time and intensity)
Muscular fitness: 20 to 30 minutes of weight lifting (increase time)
Flexibility: 5 to 10 minutes of stretching before/after cardiovascular and muscular workouts

BASIC NUTRIENTS AND PHYSICAL FITNESS

Basic nutrients fuel the body on a daily basis. If a person skips a meal, their body may still be able to function. The same basic nutrients are critical during physical activities. If they run out, an athlete can "hit the wall." Performance and health may suffer.

Carbohydrates, lipids, and protein help supply cardiovascular and muscular energy for exercise. Vitamins and minerals support their metabolism into energy. Water is the medium that transports these nutrients to cells for energy and excretes their by-products. Water also helps cool the body from all the heat that is produced from exercise. It may be the most important nutrient for physical fitness.

AEROBIC AND ANAEROBIC METABOLISM

Every time we eat a meal, drink a beverage, and then breathe deeply to relax and enjoy the meal, we use the calories, liquid, and oxygen to create energy. *Metabolism* is the process by which the body uses these substances to create energy. *Aerobic metabolism* occurs in the presence of oxygen. *Anaerobic metabolism* occurs without oxygen. Understanding how both types of metabolism interact to fuel the body is fundamental for maximum energy, muscular strength, and overall fitness.

When the body is at rest, most of the energy it requires is supplied by lipids. When exercising, the energy that the body needs is dependent on available fuel and oxygen. In aerobic metabolism, oxygen is available for moderate exercise as long as it is within one's target heart rate. A good measure is the ability to talk to someone while exercising.

455

When exercise exceeds this moderate level and less oxygen is available compared to energy demands, the muscles convert to anaerobic metabolism and rely on a special type of stored carbohydrate for fuel. This carbohydrate is immediately available—probably the result of ancient humans' need to quickly run away from dangerous situations. Today we might use it to sprint up a flight of stairs or run for a bus. Only about 5 percent of stored carbohydrates are used in this manner.

The aftermath of anaerobic metabolism is a by-product called *lactic acid.* Lactic acid can cause muscles to burn or fatigue. Cooling down after hard, anaerobic activities permits the blood to transport lactic acid to the liver, where it is changed back into glucose and brings oxygen back to the muscles for aerobic metabolism.

Aerobic and anaerobic metabolisms work together to supply the body with energy. In order to lose weight, one must first consume enough carbohydrates to supply energy for the working muscles. Then one needs to exercise aerobically to burn excess body fat and preserve carbohydrates for vital energy needs. And enough protein must be consumed to maintain muscle as one loses fat.

Making the best use of carbohydrates, lipids, and protein for optimal sports performance is explained by the science of *sports nutrition.* Translating this science into practice—into healthful recipes, meals, and menus—is the challenge of culinary specialists who specialize in feeding athletes. An examination of fuels for sports is fundamental to help meet this challenge.

CARBOHYDRATES

Glucose, a simple carbohydrate or sugar, is one of the most important fuels for most types of exercise. It comes from carbohydrate-containing foods, such as breads, fruits, legumes, milk, and vegetables, and also from blood, liver, and muscle stores. Carbohydrates in the blood are called *blood glucose.* Carbohydrates in the liver and muscle stores are called *glycogen.*

When a person exercises, glycogen in the muscles and liver is broken down to supply blood glucose (sugar) for energy. Short-term exercise of 30 minutes or less generally uses blood glucose for energy. Longer-term exercise relies more on muscle and liver glycogen.

Very intense exercise done for a very short duration, such as sprinting or power lifting, relies on a unique energy system fueled by specialized stored carbohydrates. Regular training maximizes these stores. Dieting, fasting, and inactivity minimize these stores.

Once blood glucose is depleted, if glycogen stores are not ample and if a person has not trained well, they can "hit the wall." This is because the body diverts available glucose to maintain its vital functions, such as the brain and heart. With less available glucose to fuel the working muscles, a person cannot continue to exercise. The central nervous system, especially the brain, prevails.

Trained athletes use less blood glucose than untrained people who exercise for health or weight loss. When a person first begins an exercise program, her muscles rely heavily on blood glucose for fuel. As the person trains, she becomes more adept at conserving glucose and relies more on stored lipids for fuel. The result is fat loss.

CARBOHYDRATE LOADING

Some athletes use a special technique called *carbohydrate loading* to pack their muscles with glycogen before important events. It is generally used for activities that last more than 90 minutes, such as marathons, triathlons, cross-country bike races, and so forth. The supply of muscle glycogen is roughly 1,800 kilocalories—about the amount that supplies fuel for 1½ to 2 hours' worth of activities. Carbohydrate loading "tops" this amount with more available carbohydrates.

Carbohydrate loading requires a program of intense exercise with an adequate carbohydrate intake (40 to 50 percent of total calories), then restricted exercise with a high carbohydrate intake (60 to 70 percent of total calories). The idea is that the muscles will be close to depleted from the intense exercise and will take up extra carbohydrates when exercise is restricted.

The drawbacks of carbohydrate loading include blood sugar changes, digestive discomfort, lightheadedness and weakness, and weight gain from the water that is inside carbohydrates. This actually works like an internal hydration system, since water is released when carbohydrates break down.

Recipe: Roasted Beet Soup

Beets are rich in carbohydrates and fiber. Beet fiber, like carrot fiber, has potential gastrointestinal and cardiovascular benefits, which may be due to its pectin polysaccharides. These substances act as gelling and thickening agents in foods and as stabilizers. In this recipe for Roasted Beet Soup in the Recipe file which is located within the Culinary Nutrition website at www.culinarynutrition. elsevier.com, beets help to provide the body with needed carbohydrates for energy, fullness and satisfaction." The finished dish is shown within the centerfold Photo file in Plate 10.1.

PROTEIN

Protein contributes only about 5 to 10 percent of energy requirements if carbohydrates and lipids are not available and if a person is untrained. Some physical activities may require even more protein to replace what is used for energy or to build muscle mass. This is because muscles require more red blood cells and enzymes to increase in size and use fuel effectively.

The RDA for protein is 0.8 grams per kilogram (0.4 grams per pound) of protein daily. Endurance athletes require 1.2 to 1.4 grams per kilogram (0.6 to 0.7 grams per pound) of protein daily and weight lifters require 1.6 to 1.7 grams per kilogram (0.8 to 0.85 grams per pound) of protein daily. For example, a 200-pound man requires 80 grams of protein daily; a 115-pound female runner requires 69 to 80.5 grams of protein daily; and a 150-pound male weight lifter requires 120 to 127.5 grams of protein daily [39–42].

Muscles are like sponges right after heavy exercise. They seek available amino acids to repair and rebuild, so their growth actually increases after exercise, assuming that these amino acids are available. A trained athlete is conditioned for this regrowth to occur. Consuming one to two (3-ounce) servings of protein after a heavy muscular workout should be sufficient in most cases. Excess protein will be excreted in the urine, or it could be converted into fat.

457

Recipe: Grilled Flank Steak

Flank steak is considered a lean cut of beef. This is not surprising, since flank steak comes from a strong, well-exercised section of beef. Grilled just to doneness, then cut across the grain, as this recipe for Grilled Flank Steak requires. It is found in the Recipe file which is located within the Culinary Nutrition website at www.culinarynutrition.elsevier.com. The finished dish is shown within the centerfold Photo file in Plate 10.2.

LIPIDS

The fats and oils consumed daily are used for energy, stored in fat deposits all over the body, and as intramuscular fat. Blood is the vehicle that delivers fatty acids to the muscles so they can be stored and converted into energy as needed.

One of the goals in a weight-loss program is to lose body fat from nonessential body stores. This is also one of the goals in physical fitness. Some activities, such as cross-country running or biking, require having the least amount of fat and the most amount of energy. They rely on glycogen stores. Other activities, such as swimming or soccer, have higher fat needs for optimal performance. This is because intramuscular fat is the primary energy source for moderate exercise. Trained athletes use fat for energy more efficiently than untrained athletes.

Average fat stores are between 25 and 30 pounds, so there is a significant amount available for routine activities and the demands of exercise. In comparison, only about 1 pound of carbohydrate is stored. A fit body spares this carbohydrate and makes excellent use of stored fats for energy. Athletes should strive for about 25 percent of calories from fat, or about 56 grams on a 2,000-calorie daily diet.

Recipe: Pork Tenderloin with Root Vegetables

*Pork has been called "the other white meat," since many cuts of lean pork are similar in nutrients to a skinless chicken breast. This recipe for **Pork Tenderloin with Root Vegetables** in the **Recipe file** which is located within the* Culinary Nutrition *website at www.culinarynutrition.elsevier.com, is one of the lean cuts that earn this slogan. Stuffed with garlic and surrounded by roasted root vegetables of choice, this recipe makes a lean yet filling entree. The finished dish is shown within the centerfold* **Photo file** *in Plate 10.3.*

WATER AND OTHER FLUIDS

Perhaps the most important nutrient for exercise is water. Inadequate hydration could cause cramping, headaches, increased heat-related injuries, muscular aches and pains, poor performance, and, in extreme cases, death. Dehydration and its potentially life-threatening effects on the body are discussed in Chapter 8. People who exercise and those who are physically active in heat and humidity most likely will need more than 4 cups of water per 1,000 calories. It is not uncommon for athletes to lose 8 cups of fluid through respiration and sweat in as little as one hour. To replace this amount of fluid, athletes must prehydrate, hydrate during exercise, and posthydrate. A good rule of thumb is to consume 2 to 3 cups of fluid two to three hours before exercise; 6 to 12 ounces of fluid about every 15 minutes during exercise; and two (8-ounce) cups of cool fluid for each pound lost after exercise. The athlete should be able to urinate, and the urine should be clear.

For endurance events that are 60 minutes or longer, sports drinks with glucose, electrolytes and fluid in an optimal formulation for exercise should be considered for rehydration (see Chapter 8). If people participate in shorter-duration activities, sports drinks may be unnecessary. They may contribute extra calories and cause weight gain or gastrointestinal distress.

VITAMINS AND MINERALS

458

Under normal conditions, people who exercise for overall health can probably meet their vitamin and mineral needs with a well-planned diet. Competitive athletes, who expend two to three times more calories than usual, would have to eat a massive amount of food to meet their nutrient needs. That is why vitamin and mineral status in competitive athletes requires scrutiny. If there are gaps, certain vitamin and mineral supplements should be considered.

The B-complex vitamins do not provide energy—they support it. If enough carbohydrates are consumed for energy, then B vitamins should accompany them. If not, then a B-complex supplement may be warranted. Muscle-building athletes should ensure that their copper, folate, vitamin B6, vitamin B12, iron, and zinc consumptions are adequate. Most of these vitamins and minerals also guard against sports anemia, which is prevalent in female athletes and men in contact sports. The antioxidant vitamins A, C, and E and the mineral selenium help guard against exercise-induced oxidative stress injuries. Vitamins and minerals that build blood, bones, and tissues, including calcium, vitamins A and D, magnesium, and phosphorus, are essential for growing children and teenage athletes. Magnesium, a mineral that assists heart function, and chromium, a mineral that supports glucose metabolism, may be needed in increased amounts because of the major roles they play in energy production and utilization.

IRON AND SPORTS ANEMIA

Sports anemia is low hemoglobin as a result of adaptation to physical training. It occurs early in training when athletes temporarily develop low blood hemoglobin. Aerobic activities enlarge the blood volume. When this condition is accompanied by added fluids, the red blood cell count drops. Sports anemia should disappear on its own with continued training, unless iron intake is poor.

Iron is crucial to physical performance because it is critical in oxygen transport. If oxygen cannot get to the working muscles, this can cause fatigue and decrease the muscles' capacity to perform. Vegetarians and menstruating women are at risk of iron deficiency because red meat is an excellent source of iron, and iron is lost during menses.

Iron can also be lost in sweat, although less is lost in trained athletes than untrained athletes. Athletes who participate in contact sports may also develop sports anemia from red blood cell destruction around the contact area and in the digestive tract. It is then lost in the urine and feces.

THE FEMALE TRIAD

The *female triad* is a combination of three conditions in female athletes: *amenorrhea, disordered eating,* and *osteoporosis*. **Amenorrhea** is the loss of menstrual periods. When too little energy is available for exercise, a female athlete's body conserves energy by curtailing other functions. For one, it suppresses menstrual function. Some female athletes display a range of infertility problems. In very young female athletes, low-energy intake and high-energy usage may also delay the onset of menstruation.

Disordered eating is another feature of the female triad. In an effort to improve performance, some female athletes may try to lose weight or body fat through anorexia nervosa, bulimia nervosa, or a combination of the two. Coupled with hard training, physical problems like hypotension and hypoglycemia may result. Without intervention, disordered eating in athletes could cause death.

When too little energy is available after exercise, an athlete's body may slow bone tissue turnover (the resorption of old bone and the formation of new bone). As a result, resorption of old bones exceeds formation of new bones, and there may be progressive, irreversible reduction in bone density. This condition may be harmful to young athletes because 50 percent of bone mass is created during adolescence. With intense exercise, it can increase the risk of stress fractures and other bone disorders. It may also promote early *osteoporosis*—a condition that is usually seen in the elderly.

ERGOGENIC AIDS

Ergogenic aids are mechanical, nutritional, pharmacological, physiological and psychological tools that athletes use to increase energy, performance and recovery. Commonly used ergogenic aids include dried adrenal glands, amino acids, bee pollen, caffeine, carnitine, chromium, creatine, ginseng, glucosamine and protein powders. Side effects from high doses may include allergic reactions, central nervous system and gastrointestinal disorders, and kidney damage.

Anabolic steroids, androstenedione (andro) and DHEA , beta-hydroxy-beta-methylbutyrate (HMB), gamma hydroxybutyric acid (GHB) and human growth hormone (HGH) may cause significant side effects, and, in some cases, death. The International Olympic Committee has banned androstenedione and human growth hormone, and the National Collegiate Athletic Association (NCAA) has banned caffeine at the 600-milligram level (six to eight 8-ounce cups of brewed coffee daily) [43–46].

Consistent sport-specific training; well-designed sport-specific diets supported by adequate fluids, vitamin and mineral supplements; and rest are still the safest strategies for sports performance. The field of sports nutrition is growing to address these and other strategies. But so are ergogenic aids, especially through the Internet.

SPORTS NUTRITION

Planning diets and cooking for sports teams or individual athletes are growing trends in the food service industry at academic institutions, fitness and training centers, and for professional teams and individual athletes.

Sports and Cardiovascular Nutritionists (SCAN) is a dietetic practice group of the American Dietetic Association who specialize in cardiovascular health, disordered eating prevention and treatment, sports performance, weight management, and wellness. Sports nutritionists team with culinary specialists to design and execute recipes, meals, and menus for collegiate athletics to Olympians. The benefit of this collaboration is that nutritious diets can be designed to meet individualized athletes' needs and then converted into tasty and appealing foods and beverages.

This is accomplished by customizing the right amount of calories, carbohydrates, protein, and fat for individual athletes and sports. A number of variables are taken into account, such as age, gender, height, weight, and special dietary needs. Computerized dietary programs are used to generate daily diets. Meals are broken down into nutrients to ensure the right amounts of fuel throughout the day. These nutrients are converted into food servings. Culinary specialists create recipes and meals that meet these servings. Computerized dietary analysis programs compare these recipes and meals to nutrient requirements. A sample sports nutrition case study with food choices is shown in "Bite on This: a sports nutrition case study with food choices." It is filled with low-fat, carbohydrate-rich foods from grains, fruits and vegetables for endurance athletes, such as long distance runners, swimmers or cyclists. More information about sports nutrition diet planning and sports nutrition–culinary specialist collaborations can be found in "Hungry for more?"

Bite on This: a sports nutrition case study with food choices

Personal data: 150-pound lacto-ovo vegetarian teenage male cross-country runner
Nutritional guidelines: 3,000 kilocalories, 60 percent carbohydrates (to meet energy needs), 25 to 30% fat (to meet energy needs), 10–15% protein (to meet energy needs and preserve muscle). Ranges provide individual variance.

Food and Fluid Servings
Protein: 3 dairy servings, 1 meat/meat alternative serving
Carbohydrates: 23 grain servings, 4 fruit servings, 3 vegetable servings
Fluids: 12 (8-ounce) servings

Foods and Beverages
Dairy products: 1 cup dairy skim milk, 1 cup low-fat yogurt, 2 slices low-fat cheese
Meat/meat alternatives: ¾ cup cooked beans, 3 tablespoons peanut butter
Grains: 3 cups cooked whole-grain pasta, 3 slices whole-grain bread, 1 cup cooked brown rice, 1 large whole-grain roll, 2 cups whole-grain cereal, 8 graham crackers, 2 bagels, 1 (1-ounce) bag pretzels
Fruits: 1 banana, 1 orange, 1 dried fruit roll-up, 1 cup fruit juice
Vegetables: ½ cup tomato sauce, 1 medium sweet potato, 1 cup lightly steamed broccoli
Snacks: 1 energy bar, 1 cup fruit punch

Sample Menu in Servings
Breakfast: 1 dairy, 1 fruit, 5 grains
Lunch: 1 dairy, 1 fruit, 1 vegetable, 5 grains
Dinner: 1 meat, 5 grains, 2 vegetables, 1 fruit
Snacks between meals: 1 dairy, 1 fruit, 5-8 grains

Sample Menu in Foods and Beverages
Breakfast: 1 cup dairy skim milk, 2 cups whole-grain cereal, 3 slices whole-grain bread, 3 tablespoons peanut butter, 1 small banana
Lunch: 1 cup cooked brown rice, ¾ cup cooked beans, 1 medium sweet potato, 2 slices low-fat cheese, 1 large whole-grain roll, 1 orange
Dinner: 3 cups cooked whole-grain pasta, ½ cup tomato sauce, 1 cup lightly steamed broccoli, 1 cup fruit juice
Snacks: 1 cup low-fat yogurt, 1 dried fruit roll-up, 2 bagels, 8 graham crackers, 1 energy bar, 1 (1-ounce) bag pretzels

460

COOKING FOR WEIGHT LOSS: HOW TO REDUCE CALORIES IN RECIPES

Classic cooking training provides a foundation for contemporary cuisine, just like classic ballet provides a foundation for modern dance. Classic cooking requires a supreme reverence to ingredients and their functions in recipes. Little compares to beautifully executed food and drink, replete with all the calories that these recipes require to taste great.

However, there are times when it is necessary to cut back on calories, but hopefully not in taste. It may be to reduce calories for weight loss, disease, sports potential or some combination of factors. Eliminating favorite foods and beverages or substituting strange ingredients may not be the solution: cutting back may be the answer. Following are some tried-and-true techniques to turn restriction into renovation and celebration.

Morsel "In general, mankind, since the improvement of cookery, eats twice as much as nature requires." —Benjamin Franklin (Author, civic activist, diplomat, inventor, musician, political theorist, politician, postmaster, printer, satirist, scientist and statesman, 1706–1790)[47]

LOOK AT THE OVERALL RECIPE TO DETERMINE WHERE REDUCTIONS CAN BE MADE

Can one reduce the amount of total fat, total carbohydrates, sugar? In many recipes, this may be possible without too much flavor loss. The question is "How much?" Cutting *total fat* by one-half is often too drastic of a measure. Instead, start by cutting recipes by one-quarter where fat appears to be nonessential to the success or failure of a recipe. For example, if 4 tablespoons of butter are called for to saute onions and garlic, cut this amount by ¼ to 3 tablespoons. If this amount is reduced to 2 tablespoons at the beginning of the recipe, then some oil may need to be added later in the recipe—especially for ingredients that absorb a lot of fat or oil, such as eggplant or squash. Other ideas for cutting back total fat and calories in cooking include using the following substitutions. See Chapter 6 for more ideas.

Dairy products
- Low-fat cheese with no more than 5 grams of fat per ounce
- ¾ cup sharp low-fat cheese for 1 cup full-fat cheese
- 4 ounces cream, feta, or goat cheese *plus* 4 ounces reduced-fat ricotta or cottage cheese for 1 cup full-fat cheese
- 1 cup pureed reduced-fat cottage cheese pureed with 1 tablespoon lemon juice for 1 cup sour cream
- 1 cup skim, reduced-fat dairy milk or evaporated skim milk for 1 cup whole milk, half-and-half, or cream (if richness needed, add 1 tablespoon neutral oil like canola)
- 1 cup skim milk *plus* 1 tablespoon lemon juice, or 1 cup plain nonfat yogurt for 1 cup regular buttermilk

Fats and oils
- $^7/_8$ cup vegetable oil for 1 stick butter
- 3 tablespoons clarified butter for 4 tablespoons butter
- 1 to 2 tablespoons wine or chicken broth for 2 tablespoon oil for sauteing (or use nonfat vegetable oil spray and nonstick pan)
- ½ to 1 cup citrus juice, defatted chicken stock, flavored vinegar, low-fat yogurt, or wine per pound of meat or vegetables for ½ cup of oil in marinades

461

FOOD BYTE

To reduce oil in a salad dressing, use defatted chicken or vegetable stock, tomato or vegetable juice, or wine for one-third of the vegetable oil. Combine all the other salad dressing ingredients first, and then whisk in the liquid. Or combine all of the ingredients and one ice cube in a screw-top jar and shake vigorously. Once the salad dressing is extra-smooth, discard any remains of the ice cube. Use immediately on chilled salad greens and/or fresh vegetables.

Eggs, fish, poultry, meats
- 2 egg whites *plus* ½ to 1 egg yolk or 1 tablespoon neutral oil for 1 whole egg
- 3 ounces orange roughy, perch, snapper, or sole for 3 ounces bluefin tuna, mackerel, or salmon
- 3 ounces cooked skinless chicken breast for 3 ounces eye of round, top round, round tip, top sirloin, bottom round, top loin, tenderloin, or chicken thigh (total fat, saturated fat, and calories increase in each cut of beef and chicken thigh)
- 1 pound 95% lean ground beef, ground chicken or turkey breast, or ground pork tenderloin for 1 pound ground 80% lean ground beef
- 1 slice lean ham, Canadian bacon or smoked turkey for 1 slice pork bacon for smoky flavor

Recipe: Smoked Salmon Rolls

Smoked salmon (lox) is considered a medium-fat protein with 7 grams of protein, 4 to 7 grams of total fat, and 75 calories per one ounce. By using just ⅓ pound of smoked salmon, reduced-fat sour cream and whole-grain tortillas with plenty of fresh herbs, this recipe for **Smoked Salmon Rolls** *in the* **Recipe file** *which is located within the* Culinary Nutrition *website at www.culinarynutrition.elsevier.com, stretches to make six servings—or more as appetizers. The finished dish is shown within the centerfold* **Photo file** *in Plate 10.4.*

Cutting back fat that is essential to a recipe's success is more difficult. Baked goods are trickier than some cooked foods because they depend on particular formulas for baking success. Cutting fat in half may cause a recipe to be too dry. Solid fats, like butter and vegetable shortening, retain air bubbles carried by sugar crystals, lending a light texture. Fat replacers can mock the moistening and tendering effects of fats, but they do not do such a good job aerating baked products.

In baked goods, using half butter, shortening, or oil, and replacing the other half with unsweetened applesauce, mashed banana, or concentrated fruit purees, such as apple, apricot, pear, or prune, will help cut fat calories and create moisture and tenderness, but the final products may be dense. Commercially prepared fruit-based fat replacers produce similar effects. Generally, 2 tablespoons of fat per cup of flour works best to retain some taste and texture. Other reductions or substitutions follow:

- $7/8$ cup vegetable oil for 1 cup solid fat
- $1/4$ cup liquid egg substitute for 1 egg
- $1/2$ cup fruit puree for 1 cup of oil
- $1/2$ cup dried fruit *plus* $1/2$ cup nuts for 1 cup nuts
- 3 tablespoons good-quality cocoa power *plus* 1 tablespoon neutral oil like canola for 1 ounce unsweetened baking chocolate
- $3/4$ cup semisweet chocolate chips for 1 cup milk chocolate chips
- $1/2$ cup shredded coconut *plus* 1 teaspoon coconut flavoring for 1 cup shredded coconut
- Marshmallow creme can be substituted for butter in some frosting recipes.
- Substitute a graham cracker crust for a traditional lard or shortening piecrust.

> **FOOD BYTE**
>
> Too much grease on a pan may cause foods to overbrown. Too much flour and grease may become cakey. Grease a pan lightly to save fat calories, sprinkle with a small amount flour, and then tap to remove any excess. Or beat together $1/2$ cup each trans-free vegetable shortening, vegetable oil and all-purpose flour, and use this mixture gingerly to coat bread pans, cake pans, cookie sheets, or muffin tins. Refrigerate this mixture in an airtight container for up to six months.

Table 10-6 shows foods that are higher or lower in fats by category. Table 10-7 shows the calories and fat saved by making some of the substitutions just provided.

Reduce the amount of *sweeteners* in cooking first by one-quarter, and then by one-third to one-half. Consider using sweet spices like allspice, cardamom, cinnamon, cloves, coriander, ginger, mace, or nutmeg or sweet extracts like almond or vanilla to enhance the inherent sweetness of foods and beverages.

Reducing sweeteners in baking is more difficult than in cooking. Sugar is important for incorporating air into baking mixtures and for lightening the texture in cakes. In cookies, sugar contributes hardness and crispness. Other sweeteners, such as corn syrup, honey, and molasses, while more intense in sweetness, tend to absorb fluids in recipes rather than crystallize. The final products may be moist and chewy rather than crisp. That is why it is important to consider the texture of a recipe before substituting sweeteners.

Try using no less than $1/2$ cup of sugar per 1 cup of flour in cakes and cake-like cookies made with juice, milk, or water. For quick breads and muffins, try using no less than 1 tablespoon of sugar per 1 cup of flour. In quick breads, use no less than 1 teaspoon of sugar per 1 cup of flour.

If substituting honey for granulated sugar in recipes, reduce any liquid by $1/4$ cup for each cup of honey used; add $1/2$ teaspoon baking soda for each 1 cup honey, and reduce the oven temperature by $25°$.

TABLE 10-6 Foods That Are Higher and Lower in Fat and Calories by Category

Higher-Fat and Higher-Calorie Foods	Lower-Fat and Lower-Calorie Foods
Baked goods	
Buttery crackers	Whole-grain crackers, pretzels, popcorn
Cake	Angel food, gingerbread
Cookies	Graham crackers, gingersnaps, fig cookies
Croissants, brioches	Dinner rolls
Donuts	Bagels, English muffins
Cereals and grains	
Pasta with cheese sauce	Pasta with olive oil and garlic
Pasta with meat sauce	Pasta primavera
Pasta with white sauce	Pasta with red sauce
Granola	Oatmeal
Dairy products	
Cheese	2% (reduced-fat) cheese
Coffee cream (half-and-half)	Reduced-fat milk
Evaporated whole milk	Evaporated skim or reduced-fat
4% cottage cheese	2% (reduced-fat) cottage cheese
Ice cream	Reduced-fat or frozen yogurt, frozen fruit bars
Sour cream	Plain, low-fat yogurt
Whipped cream	Chilled, whipped evaporated skim milk
Whole milk cheese	Part-skim cheese
Whole milk	1%, 2% or skim milk
Fats and oils	
Butter	Whipped butter
Coconut milk	Reduced-fat coconut milk
Lard	Trans fat–free shortening
Mayonnaise	Light mayonnaise
Salad dressing	Reduced-calorie
Shortening	Vegetable oil
Vegetable oil	Nonfat cooking spray
Fish, meat, and poultry	
Bacon	Canadian bacon or prosciutto
Beef hot dogs	Chicken or turkey dogs
Beef (brisket, chuck, rib)	Beef (flank, shank, rump, round)
Frozen breaded fish	Lightly coated fish fillets
Luncheon meats	95 to 97% fat-free luncheon meats
Oil-packed fish	Water-packed, except for sardines in light olive oil
Pork sausage	Poultry or vegetarian sausage
Pork spareribs	Pork tenderloin or lean ham
Snacks	
Fudge	Chocolate syrup
Potato chips	Rice cakes
Pudding	Low-fat pudding
Other	
Beer	Light beer or wine spritzer (alcohol is metabolized as fat)
Canned cream soup	Defatted stock or broth
Specialty coffees	One-half lower-fat milk

463

FOOD BYTE

Simple syrups (also called *sugar syrups*), can be made in various densities. The amount of sugar compared to the amount of water varies. A heavy or dense solution is equal parts water and sugar; a medium-dense solution is two parts water to one part sugar; a thin solution is three parts water to one part sugar; and a light solution is five parts water to one part sugar. Use a *thin* solution with flavor extracts or sweet spices to dribble over simple cakes, glaze baked goods, marinate fresh fruit, or poach fruit to boost taste and save sugar calories.

TABLE 10-7 Calories and Fat Saved by Making Substitutions

Foods/Beverages	Substitutes	Calories Saved (cal)	Fat Saved (grams)
8 ounces cream cheese	8 ounces light cream cheese	305 cal	39 g
1 cup heavy cream	1 cup evaporated skim milk	621	87
1 cup sour cream	1 cup nonfat plain yogurt	366	48
1 cup dairy whole milk	1 cup dairy skim milk	64	8
1 pound 80% lean ground beef	1 pound 95% lean ground beef	350	27
3 ounces roasted chicken thigh with skin	3 ounces roasted chicken breast without skin	70	10
1 whole egg	2 egg whites *plus* 1 egg yolk	negligible	5
3 slices bacon	3 slices turkey bacon		
2 tablespoons butter for greasing plans	Nonfat cooking spray	216	19–24
2 tablespoons butter for sauteing	2 ounces stock	200	trace

Source: *[48]*

Other substitutions for sweeteners are ⅞ cup honey for 1 cup granulated sugar and ⅞ cup granulated sugar *plus* 1 tablespoon light or dark molasses for 1 cup brown sugar. More ideas, including the pros and cons of sugar substitutes, can be found in Chapter 4.

Sodium reductions are discussed in Chapter 7 [49,50].

Delete Ingredients

Ingredients can be deleted altogether in some recipes, such as a knob of butter, dollop of sour cream, or pool of oil. Potatoes may be fine without fat- and caloric-laden toppings; poultry can be lighted dusted instead of dredged; and layered cake can be prepared with a fresh fruit filling instead of pastry cream. Any visible fat from chops, poultry skin, roasts, and steaks should be trimmed or removed whenever possible.

Eliminating ingredients in other recipes may be unsatisfactory. For example, butter is integral in emulsions and pastries. Sweeteners balance acidic ingredients. White bread flour creates the highest and lightest loaves. While whole grains are tasty, they make denser breads, and the calories may be higher than refined wheat breads.

Add Ingredients

This approach sounds as though total calories will increase. Healthy substitutions may actually reduce the amount of fat, calories, and sodium in recipes, plus boost the nutritional content. For example, if whole wheat pasta is substituted for enriched white pasta, it will triple the fiber and may reduce total calories, depending on the brand. Legumes can be added to salads, and higher-fat meats can be reduced. Grated, shredded or chopped vegetables can extend ground meats, starches such as mashed potatoes or rice, and baked goods such as sweet breads. If foods become too dry, a little chicken stock, broth or olive oil can bring back moisture and flavor. Use flavorful ingredients such as these in moderation instead of as mainstays.

FOOD BYTE

While salt is essential to add taste and bring out the flavor in recipes, too much salt can be overpowering. From a weight-control standpoint, excess salt may lead to water retention, or water weight. If a sauce is to be reduced in a recipe, do not salt it until the end of cooking. As the liquid evaporates, the salt concentrates and the sauce may be too salty. This is why many recipes read "adjust seasonings" at the end of the recipe or "salt to taste." Add just enough for taste and enhancement of recipes without overdoing sodium.

Boost the Flavor

Fat tastes good, and when it is reduced or eliminated from foods and beverages, flavor can suffer. This is because fat contributes taste and mouthfeel and acts as a carrier of other flavors. Sweetness is synonymous with pleasure, be it in cooked or baked foods. Carrots, corn, sweet peas and potatoes are naturally sweet, especially when at their peak. Sweetness is also found in animal protein, dairy products, fruits, grains and nuts. Just taste them "as is" without other ingredients. As sauces and dressings are minimized to save calories, the sweetness of these foods may come through.

A pinch of salt emphasizes sweetness, such as toast with a *little* salted butter, plus a *little* fruit preserves. Umami heightens sweetness, too: consider a touch of soy sauce on sweet-and-sour seafood. The sweetness enhances other sweet tastes, so putting syrup on waffles intensifies the sweetness in the eggs, flour, and milk of the batter. This means one can manage with less and still perceive the desirable sweetness. Here are some cooking techniques that boost flavor without extra fat and calories:

- *Caramelizing* to bring out natural sweetness and intensify flavors and aromas
- *Degreasing gravies, pan juices, and soups* with a wide-mouthed spoon or fat-separating pitcher; refrigerate to congeal fat, then discard; or add ice cubes (the fat will rise to the top of the liquid and harden)
- *Poaching* delicate fish and seafood or poultry in stock or wine, flavored with citrus, herbs, and spices, then reducing the poaching liquid
- *Roasting* meats, vegetables, and fruits; reserving the browned bits in the bottom of the roasting pan; deglazing the pan with stock or wine, then adding herbs and spices
- *Rubbing herbs, spices, and seeds* onto protein foods, then browning or searing, and oven finishing
- *Toasting* grains, nuts, and whole spices to release natural oils and enhance flavor
- *Slow cooking* most foods, except searing or boiling water, to intensity natural flavors

Other ways of enhancing flavor without extra fat, sugar, or salt are provided in Chapters 4, 6 and 7.

Change the Preparation Methods

Healthy cooking techniques are described in Chapter 3. These include braising, broiling, grilling, poaching, roasting, sauteing, and steaming. Nutrients and flavor can be captured without adding fats or oils. For example, one-half of a fried chicken breast with skin has 364 calories, 18 grams of total fat, and 5 grams of saturated fat. If roasted, this reduces the chicken breast to 193 calories, 8 grams of total fat, and 2 grams of saturated fat. If the chicken skin is removed first and then the chicken breast is roasted, the chicken breast then contains only 86 calories, 3 grams of total fat, and 1 gram of saturated fat.

Wine, fruit juice, vegetable juice, and fat-free stock or broth can be used for basting rather than butter, drippings, or oil. Using nonstick cookware and nonstick vegetable spray helps ingredients to sweat and create their own cooking liquids.

> **Morsel** "We never repent of having eaten too little." —Thomas Jefferson (US founding father and president, 1743–1826)

Change the Portion Sizes

If it is true that we eat with our eyes, then our eyes are too big for our stomachs. Portion sizes have increased steadily, as discussed in Chapter 1. A half-sized portion of restaurant meals may still provide too many calories for sedentary people. Cutting back *each* serving allows us to have an array of carbohydrates, fats, and protein at each meal and not feel deprived. A variety of foods, in sensible amounts, still prevails as the wisest diet strategy [51]. Behavior modification techniques can be found in "Hungry for more?" [51].

Create a New Recipe Altogether

Sometimes it is nearly impossible to successfully adapt a recipe. For example, some low-fat cheese is tasteless on its own and adds little to recipes. Low-fat salad dressing and dips may have a "plastic" mouthfeel from fat replacers. Sugar substitutes may taste metallic. The recipes that rely on these ingredients may taste nothing like the recipes they try to replicate. It may be time to just simplify the recipe or take it in a different direction. If Turkey Tetrazzini is too difficult to replicate with fewer calories and fat, then maybe turkey with pasta in a light garlic and oil sauce with Parmesan cheese will suffice.

465

SERVE IT FORTH

1a. School lunches are being scrutinized as obesity and diabetes grow nationwide. In some states, high-fat and high-sugar foods and beverages are restricted in elementary and middle schools, and soft drink sales are limited. Some school districts allow local restaurants to sell healthy lunches, but high school students seem to prefer junk food.

The Goody Cafe and Bakery has received a contract for the local high school lunch program. The number one issue to be addressed is teenage obesity. The students would like a food court with fast-food options, but the parents and school district are in opposition.

The current daily lunch menus follow [52]. Your job as the executive chef for the bakery is to remake these five lunch menus to satisfy the students, parents and school administration. Some highlighted menu items are standard for vegetarians for religious purposes. What would you recommend to be added? Deleted? How would you address the concerns about teenage obesity? Support your recommendations.

CHOICE OF ONE	CHOICE OF ONE	CHOICE OF ONE	CHOICE OF ONE	CHOICE OF ONE
Cheese quesadilla	Chicken tenders with mustard sauce	Hamburger or cheeseburger on wheat bun	Spaghetti with meat or marinara sauce and breadstick	Fried chicken and biscuits
Chicken bites with corn muffin	Pork egg roll with white rice	Beef or turkey Hot dog on wheat bun	Teriyaki chicken fillet on rice	Fish fillet on wheat bun
B-B-Q ribs tips on wheat bun	Ham and cheese on Italian roll			Cheesesteak sub
Peanut butter and jelly sandwich Yogurt with veggies Hummus/pita	Peanut butter and jelly sandwich Yogurt with veggies Hummus/pita	Peanut butter and jelly sandwich Yogurt with veggies Hummus/pita	Peanut butter and jelly sandwich Yogurt with veggies Hummus/pita	Peanut butter and jelly sandwich Yogurt with veggies Hummus/pita
CHOICE OF TWO	**CHOICE OF TWO**	**CHOICE OF TWO**	**CHOICE OF TWO**	**CHOICE OF TWO**
French fries Minestrone soup	Hash browns Mixed vegetables	French fries Lettuce, tomato, pickle	Tater tots Green peas	Potato wedges Green beans
Orange	Celery/carrots with ranch dip	Cole slaw	Tossed salad with dressing	Chips and dip
Canned peaches Raisins	Applesauce Fruit salad	Banana Apple	Chilled pears Fruit crisp Chocolate chip cookie	Pineapple tidbits Ice cream

Source: [52]

2a. The Jumping Jacks, a semiprofessional basketball team is getting—*larger!* The team is moving slower and having trouble with their jump shots. You have been hired as their team chef to collaborate with a sports nutritionist to create a healthy training table. A *training table* is a buffet with carefully chosen foods and beverages that allows coaches to ensure that athletes eat enough food for their energy and muscular needs and eat healthfully.

The daily training tables include the following foods and beverages at breakfast, lunch and dinner. What would you add, delete, or change at each training table to help slim down these athletes? What type of nutritional advice would you supply at these meals? Support your recommendations.

Breakfast

Bacon, chipped beef, cold cereal, corned beef hash, cream of rice and wheat cereals, Danish pastry, donuts, eggs to order, fresh fruit, grits, hash brown potatoes, oatmeal, pecan pancakes or waffles, sausage links with gravy

Lunch

Beef enchiladas, chicken noodle soup, cheeseburgers, cold cuts, curly fries, fruit and yogurt bar, grilled chicken breast with cheese, hamburgers, hot dogs, macaroni and cheese, rice pilaf, pasta bar, potato salad, taco bar, tortellini soup, tuna salad

Dinner
Bean soup, cheddar cheese soup, carved prime rib, corn on the cob, grilled mahi-mahi, pork roast, salad bar with toppings and dressings, stir-fry vegetables, sweet potatoes, turkey breast, walnut dressing, whipped potatoes with gravy
Also:
Coffee, juices, milk, sport drinks, tea, and water at each meal
Cakes, cookies, fruit cobbler, ice cream at lunch and dinner

3a. The Oracle, a health and wellness spa for women, is interested in developing a higher-protein and lower-carbohydrate diet for weight loss. They want to base this diet on the *2010 USDA Dietary Guidelines for Americans* (see Chapter 1). You have been hired as the research chef to work with a registered dietitian to create the Oracle Diet for this spa.

According to the *2010 USDA Dietary Guidelines for Americans*, the daily calorie intake for moderately active women aged 19 to 30 years is 2,000 to 2,200 calories daily. The spa has selected a daily calorie level of 1,500 calories, which should create a one- to two-pound loss after about one week. The DRI for protein is 10 to 35 percent of total calories, and the DRI for carbohydrates is 45 to 65 percent of total calories. A higher-protein, lower-carbohydrate diet is 35 percent protein (525 calories) and 45 percent carbohydrates (675 calories). The remaining 20 percent of the calories are from fat (300 calories).

Using the information in http://www.caloriecountercharts.com/chart1a.htm to create a day's worth of foods and beverages in the amounts that meet these calorie, protein, carbohydrate and fat levels. Support your choices [53–56].

WHAT'S COOKING?

1. **Creating your own soft drinks**
   Objectives
   ○ To see how soft drinks are created
   ○ To understand why certain substances are better suited for soft drink production
   ○ To create soft drinks that are lower in sugar and calories
   Materials
   Baking soda; apple, grape, lemon, and orange juice; water; superfine (castor) sugar; 5 glasses; measuring spoons; spoon
   Procedure
   Fill each glass full of juice; fill one glass with water.
   Add 1 teaspoon baking soda to each glass; stir.
   Observe and note reactions of each mixture.
   Taste each mixture for sweetness; note.
   Add 1 teaspoon castor sugar to each juice/baking soda mixture; stir; taste for sweetness; note.
   Continue adding 1 teaspoon sugar until desired sweetness.
   Which of the mixtures require more sugar? Note.
   Evaluation
   There should be no reaction in the water/baking soda mixture. It may require considerable sugar to taste appealing. Bubbles should form in the orange juice and lemon juice/baking soda mixtures. Orange juice and lemon juice are acids. When baking soda is added, carbon dioxide is released. This is the bubbly gas that is common in soft drinks. Apple juice and grape juice have less acid; their reactions should be different.The amount of sugar needed for sweetening reflects the acidity of the juice and the sugar needed to balance this acidity. It also reflects your individual sense of the sweet taste.
   Culinary applications
   How can this information be applied to beverage production and recipe development?

2. **Breakfast satiety**
   Objectives
   ○ To compare three different types of breakfast for satiety (satisfaction)
   ○ To create a new breakfast meal that provides satisfaction with fewer calories than typical US breakfasts

467

Materials

1 slice white toast, 2 slices whole-grain toast, 1 cup apple juice, 1 teaspoon peanut butter (or butter if allergic), 2 cups dairy skim milk

Procedure

Day 1: Eat the white toast and drink 1 cup apple juice. Note the time you eat this meal and your satisfaction/lack of satisfaction with this meal. Also note the first signs and time of hunger before you sense that you need to eat again.

Day 2: Eat 1 slice whole wheat toast and drink 1 cup dairy skim milk. Note the time you eat this meal and your satisfaction/lack of satisfaction with this meal. Also note the first signs and time of hunger before you sense that you need to eat again.

Day 3: Eat 1 slice whole wheat toast with 1 teaspoon of peanut butter or butter, and drink 1 cup dairy skim milk. Note the time you eat this meal and your satisfaction/lack of satisfaction with this meal. Also note the first signs and time of hunger before you sense that you need to eat again.

Evaluation

Compare/contrast your satisfaction level of each meal and the time of hunger before you sense that you need to eat again. What can you conclude about the composition of these meals and satiety?

Based on this experiment, suggest a breakfast that reflects your conclusions. Provide types of foods and serving sizes. Support your suggestions.

Culinary applications

How can this information be applied to food production and recipe development?

3. **Effects of cooking on fat and calories**

   Objectives

   ○ To determine the nutritional difference between burgers made with extra-lean, lean, and regular ground beef

   ○ To compare the price and flavor differences between burgers made with extra-lean, lean, and regular ground beef

   ○ To choose ground beef with the most taste and least fat and calories for everyday use

   Materials

   4 ounces each extra-lean (17% fat), lean (21% fat), and regular (27% fat) ground beef; oven or grill, rack, drip pan, nonstick spatula, measuring cup, food scale

   Procedure

   Cook each burger separately until well done; collect and weigh the drippings; record.

   Compare the calories and fat in each of the burgers, both raw and well done.

   This information is available at

   http://www.nutritiondata.com/foods-ground%20beef00000000000000000000.html

   Evaluation

   When broiled to well done, regular ground beef loses about 2 ounces of fat. Lean meat also loses about 2 ounces, but part of this loss is water, since it is less fat. There should be less fat and more water loss with the extra-lean ground beef, but the total loss should also be similar.

   Compare and contrast the calories and grams of fat in the raw and cooked burgers. You should notice that in the raw ground beef, the difference in calories and fat is significant, while in the well-done ground beef, the calories and fat are similar. Your calculations should show that in 4 ounces of regular ground beef that is cooked well done, there are only 12 more fat calories than extra-lean ground beef and almost the same number of calories as lean ground beef.

   Culinary applications

   How can this information be applied to food production and recipe development?

OVER EASY

Weight management may be the most important focal area for nutrition and culinary specialists today. This is because the predictions for global overweight and obesity continue to rise, driving more opportunities. Weight loss is complex with so many variables that interfere with success, including dieting itself. Knowing the particulars of getting and keeping weight off provides the framework for well-designed, realistic, and satisfying diets, recipes, meals and menus.

Diets taken to the extreme become disordered eating. Anorexia and bulimia nervosa strike women and men of all ages. Eating more is not the answer. Working in tandem, nutrition and culinary professionals can team together at treatment facilities to ensure that even the smallest portions are rewarding.

Medical and destination spas offer controlled-calorie diets to lose weight fast. The metabolism of speedy weight loss requires a different approach than slow and steady. Understanding what happens to the body when the basic nutrients are maneuvered is foremost for spa cooking and baking.

Fueling everyday and professional athletes is a science; feeding them is an art. Cooking and baking for health clubs, sports teams, or Olympic athletes require a special set of sports nutrition fundamentals. Personal chefs may discover niche opportunities to team with sports nutritionists or athletic trainers. Many professional sports teams have developed training diets and training tables as a result of these collaborations.

The chapter ends with tips and techniques for cooking for weight loss. These barely rely on diet substitutes; instead, portion control and ingenious use of ingredients are featured.

CHECK PLEASE

1. The type of exercise that relies on oxygen is called:
   a. anabolic
   b. anaerobic
   c. aerobic
   d. anaphylaxis
   e. alkalosis
2. The type of exercise that occurs in oxygen debt is called:
   a. anabolic
   b. anaerobic
   c. aerobic
   d. anaphylaxis
   e. alkalosis
3. Overweight is defined as:
   a. 5 to 10 percent above desirable weight
   b. 10 to 20 percent above desirable weight
   c. 20 to 30 percent above desirable weight
   d. 20 percent or greater above desirable weight
   e. none of the above

Essay Question

1. Describe two causes of overweight and/or obesity that *are not* in a person's control? What can overweight or obese people do to try to combat each of these factors?

For additional questions, please see the Culinary Nutrition website at www.culinarynutrition.elsevier.com.

HUNGRY FOR MORE?

Sports Nutrition

American College of Sports Medicine   http://www.acsm.org/AM/Template.cfm?Section=Home
Calorie Control Council   http://www.caloriecontrol.org/index.html
FitDay (Diet and Exercise Tracker)   http://www.fitday.com/
National Eating Disorders Association   www.nationaleatingdisorders.org
Nancy Clark's Sports Nutrition Guide Book, 4th ed., 2008 Human Kinetics, Champaign, IL,   http://www.humankinetics.com/products/all-products/nancy-clarks-sports-nutrition-guidebook-4th-edition
Shape Up America   http://www.shapeup.org/

Weight Management

Body Mass Index Calculator National Heart, Lung, and Blood Institute   http://www.nhlbisupport.com/bmi/bmicalc.htm

Get Moving Calculator *Calorie Control Council*   http://www.caloriecontrol.org/exercalc.html
http://www.choosemyplate.gov/weight-management-calories.html
http://www.choosemyplate.gov/weight-management-calories/calories.html
http://www.choosemyplate.gov/weight-management-calories/resources.html
http://www.cdc.gov/healthyweight/assessing/bmi/index.html
http://www.choosemyplate.gov/supertracker-tools/supertracker.html
The LEARN Program for Weight Management   http://www.thelifestylecompany.com/wloss/wm10thed.asp
Weight Control Information Network (WIN)   http://win.niddk.nih.gov/index.htm
Weight Watchers International, Inc.   http://www.weightwatchers.com/index.aspx

TAKE AWAY
Eating Right When Eating Out

The number of meals that are consumed away from home may foil a diet unless they are chosen wisely. Most restaurants are taking steps to provide healthy menu options. The responsibility for healthy eating when eating out ultimately lies with the customer.

Before you go, have a small, healthful snack to quell hunger. Choose restaurants with widely varied menus. Be wary of buffets where the variety is daunting. Provided with more choices, people tend to select and eat more of the wrong foods. Ask about food preparation methods and ingredients.

Start a meal with a filling noncaloric bubbly beverage, such as sparkling water, and then move on to a volume food, such as a salad with raw vegetables or a clear soup. Ask that bread and butter be removed from the table if they are too irresistible. Order from the appetizer menu; stick to choices that are lower in fat and calories, such as fresh seafood, lean meats, or small portions of pasta.

For entrees, order protein foods with the least calories and fat. Stick with those that are baked, broiled, grilled, poached, roasted, or steamed, or ask for them to be prepared to order. Be leery of menu items that include terms such as *au gratin, battered, breaded, cream, fried,* or *gravy*. Inquire about side dishes; do not take them for granted. Eat half of *all* the portions—not just the entrees.

The following restaurant meals can be trimmed in calories by making these healthier choices:

MEXICAN RESTAURANT

Typical: 25 corn chips with hot sauce, 1 large beef enchilada, 1 cup refried beans, 1 Margarita
= about 1,600 calories
Trimmed: 2 chicken fajitas with lettuce, tomato, onion, and pico de gallo; ½ cup Spanish rice; iced tea
= about 700 calories

SEAFOOD RESTAURANT

Typical: 6 ounces fried fish fillet, 3 fried potato cakes, ½ cup creamy coleslaw, 1 large french fries, 12-ounce regular soft drink
= about 1,300 calories
Trimmed: 6 ounces broiled fish, 1 cup green beans, ½ cup rice, 1 wheat roll with 1 teaspoon butter, 1 cup diet lemonade
= about 600 calories

ITALIAN RESTAURANT

Typical: 1½ cups lasagna, 1 slice garlic bread with 1 tablespoon butter, 1 cup dinner salad with 2 tablespoons oil and vinegar salad dressing and 2 tablespoons Parmesan cheese, 1 (1/8 piece of 18-ounce) chocolate cake, 6 ounces red wine
= about 1,400 calories
Trimmed: 1 cup pasta with Marinara sauce, 2 slices Italian bread with 1 tablespoon flavored olive oil, 1 cup cooked greens, 1 cup fresh fruit
= about 500 calories

TRADITIONAL US STEAK HOUSE

Typical: 9-ounce rib-eye steak, 15 steak fries, 1 dinner roll with 1 teaspoon butter, 1½ ounces hard liquor = about 1,600 calories

Trimmed: 6-ounce filet steak, ½ cup broccoli, 1 medium baked potato with 2 teaspoons light butter, 1 cup tossed salad with 1 tablespoon Italian dressing, 12 ounces sparkling water with lemon = about 800 calories

Source: [57,58].

Morsel "One should eat to live, not live to eat." —Cicero (Roman constitutionalist, consul, lawyer, orator, philosopher, political theorist and statesman, 106-43 BC)

Behavior Modification and Weight Management

A well-constructed calorie-deficit diet coupled with a well-designed exercise program that includes cardiovascular and muscular fitness should result in weight loss. Yet, behaviors interfere that sabotage even the best diet and exercise regimens. Behavior modification gets to the heart of these behaviors to initiate and sustain changes for successful weight loss and weight maintenance.

Behavior modification is the use of behavior change techniques to improve a person's eating behavior. It involves modifying old eating habits and developing better eating habits. This is done through a series of steps that focus on environmental or situational control of routines.

The steps reduce the exposure, susceptibility, and responses to environmental situations that cause overeating and underexercising. They are based on self-monitoring and self-management. By overseeing and charting daily behaviors, negative eating behaviors and exercise habits can be replaced with positive ones. These behavior modification guidelines can be individualized to target specific behaviors:

- **Control the types of food eaten.** A well-balanced diet that is consumed in moderation, without forbidden foods and beverages, is the most sensible and realistic approach. Do not label foods "good" or "bad." Instead, consider grouping foods "always," "sometimes," and "almost never."
- **Control quantity of food eaten.** The correct serving sizes of foods and beverages teach moderation and control. Follow the portion size guidelines in Chapter 1.
- **Use a small plate.** Use a salad plate instead of a dinner plate for entrees. Develop the habit of leaving at least one bite of each item on the plate. By using a smaller plate, it will become easier to stop eating when full to leave food behind. Do not serve family style or put serving dishes on the dinner table. When out of sight, second servings are out of mind.
- **Eat three daily meals and planned snacks at regular times throughout the day.** Eating regularly helps a person develop awareness of his or her internal hunger cues; respond to them, and stop when satiety is reached.
- **Eat slowly and consciously.** It takes about 20 minutes for the brain to know that the stomach has been fed and satisfied, plus it provides opportunities to truly savor food and drink. Put down an eating utensil between bites, and do not pick up an eating utensil until you have swallowed the bite.
- **Choose one specific location to eat.** Unconscious eating while cooking, driving, standing, or watching television or a movie can cause mindless eating and overeating. Do not keep food in any room except the kitchen.
- **Make eating a singular activity.** Talking on the phone, reading, or watching television may lead to unconscious eating and overeating. Dish out set amounts of food and beverage, and then focus on eating and drinking deliberately, without distractions.
- **Become aware of social influences.** Family, friends, and work associates may disrupt diet and exercise plans. Developing confidence in managing these relationships promotes long-term weight management success.

471

- **Substitute another activity for between-meal snacking.** Delay going to a vending machine or to the kitchen until the desire to eat is gone. Vigorous exercise will dull hunger. So will slow-up liquids, such as a big glass of flavored noncalorie water, like the ones that are featured in this chapter.
- **Control emotional eating.** Eating when angry, bored, happy, or sad sets up triggers for eating the wrong foods at the wrong times. Learning how to recognize and replace emotional overeating with alternative activities may be the most important behavior change of all.
- **Add pleasure to meals.** Dieting does not have to mean denial. Foods and beverages should be attractive and flavorful, and the meal settings should foster enjoyment. Remove foods from containers. Garnish plates with fresh fruits and vegetables. Eat hot foods hot and cold foods cold. Make every meal and snack a celebration rather than a punishment.

References

[1] Ebbell B, Banov L. In: The Papyrus ebers—the greatest Egyptian medical document. Copenhagen: Levin & Munksgaard; 1937.

[2] Timetoast. Perceptions of body image throughout history. <http://www.timetoast.com/timelines/40315/>; [accessed 02.09.08].

[3] Haslam D. Obesity: a medical history. Obes Rev 2007;8:31–6.

[4] Kromhout D, Keys A, Aravanis C, et al. Food consumption patterns in the 1960s in seven countries. Am J Clin Nutr 1989;49:889–94.

[5] University of Florida. Food pyramid history. <http://iml.jou.ufl.edu/projects/fall02/greene/history.htm>; [accessed 02.09.08].

[6] http://www.nhlbi.nih.gov/health/health-topics/topics/obe/

[7] http://www.cdc.gov/obesity/causes/index.html/

[8] Wyatt SB, Winters KP, Dubbert PM. Overweight and obesity: prevalence, consequences, and causes of a growing public health problem. Am J Med Sci 2006;331(4):166–74. Bariatric Surgery.

[9] http://win.niddk.nih.gov/publications/understanding.htm/

[10] <http://www.acefitness.org/> ACE Lifestyle & Weight Management Coach Manual.

[11] Hargrove JL. History of the calorie in nutrition. Am Soc Nutr J Nutr 2006;136:2957–61.

[12] http://krupp.wcc.hawaii.edu/BIOL100L/nutrition/energy.pdf/

[13] http://www.rd411.com/index.php?option=com_content&view=article&id=96:energy-expenditure-rmr-and-thermal-effect-of-food&catid=74:nutrition-assessment&Itemid=353

[14] <http://www.ajcn.org/content/63/2/164.short>. Am J Clin Nutr Vol 63: 164-169. GW Reed and JO Hill. Measuring the thermic effect of food.

[15] http://www.nal.usda.gov/fnic/foodcomp/search/

[16] Bray GA. Dietary therapy for obesity. <http://www.uptodate.com/home/index.html/>.

[17] Gardner CD, et al. Comparison of the Atkins, Zone, Ornish, and LEARN diets for change in weight and related risk factors among overweight premenopausal women: the A to Z weight loss study: a randomized trial. JAMA 2007;297:969.

[18] Liu S, et al. Dietary carbohydrates. <http://www.uptodate.com/home/index.html/>.

[19] Sacks F, et al. Comparison of weight-loss diets with different compositions of fat, protein, and carbohydrates. N Engl J Med 2009;360:859.

[20] Shai I, et al. Weight loss with a low-carbohydrate, Mediterranean, or low-fat diet. N Engl J Med 2008;359:229.

[21] Stephen AM, Seiber G, Gerster Y, Morgan D. Intake of carbohydrate and its components— international comparisons, trends over time, and effects of changing to low-fat diets. Am J Clin Nutr 1995;62(4):851S–67S. A well-planned diet can healthfully induce weight and fat loss and preserve muscle mass.

[22] http://www.mayoclinic.com/health/healthy-diet/NU00200/

[23] http://www.theatlantic.com/life/archive/2011/08/why-does-the-fda-recommend-2-000-calories-per-day/243092/

[24] http://www.fda.gov/food/dietarysupplements/default.htm/

[25] http://www.fda.gov/RegulatoryInformation/Legislation/default.htm/

[26] http://www.consumerreports.org/health/free-highlights/manage-your-health/supplements_questions.htm/

[27] Walter L, Larimore MD, Dónal P, O'Mathúna MA. Quality assessment programs for dietary supplements. Ann Pharmacother 2003;37(6):893–8.

[28] http://www.ext.colostate.edu/pubs/foodnut/09363.html/

[29] http://www.mayoclinic.com/health/weight-loss/HQ01160/

[30] Kernt P, Naughton J, Driscoll C, Loxterkamp D. Fasting: the history, pathophysiology, and complications. West J Med 1982;137:379–99.

[31] Bulik CM, et al. Diagnosis and management of binge eating disorder. World Psychiatry 2007;6:142.

[32] Anderluh M, Tchanturia K, Rabe-Hesketh S, Collier D, Treasure J. Lifetime course of eating disorders: design and validity testing of a new strategy to define the eating disorders phenotype. Psychol Med 2009;39:105–14.

[33] Winkelman JW. Sleep-Related Eating Disorder and Night Eating Syndrome: Sleep Disorders, Eating Disorders, or Both? SLEEP 2006;29(7):949–54.

[34] http://www.nationaleatingdisorders.org/

[35] http://www.nationaleatingdisorders.org/nedaDir/files/documents/handouts/WhatIsEd.pdf/

[36] http://www.renfrewcenter.com/for-you/signs-symptoms.asp/

[37] http://www.sleepfoundation.org/articles/hot-topics/

[38] American Council on Exercise. ACE fitness. <http://www.acefi/tness.org/healthandfitnesstips/default.aspx/>; [accessed 10.28.12]. < http://www.acsm.org/about-acsm/media-room/news-releases/2011/08/01/acsm-issues-new-recommendations-on-quantity-andquality-of-exercise/>.

[39] http://www.aces.edu/pubs/docs/H/HE-0748/

[40] http://btc.montana.edu/olympics/nutrition/eat11.html/

[41] http://www.ncbi.nlm.nih.gov/pubmed/17213878/

[42] http://www.acefitness.org/fitnessqanda/fitnessqanda_display.aspx?itemid=271/

[43] Ellender L, Linder MM. Sports pharmacology and ergogenic aids. Prim Care 2005;32:277–92.

[44] Sinclair CJ, Geiger JD. Caffeine use in sports. A pharmacological review. J Sports Med Phys Fitness 2000;40:71–9.

[45] http://www.medscape.com/viewarticle/487473_6/

[46] http://sportsanddrugs.procon.org/view.resource.php?resourceID=002366/

[47] <www.quotegarden.com/dieting.html/>; The Quote Garden: A Harvest of Quotes for Word Lovers; <www.quotegarden.com/> Copyright © 1998–2008.

[48] http://nutritiondata.self.com/

[49] http://allrecipes.com/HowTo/baking-with-sugar-and-sugar-substitutes/detail.aspx

[50] http://www.mayoclinic.com/health/healthy-recipes/NU00585/

[51] http://www.mayoclinic.com/health/calories/WT00011/NSECTIONGROUP=2/

[52] Fairfax County Public Schools. <http://www.fcps.edu/index.shtml/>; [accessed 02.09.08] Adapted from <http://www.fcps.edu/parents/HS%20August%202008%20Menu.pdf/>.

[53] Diet analysis: <http://nutritiondata.self.com/mynd/mytracking/welcome?returnto=/mynd/mytracking/>.

[54] Healthy diet guidelines: <http://www.mayoclinic.com/health/healthy-diet/NU00200/>.

[55] http://www.cnpp.usda.gov/Publications/DietaryGuidelines/2010/PolicyDoc/Chapter2.pdf/

[56] http://www.iom.edu/Activities/Nutrition/SummaryDRIs/~/media/Files/Activity%20Files/Nutrition/DRIs/5_Summary%20Table%20Tables%201-4.pdf/

[57] http://www.heart.org/HEARTORG/GettingHealthy/NutritionCenter/DiningOut/Tips-by-Cuisine_UCM_308333_Article.jsp/

[58] http://fnic.nal.usda.gov/nal_display/index.php?info_center=4&tax_level=3&tax_subject=358&topic_id=1611&level3_id=5972&level4_id=0&level5_id=0&placement_default=0/

473

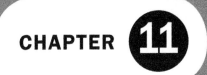

Life Cycle Nutrition:
Healthful Eating Throughout
the Ages

Practical Applications for Nutrition, Food Science and Culinary Professionals

OBJECTIVES

1. Identify the nutritional needs before, during and after pregnancy and lactation
2. Plan recipes, meals and menus for pregnant and lactating women
3. Discriminate among food and nutrition choices for infants and children
4. Apply knowledge of food allergies to infant and child nutrition

Culinary Nutrition. DOI: http://dx.doi.org/10.1016/B978-0-12-391882-6.00011-X

5. Plan recipes, meals and menus for infants and children

6. Determine healthy food choices for toddlers and school-age children

7. Assess teenage food choices compared to nutrient needs

8. Develop foods, recipes and menus for normal teenage diets

9. Create foods, recipes and menus for specialized teenage diets

10. Recognize physiological changes of aging and corresponding nutrient needs; plan recipes, meal and menus for changing tastes due to aging; and evaluate foods and beverages designed for each stage of the life cycle

Morsel "Food is a central part of our lives. It provides the body with fuel and raw materials for maintenance, growth and repair. It draws together family and friends, anchors celebrations and rites of passage, and sometimes soothes the soul." —Ethan Becker (Author of *The Joy of Cooking*, 1997 version)

INTRODUCTION: NORMAL AND SPECIALIZED LIFE CYCLE NUTRITION

Life is a succession of birth, life and death. Making the most of one's life through proactive life choices—consuming nutritious foods and beverages, exercising, refraining from smoking, consuming alcohol in moderation, if at all, and practicing overall body maintenance—should be lifetime goals. By making wise nutrition and diet choices throughout the life cycle, the quality and quantity of one's life may improve.

476

This chapter begins with life in utero and focuses on maternal nutrition. It continues with infant nutrition and the choices between breastfeeding and commercial infant formulas. As infants develop into toddlers and throughout childhood, their food and nutrition needs change—from higher to meet toddlers' active lifestyles to lower as children settle into school.

While early childhood seems busy, children generally do not accelerate in growth until their middle years. Then prepuberty brings a host of increased food and nutrition needs, including calories for energy and healthy fats for hormone formation.

Teenage years bring tremendous growth and development, with parallel needs for wide-ranging nutrients. Teenage athletes require increased energy and nutrients, including the B vitamins, vitamin D, calcium, iron and zinc, to name a few. Eating disorders may become noticeable at this age and require the health professional intervention. Obesity is as much an eating disorder as anorexia or bulimia. Obesity interventions should start much earlier, since childhood obesity is on the rise.

The years between 20 and 50 years of age are a period of maintenance and health promotion, rather than growth. During these years, it is best to consume the right amount of calories and other nutrients for weight and health maintenance.

When the older years begin after age 50, many nutrient requirements actually decrease because the body's systems are slowing down. By keeping active and eating right, one may be able to offset some of the profound changes that occur throughout aging. Changes in taste and smell might offer some of the most challenging tasks for choosing and consuming healthy foods and beverages.

Many opportunities exist for nutrition, food science and culinary professionals in the realm of life cycle nutrition. Whether it is at the start of life or toward its end, the challenges of infant, children, adolescent and senior nutrition are ever-present. Developing nutritious, age-appropriate foods and beverages, and positioning them within healthy lifestyle stages are some of the most important roles that food and nutrition professionals may have.

MAIN COURSES
Pregnancy and Lactation

A HEALTHY START: NOURISHMENT BEFORE, DURING AND AFTER PREGNANCY

Creating a new life begins from the ground up, much like the construction of a new building. A building complex demands high-quality building materials, an intricate working structure, and a finely tuned communication network, among other systems. A building of this nature can take many months in execution.

A human body requires high-quality nutrients (building materials); a complex maze of cells, organs and systems (intricate working structure); and countless signals from chemical messengers about the blood levels of nutrients, hormonal balance, sensory signals and more (finely tuned communication network). That is why the creation of a new human body requires nine months.

If a woman is at her nutritional best before she conceives, this may increase her chances of birthing a healthy infant who will be able to grow and thrive. If there are any weak links along the way, the mother, infant or both may suffer—much like the flaws in a complex building structure.

The childbearing years, which may include pregnancy and lactation, present a unique set of nutritional needs for women. A woman must ready her body to ensure a healthy start for an infant. This means abstaining from certain substances and ingesting others—sometimes well in advance of pregnancy. Nutrition and culinary specialists who create food for women of childbearing years should learn the right nutritional and lifestyle approaches for healthy pregnancies and translate this information into healthy recipes, meals and menus.

A pregnant woman's heightened nutritional needs undergo additional changes during *lactation*, or milk production. These additional nutritional needs also require skilled diet design and culinary interpretations by trained nutrition and culinary specialists.

THE CHANGES AND CHALLENGES OF PREGNANCY

Pregnancy is the period of time from conception to birth when a woman carries a developing embryo or fetus in her uterus. An *embryo* is a developing human being from the time of implantation to the end of the eighth week after conception (when the major body structures have formed). A *fetus* is an unborn offspring from the end of the eighth week after conception until birth.

The lifeline between a mother and a fetus is an organ that is called the *placenta.* During pregnancy, the placenta delivers oxygen and nutrients to the fetus and removes wastes. It is attached to the fetus by the *umbilical cord*, which is cut after birth, after which the placenta is expelled.

The fetus is surrounded by the *uterus*, also called the *womb*. When a woman is pregnant, the baby grows inside of the uterus until birth. The *amniotic sac* is a bag of fluid within the womb where the fetus develops and grows. It is filled with clear fluid in which the fetus floats and moves. The amniotic sac cushions the fetus from injury, provides it with fluids that it can swallow, and helps to maintain a constant temperature. Everything a pregnant woman takes into her body may affect the growth and development of the fetus, in addition to these structures that support the fetus.

PRENATAL NUTRITIONAL NEEDS

The *prenatal* period is the period of time before birth. A woman's nutritional needs are high during this time. Because a woman may not know that she is pregnant, she may be poorly nourished. She may also consume alcohol or caffeine in excess, which may affect the growing embryo or fetus.

A woman should be at nutritional readiness for pregnancy during her childbearing years. Her body weight should be at a desirable level. She should consume a wide range of foods and beverages that contain a variety of nutrients, including an assortment of fruits and vegetables—particularly those that are rich in iron and folate to help prevent anemia and neural tube defects—and calcium for growth, development and repair. She should be at her peak of physical fitness to handle the tremendous physical stresses of pregnancy. Yet, even nutritional and physical readiness does not ensure a healthy, risk-free pregnancy or birth.

477

The risk factors of pregnancy include alcohol intake, chronic disease such as diabetes or hypertension, drug intake, eating disorders, excessive dieting, folic acid deficiency, iron deficiency, lack of health care, multiple pregnancies, nicotine use, overweight, poor education, poor pregnancy outcomes, poverty, previous abortions, teenage pregnancy and/or underweight.

THE NUTRITIONAL NEEDS OF PREGNANCY

A normal human pregnancy consists of three trimesters of three months each, for a total of nine months. The nutritional needs of the mother and the fetus increase during each trimester.

Calories

A pregnant woman needs about 150 to 200 additional calories daily during the first trimester. During the second trimester, she requires about 350 calories daily, and during the third trimester, about 450 additional calories. The third trimester is when the fetus is doing most of its growth. Based on the Daily Value (DV) of 2,000 calories daily for most healthy adults over the age of 18 years, this amounts to about 2,350 calories daily during the second trimester and 2,450 calories daily during the third trimester.

Protein

The Dietary Reference Intake (DRI) for a nonpregnant adult woman is 46 grams of protein daily, and the DRI for a pregnant woman is 71 grams of protein daily. This is an increase of about 20 grams of protein daily. This protein requirement is based on body weight (see Chapter 5). A woman's body weight increases to support the growing fetus and maternal nutrient stores [1].

Carbohydrates

Also based on the DRIs, a pregnant woman requires about 175 grams of carbohydrates daily. This amounts to about 700 calories' worth of carbohydrates daily (175 grams of carbohydrates × 4 carbohydrate calories per gram = 700 daily calories). At least half of these carbohydrates should be from whole grains for fiber and nutrients. The Adequate Intake (AI) for fiber for pregnant women is 28 grams daily.

Lipids

While a recommended level of lipids during pregnancy has not been determined, an AI level of the essential fatty acids linolenic and alpha-linolenic acids have been established. These are 13 grams/day of linolenic acid, and 1.3 grams/day of alpha-linolenic acid. Both are important to consume in balance for fetal brain development. Linolenic acid is found in plant oils such as corn oil, safflower oil and sunflower oil. Alpha-linolenic acid is found in seed oils, such as flaxseed, soybean and walnut oils.

Vitamins

By consuming a wide range of foods and beverages and the right amount of calories, most vitamin requirements during pregnancy should be met. The need for folate is exceptional.

Folate (folic acid, folacin) is a B vitamin that is naturally found in broccoli, citrus fruits and juices, green leafy vegetables, and legumes. Folic acid is the synthetic form of this B vitamin that is used in supplements and in fortified foods. Folate is only partially absorbed by the body, while folic acid is almost completely absorbed. Folacin is another term for this B vitamin. Folate, folic acid and folacin are often used interchangeably.

A pregnant woman's need for folate increases by 50 percent over her prepregnancy folate needs due to an increase in her blood volume and fetal growth. Folate also helps prevent *neural tube defects*—birth defects that affect the fetal brain and spinal cord that can cause disorders in the central nervous system of the developing fetus. The two main types of central nervous system disorders include *spina bifida*, and *anencephaly*.

Spina bifida is a central nervous system disorder that is characterized by the incomplete closure of the bony casing around the spinal cord. *Anencephaly* is distinguished by a partial brain or no brain.

The neural tube closes before the sixth week of pregnancy, so sufficient folate is recommended during the first trimester, as well as three months prior to conception. Since so many pregnancies are unplanned, this is why women of childbearing years should have a regular intake of folate.

The AI for folate for women of childbearing years is 400 micrograms daily, which increases to 600 micrograms daily during pregnancy to help decrease the risk of birth defects. A high intake of folate can mask a vitamin B12 deficiency, so folate intake during pregnancy should be carefully monitored.

Since 1999, all refined grain products, such as breads, cereals, cornmeal, farina, flour, grits, pasta and rice, must be fortified with folic acid. This form may be better absorbed than the naturally occurring folate in citrus fruits and green leafy vegetables. Some fruit juices and fruit juice beverages are also fortified with folic acid in various amounts.

Minerals

A varied diet that meets the caloric needs of pregnancy should also meet daily mineral requirements. Calcium and iron deserve special attention.

The AI for *calcium* for women of childbearing years is 1,000 milligrams daily. It increases to 1,300 milligrams daily for pregnant teenagers aged 14 to 18 years. Calcium absorption in the intestine doubles during pregnancy. This calcium is transported by the bloodstream to the mother's bones, where it is stored until the last trimester when fetal needs for calcium are high. Calcium is then released back into the mother's bloodstream, where it is transferred by the placenta and umbilical cord to the fetus. About 300 milligrams of calcium are transferred daily between the mother and the fetus in this manner.

Dairy products provide calcium, vitamins A and D, and riboflavin. One cup of reduced-fat, vitamin A–fortified dairy milk supplies about 286 milligrams of calcium, 461 IU of vitamin A, 105 IU of vitamin D, and 0.5 milligrams of riboflavin. Besides dairy milk, good sources of calcium include cheese, fortified cereals, fortified fruit juices, fortified soy foods, green leafy vegetables and legumes. Vitamin D is also available in eggs and fish, and riboflavin can be found in leafy green vegetables, fortified breads and cereals and whole grains.

A pregnant woman stockpiles *iron* during pregnancy. This is because she is no longer menstruating, and iron absorption increases to three times as normal. Additionally, from months three to six, the fetus creates its own iron stores, so while iron absorption increases dramatically, so does a mother's need for iron. Iron-poor blood can lead to anemia and its symptoms, which may include excessive tiredness, dizziness, fast or irregular heartbeat, fainting, pale skin and/or shortness of breath.

The DRI for iron is 15 milligrams daily for teenage girls aged 14 to 18 years and 18 milligrams daily for women aged 19 to 50 years. The DRI for iron increases to 27 milligrams daily for women aged 14 and older during pregnancy.

An iron supplement is common during pregnancy to help meet these requirements. Even more iron may be necessary for vegetarian women or women with a history of anemia. Iron is best absorbed along with a source of vitamin C, such as citrus juice or tomato products, and between meals, so that it does not compete with other supplements, foods or beverages.

Other Vitamins and Minerals: Vitamin C, Thiamin, Niacin and Iodine

Other vitamin and mineral requirements that increase during pregnancy include *vitamin C, thiamin, niacin* and *iodine*. The DRIs for these vitamins for females 14 to 18 years and 19 through 50 years of age are shown here.

Vitamin/Mineral	Female DRI	Pregnancy DRI
	14–18 years/19–50 years	*14–18 years/19–50 years*
Vitamin C	65/75 milligrams	80/85 milligrams
Thiamin	1.0/1.1 milligrams	1.4 milligrams
Niacin	14 milligrams	18 milligrams
Iodine	150 micrograms	220 micrograms

A diet that includes brightly colored, fresh fruits and vegetables; lean proteins; and whole-grain and enriched and fortified breads and cereals should supply these vitamins and minerals. While prenatal vitamins and minerals are often prescribed during pregnancy, they should only be taken under the care of a health professional. Prenatal supplements do not make up for a poor diet; they *supplement* the diet.

TABLE 11-1 Components of Normal Weight Gain during Pregnancy	
Factors	**Weight Gain (pounds)**
Size of infant at birth	6½–8 pounds
Mother's fat stores	6–8
Increase in mother's:	
Fluid volume	3–4
Blood volume	3–4
Uterus and uterine muscles	2–3
Breasts	2–3
Fluid in amniotic sac	2–3
Placenta	2–3
Total range	25–35 pounds

Fluids

The recommended amount of fluid intake for pregnant women is four (8-ounce) cups per 1,000 calories, similar to a nonpregnant woman. Because fluid volume increases during pregnancy, adequate fluid consumption is vital.

Weight Gain

Maternal weight gain is normal and expected during pregnancy. Normal weight gain is about 25 to 35 pounds, as shown in Table 11-1.

If a woman is considered underweight before she conceives, her recommended weight gain is about 28 to 40 pounds. If she is considered overweight, her recommended weight gain is about 15 to 25 pounds. And if she is considered obese, her recommended weight gain is about 15 pounds. A pregnant teenager should aim for the weight at the higher end of each of these ranges to account for her higher nutrient needs.

Weight gain should be modest during the first trimester—only 3 to 4 pounds, with about a 1-pound weekly gain in weight throughout the course of pregnancy. The "normal" weight for an infant is considered to be about 6½ to 8 pounds at birth. The rest of maternal weight gain during pregnancy is due to increased fluid volume, muscles and tissues, with a small increase in fat stores. Much of maternal weight gain is lost at delivery or soon thereafter, with the bulk of weight lost after a few months when maternal blood volume returns to normal. If excessive weight is gained during pregnancy, then a woman may have a more difficult time returning to her prepregnancy weight.

If a woman does not gain as much weight as recommended, she may run the risk of a low-birth-weight (LBW) infant, often indicative of future health problems. An LBW infant is considered to be 5½ pounds or less. They may be born prematurely or suffer growth failure.

Conversely, if a woman gains too much weight during her pregnancy, this may be indicative of labor and delivery complications, gestational diabetes, hypertension, or postpartum obesity. A high-birth-weight baby (over 9 pounds at birth) may be at increased risk of health problems later in life, such as diabetes [2–4].

HEALTH CONCERNS OF PREGNANCY

Factors such as alcohol, anemia, caffeine, food cravings, exercise, fatty fish/mercury, gastrointestinal disturbances, gestational diabetes, lead, morning sickness, pregnancy-induced hypertension, teenage pregnancy and tobacco may contribute to the health and well-being of both the mother and the child.

Alcohol

Consuming alcoholic beverages during pregnancy may lead to a serious condition called *fetal alcohol syndrome (FAS)*. FAS is a group of symptoms that become apparent after birth in an infant or child. These may include facial malformations, impaired central nervous system development and retarded growth. *Fetal alcohol effect (FAE)* may not be as severe. It may result in impaired learning. As little as 2 ounces of alcohol daily may be enough to cause birth defects, low birth weight, and/or spontaneous abortions. (A standard shot contains 1.5 ounces of alcohol [ethanol].)

Since there is no known safe amount of alcohol consumption during pregnancy, the American Academy of Pediatrics advises abstinence from alcohol for women who are planning a pregnancy or who are pregnant. In unplanned pregnancies, this warning may be too late to prevent FAS or FAE [5].

Anemia

A pregnant woman's blood volume increases 40 to 50 percent of normal, but her red blood cells only increase 20 to 30 percent of normal. Due to this condition, *physiological anemia* (a lower proportion of red blood cells compared to fluid) may occur. Physiological anemia is normal during the first trimester. It usually corrects itself as the pregnancy progresses into the second trimester. An early symptom of physiological anemia is general tiredness. Extreme signs of anemia may include fast or irregular heartbeat, fainting and/ or shortness of breath. A woman may feel tired again during the third trimester, but this may be the sign of a rapidly growing fetus and extra body weight.

Caffeine

While caffeine is considered to be one of the oldest drugs, the safety of its consumption during pregnancy is not confirmed. If a woman chooses to consume caffeinated beverages during her pregnancy, she should probably cut back. Caffeine does cross the placenta and enter the fetus where it could affect its heart and respiration rates. The March of Dimes recommends that women who are pregnant or trying to become pregnant limit caffeine to no more than 200 milligrams daily (about one 12-ounce cup of coffee). More information about caffeine can be found in Chapter 8 [6].

Cravings

Pregnant women are known to crave a number of food and nonfood items, probably due to the multitude of chemicals and hormones that cascade through their bodies during pregnancy. Some food cravings may be provoked by swings in blood sugar. If there are blood sugar irregularities, then women should have a glucose tolerance test to rule out gestational diabetes—especially if there is a family history of diabetes.

A craving for salt may be the result of a pregnant woman's expanding blood volume and the electrolytes that salt provides. Some food and/or beverage cravings could be the result of sensory changes—particularly in taste and smell. These sensory changes in the mother help to protect the unborn child from harmful substances.

Nonfood cravings are called *pica*. Pregnant women and children may eat clay, coffee grounds, dirt, ice, laundry starch, wallpaper or other nonfood items. Pica often masks a more serious problem, which may result in intestinal obstruction, malnutrition, obesity or poisoning. Pica sometimes indicates iron deficiency, which may be common to both pregnant women and their children.

Exercise

If a pregnant woman has been exercising regularly before conception, she should be able to maintain her exercise program during her pregnancy. However, she should first discuss her exercise protocol with her health care provider. Exercise during pregnancy may help manage mood swings brought about by changing hormones, edema from water retention and irregular sleep, especially in the last trimester, when the growing fetus can become uncomfortable. Exercise helps tone the muscles, which help to burn calories postpregnancy and promote a speedy return to a desirable body weight.

Fatty Fish and Mercury

Mercury is an environmental contaminant, much like iron. Most fish and shellfish contain some degree of mercury, which is probably safe for healthy adults. Some fish and shellfish contain higher levels that may be potentially dangerous—especially to the growing fetus.

The US Food and Drug Association and Environmental Protection Agency recommend that pregnant and nursing women not exceed 12 ounces (two average meals) of certain fish and shellfish weekly. These include canned light tuna, catfish, pollock, salmon and shrimp. King mackerel, shark, swordfish and tilefish should be avoided due to their high mercury content. Since an infant's central nervous system is still developing after birth, fish and shellfish with high amounts of mercury are not recommended for infants [7].

Gastrointestinal Disturbances

Due to the hormonal changes of pregnancy, the smooth muscles that line the gastrointestinal tract relax and movements slow down, which may cause constipation. This condition is worsened by iron supplements and inadequate fluid intake. Adequate fiber and fluid intake and regular activity help to stimulate the gastrointestinal tract.

As the fetus grows inside the mother's womb in the last trimester, the uterus pushes upward into the mother's abdomen and causes pressure on her stomach. Stomach acid may back up into the esophagus, causing rebound acidity, or *heartburn*. Rather than take antacids, a pregnant woman should consume smaller meals, avoid spicy and/or fatty foods, and avoid lying down after meals.

Gestational Diabetes

Midway through pregnancy, many health providers test pregnant women for *gestational diabetes*, a form of Type II diabetes that may disappear once pregnancy is completed. Sometimes women with gestational diabetes must inject insulin until their blood sugar returns to normal after birth. Women who have experienced gestational diabetes may be more likely to develop Type II diabetes later in life.

Women with a family history of diabetes should monitor their weight gain and manage their food and beverage intake, especially carbohydrates and fats. If glucose cannot enter the mother's cells for energy, then it may travel to the fetus and be converted into fat. Babies born to women with gestational diabetes may be heavy at birth (over 9 pounds) and are usually tested for diabetes soon after birth.

Lead

Like mercury, lead is a contaminant in the environment that can leach into our food supply. Untreated ceramic cups and lead crystal should not be used for hot food or beverages or on a regular basis. It is best to check the manufacturer for more information about their composition and construction.

It is important to know the source of and production of drinking water. Unlined lead water pipes may leach lead into drinking water and be hazardous to the developing nervous system of the growing fetus.

Morning Sickness

Morning sickness is a condition that can happen at any time of day, but it frequently occurs early in the morning. It can range from general ill feelings to nausea and vomiting, which may be caused by fluctuating hormones, emotional stress or even ordinary foods.

Morning sickness often occurs at the start of pregnancy and dissipates by the second trimester. It may be so intense that it leads to weight loss and necessitates bed rest. Some women go through pregnancy without any morning sickness. Others may have extreme cases that may require hospitalization.

Pregnancy-induced Hypertension

When pregnant women gain weight rapidly after the fifth month of pregnancy, this may be a sign of *pregnancy-induced hypertension (PIH)*, or *preeclampsia*. This condition is characterized by *edema*, swelling that is caused by fluid trapped within body tissues. Edema occurs most often in the ankles, feet and legs. Abnormal liver function, hypertension and protein "spillage" in the urine characterize preeclampsia.

If preeclampsia worsens, a woman could suffer convulsions. This condition is called *eclampsia* and may lead to coma and/or death. Excessive sodium intake, teenage pregnancy, pregnancy over 35 years of age,

482

multiple fetuses (as in twins or triplets), and a family history of diabetes or hypertension may predispose a woman to PIH. Removing the fetus by caesarean section may return maternal blood pressure to normal. However, if a fetus is surgically removed before 24 weeks of pregnancy, it may have a low birth weight or may not survive.

Blood pressure should be monitored regularly throughout pregnancy. A family history of hypertension and pregnancy-induced hypertension should be disclosed to health care providers.

Teenage Pregnancy

Countless chemicals in the body interplay during pregnancy. They may directly or indirectly affect the emotional, physical and social behaviors of the mother. It is difficult for an adult woman to successfully manage all of the highs and lows of pregnancy. The emotional "roller coaster" may be even more challenging for teenagers. Plus, teenagers may not be finished growing, so pregnancy may compromise their growth and health. Pregnant teenagers are more prone to anemia, low-birth-weight infants with failure to thrive, pregnancy-induced hypertension and premature birth.

Tobacco

Nicotine is a drug that passes through the placenta, like other drugs. Smoking restricts the flow of blood to the fetus, which may limit the nutrients that it can access and its ability to remove waste products. Tobacco may also stunt fetal growth and contribute to low birth weight, developmental retardation and spontaneous abortions.

Sudden infant death syndrome (SIDS) has been associated with smoking during pregnancy and to secondhand smoke postpregnancy. SIDS is the leading cause of death for babies between one month and one year of age [8].

THE NUTRITIONAL NEEDS OF LACTATION

The nutritional needs during lactation are very similar to the nutritional needs of pregnancy. Milk production requires about 800 calories daily. On average, mothers who breastfeed produce about 30 ounces of milk daily, which is generally covered by a modest increase in calories and fluids. One ounce of breast milk contains about 20 calories.

A nursing mother will need to consume about 400 calories daily that are over and beyond her normal needs. Based on the DV of 2,000 calories daily for most healthy women over the age of 18 years, this amounts to about 2,400 calories. The remaining 400 calories will be drawn from the mother's fat stores that were generated during her pregnancy. A pregnant or lactating woman requires about:

- 3 to 4 daily servings of dairy products or equivalents
  (1 serving = about 1 cup of dairy milk or 1 ounce or 1 slice of cheese)
- 2 to 3 daily servings of meats or vegetable proteins
  (1 serving = about 3 ounces of beef, fish or shellfish, pork, poultry or vegetarian substitute)
- 3 to 4 daily servings of fruits
  (1 serving = about 1 small piece of fruit or ½ cup of canned fruit)
- 3 to 5 daily servings of vegetables
  (1 serving = about 1 cup of fresh vegetables or ½ cup of cooked vegetables)
- 7 to 11 daily servings of breads, cereals and grains, with at least half of these servings from whole grains
  (1 serving = about 1 slice of bread or ½ cup of cooked grains, such as rice or pasta)
- 4 daily servings of fats and oils
  (1 serving = 1 teaspoon margarine or butter or 1 tablespoon salad dressing)

A guide to serving sizes can be found in Chapter 1.

A nursing mother should also consume at least four 8-ounce cups of fluid per 1,000 calories to meet her milk production needs. She should try to consume beverages whenever her infant nurses to help keep up with its demand.

HEALTHY DIET AND MEAL PLANNING FOR PREGNANCY AND LACTATION

The sample meal plan that is shown in Table 11-2 is based on the number of servings that pregnant or lactating women need daily.

TABLE 11-2 Sample Daily Meal Plan for Pregnancy or Lactation

Breakfast	Snack
1½ cups whole-grain, high-fiber cold cereal (2 servings breads/cereals/grains) 1 cup reduced-fat dairy milk or milk substitute (1 serving dairy products) 1 small banana (1 serving fruit) 1 *or more* cups water or nonsugar beverage	1 small orange (1 serving fruit) 1 *or more* cups water or nonsugar beverage
Lunch	**Snack**
High-protein and vegetable entree salad: 2 cups fresh salad greens ("free food") 1 cup raw sliced sweet peppers, carrots, and celery (1 serving vegetables) 3 ounces lean meat, skinless poultry, fish or vegetarian substitute (3 ounces protein = 1 serving protein) 1 ounce reduced-fat cheddar cheese or cheese substitute (1 ounce protein) 2 tablespoons vinegar and oil salad dressing (2 servings fats/oils) 2 small whole-grain rolls (2 servings breads/grains/cereals) 1 small apple (1 serving fruit) 1 cup reduced-fat dairy milk or milk substitute (1 serving dairy products) 1 *or more* cups water or nonsugar beverage	1 small bran muffin (1 serving breads/grains/cereals) 1 cup nonfat plain yogurt (1 serving dairy products) 1 *or more* cups water or nonsugar beverage
Dinner	**Snack**
High-protein chicken, pasta and broccoli casserole: 1½ cups cooked high-protein pasta (3 servings breads/grains/cereals) 3 ounces broiled skinless chicken breast or vegetarian substitute (3 ounces protein = 1 serving protein) 2 teaspoons butter (2 servings fats/oils) 1 cup lightly steamed broccoli (2 servings vegetables) 1 cup reduced-fat dairy milk or milk substitute (1 serving dairy products) ½ grapefruit (1 serving fruit) 1 *or more* cups water or nonsugar beverage	6 graham crackers (2 servings breads/grains/cereals) 1 cup reduced-fat dairy milk or milk substitute (1 serving dairy products) 1 *or more* cups water or nonsugar beverage

Totals
10 servings of breads/grains/cereals
7 ounces of meat (beef, fish and shellfish, pork or poultry) or vegetarian substitute
4 servings of milk or milk substitutes
4 servings of vegetables
4 servings of fruits
4 servings of fats or oils
6 *or more* cups of water or nonsugar beverages

Source: [9].

COOKING FOR PREGNANCY AND LACTATION

Calcium-rich foods and beverages, fresh fruits and vegetables, healthy fats and oils, lean proteins, wholesome grains, and plenty of nourishing liquids (especially water) provide the best nutritional foundation for pregnant and lactating women. Supplements cannot fully replace all of the nutrients that are found in these foods and beverages. There are no special foods or beverages that are designed to ensure a healthy pregnancy, but there are food safety guidelines for preparing safe cuisine.

Pregnant women need to be especially careful about three potentially dangerous substances in the food supply that can cause serious illness and/or death to the mother and her fetus: *listeria, mercury* and *toxoplasma.*

Listeria is a dangerous bacterium that can grow even in cold refrigerators. *Mercury* is a potentially harmful heavy metal that can leach into our food supply (see "Fatty fish and mercury in health concerns of pregnancy"). *Toxoplasma* is a parasite that is found in undercooked meat and unwashed fruits and vegetables. Some guidelines to help avoid these substances follow. To be on the safe side, do not prepare or serve these foods to pregnant or lactating women [10]:

- Pates or meat spreads
- Raw sprouts of any kind (including alfalfa, clover and radish)
- Raw or undercooked eggs, fish or shellfish (sushi or sashimi), meat or poultry
- Raw or unpasteurized dairy milk, or foods or beverages that contain raw or unpasteurized dairy milk
- Smoked seafood (including salmon, mackerel or whitefish), which are usually labeled "Nova-style," lox, kippered or jerky
- Soft cheeses (including brie or camembert), blue-veined cheeses, feta, queso blanco or queso fresco or panela, unless pasteurized or from pasteurized dairy milk
- Swordfish, tilefish, king mackerel or shark
- Uncured hot dogs and luncheon meats, unless they are steaming hot
- Unwashed fruits or vegetables
- Unpasteurized juices by the glass

COOKING FOR SPECIALIZED NUTRITIONAL NEEDS IN PREGNANCY

The symptoms of pregnancy, including morning sickness (also called *nausea, vomiting of pregnancy* or *pregnancy sickness*), tend to be more common in early pregnancy when a pregnant woman is tired or hungry. In some cases, however, they can last throughout the day and night. The daily diet should be kept as normal as possible. Fluids are essential. If food and beverages are refused, then medical attention should be sought.

Here are some cooking and meal planning suggestions for *morning sickness*:

- Prepare smaller meals and snacks that can be served throughout the day.
- Start a meal with plain carbohydrates, such as crackers or crusty bread.
- Create fewer foods and beverages that are high in fat.
- Make fewer spicy recipes.
- Control cooking odors. Avoid cooking odorous vegetables, such as cauliflower or Brussels sprouts, right before serving. Prepare them earlier in the day so the kitchen can air out.
- Add ginger to dishes where it seems logical. Ginger is known to relieve gastrointestinal disorders.
- Provide lemonade or ginger ale as beverages, in addition to water.

Pregnant women may have more indigestion and heartburn in the last trimester of pregnancy when the fetus is increasing in body size. *Indigestion* is characterized by chronic or recurrent pain and fullness in the upper abdomen. It is frequently due to regurgitated gastric acid. Indigestion may be accompanied by belching, bloating, heartburn or nausea. Heartburn is a painful or burning sensation in the esophagus just below the breastbone.

If a pregnant woman is plagued by indigestion or heartburn, these guidelines should be followed:

- Prepare regularly spaced smaller meals and snacks that can be served throughout the day.
- Create fewer foods that are higher in fats and oils, pickled and spicy.

- Limit acidic foods, such as citrus fruits, onions and tomatoes—particularly if they provoke symptoms. Some fruit juices may be too acidic, but there are some low-acid varieties. Whole fruit should not be avoided, unless it triggers discomfort.
- Start meals with plain carbohydrates, such as unseeded Italian or French bread or plain crackers, or serve simple broth.
- Do not consume a lot of beverages with meals.
- Minimize or eliminate alcohol, caffeinated and carbonated beverages.
- Avoid chocolate, peppermint and chamomile tea if problematic—especially at night.

Remember that pregnancy is highly individualized and that hormonal and chemical reactions vary from woman to woman. A pregnant woman's sense of taste and smell are heightened, so she may experience foods and beverages differently than before her pregnancy.

Flexibility matters: ingredients may have to be substituted and recipes may have to be modified to appeal to widely changing tastes.

Infancy

FEEDING INFANTS RIGHT FROM THE START

It cannot be overstated: there is not a wrong or a right way to feed infants "right from the start." While breast milk is considered by some to be nature's almost perfect food, dairy- or soy-based infant formulas may be nutritious options to breast milk.

There are contraindications to breastfeeding and complex psychological and emotional reasons why a woman may choose not to breastfeed. What matters the most is a positive attitude about breast- or bottle feeding and concerted bonding time between the mother and infant.

NATURE'S ALMOST PERFECT FOOD: BREAST MILK

486

The fetus has a direct and vital nutrient lifeline to the mother through the umbilical cord and placenta. Infants also have a direct and vital nutrient lifeline to the mother through lactation. When an infant suckles on its mother's breast, an impulse is sent through the mother's central nervous system to her brain to release two hormones into her bloodstream: *prolactin* and *oxytocin*. **Prolactin** stimulates her breast cells to produce breast milk, and **oxytoxin** signals a **letdown reflex** by her breast tissue to transport milk to the suckling infant. The more the infant suckles, the more milk is produced. Once a nursing mother and infant are accustomed to this cycle, just the thought of nursing or a crying infant may cause the letdown reflex to occur without the infant's suckling.

Early breast milk is not truly milk but a milk-like secretion called **colostrum**. Colostrum is rich in protective substances for the infant, which include antibodies and white cells. Colostrum helps protect an infant from infections and serves to inactivate bacteria in an infant's gastrointestinal tract.

Colostrum and early breast milk also contain **bifidus factor** that encourages the growth of the healthy bacteria *Lactobacillus bifidus* in an infant's gastrointestinal tract. Early breast milk also contains an antibacteria agent, **lactoferrin**, that helps to bind iron and improve its absorption. Lactoferrin is also a component of the immune system, and it has antimicrobial properties. In particular, lactoferrin prevents bacteria growth in an infant's intestine.

According to the American Academy of Pediatrics, human breast milk is the nourishment of choice for infants for at least the first six months of life. Furthermore, the AAP suggests that pediatricians and other health care professionals recommend human milk for all infants unless breastfeeding is contraindicated. Additional water intake may be justified for exclusively breastfed infants and during abnormal conditions, such as diarrhea, fever, hot weather or vomiting. A health care provider should be consulted [11].

The Benefits of Breastfeeding and Breast Milk

The process of breastfeeding and breast milk is considered an ideal method and form of nourishment for a newborn and developing infant. Women who are better educated, older, and more affluent are more likely to breastfeed than women who are younger and from lower-income, diverse groups.

The production of human breast milk and the process of breastfeeding are adaptable, antibacterial, connective, convenient, economical, nutritional, protective and restorative:

- Breastfeeding adapts to an infant's developing needs. Early breast milk is low in fat, while "hind milk" is higher in fat, which provides satiety.
- Depending on the sanitation of the mother, breastfeeding supplies a practically bacteria-free environment for transporting nutrients.
- Breastfeeding promotes the mother–infant relationship bond.
- Although breastfeeding is not condoned in some developed countries, it is still the most convenient method of feeding an infant worldwide.
- While it is imperative for a mother to consume a nutritionally sound diet, including plenty of fruits and vegetables, lean proteins and whole grains, breastfeeding requires no additional costs.
- Breast milk supplies these vital nutrients:
  - Easily digestible and absorbable carbohydrate in the form of *lactose*
  - Protein in the form of *alpha-lactalbumin*
  - The essential omega-6 fatty acid, *linolenic acid*
  - Vitamins and minerals, except for vitamin D. Breast milk is especially rich in calcium, magnesium, phosphorus and highly absorbable iron and zinc. Breast milk is also low in sodium.
- Breastfeeding may reduce the risks of developing diseases such as asthma, ear infections, food allergies, intestinal diseases, obesity, respiratory diseases and Type I diabetes in an infant. Breastfeeding may also decrease the risks of developing breast and ovarian cancer in the mother.
- Breastfeeding reduces postdelivery uterine bleeding, promotes the return of the uterus to normal size, and supports postpregnancy weight loss [12].

Contraindications to Breastfeeding

A mother may choose not to breastfeed for several reasons. She may not be able to breastfeed, or she may be advised not to breastfeed. Moreover, the process of breastfeeding may be contraindicated for reasons including alcohol consumption, anxiety, communicable diseases, drug use, embarrassment, emotional stress, fatigue, infections or exposure, lack of knowledge, nicotine use, pain, postpartum depression and work policies for these reasons:

- **Alcohol consumption:** Alcohol passes from the mother to the infant through her breast milk. This may adversely affect an infant's sleep and gross motor development. Additionally, maternal alcohol consumption may slightly reduce the mother's milk production.
- **Anxiety about the process of breastfeeding:** While breastfeeding is a normal biological function, the process of breastfeeding may be uncomfortable and anxiety-provoking for some mothers. The release of milk, or letdown, is affected by anxiety, while milk production is not, since different hormones control both processes.
- **Communicable diseases, such as hepatitis, HIV or tuberculosis:** Communicable diseases can pass from one human to another through direct contact and fluids, such as breast milk.
- **Drug use:** Like alcohol, drugs may pass from a mother to an infant through breast milk. Some drugs may be safe, but their safety should be determined by a health care provider. Other drugs, such as nicotine, may have both short- and long-term effects. Caffeine is excreted into breast milk in small amounts and metabolized slowly by nursing infants. Adverse effects in nursing infants are unlikely; however, irritability and poor sleep patterns have been reported.
- **Embarrassment:** Developed societies tend to be more guarded about breastfeeding than in some emergent societies where breastfeeding is common. Embarrassment, anxiety and emotional stress may all interfere with successful breastfeeding.
- **Emotional stress:** Teenage pregnancy, multiple births, complicated delivery and a host of other circumstances may increase the emotional stress of a mother and her ability to relax and enjoy the breastfeeding process. Helping a mother to initiate or continue to breastfeed may relieve stress and improve milk release (letdown).
- **Fatigue:** Postdelivery fatigue is common. Inadequate rest of a mother during the first six weeks postpartum may interfere with her ability to successfully breastfeed.

- **Infections and exposure:** Mothers who are hepatitis B–positive, infected with hepatitis C virus, and have been exposed to high levels of environmental chemical agents should avoid breastfeeding.
- **Lack of knowledge about the advantages or the process of breastfeeding:** Breastfeeding may not be advocated in certain families or societies, and it may be viewed with skepticism. International organizations help to promote breastfeeding worldwide and develop strategies to increase the number of women who exclusively breastfeed.
- **Nicotine use:** Like alcohol and drugs, nicotine passes through breast milk. Nicotine is a pharmacological stimulant that may affect the developing brain. Nicotine has been shown to cause long-term behavioral and learning deficits in infants and children. Infants are also exposed to nicotine through secondhand smoke.
- **Pain:** Pain is often cited as a common cause for abandoning breastfeeding. If a nursing mother's milk supply is perceived as low milk, then the act of breastfeeding might be painful.
- **Postpartum depression:** Anxiety, irritation, restlessness and/or tearfulness are common in some mothers for a few weeks after delivery. If severe, breastfeeding may be compromised.
- **Work policies that do not support breastfeeding:** Worksite child care, time to breastfeed in private spaces, and refrigeration of breast milk accommodate nursing mothers. Other conditions may not support breastfeeding [13].

Infant Formula: A Nutritious Option to Breast Milk

Infant formula is an alternative to human breast milk for early nourishment. It is designed to closely resemble human breast milk. If a woman decides not to breastfeed or cannot breastfeed, then she must use some form of infant formula rather than cow's milk for the first year of an infant's life. This is because dairy milk is deficient in iron, vitamin B12 and vitamin C, and it contains too much protein and sodium for an infant to handle.

An infant's digestive system is still maturing after birth, and it does not have the ability to digest an excessive amount of milk protein. Since dairy milk is deficient in iron, it may increase an infant's risk of iron-deficiency anemia. Also, since dairy milk is high in sodium, it may disturb the normal balance of fluid in an infant.

Dairy milk can be introduced after an infant's first birthday, except in allergic families, where it may not be introduced until the second year of age. A health care provider should be consulted for the exact timing.

In most cases, infant formula provides a wide array of the nutrients that an infant needs for the first four to six months. Some vitamins and minerals are of critical importance and may need to be supplemented. These include iron, vitamins D and B12, and fluoride.

Iron is essential for hemoglobin and myoglobin formation and for the use of energy. An infant's iron stores are usually low. Iron-deficiency anemia in infants is associated with long-term reduced behavioral, mental and motor functioning. Efforts to prevent iron deficiency include the complete avoidance of dairy milk under the age of one year, iron supplementation at four to six months of age in breastfed infants, and the use of iron-fortified formula when not breastfeeding [14].

Vitamin D is recommended as a supplement for breastfed babies and babies who drink less than 32 ounces of formula per day. This is because vitamin D is an essential vitamin for bone and teeth formation, and breast milk is low in vitamin D. A minimum daily intake of 400 IU of vitamin D is recommended beginning soon after birth until this amount of vitamin D is consumed through the diet.

If a woman who breastfeeds is vegetarian, then her infant may require a **vitamin B12** supplement. A health care provider should first be consulted before vitamins D and B12 supplementation [15].

Fluoride is another mineral of concern for an infant's developing teeth. Supplemental fluoride may be needed by an infant after 6 months of age, depending on the fluoridation of local water. It was once thought that fluoride supplementation caused *mottling*, or spotted tooth enamel, in developing teeth, but this is only the case if fluoride supplementation is excessive. It is best to seek the advice of a health care provider before any fluoride supplements are given.

TABLE 11-3 Comparison of the Average Nutrients in 1 Ounce of Breast Milk, Cow's Milk and Soy-Based Formula

Contents/Nutrients	Breast Milk	Cow's Milk	Soy-Based Formula
Calories	20	17	20
Carbohydrates (grams)	2	1	2
Protein (grams)	0.3	1	1
Total fat (grams)	1	1	1
Saturated fat (milligrams)	4	3	0
Cholesterol (milligrams)	5	11	7
Iron (milligrams)		0.01	0.36
Calcium (milligrams)		31.6	20.7

Source: [16].

An often criticized disadvantage of infant formula is that it is uniform in consistency and provides less satisfaction than breast milk. Also, the mother or care provider determines when the infant has "had enough," rather than the suckling infant who pulls away from its mother's breast once it is satisfied.

Nutrients in Infant Formula Compared to Human Breast Milk

Human breast milk contains about 20 calories per 1 ounce. In comparison, some varieties of soy protein-based infant formula also contain about 20 calories per ounce, and whole cow's milk contains about 17 calories per ounce—the difference is mostly in fat calories. Table 11-3 shows a comparison of other nutrients in human breast milk, whole cow's milk and infant soy formula. As shown, they are very close in nutrients.

Between the ages of 1 month and 6 months, infants that are exclusively breastfed consume an average of 19 to 30 ounces of breast milk daily. At this rate, they consume about 427.5 to 675 calories daily.

Formula-fed infants consume about 2½ ounces of formula daily for every pound of body weight. An average 3-month-old infant who weighs 13 pounds should consume about 32½ ounces of infant formula daily (13 pounds × 2.5 ounces = 32.5 ounces), or about 650 calories (32.5 ounces × 20 calories/ounce = 650 calories), which is similar to a breastfed infant's caloric intake.

Most formula-fed infants are satisfied with about 3 to 4 ounces of formula per feeding during the early months of life. Breastfed babies may be satisfied with about 3 ounces of breast milk per feeding, provided eight times throughout the day, but this amount may vary greatly.

INTRODUCING SOLID FOODS TO INFANTS

It cannot be stressed enough that infant formula and human breast milk provide all of the nourishment that an infant requires for the first 4 to 6 months of its life. Feeding any type of solid food before this age is not warranted, including the practice of mixing infant cereal with breast milk or infant formula. After 4 to 6 months, solid foods can be gradually introduced. Introducing solid foods any sooner may cause allergies, digestive problems and childhood obesity, among other issues.

Before 4 months of age, an infant tends to push its tongue against a spoon or food inside its mouth instead of pushing the contents backward and swallowing. Most babies stop thrusting their tongue and start using their tongue to swallow when they are physically ready.

An infant's energy needs begin to increase around 4 to 6 months; however, some digestive organs are still developing, such as the gastrointestinal tract and kidneys. This is why the level of protein and starch in some solid foods may be too high for an infant's immature gastrointestinal system to process.

Single-grain, iron-fortified cereals, such as rice, barley or oats, are usually introduced first for this reason. An infant's body stores of iron tend to deplete once her birth weight doubles. Early introduction of iron-fortified infant cereals such as these and later introduction of softened meats or meat substitutes helps supply needed iron for an infant.

Contrary to past recommendations, there is no medical evidence that supports the introduction of solid foods in a particular order. A suggested order of introducing solid foods is one at a time: iron-fortified infant cereals, soft vegetables, fruits and protein foods (especially with iron and zinc). Once an infant learns to eat and tolerate one food, another food can gradually be offered. Generally meats and vegetables contain more nutrients per serving than fruits, vegetables or cereals, unless they are enriched or fortified.

A good source of vitamin C like vitamin C–fortified fruit juice may be introduced at about 6 months of age in an infant cup (to distinguish it from breast milk or formula) and to help prevent dental caries in budding teeth. Only 4 to 6 ounces (about ½ to ⅔ cup) of fortified juices per day are recommended. More may add extra calories.

Some pediatricians are cautionary about highly allergic foods, such as eggs and fish, during the first year of life. However, there is no evidence that introducing these foods after 4 to 6 months of age predisposes childhood allergies. If there is a family history of food allergies, then it is best to be quite precautionary.

A strategy is to give an allergy-prone infant one new food at a time and wait at least two to three days before introducing another new food. (Allergy-prone infants may have a strong genetic predisposition to food allergies.) After the introduction of each new food, observe the infant closely for any allergic reactions, such as breathing problems, diarrhea, rash or vomiting. Immediately contact a health care provider if any symptoms develop.

After one year of age, an allergy-free infant should be consuming a wide variety of foods, including breast milk, infant formula or whole dairy milk; meats (including beef, eggs, fish and poultry) or meat substitutes (including soy products and cooked legumes); fortified cereals and whole grains; vegetables; fruits; and healthy fats and oils. Allergic children should be following diets prescribed by registered dietitians and other health professionals that eliminate allergens and are balanced in other foods and nutrients [17].

FEEDING THE ALLERGIC INFANT OR CHILD

The American Academy of Pediatrics (AAP) and the American College of Asthma, Allergy & Immunology (ACAAI) have established guidelines to help prevent or delay food allergies in high-risk children. These guidelines state that the timing of introducing foods with common allergens (such as dairy products, eggs or nuts) is no longer thought to affect a child's probability of developing food allergies later in life. There is no proven way to prevent food allergies, but these guidelines are believed to be good practices for reducing the risk of developing food allergies, especially in high-risk families.

The ACAAI recommends that *all foods*, even those with a low probability of causing allergies (such as some fruits, grains and vegetables), should be introduced *one at a time* and in their cooked form (some are less allergenic when cooked). They should not be combined until the individual ingredients are well tolerated. Mixed commercial infant foods may include potentially allergic ingredients, so label reading is crucial [18–20].

NUTRITIONAL NEEDS DURING THE FIRST TWO YEARS OF LIFE

As previously stated, the amount of breast milk or infant formula that a 1- to 2-year-old should consume is about 32 ounces daily. Any more breast milk or infant formula at this age may discourage the consumption of solid foods with their essential nutrients.

Besides breast milk and infant formula, infants need water as a beverage. Most of an infant's body weight is water. Because an infant's kidneys are not fully functional, water loss is easy. Conditions such as diarrhea or vomiting may cause dehydration, electrolyte loss, fever or even death.

An array of commercial or homemade infant foods with a broad spectrum of nutrients should ensure a healthy diet and a thriving infant. The exceptions are iron and vitamin C. This is why many commercial infant foods are fortified with either one or both of these nutrients. Infant foods should have little to no added fat, sodium and sugars to help control these substances in an infant's diet. The following are some simple guidelines for infant food preparation and feeding:

Do:

- Hold or prop an infant in an upright position for easy swallowing and to prevent choking.
- Match food with physical readiness. An infant's ability to swallow food varies between 4 to 6 months. An infant may gag or choke even on pureed foods if they are introduced any sooner. Place an infant spoon-sized serving on the tip of an infant's tongue and let it naturally slide back into the oral cavity (entire mouth) to determine if the infant is ready to eat. An infant's *gag reflex* should be desensitized by proceeding slowly in this manner. The *extrusion reflex* causes an infant to thrust its tongue forward and extrude or force food out of its mouth. Mostly an infant is investigating the new food. Sometimes an infant has had enough to eat, and it uses this reflex to signal this to the care provider.
- Note an infant's physical developments in self-feeding, such as the palmer grasp and the pincer grasp. In the *palmer grasp*, food is palmed by an infant and moved into the mouth, and in the *pincer grasp*, an infant's thumb and forefinger pinch little pieces of food that are then brought to its mouth. Both grasps promote manual dexterity, jaw muscle development and control.
- Moisten foods with a little infant formula or expressed breast milk.
- Offer just a few mouthfuls of food at one time. This is all that is required across the food groups to satisfy most of an infant's early nutritional needs. (See "Healthy diet and meal planning for infants".) If food is spit out of an infant's mouth, this may indicates that the infant is satiated, it is too much food in the infant's mouth, and/or the infant is no longer interested. Try again with the same food during the next meal.
- Take food texture into consideration, and match the textures of foods with the infant's developmental abilities, especially teeth to tear and grind.
- Use infant-sized cups, eating utensils and plates.

Do not do or use:

- Anything other than infant formula in baby bottles, which may discourage self-feeding skills, contribute to overfeeding and/or cause choking.
- Candy, gelatin and soft drinks, which may contain too much sugar and too few nutrients.
- Canned fruits with added sugars.
- Canned vegetables with added sodium.
- Excessive fruit juices, especially apple or pear. They may contain too much sugar in the form of fructose and sorbitol, a sugar alcohol that can lead to diarrhea.
- Goat's milk, which is low in folate, iron, and vitamins C and D.
- Honey, which may contain *Clostridium botulinum* spores with a potentially fatal toxin.
- Foods that are bite-sized, such as carrots, cut-up hot dogs, grapes, hard candies, nuts, olives, popcorn, or raisins, to help prevent choking.
- Sticky foods, such as jam or peanut butter, to help prevent choking.
- Unpasteurized (raw) dairy milk, which may contain bacteria or viruses.
- Unfortified vegetable and nut "milks," such as soy or almond.

NORMAL INFANT GROWTH AND DEVELOPMENT

Health care providers typically measure an infant's height, weight and head circumference to determine normal infant growth. Then these figures are compared to percentiles that rank an infant's growth compared to the average infant population. They are also used as standards for future measurements. An infant's head is measured because this measurement indicates brain growth, which should be rapid during the first 18 months of an infant's life. Typical infant percentile growth charts can be found at the National Center for Health Statistics at http://www.cdc.gov/growthcharts/.

INFANT DIET AND HEALTH CONSIDERATIONS AND CONCERNS

A number of nutrition-related reasons help to explain why some infants fail to thrive. These include diabetes, gluten intolerance, iron-deficiency anemia and/or lactose intolerance. Other diet and health concerns and considerations of infants include dental caries, obesity, weaning and dairy whole milk/dairy milk choices.

- *Diabetes:* If diabetes runs in a family, a woman develops gestational diabetes during her pregnancy, or if an infant is over 9 pounds at birth, then an infant may have an increased risk of developing diabetes.
- Care providers should be aware of the following signs of diabetes in infants: constant hunger and/or thirst, diaper rash that does not quickly disappear or keeps recurring, excessive wet diapers, irritability or fussiness that is not related to colic, and more sleep than usual. Medical attention should be immediately sought.
- *Gluten intolerance:* Like diabetes, gluten intolerance (celiac disease) tends to run in families. Celiac disease may develop in infants shortly after cereals are introduced. If the cereal contains gluten, an infant might have diarrhea, stomach pains or stop gaining weight at a normal rate. Skin rashes might also appear around the buttocks, elbows and knees, among other places. Over time, an infant might develop anemia, irritability or mouth sores.
- *Iron deficiency:* The most typical signs of anemia in infants are brittle nails, loss of appetite, irritability, pale skin, rapid heartbeat, tiredness and a sore or swollen tongue. It is common for an anemic infant not to have any symptoms at all. Look for anemia in:
  - premature and low-birth-weight infants, 2 months of age or older, whose iron stores may be nearly depleted.
  - full-term, formula-fed infants who are not fed iron-fortified formula.
  - breastfed infants who are not fed iron-fortified foods after 4 to 6 months of age.
  - infants who are fed cow's milk before 1 year of age. Cow's milk is low in iron; it interferes with the body's absorption of iron, replaces iron-rich foods in the diet, irritates the intestinal lining, and can cause slow blood loss.
- *Lactose intolerance:* Lactose intolerance is not common in infants, although they may have a milk allergy, which is different from a sensitivity to the milk sugar lactose. Chronic colic, crying, eczema, ear infections, gas, loose stools and reflux (vomiting) may indicate a milk allergy. The milk enzyme lactase reaches its maximum level in the small intestine soon after birth, and then declines after about 3½ years of age. Symptoms of inadequate lactase may not show up until much later.

492

Other Diet and Health Considerations

While these diet and health considerations may not become significant enough to cause failure to thrive, they may still be problematic on their own.

- *Dental caries:* Emerging teeth may suffer from constant exposure to baby bottles that are filled with infant formula, fruit juice or other sugary beverages. Infants should not be put to bed with a bottle; rather, the bottle should be removed soon after the infant falls asleep. Sugar bathes the gums and promotes a medium for oral bacteria. These bacteria produce an acid that dissolves tooth enamel on erupting teeth. Water does not produce **baby bottle caries (cavities)** like sugar, so between infant formula feedings, water should be the beverage of choice.
- *Obesity:* It stands to reason that infants should become thinner as their activity level increases. Most infants who follow their growth curve double their birth weight in about 5 to 6 months. If an infant gains more weight, then the infant's eating patterns should be assessed. Putting an infant "on a diet" or limiting its intake of breast milk or infant formula is not recommended. Examining the components and amounts of an infant's diet is advised.

As the infant transitions from toddlerhood to childhood, the average daily intake of breast milk or infant formula should still be 32 ounces daily. Once fruit juice is introduced into an infant's diet, it should be limited to only 4 to 6 ounces of 100 percent pure fruit juice. Fruit drinks and soda should be avoided.

If an infant doubles its birth weight at 3 to 4 months, is fed infant cereal and/or juice earlier than 4 months, or is given more than 32 to 40 ounces of breast milk or formula daily, and the infant still seems hungry and/or inconsolable, a health care provider should be consulted.

- *Weaning:* When an infant makes the transition from breast milk to other sources of nourishment, this is called **weaning**. There is no specific time to wean. It is usually a decision between the mother and the child. Weaning may be easier if an infant has consumed milk from another source, supplementary infant formula or a water bottle.

- After an infant's first birthday may be a good time to wean, since infants of this age are adaptable to change and are consuming more solid foods, so they may naturally lose their interest in nursing. If an infant seems very distractible when it is nursing, and it takes an excessive amount of time to nurse, these behaviors could indicate a readiness to wean.
- *Dairy whole milk/dairy milk choices:* An infant without a food allergy can begin to drink cow's milk once he or she is 1 year old. The AAP recommends that children over the age of 1 year consume dairy whole milk until they are 2 years old. This is because children under 2 years of age need the calories from fat for growth and brain and nerve development.

If a child has a milk allergy, he or she can use a fortified soy beverage that approximates the composition of dairy whole milk, as shown in Table 11-3. In this example, the formula contains slightly more carbohydrates and iron than whole cow's milk and less protein and calcium, without any cholesterol. These differences should be discussed with a health care provider.

HEALTHY DIET AND MEAL PLANNING FOR INFANTS

By the time an infant is about 1 year of age, he should be consuming the amounts of foods and beverages daily that are shown in Table 11-4. Exact amounts are dependent on an infant's body weight and height, growth and activity level. A general guideline for adequate portion sizes is about 1 tablespoon of food from each food group for each year of age.

A sample meal plan for infants at least 1 year of age that is based upon these daily servings of foods and beverages is shown in Table 11-5.

493

TABLE 11-4 Daily Servings of Foods and Beverages for Infants at Least 1 Year of Age

Food Groups	Daily Servings	Serving Sizes	Typical Servings
Dairy milk and milk products or substitutes	16 to 20 ounces of whole milk or fortified soy milk	2 to 4 ounces	¼ cup of yogurt = 2 ounces of milk ½ to ¾ ounce of cheese = 4 ounces of milk
Fruits and nonstarchy vegetables	5 or more servings daily	1 tablespoon pureed, mashed or cubed fruits or vegetables	1 tablespoon no-sugar-added applesauce 1 tablespoon cooked spinach
Breads, cereals, grains or starchy vegetables	3 to 4 servings daily	¼ cup of cooked or dry cereal, cooked pasta or rice, or starchy vegetables (such as potatoes or winter squash); ½ tortilla or slice of bread 2 to 3 crackers	¼ cup cooked oatmeal ½ slice gluten-free bread (for allergic infants)
Protein: eggs, fish, legumes, poultry or meats	2 servings daily	½ cooked egg 1 ounce of fish, lean beef, poultry or pork 1 tablespoon of peanut butter 2 to 3 tablespoons of cooked pureed or mashed legumes	½ scrambled large egg 2 tablespoons pureed vegetarian baked beans

TABLE 11-5 Sample Meal Plan for Infants at Least 1 Year of Age

Meals	Food Groups
Breakfast	
¼ cup iron-fortified oat cereal 1 tablespoon mashed bananas 4 ounces dairy whole milk or substitute	1 serving breads, cereals, grains or starchy vegetables 1 serving fruits and nonstarchy vegetables 4 ounces dairy milk or milk products and substitutes

(Continued)

TABLE 11-5 (Continued)	
Meals	**Food Groups**
Morning Snack	
2 graham crackers	1 serving breads, cereals, grains or starchy vegetables
4 ounces dairy whole milk or substitute	4 ounces dairy milk or milk products and substitutes
Lunch	
1 ounce chopped cooked chicken breast	1 serving protein
¼ cup cooked macaroni noodles	1 serving breads, cereals, grains or starchy vegetables
1 tablespoon cooked pureed broccoli	1 serving fruits and nonstarchy vegetables
4 ounces dairy whole milk or substitute	4 ounces dairy milk or milk products and substitutes
Afternoon Snack	
4 ounces plain whole milk yogurt	4 ounces dairy milk or milk products and substitutes
1 tablespoon mashed skinless pears	1 serving fruits and nonstarchy vegetables
Dinner	
1 ounce well-cooked ground beef	1 serving protein
¼ cooked mashed potato	1 serving breads, cereals, grains or starchy vegetables
1 tablespoon cooked pureed carrots	1 serving fruits and nonstarchy vegetables
1 tablespoon mashed skinless peaches	1 serving fruits and nonstarchy vegetables
4 ounces dairy whole milk or equivalent	4 ounces dairy milk or milk products and substitutes
Totals	
Dairy milk or milk products and substitutes: 20 ounces	
Fruits and nonstarchy vegetables: 5 servings	
Breads, cereals, grains or starchy vegetables: 4 servings	
Protein (eggs, fish, legumes, poultry or meats): 2 servings	

Source: [21–23].

Bite on This: preparing homemade infant foods

Commercial or homemade infant food can be introduced into the diet of a 4- to 6-month-old infant as recommended by a health care provider. Homemade infant food may help cut food costs, provide an infant with nutritious foods, and help an infant become accustomed to family foods.

A blender, food grinder or food mill, plastic-type ice cube trays, freezer-proof bags or containers, potato masher, sieve or strainer, and a spoon and fork are simple and useful equipment for making homemade infant foods.

- Blenders are useful for larger batches of food that can be poured into plastic ice cube trays. Immersion blenders are particularly useful for smaller quantities.
- A small-sized baby food mill can be used for cooked and soft-fleshed fruits and vegetables. Larger food grinders and mills are handy for soft meats.
- Plastic-type ice cube trays are practical for freezing pureed foods. After the food is frozen, the cubes can be removed and stored in freezer-proof bags or containers.
- Potato mashers, forks, and spoons can be used to mash soft and peeled foods, such as bananas, canned fruits, cooked egg yolks and potatoes.
- A sieve or strainer should have a small mesh. Soft fruits and vegetables can be pressed through the mesh with the back of a spoon. Meats should not be sieved or strained this way, since hard pieces may pass through the mesh.

Fresh fruits and vegetables should be cooked without added fat, salt or sugar before pureeing. Canned or fresh-frozen fruits and vegetables without added fat, salt or sugar may also be used or blended with fresh fruits and vegetables. The purees should be liquid-like and smooth in texture. Some foods, such as ripe bananas or pears, do not need precooking. They can be peeled or skinned and mashed with the tines of a fork. It may be necessary to add some fluid (breast milk, cooking water, infant formula or water) to create the right consistency.

Peeled or skinned apples, bananas, peaches, pears, plums and dried prunes are generally well favored by infants. Acceptable vegetables include acorn and butternut squash, asparagus, carrots, green and wax beans, green peas and sweet and white potatoes. When an infant is 8 to 11 months of age, **table food** (age-appropriate food that has not been pureed) may be added to its diet. At this age, infants will likely be able to move their tongue from side to side, gum or chew food with their budding teeth, feed themselves with their fingers, spoon-feed themselves with some help, and/or drink from a cup with help. If an infant is not at this developmental point, then this situation should be discussed with a health care provider *before* table food is added.

Mashed or diced softened fruit; finely chopped and soft-cooked or mashed vegetables; mashed, cooked egg yolk; strained fish, meats or poultry; mashed, cooked and strained dry beans, lentils and peas; cottage cheese or soft cheese slices; and soft breads may be enjoyed independently by the time an infant is 1 year old.

High-nitrate vegetables such as beets, broccoli, cabbage, carrots, celery, collard greens, lettuce, spinach and turnips should not be fed to infants of this age in large quantities. The nitrates can change into nitrites, which may bind iron in an infant's blood and interfere with its oxygen-carrying ability. This may prevent oxygen from reaching the cells, make it difficult for an infant to breathe, and cause its skin to turn blue in color.

The following are some general guidelines for preparing homemade infant foods. Precautionary safety and health measures are noted.

- Follow immaculate personal and food sanitation practices, since infants have immature immune systems.
- *Thoroughly wash* any fresh fruits or vegetables to remove any dirt and chemicals.
- Prepare fresh fruits and vegetables by *scrubbing, peeling, paring and removing seeds or pits.*

CAUTION: *Remove all bones, connective tissue, fat, gristle and skin from fish, meats and poultry to prevent choking.*

495

- Separate infant portions of family meals before adding any additional fat, salt or sugar.
- Cook fruits and vegetables in a small saucepan with little water; cover and steam until tender. The texture should be mushy to liquid-like for an infant that has just started eating solid foods or a texture that can be easily pierced with a fork if an infant has been eating solid foods for a few months.
- Puree foods with a clean blender, food processor, infant food grinder, or mill, or mash well with the back of a fork or spoon.

CAUTION: *Grind tough foods and remove any hard pieces.*

- Rub a small amount of food between your fingers to test for *smoothness*; add a little breast milk, fruit juice, infant formula or water for desired consistency.
- Cut food into *small pieces or thin slices*.

CAUTION: *While infants have very tiny mouths with very few teeth, do not cut food too small because it can lodge inside an infant's esophagus.*

- Remove portions of pureed or cut-up foods and *serve immediately. Refrigerate or freeze* remaining foods in refrigerator or freezer-safe containers.
- To freeze, pour cooled, pureed foods into *clean* plastic-type ice cube trays or miniature muffin tins; then *wrap tightly* in *freezer-safe food wrap* and place in the freezer.
- Once frozen, remove food cubes from trays *with clean, washed hands or utensils*; place in *freezer bags or freezer-proof containers* and return to the freezer.
- Infant foods that are *well wrapped for freezing* will probably retain their quality about one month.

CAUTION: *Freeze infant foods in the coldest part of a stocked freezer that maintains consistent temperature.*

- Frozen, homemade infant foods can be thawed in the refrigerator or in a microwave oven on the defrost setting.

CAUTION: *Infant foods that have been thawed should never be reheated.*

- Reheat frozen food cubes in a *heat-resistant container* that is placed in a saucepan of hot water. *Slowly warm over low heat and stir often.* Frozen food cubes can also be reheated in a microwave oven.

CAUTION: *The center of food that is reheated or cooked in a microwave oven may be hotter than the exterior. A microwave oven heats food unevenly and may cause hot spots that are deceiving in consistency.*

- To reheat in a microwave oven, place frozen food cubes in a *microwave-safe dish and heat only a few seconds. Stir food well*; let stand about one minute. *Test the temperature*; it should be about room temperature throughout.

CAUTION: *Each type of frozen food cubes will vary in the time and temperature it takes for reheating in a microwave oven. Pureed meats should not be reheated in the microwave oven.*

CHILDHOOD

Growing Up: Toddler and Childhood Nutrition

The rapid growth and development that an infant undergoes during their first year of life slows down during early and middle childhood. What this means to nutrition and culinary specialists is that children need less food after their first year of life, and especially after two years of age. Children should grow at a rate of 2 to 3 inches and gain about 5 pounds annually between the ages of 1 year and adolescence. Most importantly, a child should follow his or her individual growth curve.

Normal Toddler and Child Growth and Development

Between ages 1 and 2, toddlers may gain between 3 and 5 pounds. An average 15-month-old girl may weigh about 22 pounds and be about 31 inches in height. Boys average about a pound heavier than girls and the same height at 15 months of age.

By age 2, both girls and boys stand about 34 inches tall and weigh, on average, about 27 to 28 pounds. Head size (also a measure of growth) increases by about 1 inch in circumference from year one.

During the third year of life, children gain about 4 pounds and grow about 2 to 3 inches. Children 4 to 5 years of age typically gain about 4 pounds and grow about 2 inches, which indicates that growth slows down.

Childhood Obesity

If too much weight is gained compared to height, then a health care provider should be consulted. Childhood obesity is an increasing public health concern. Childhood obesity has tripled over the last 30 years due to "caloric imbalance"—too many calories consumed versus too few calories expended—as well as several behavioral, environmental and genetic factors.

Short term, obese children are at greater risk of developing such conditions as bone and joint problems and sleep apnea, in addition to poor self-esteem and the shame of feeling different from other children. Children who become obese by age 2 are more likely to be obese adults.

Long term, obese children may mature earlier than normal-weight children and develop adult health problems that may result from the complications of obesity. These include osteoarthritis, cardiovascular (heart and vessels) and cerebral vascular (brain and vessels) disease, different types of cancers, and Type II diabetes. Consuming the right types and amounts of foods and beverages, engaging in regular physical activity, and participating in other health-promoting lifestyle habits may help to lower the risk of childhood obesity.

In 2010, Michelle Obama announced an ambitious national goal to solve the challenge of childhood obesity. To help meet this goal Mrs. Obama unveiled a nationwide campaign called *Let's Move. Let's Move* is a comprehensive, collaborative, and community-coordinated effort to reduce US childhood obesity. It encompasses effective strategies that utilize both public and private-sector resources to impact children's wellness. It fosters collaboration among leaders in athletics, business, community, education, government, medicine and science. It provides communities, families, and schools with practical and doable tools to help children eat better, be more active and become healthier.

The Obama administration and public and private efforts are designed to help reach the First Lady's national goal of solving childhood obesity, including the following [24–28]:

1. Help parents make healthy family choices.
2. Provide parents with a prescription for healthier living.
3. Serve healthier food in school.
4. Step up school leadership.
5. Access healthy, affordable food.
6. Increase physical activity.
7. Partner for a healthier America.

NUTRITIONAL NEEDS OF TODDLERS AND CHILDREN

A young child who is learning to walk or "toddle" is considered a *toddler*, the second stage of human development after infancy. This stage occurs at around 1 to 3 years old. Most fine motor skills required for eating and drinking have developed by this time. Toddlers have larger body mass, greater bone density and denser muscle tissues than infants. By the time a child is 2 years old, much of her baby fat has been lost. A diet with a wide variety of foods and beverages that represents all of the food groups is the best assurance for nutrition and health for toddlers of this age range.

Daily Nutrients for Children Ages 1 to 3 Years Old

According to the DRIs, children 1 to 3 years of age require the nutrients that are shown in Table 11-6. Also according to the DRIs, children this age require about 130 grams (1,200 calories) of carbohydrates daily, 19 grams of fiber*, and 13 grams (54 calories) of protein, depending on their BMI and activity level.

Adequate Intakes

A child may not consume the nutrients in Table 11-6 daily through foods and beverages, but she may consume them over a few days. Also, a child's appetite might vary according to its activity level. On very active days, a child may consume more foods and beverages that supply these nutrients, and on inactive days, he may consume much less. Children may also experience *food jags*, which are excessive preferences for only one or a few foods. They may also fear new foods and/or refuse to eat what is served to them.

497

TABLE 11-6 Daily Nutrients Required by Children Ages 1 to 3 Years Old

300 mcg/d vitamin A	700 mg/d calcium
15 mg/d vitamin C	11 mcg/d chromium*
15 mcg/d vitamin D	340 mcg/d copper
6 mg/d vitamin E	0.7 mg/d fluoride*
30 mcg/d vitamin K*	90 mcg/d iodine
0.5 mg/d thiamin	7 mg/d iron
0.5 mg/d riboflavin	80 mg/d magnesium
6 mg/d niacin	1.2 mg/d manganese*
0.5 mg/d vitamin B6	17 mcg/d molybdenum
150 mcg/d folate	460 mg/d phosphorus
0.9 mcg/d vitamin B12	20 mcg/d selenium
2 mg/d pantothenic acid*	3 mg/d zinc
8 mcg/d biotin	1,000 mg/g sodium*
200 mg/d choline	3,000 mg/d potassium*
	1,500 mg/d chloride*

Source: [29].
Note: Adequate Intake levels (AIs) are marked by an asterisk (*).

FOOD BYTE

Though newborns are born with a preference for sweet tastes, they are not born with a preference for bitter, spicy or irritating substances. Preference for spicy foods develops over time in response to environmental and social factors. It may never develop in some children for complex and unidentified biological reasons. **Food preferences** are determined by many factors—mostly by age. Studies that examine the relationship between food preferences among parents and children sometimes neglect this factor and focus more on the parent–child relationship. Children often grow out of food jags as long as patience, persistence and care prevail [30].

Bite on This: feeding the picky eater

Eating habits are established in the first three years of life, and they may last a lifetime. Children may be picky eaters for a variety of reasons, including a heightened sensitivity to smell, taste and texture; an imitation of parent's selective eating habits; or a power struggle between a child and parents or care providers.

Parents and care providers are responsible for creating and serving healthy foods and beverages at appropriate times throughout the day. Children are responsible for selecting these foods and beverages in the amounts that satisfy their hunger. If vegetables, whole grains, lean proteins, dairy products and healthy fats are served, then children have wholesome choices from which to make their selections. If highly processed foods and sugar-laden foods and beverages are regularly served, then healthy foods may be rejected.

The family menu should not be limited to a child's favorite foods. Nor should a separate meal be prepared for each family member. This sets up incorrect expectations for a child and its family. If a child refuses to eat, he or she should still be expected to participate in the family meal. Distractions should be limited, including television.

Hungry children are not patient. Two-year-olds may stay at the table only 10 minutes, while 4-year-olds may be ready to leave the table after 20 minutes. Children generally eat better when an adult joins them. Be patient with slower eaters who play with their food or dawdle due to lack of hunger.

If a child refuses a family meal, he might be snacking too close to dinnertime. Limit the size of snacks and beverages about one to two hours before dinner. Too many calories from fruit juice, milk or soda may cause fullness and an inability to eat. The quantity of these beverages should be limited, except for milk or milk substitutes—no more than about 24 ounces daily. After age 1, milk should be considered more of a beverage than an infant "food" like breast milk or infant formula supplied during the first year of life.

A set schedule of breakfast, midmorning snack, lunch, afternoon snack, dinner and bedtime snack where warranted may help to regulate a child's hunger and appetite. If a child skips a meal or a snack, she can wait until the next meal or snack and not eat or drink impulsively.

When a new food is served to a child, it should be accompanied by a familiar and well-liked food. Encourage a child to taste a new food, but do not anticipate that a child will accept it. Two-year-olds are particularly apprehensive. Be patient about a child's food idiosyncrasies. Children often develop food fads that typically pass over time.

Serve "finger foods" rather than mixed dishes, such as casseroles or stews, because some children may be suspicious of what they do not recognize. A child may react differently to the same food that is served in different ways, such as plain, steamed broccoli, and broccoli au gratin. Respectfully remind a child about the last time he ate and enjoyed broccoli, and he may agree to try it again.

Arrange food attractively on small plates, and keep the portions small. Allow a child to ask for a second portion only after he has finished the first serving. If a child is forced to eat more than he would like, it may interfere with his ability to determine when he is full, which may lead to overweight or obesity.

Do not offer dessert as a reward or incentive for eating a new food. Moreover, dessert does not need to be offered with every meal or every day. If a child refuses to eat a meal, withholding dessert is not the solution. A child may then place a higher value on dessert than other foods. This yearning for sweets may continue to plague the child as it grows. Fresh fruit, lower-fat dairy confections, pudding and/or flavored or fruited yogurt can provide a sweet finale to a meal without excessive sugar.

Recipe: Grilled Fruit Skewers with Tropical Yogurt Sauce

*This recipe for **Grilled Fruit Skewers with Tropical Yogurt Sauce** in the **Recipe file** which is located within the Culinary Nutrition website at www.culinarynutrition.elsevier.com, capitalizes on the flavor and nutrients in fresh fruit and tangy yogurt. Grilling fruit caramelizes the sugars so they are dark, deep and toasty in flavor. The mixed fruit sugars balance with the tanginess of the yogurt sauce for a unified finish. Children like finger food such as these fruit chunks, and they can dip them into the flavorful yogurt sauce. Make sure to carefully remove the skewers before serving.*

HEALTHY DIET AND MEAL PLANNING FOR TODDLERS AND CHILDREN

> **Morsel** "As a child my family's menu consisted of two choices: take it or leave it." —Buddy Hackett (American actor and comedian, 1924–2003)

The portion sizes that are detailed in Chapter 1 are designed mainly for adults, Different portion sizes should be used for toddlers and children. A useful rule of thumb is to provide about one-quarter of an adult portion per year of age, depending on the food or beverage. For example, a 2-year-old should be offered about half of a hamburger (¼ of 1 hamburger × 2 years of age = ½ of 1 hamburger), with about 2 tablespoons of chopped cooked green beans (¼ of ½ cup [8 tablespoons] of cooked green beans = about 2 tablespoons of cooked green beans).

Emphasis should be placed on nutrient-dense foods, such as lower-fat dairy products (or dairy substitutes for allergic children); lean meats (or meat substitutes for vegetarians); enriched and fortified breads, cereals and grains (with one-half of them whole grains); fresh fruits and vegetables; and healthy fats

Fats should emphasize nut, olive and seed oils, and the essential fatty acids from fish (with a limitation on high-mercury fish like bluefin tuna, barramundi, ray, roughy, shark and swordfish). Once these nutritionally dense foods fill a child's diet, then extra calories may be added with moderation. Withholding calories or sugary foods may lead to food fights, food jags and/or negative feelings about food and the eating experience. It is important for the care provider to have a positive attitude about food, embrace the concept that all food fits in a healthy diet, and that there is room for "fun foods" as long as the basic diet is sound.

Daily Servings of Foods and Beverages and a Sample Meal Plan for Children 2 to 3 years of Age

Based on the USDA MyPlate recommendations, children 2 to 3 years of age require about *1,000 calories daily*. Daily servings of foods and beverages for children 2 to 3 years of age are shown in Table 11-7.

A sample meal plan for children 2 to 3 years of age that is based upon these daily servings of foods and beverages is shown in Table 11-8.

Recipe: Cream of Tomato-Basil Soup with Grilled Cheese Croutons

*A long-standing child favorite meal is tomato soup with a grilled cheese sandwich. This updated recipe for **Cream of Tomato-Basil Soup with Grilled Cheese Croutons** in the **Recipe file** which is located within the Culinary Nutrition website at www.culinarynutrition.elsevier.com, is a takeoff on this popular combination. Basil has a particular affinity to tomatoes, and child-size grilled cheese croutons are used for garnish and become laden with the antioxidant-rich tomato-based soup. Add just one minisandwich for smaller appetites and more for older children. Use a reduced-fat cheese to keep total fat and calories under control. The finished dish is shown within the centerfold **Photo file** in Plate 11.1.*

499

TABLE 11-7 Daily Servings of Foods and Beverages for Children 2 to 3 Years of Age

Food Groups	Daily Servings
3 ounces or slices of breads, cereals, cooked grains or starchy vegetables with one-half (1½ ounces or slices) from whole grains	In general, 1 slice of bread, 1 cup of ready-to-eat cereal, or ½ cup of cooked cereal, pasta or rice are considered 1 ounce of bread, cereal, cooked grains and starchy vegetable equivalents.
1 cup of vegetables	In general, 1 cup of raw or cooked vegetables, 1 cup of vegetable juice, or 2 cups of raw leafy greens are considered 1 cup of vegetable equivalents.
Weekly recommendations: ½ cup dark green vegetables 2½ cups red and orange vegetables ½ cup cooked beans and peas 2 cups starchy vegetables 1½ cups other vegetables	
1 cup of fruit	In general, 1 cup of fruit or 100% fruit juice or ½ cup of dried fruit are considered 1 cup of fruit equivalents.
2 cups of dairy milk and milk products or substitutes	In general, 1 cup of dairy milk, yogurt or soymilk, 1½ ounces of natural cheese, or 2 ounces of processed cheese are considered 1 cup of dairy milk or milk substitute equivalents.
2 ounces of meat or meat substitutes	In general, 1 ounce of meat, poultry or fish, ¼ cup of cooked beans, 1 egg, 1 tablespoon of peanut butter, or ½ ounce of nuts or seeds are considered 1 ounce of meat or meat substitute equivalents.
3 teaspoons of additional fats or oils	In general, 1 teaspoon of oils (canola, olive, peanut or safflower), butter or margarine are considered 1 teaspoon fat or oil equivalents.

Source: [31].

500

TABLE 11-8 Sample Meal Plan for Children 2 to 3 Years of Age

Breakfast	Morning Snack
½ slice whole-grain wheat toast (½ serving of breads, cereals, grains or starchy vegetables) 1 egg (1 ounce of meat or meat substitutes) 1 teaspoon light butter or margarine (1 serving of fats or oils) ¼ cup banana slices (¼ serving of fruit)	2 graham crackers (½ serving of breads, cereals, grains or starchy vegetables) ¼ cup apple slices (¼ serving of fruit)

Lunch	Afternoon Snack
½ slice whole-grain bread (½ serving of breads, cereals, grains or starchy vegetables) 1 teaspoon reduced-fat mayonnaise (1 serving of fats or oils) 1 ounce turkey breast (1 ounce of meat or meat substitutes) 1 cup dairy reduced-fat milk (1 serving of dairy milk or milk substitutes) ½ cup carrot and sweet bell pepper slices (½ serving of vegetables)	2 whole-grain pretzels (½ serving of breads, cereals, grains or starchy vegetables) ½ cup 100% fruit juice (1 serving of fruit)

Dinner

Stuffed Baked Potato
1 small baked potato (1 serving of breads, cereals, grains or starchy vegetables)
1 teaspoon light butter or margarine (1 serving of fats or oils)
1 cup low-fat yogurt (1 serving of dairy milk or milk substitutes)
½ cup broccoli florets (½ serving of vegetables)

Daily Nutrients for Children Ages 4 to 8 years Old

According to the DRIs, children aged 4 to 8 years require the nutrients that are shown in Table 11-9. Also according to the DRIs, children in this age range require about 130 grams (520 calories) of carbohydrates daily, 25 grams of fiber, and 19 grams (76 calories) of protein, depending on their BMI and activity level.

TABLE 11-9 Daily Nutrients Required by Children 4 to 8 Years of Age	
400 mcg/d vitamin A	1,000 mg/d calcium
25 mg/d vitamin C	15 mcg/d chromium*
15 mcg/d vitamin D	440 mcg/d copper
7 mg/d vitamin E	1 mg/d fluoride*
55 mcg/d vitamin K*	90 mcg/d iodine
0.6 mg/d thiamin	10 mg/d iron
0.6 mg/d riboflavin	130 mg/d magnesium
8 mg/d niacin	1.5 mg/d manganese*
0.6 mg/d vitamin B6	22 mcg/d molybdenum
200 mcg/d folate	500 mg/d phosphorus
1.2 mcg/d vitamin B12	30 mcg/d selenium
3 mg/d pantothenic acid*	5 mg/d zinc
12 mcg/d biotin*	1,200 mg/d sodium*
250 mg/d choline*	3,800 mg/d potassium*
	1,900 mg/d chloride*

Source: [29].
Note: Adequate Intake levels (AIs) are marked by an asterisk (*).

Note that these requirements are higher than those for a child aged 1 to 3 years to account for growth and development.

Daily Servings of Foods and Beverages for Children 4 to 8 years of Age

Based on the USDA MyPlate recommendations, children 4 to 8 years of age require a range of 1,200 calories daily (girls) to 1,400 calories daily (boys). Daily servings of foods and beverages for this age group follow. Refer to Table 11-7 for portion sizes and equivalents.

- 5 ounces of breads, cereals, cooked grains or starchy vegetables with one-half (2½ ounces) whole grains
- 1½ cups of vegetables
- 1 to 1½ cups of fruit
- 2½ cups of dairy milk and milk products or substitutes
- 4 ounces of meat or meat substitutes
- 4 teaspoons of additional fats or oils

A sample meal plan for children 4 to 8 years of age is shown in Table 11-10. It resembles the sample meal plan for children ages 1 to 3 years of age that is shown in Table 11-8, with additional servings for older children.

THE SCHOOL-AGE YEARS: DIET AND HEALTH CONSIDERATIONS AND CONCERNS

From 1 to 5 years of age, children need to follow their individual growth curves for height and weight, as determined by their health care provider. Growth slows down after the age of 5, plus school-age children are more sedentary, so they do not require significantly more calories.

Morsel "The cold truth is that family dinners are more often than not an ordeal of nervous indigestion, preceded by hidden resentment and ennui, and accompanied by psychosomatic jitters." —M.F.K. Fisher (American food writer, 1908–1992)

Children should not be put on diets, but their diet should be rich in nutrient-dense foods instead of calorie-dense foods. If children weigh too much for their height, excessive fats and refined carbohydrates should be limited and activity should be encouraged.

Generally, when a child reaches school age, his or her diet evolves into one that is nutritionally adequate—unless a child was a picky eater and then her idiosyncrasies may remain. Some schools provide breakfast at school. The School Breakfast Program (SBP) provides cash assistance to states to operate nonprofit breakfast programs in schools and residential child care institutions. It is not uncommon for children to skip breakfast, one of the most important meals of the day (see "Take away").

501

TABLE 11-10 Sample Meal Plan for Children 4 to 8 Years of Age

Breakfast	Morning Snack
1 slice whole-grain wheat toast (1 serving of breads, cereals, grains or starchy vegetables) 1 egg (1 ounce of meat or meat substitutes) 1 teaspoon light butter or margarine (1 serving of fats or oils) ½ cup banana slices (½ serving of fruit)	2 graham crackers (½ serving of breads, cereals, grains or starchy vegetables) ½ cup apple slices (½ serving of fruit)
Lunch	**Afternoon Snack**
1 slice whole-grain bread (1 serving of breads, cereals, grains or starchy vegetables) 1 teaspoon reduced-fat mayonnaise (1 serving of fats or oils) 1 ounce turkey breast (1 ounce of meat or meat substitutes) 1 cup dairy reduced-fat milk (1 serving of dairy milk or milk substitutes) ½ cup carrot and sweet bell pepper slices (½ serving of vegetables)	2 whole-grain pretzels (½ serving of breads, cereals, grains or starchy vegetables) ½ cup 100% fruit juice (1 serving of fruit)
Dinner	**After-dinner Snack**
Stuffed Baked Potato 1 small baked potato (1 serving of breads, cereals, grains or starchy vegetables) 1 teaspoon light butter or margarine (1 serving of fats or oils) 1 cup low-fat yogurt (1 serving of dairy milk or milk substitutes) ½ cup broccoli florets (½ serving of vegetables) 2 ounces diced chicken (2 ounces of meat or meat substitutes) **Small Salad** ½ cup lettuce and tomato (½ serving of vegetables) 1 teaspoon vinaigrette-style salad dressing (1 serving of fats and oils)	3 cups popcorn (1 serving of breads, cereals, grains or starchy vegetables) 4 ounces smoothie made with dairy skim milk (½ serving of dairy milk or milk substitutes)

502

TABLE 11-11 Daily Nutrients Required by Children 9 to 13 Years of Age

600 mcg/d vitamin A	1,300 mg/d calcium
45 mg/d vitamin C	21 (girls) and 25 (boys) mcg/d chromium*
15 mcg/d vitamin D	700 mcg/d copper
11 mg/d vitamin E	2 mg/d fluoride
60 mcg/d vitamin K*	120 mcg/d iodine*
0.9 mg/d thiamin	8 mg/d iron
0.9 mg/d riboflavin	240 mg/d magnesium
12 mg/d niacin	1.6 (girls) and 1.9 (boys) mg/d manganese[a]
1.0 mg/d vitamin B6	34 mcg/d molybdenum
300 mcg/d folate	1,250 mg/d phosphorus
1.8 mcg/d vitamin B12	40 mcg/d selenium
4 mg/d pantothenic acid*	8 mg/d zinc
20 mcg/d biotin*	1,500 mg/d sodium*
375 mg/d choline*	4,500 mg/d potassium*
	2,300 mg/d chloride*

Source: [29].
Note: Adequate Intake levels (AIs) are marked by an asterisk (*).

Daily Nutrients for Children Ages 9 to 13 years Old

According to the US DRIs, children 9 to 13 years of age require the nutrients that are shown in Table 11-11. Also according to the DRIs, children in this age range require about 130 grams (520 calories) of carbohydrates daily, 26 grams of fiber for girls and 31 grams of fiber for boys, and 34 grams (136 calories) of protein, depending on their BMI and activity level.

Daily Servings of Foods and Beverages for Children 9 to 13 years of Age

Based on the USDA MyPlate recommendations, children 9 to 13 years of age require a range of 1,400 to 2,200 calories daily for girls, and 1,600 to 2,600 calories daily for boys, depending on growth and activity level. Daily servings of foods and beverages for this age group follow. Refer to Table 11-7 for portion sizes and equivalents.

- 5 ounces of breads, cereals, cooked grains or starchy vegetables for girls, and 6 ounces of breads, cereals, cooked grains or starchy vegetables for boys with one-half (2½ to 3 ounces) whole grains
- 2 cups of vegetables for girls
- 2½ cups of vegetables for boys
- 1½ cups of fruit for girls and boys
- 3 cups of dairy milk and milk products or substitutes for girls and boys
- 5 ounces of meat or meat substitutes for girls and boys
- 5 teaspoons of additional fats or oils for girls and boys

Vitamin and mineral supplements should not be necessary if these daily servings are followed. If any of the food groups are omitted due to allergies, religious reasons or vegetarian or vegan diets, then supplements may be warranted as determined by a health care provider.

A sample meal plan for children 9 to 13 years of age is shown in Table 11-12. It is basically the same meal plan as shown for younger children with additional servings based on age. This demonstrates that most children can consume a similar meal plan with modifications in the numbers of servings.

TABLE 11-12 Sample Meal Plan for Children 9 to 13 Years of Age

503

Breakfast	Morning Snack
1 slice whole-grain wheat toast (1 serving of breads, cereals, grains or starchy vegetables) 1 egg (1 ounce of meat or meat substitutes) 1 teaspoon light butter or margarine (1 serving of fats or oils) ½ cup banana slices (½ serving of fruit)	2 graham crackers (½ serving of breads, cereals, grains or starchy vegetables) ½ cup apple slices (½ serving of fruit)
Lunch	**Afternoon Snack**
1 slice whole-grain bread (1 serving of breads, cereals, grains or starchy vegetables) 1 teaspoon reduced-fat mayonnaise (1 serving of fats or oils) 1 ounce turkey breast (1 ounce of meat or meat substitutes) 1 cup dairy reduced-fat milk (1 serving of dairy milk or milk substitutes) ½ cup carrot and sweet bell pepper slices (½ serving of vegetables)	2 whole-grain pretzels (½ serving of breads, cereals, grains or starchy vegetables) ½ cup 100% fruit juice (1 serving of fruit)
Dinner	**After-Dinner Snack**
Stuffed Baked Potato 1 small baked potato (1 serving of breads, cereals, grains or starchy vegetables) 1 teaspoon light butter or margarine (1 serving of fats or oils) 1 cup low-fat yogurt (1 serving of dairy milk or milk substitutes) ½ cup broccoli florets (½ serving of vegetables) 3 ounces diced chicken (3 ounces of meat or meat substitutes) **Small Salad** 1 to 1½ cups lettuce and tomato (1 to 1½ servings of vegetables) 2 teaspoons vinaigrette-style salad dressing (2 servings of fats and oils)	3 cups popcorn (1 serving of breads, cereals, grains or starchy vegetables) 1 cup smoothie made with dairy skim milk (1 serving of dairy milk or milk substitutes)

Bite on This: healthful snacks for children

As long as the DRI or AI levels are met and a child is active, most foods and beverages can fit into a child's diet. While some snacks with sugar, fat and sodium are criticized for their place in a child's diet, they still may have a place in it.

Snacks have calories that children need for energy, and many contain an array of vitamins and minerals. While critics claim these nutrients are not natural sources, they may be deficient in a child's diet.

Young children have a limited stomach capacity, and some children cannot consume enough foods and beverages to meet their nutritional needs. Healthful, well-planned morning and afternoon snacks can be both filling and fueling.

Snacks should be considered as complements to meals, not meal replacers. In total, snacks should contribute only one-quarter of a child's total daily calorie intake. By offering only two or three healthy snack options, the care provider can set the nutritional standards, while a child can still have both choice and control in his selections. Some healthy snacks follow.

- *Fruits and vegetables:* Fruits should be well scrubbed and served whole or sliced into halves, cubes or wedges. Canned fruit in its own juice, fresh-frozen fruits or dried fruits are other options. The sugars in fruits, particularly dried fruits, adhere to young teeth. It is recommended that a nonsugary liquid be consumed to swish away the sugary residue.

  Aside from whole fruit, healthy fruit options include applesauce, apple slices, frozen bananas or blueberries, dried fruit such as cranberries or raisins, fruit leathers (without added sugar), all-fruit popsicles, and fruit smoothies. Fruits can be served with dips, such as yogurt, peanut or other nut butters or chocolate-hazelnut spread.

  Fresh, raw vegetables can be served on their own or with dips, such as hummus and other bean dips, reduced-fat salad dressing or yogurt. Broccoli, cauliflower, celery, cucumbers, jicama, sweet peppers, sugar snap peas, sweet peppers and others provide a wide range of phytonutrients and are generally well liked. Vegetables in the cruciferous family (broccoli, cauliflower, cabbage) are better accepted with a dip or sauce to temper their bitter taste.

- *Whole grains low in fat and sugar:* Child-friendly healthy whole-grain snacks include breadsticks, cold breakfast cereal, cereal bars, cornbread, crackers, English muffins, flatbreads, gingersnaps, graham crackers, granola, muffins, pita, popcorn, pretzels, rice cakes, tortillas and unsalted tortilla chips. Whole grains are hearty, and they tend to be less rich-tasting than some refined-grain products. When paired with dairy reduced-fat milk or dairy products or pureed legumes such as hummus, whole grains contribute an earthy nuttiness. Consumed with proteins and not on their own, they transform into minimeals.

- *Lean protein:* One or two slices or ounces of lean protein, such as chicken or turkey breast or ham, rolled around crisp vegetables, such as carrots, celery or sweet bell pepper strips, make a handy and fun snack for children. Slices or cubes of reduced-fat cheese also supply good-quality protein, calcium, riboflavin and vitamin D. Reduced-fat dairy products and dairy substitutes, including plant and nuts "milks," pudding and yogurt also supply protein, vitamins and minerals—some more than others.

  For older children who chew well, trail mixes with nuts, whole-grain cereal and dried fruit supply protein, fiber and iron. Have soy products on hand for vegetarian children or those with milk allergies, including bite-sized cubes of tofu, fresh soybeans (edamame), individual boxes of soy milk fortified with calcium and vitamin D, meat analogs, soy ice cream and soy yogurt. Gluten, the protein in grains, is responsible for intolerance in some sensitive individuals. Some gluten-free grain products may be lower in protein. This can be compensated by the addition of gluten-free milk powder or nut and soy flours.

- *Healthy beverages:* Water should be the main beverage to accompany snacks. It can be plain or sparkling, flavored or unflavored. Dairy reduced-fat and fat-free milk and milk substitutes help to meet fluid needs and daily nutrient requirements; however, even these can be consumed in excess, contributing too many calories.

  If fruit juice is consumed, choose only 100 percent fruit juice and not fruit drinks, but limit the servings. According to the AAP, fruit juice should never be fed to small children in a bottle. When children are able to drink from a cup and up through 6 years of age, 4 to 6 ounces of 100 percent fruit juice can be offered daily. Children and teenagers aged 7 to 18 years should not exceed 8 to 12 ounces of 100 percent fruit juice daily.

The *2010 Dietary Guidelines for Americans* recognize how 100 percent fruit juice can fulfill a part of the daily fruit allowance for children and teenagers. According to the US Centers for Disease Control and Prevention (CDC), the majority of US children and teenagers are currently consuming 100 percent fruit juices in the amounts that are recommended by health professionals. Beyond these amounts, children and teenagers should be encouraged to consume whole fruits instead [32,33].

School lunch is an important time of day to help nourish a child for academics and after-school activities. Very often, and unfortunately so, school lunch is the only true meal for some children. However, all too often children skimp on important foods at lunch and consume sugary or fat-filled snack foods.

A typical lunch for school-aged children should contain about one-third of the day's calories—about 300 calories per lunch for a more sedentary and light eater; about 500 calories per lunch for a more active and moderate eater; and about 700 calories per lunch for a very active and hearty eater, as shown in Table 11-13.

Like school breakfast, school lunch is provided in many US schools. The National School Lunch Program (NSLP) is a federally assisted meal program that operates in public and nonprofit private schools and in residential child care institutions.

TABLE 11-13 School Lunches at 300, 500 and 700 Calories Daily		
Light Lunch: **300 Daily Calories**	**Moderate Lunch:** **500 Daily Calories**	**Hearty Lunch:** **700 Daily Calories**
½ turkey sandwich: 2 ounces lean turkey breast 1 slice whole-grain bread Lettuce, tomato 1 medium apple 1 cup nonfat milk	1 turkey sandwich: 2 ounces lean turkey breast 2 slices whole-grain bread Lettuce, tomato 1 teaspoon mayonnaise 1 cup carrot sticks 1 small apple 1 cup nonfat milk	1 turkey sandwich: 3 ounces lean turkey breast 2 slices whole-grain bread Lettuce, tomato 2 teaspoons mayonnaise 1 cup carrot sticks 1 large apple 1 cup nonfat milk 1 oatmeal cookie
Servings		

1 slice whole-grain bread—
  1 serving breads, cereals, cooked grains or starchy vegetables (80 calories)
2 ounces lean turkey breast—
  2 servings meat or meat substitutes (90 calories)
(Can substitute 2 ounces lean beef, ham, reduced-fat cheese or canned tuna fish)
1 cup lettuce and tomato slices—
  1 serving vegetables (25 calories)
1 small apple—
  1 serving fruit (60 calories)
	2 slices whole-grain bread—
	  2 servings breads, cereals, cooked grains or starchy vegetables (160 calories)
	2 ounces lean turkey breast—
	  2 servings meat or meat substitutes (90 calories)
	(Can substitute 2 ounces lean beef, ham, reduced-fat cheese or canned tuna fish)
	1 cup lettuce and tomato slices—
	  1 serving vegetables (25 calories)
	1 teaspoon mayonnaise—
	  1 serving fats and oils (45 calories)
	1 cup carrot sticks
	  1 serving vegetables (25 calories)
	1 small apple—
	  1 serving fruit (60 calories)
		2 slices whole-grain bread—
		  2 servings breads, cereals, cooked grains or starchy vegetables (160 calories)
		3 ounces lean turkey breast—
		  3 servings meat or meat substitutes (135 calories)
		(Can substitute 3 ounces lean beef, ham, reduced-fat cheese or canned tuna fish)
		1 cup lettuce and tomato slices—
		  1 serving vegetables (25 calories)
		2 teaspoons mayonnaise—
		  2 servings fats and oils (90 calories)
		1 cup carrot sticks
		  1 serving vegetables (25 calories)
		1 large apple—
		  2 servings fruit (120 calories)

(Continued)

TABLE 11-13 (Continued)

Light Lunch: 300 Daily Calories	Moderate Lunch: 500 Daily Calories	Hearty Lunch: 700 Daily Calories
1 cup dairy nonfat milk— 1 serving dairy milk or milk substitute (85 calories)	1 cup dairy nonfat milk— 1 serving dairy milk or milk substitute (85 calories)	1 cup dairy nonfat milk— 1 serving dairy milk or milk substitute (85 calories) 1 oatmeal cookie— 1 serving breads, cereals, cooked grains or starchy vegetables (80 calories)

Totals

Light Lunch: 300 Daily Calories	Moderate Lunch: 500 Daily Calories	Hearty Lunch: 700 Daily Calories
1 serving breads, cereals, cooked grains or starchy vegetables 2 servings meat or meat substitutes 1 serving vegetables 1 serving fruit 1 serving dairy milk and milk products or substitutes	2 servings breads, cereals, cooked grains or starchy vegetables 2 servings meat or meat substitutes 2 servings vegetables 1 serving fruit 1 serving dairy milk and milk products or substitutes 1 serving fats and oils	3 servings breads, cereals, cooked grains or starchy vegetables 2 servings meat or meat substitutes 2 servings vegetables 2 servings fruit 1 serving dairy milk and milk products or substitutes 2 servings fats and oils

Note: Total calories are approximate

The NSLP provides nutritionally balanced, low-cost or free lunches to school children daily. About 517 calories per lunch are provided at the preschool level, 664 calories for kindergarten through sixth grade, and about 825 calories for grades 7 to 12.

Several menu planning approaches for healthful and appealing meals provide food service professionals with flexibility. Local school districts can determine which foods are to be served, including their preparation and presentation. Check out www.fns.usda.gov/cnd/menu/menu_planning.doc for traditional and enhanced food-based menu planning approaches for school lunches.

Some school districts design their own menus that are independent of government funding. Others use commercial food service operations, including some fast-food corporations. For some revolutionary approaches to school lunch programs and integrated food and nutrition programs in schools, see "Serve it Forth" later in this chapter.

Adolescence

EATING FOR CHANGE: TEENAGE NUTRITION, DIET AND HEALTH

Adolescence, the *teenage* years between ages 13 and 19, is a period of rapid growth and development with demanding nutritional needs. The changes in body images are unparalleled because adolescents transform from childlike physiques into young men and women.

Puberty is a period of rapid physical growth and sexual maturation that signals the start of adolescence. *Prepubescence* marks the start of secondary sexual characteristics—features that distinguish between boys and girls but are not directly part of the reproductive system.

Due to an increase in body fat, prepubescent girls may begin to develop as early as 8 years old, with full sexual development from 12 to 18 years of age. *Menarche*, the beginning of menstrual periods, occurs on the average about 2 years after prepubescence—as early as 10 years old or as late as 15 years old. Rapid growth in height in girls occurs between the ages of about 9½ and 14½ years, and peaks about 12 years. Adolescent girls may continue to grow in height about two years after menarche.

Boys may begin to develop secondary sexual characteristics as early as 9 years of age, with full sexual development around 16 to 17 years of age. Puberty is not marked with a sudden incident like menstruation

TABLE 11-14 Daily Nutrient Recommendations for Girls 14- to 18-Years of Age

700 mcg/d vitamin A	1,300 mg/d calcium
65 mg/d vitamin C	24 mcg/d chromium*
15 mcg/d vitamin D	890 mcg/d copper
15 mg/d vitamin E	3 mg/d fluoride*
75 mcg/d vitamin K*	150 mcg/d iodine
1.0 mg/d thiamin	15 mg/d iron
1.0 mg/d riboflavin	360 mg/d magnesium
14 mg/d niacin	1.6 mg/d manganese*
1.2 mg/d vitamin B6	43 mcg/d molybdenum
400 mcg/d folate	1,250 mg/d phosphorus
2.4 mcg/d vitamin B12	55 mcg/d selenium
5 mg/d pantothenic acid*	9 mg/d zinc
25 mcg/d biotin*	1,500 mg/d sodium*
400 mg/d choline*	4,700 mg/d potassium*
	2,300 mg/d chloride*

Source: [29].

Note: Adequate Intake levels (AIs) are marked by an asterisk (*).

TABLE 11-15 Daily Calories and Major Nutrient Needs for 13- and 14- to 18-Year Old Girls

Estimated Daily Calorie and Nutrient Needs for 13-year-old Girls (at 1,600 Calories)	Foods and Beverages that Meet Nutrient Requirements
1,600 calories	5 ounces of breads, cereals, cooked grains or starchy vegetables with one-half (2½ ounces) whole grains
130 grams of carbohydrates (520 calories)	2 cups of vegetables
22* grams of fiber	1½ cups of fruit
34 grams of protein (136 calories)	3 cups of dairy milk and milk products or substitutes
	5 ounces of meat or meat substitutes
	4½ teaspoons of additional fats or oils
Estimated Daily Calorie and Nutrient Needs for 14- to 18-Year-Old Girls (at 1,800 Calories)	**Foods and Beverages that Meet Nutrient Requirements**
1,800 calories daily	6 ounces of breads, cereals, cooked grains or starchy vegetables with one-half (3 ounces) whole grains
130 grams of carbohydrates (520 calories)	2½ cups of vegetables
25* grams of fiber	1½ cups of fruit
46 grams of protein (184 calories)	3 cups of dairy milk and milk products or substitutes
	5 ounces of meat or meat substitutes
	5 teaspoons of additional fats or oils

Note: Adequate Intake levels (AIs) are marked by an asterisk (*).

507

as it is in females. Rapid growth in height in boys occurs between the ages of 10½ and 18, and peaks about age 14. Adolescent boys may continue to grow in height throughout their early twenties.

Growth may not be smooth and continual; rather, prepubescent and adolescents may experience *growth spurts*, which are rapid increases in height and weight. Teenage girls accumulate both lean and fat tissue during these growth spurts, and teenage boys accumulate mostly lean tissue. This is because body fat is needed for future reproductive purposes, and the adult male body will eventually carry more muscle tissue in proportion to fat.

NUTRITIONAL NEEDS OF TEENAGERS

During the teenage years caloric needs parallel growth and development. The daily nutrient recommendations according to the *2010 USDA Dietary Guidelines* for girls aged 14 to 18 years are shown in Table 11-14. The daily calories and major nutrient needs for 13 year old girls, who require less, and for 14- to 18-year-old girls, are shown in Table 11-15.

During the teenage years, the nutrient needs of boys differ in key nutrients from girls to cover their growth, increased energy and muscular needs. Table 11-16 shows the daily nutrition goals for 14- to 18-year-old boys, and Table 11-17 shows the daily calories and major nutrient needs for 13-year-old boys, who require less, and for 14- to 18-year-old boys.

TABLE 11-16 Daily Nutrient Recommendations for Boys 14- to 18-Years of Age

900 mcg/d vitamin A	1,300 mg/d calcium
75 mg/d vitamin C	35 mcg/d chromium*
15 mcg/d vitamin D	890 mcg/d copper
15 mg/d vitamin E	3 mg/d fluoride*
75 mcg/d vitamin K*	150 mcg/d iodine
1.2 mg/d thiamin	11 mg/d iron
1.3 mg/d riboflavin	410 mg/d magnesium
14 mg/d niacin	2.2 mg/d manganese*
1.2 mg/d vitamin B6	43 mcg/d molybdenum
400 mcg/d folate	1,250 mg/d phosphorus
2.4 mcg/d vitamin B12	55 mcg/d selenium
5 mg/d pantothenic acid*	9 mg/d zinc
25 mcg/d biotin*	1,500 mg/d sodium*
550 mg/d choline*	4,700 mg/d potassium*
	2,300 mg/d chloride*

Source: [29].
Note: Adequate Intake levels (AIs) are marked by an asterisk (*).

TABLE 11-17 Daily Calories and Major Nutrient Needs for 13- and 14-to 18-Year Old Boys

Estimated Daily Calorie and Nutrient Needs for 13-year Old Boys (at 2,000 Calories)	Foods and Beverages that Meet Nutrient Requirements (at 2,000 Calories Daily)
2,000 calories daily	6 ounces of breads, cereals, cooked grains or starchy vegetables with one-half (3 ounces) whole grains
130 grams of carbohydrates (520 calories)	2 ½ cups of vegetables
25* grams of fiber	2 cups of fruit
34 grams of protein (136 calories)	3 cups of dairy milk and milk products or substitutes
	5 ounces of meat or meat substitutes
	5 ½ teaspoons of additional fats or oils
Estimated Daily Calorie and Nutrient Needs for 14- to 18-Year-Old Boys (at 2,000-2,400 Calories)	**Foods and Beverages that Meet Nutrient Requirements (at 2,000/2,200/2,400 Calories Daily)**
2,000–2,400 calories daily	6/7/8 ounces of breads, cereals, cooked grains or starchy vegetables with one-half (3 ounces/3½ ounces/4 ounces) whole grains
130 grams of carbohydrates (520 calories)	2½/3/3 cups of vegetables
31* grams of fiber	2/2/2 cups of fruit
52 grams of protein (208 calories)	3/3/3 cups of dairy milk and milk products or substitutes
	5½/6/6½ ounces of meat or meat substitutes
	5½/6/6½ teaspoons of additional fats or oils

Note: Adequate Intake levels (AIs) are marked by an asterisk (*).

FOOD BYTE

Many studies have supported the value of family meals. Two in particular have correlated family meals with better nutrition. The first study concluded that the frequency of family meals is related to better nutritional intake and decreased risk of unhealthy weight-control practices and substance abuse. The second study showed that eating family dinners together most or all of the days of the week was associated with eating more healthfully; consuming higher amounts of calcium, fiber, iron, and vitamins B6, B12, C and E; and smaller amounts of fats than families who "never" or "only sometimes" ate meals together [1,34–36].

TEENAGE EATING HABITS

Teenage boys and girls require at least a 20 to 30 percent increase in daily requirements of many vitamins and minerals as they grow from preteens to teenagers. Instead, teenagers are consuming fewer fruits and vegetables today than they did 10 years ago, as recommended by the US Department of Health and Human Services' *Healthy People 2010* objectives and the *2010 Dietary Guidelines for Americans*. Fruits and vegetables have important phytonutrients and fiber for optimal health and chronic disease prevention. By not consuming the recommended daily servings of fruits and vegetables, teenagers may be establishing unhealthy lifelong practices.

The most significant drop in fruit and vegetable intake in teenagers is between the middle school and high school years. The next major drop in fruit and vegetable intake is between high school and adulthood. Simply learning about the importance of fruits and vegetables may not be enough to encourage teenagers to select them. The school environment should also be supportive by providing healthier food options. The frequency of family meals may also promote healthier food choices among adolescents.

International studies of teenage eating habits also reveal poor fruit and vegetable intake. For example, a study of Irish teenagers concluded that one in three teens studied did not eat any fruit at all, and over 50 percent ate too much fat. Vegetable consumption was well below international recommendations. Four out of five teenagers did not consume enough fiber, and daily salt intake from processed meats and breads was higher than recommended levels.

Many factors contribute to poor teenage eating habits. For one, teenagers consume more of their meals away from home at school and fast-food outlets, where selections may be higher in calories, fats, sugars and sodium. Body image is also a contributing factor. Some teenage boys may emulate professional athletes and "bulk up," while some girls may equate model-like slenderness with beauty. It is true that teenage boys need more protein than preteen boys—52 grams of protein daily for 14- to 18-year-olds versus 34 grams of protein daily for 9- to 13-year-olds. Teenage girls generally need less daily protein than boys; 14- to 18-year-olds require 46 grams of protein daily, while 9- to 13-year-olds require 34 grams of protein daily.

According to the DRIs, the Recommended Dietary Allowance (RDA) for carbohydrates for 14- to 18-year-old girls and boys is similar: 130 grams of carbohydrates daily, or 520 calories. Some teenagers barely eat this amount of calories if they are dieting. The DRI Acceptable Macronutrient Distribution Range for carbohydrates is 45 to 65 percent of total calories for children through teenagers, 4 to 18 years of age. Based on an average intake of 2,000 calories daily for teenagers, this amounts to about 900 to 1,300 calories, or 225 to 325 grams of carbohydrates daily. Once again, some teenagers do not come close to consuming this amount.

509

The sense of taste changes at puberty when hormones are shifting. Blood sugar levels may be erratic, causing greater intake of calories, fats and carbohydrates. Boys may crave more protein-rich foods for muscle, while girls may crave more sweets before menstruation.

Menstruation also increases monthly iron loss and requires replacement by iron-rich foods and beverages. Teenage girls need almost twice as much daily iron once they begin to menstruate (15 grams of iron daily for 14- to 18-year-olds versus 8 grams of iron daily for 9- to 13-year-olds). Boys need around one-third more daily iron during rapid muscle growth (11 grams of iron daily for 14- to 18-year-olds versus 8 grams of iron daily for 9- to 13-year-olds).

Both teenage boys and girls also need more zinc—a mineral that is required during growth and development. Teenage boys need about one-third more zinc daily, and teenage girls need about 10 to 15 percent more zinc daily than in the preteen years. Both teenage boys and girls need around 1,300 milligrams of calcium daily for strong bones and teeth—this is the same amount that is needed for preteens daily.

Though the brain has completed most of its growth and changes by adolescence, it relies on healthy fats for its vital functions. Teenagers may either restrict their fat intake or consume too much fats and oils. Healthy fats are particularly essential to young women during their childbearing years [37–39].

Healthy Diet and Meal Planning for Teenagers

Nutritionally balanced meals and snacks can be planned for teenage girls and boys based on the calorie and nutrient recommendations in Tables 11-14 to 11-17. The first meal plan in Table 11-18 is for a 14- to 18-year-old teenage girl. It is followed by the same meal plan with additional servings for a 14- to 18-year-old teenage boy in Table 11-19. This shows how the same foods and beverages can be served with minimal adjustments for calories and nutrients.

FOOD BYTE

The exact cause of acne is unknown. Heredity is a known factor, as are allergies or sensitivities to chemicals, cosmetics, foods and molds. Central nervous system disorders, hormonal imbalances, and some medications are also suspect. Some research indicates that some carbohydrates with a high glycemic index may affect the development of acne and its severity. A diet high in protein and carbohydrates with a low glycemic index may improve acne breakouts. The results suggest that a healthy diet with less sugar may be preventive in acne treatment. Fewer refined carbohydrates make room for healthier carbohydrates from fruits, vegetables and whole grains with their array of vitamins, minerals and phytonutrients—many of which are skin enhancing [40,41].

TABLE 11-18 Meal Plan for a 14–18-Year-Old Teenage Girl (with Servings)

Breakfast	Morning Snack
½ cup of cooked oatmeal (1 serving of breads, cereals, grains or starchy vegetables)	1 small whole-grain bagel (1 serving of breads, cereals, grains or starchy vegetables)
1 cup of dairy skim milk (1 serving dairy milk or milk substitutes)	1 tablespoon of cream cheese (1 serving of fats or oils)
1 extra-small banana (1 serving of fruit)	

Lunch	Afternoon Snack
2 slices of whole-grain bread (2 servings of breads, cereals, grains or starchy vegetables)	3 graham crackers (1 serving of breads, cereals, cooked grains or starchy vegetables)
2 ounces of turkey breast (2 ounces of meat or meat substitutes)	1 cup of yogurt (1 serving of dairy milk or milk substitutes)
½ cup of sliced tomatoes and lettuce for sandwich (½ serving of vegetables)	
2 teaspoons of mayonnaise (2 servings of fats or oils)	

Dinner	After-dinner Snack
½ cup of cooked brown rice (1 serving of breads, cereals, cooked grains or starchy vegetables)	1 cup of yogurt smoothie (1 serving of dairy milk or milk substitutes)
3 ounces of skinless chicken breast (3 ounces meat or meat substitutes)	1 small orange (1 serving of fruit)
1 cup of tossed salad (1 serving of vegetables)	
2 teaspoons of vinaigrette salad dressing (2 servings of fats or oils)	
½ cup of cooked broccoli (1 serving of vegetables)	

Totals

6 ounces of breads, cereals, cooked grains or starchy vegetables with one-half (3 ounces) whole grains
2½ cups of vegetables
1½ cups of fruit
3 cups of dairy milk and milk products or substitutes
5 ounces of meat or meat substitutes
5 teaspoons of additional fats or oils

TABLE 11-19 Meal Plan for a 14–18-Year-Old Teenage Boy (with Servings)

Breakfast	Morning Snack
1 cup of cooked oatmeal (2 servings of breads, cereals, grains or starchy vegetables) 1 cup of dairy skim milk (1 serving of dairy milk or milk substitutes) 1 medium banana (1½ servings of fruit)	2 small whole-grain bagels (2 servings of breads, cereals, grains or starchy vegetables) 1 tablespoon of cream cheese (1 serving of fats or oils)
Lunch	**Afternoon Snack**
2 slices of whole-grain bread (2 servings of breads, cereals, grains or starchy vegetables) 3 ounces of turkey breast (3 ounces meat or meat substitutes) ½ cup of sliced tomatoes and lettuce for sandwich (½ serving of vegetables) 4 black olives (½ serving of fats or oils) 2 teaspoons of mayonnaise (2 servings of fats or oils)	1 cup of yogurt (1 serving of dairy milk or milk substitutes) 3 peanut butter graham crackers (1 serving of breads, cereals, cooked grains or starchy vegetables *plus* about ½ serving of meat or meat substitutes)
Dinner	**After-dinner Snack**
½ cup of cooked brown rice (1 serving of breads, cereals, cooked grains or starchy vegetables) 3 ounces of skinless chicken breast (3 ounces of meat or meat substitutes) 1½ cups of tossed salad (1½ servings of vegetables) 2 teaspoons of vinaigrette salad dressing (2 servings of fats or oils) ½ cup of cooked broccoli (1 serving of vegetables) 1 teaspoon of margarine (1 serving of fats or oils)	1 cup yogurt smoothie (1 serving of dairy milk or milk substitutes) 1 small orange (1 serving of fruit)

Totals

8 servings of breads, cereals, cooked grains or starchy vegetables with one-half (4 servings) whole grains
3 servings of vegetables
2 servings of fruit
3 servings of dairy milk and milk products or substitutes
6½ ounces meat or meat substitutes
6½ servings of additional fats or oils

FAST FOOD AND FAST FOOD SUBSTITUTIONS

Teenagers are notorious for their erratic eating habits. Skipping meals, eating on the run, and overindulging are common. In some cases, the teenage body is forgiving. Other teenagers may eat too little and suffer eating disorders, such as anorexia nervosa or bulimia nervosa. Or they may suffer from obesity and even the early stages of diabetes or atherosclerosis that are normally found in adults. Diets high in cholesterol and saturated fats, common in fast food, may contribute to these and other chronic diseases.

Consuming fast food is a modern way of life. Fast food is a relatively affordable and quick way of eating. It delivers a lot of taste with all of its fat, sodium and sugar. Fast food can fit into a teenager's diet as long as calories permit and the rest of their diet supplies their daily nutrient needs.

Some fast foods can be substituted or "exchanged" for some of the foods and beverages in the teenage meal plans that are shown above. For example, a fast-food "junior" hamburger may contain about 322 calories, 17 grams of fat and 486 milligrams of sodium. This is the equivalent of about two servings of breads, cereals, cooked grains or starchy vegetables; 2 to 3 ounces of meat or meat substitutes; and 1 serving of fats or oils. These servings are very similar to the types of foods and the number of servings at lunch in the meal plan of the 14- to 18-year-old teenage girl. On occasion, she can "exchange" the fast-food junior hamburger for the turkey breast sandwich.

The amount of sodium per serving is high. The tolerable upper limit (UL) of sodium in this age group is 2,300 milligrams daily. If the fast-food junior hamburger is consumed at lunch, then it is advisable that sodium be cut back at other meals or snacks. A quarter-pound hamburger may contain about 414 calories, 22 grams of fat and 730 milligrams of sodium. This is the equivalent of about two servings of breads, cereals, cooked grains or starchy vegetables; 3 to 4 ounces of meat or meat substitutes; and 1 serving of fats or oils. These servings are very similar to the types of foods and the number of servings at lunch in the meal plan of the 14- to 18-year-old teenage boy. On occasion, he can "exchange" the fast-food quarter-pound hamburger for the turkey breast sandwich. The amount of sodium in the quarter-pounder is even higher than in the junior hamburger, so this substitution will require an even greater reduction of sodium throughout the rest of the day.

Other fast food choices, as shown in Table 11-20, may occasionally be substituted or "exchanged" according to equivalent servings. Vegetables servings may vary according to how fast foods are ordered (such as with or without lettuce and tomatoes).

TABLE 11-20 Sample Fast Food Nutrients and Equivalent Servings

Chicken tenders (4 pieces)

170 calories	This entree is the equivalent of about:
10 grams of carbohydrates	½ to 1 serving of breads, cereals, cooked
10 grams of protein	grains or starchy vegetables
10 grams of fat	1½ ounces of meat or meat substitutes and
25 milligrams of cholesterol	2 servings of fats or oils.
450 milligrams sodium	

Breakfast sandwich with egg

290 calories	This breakfast sandwich is the equivalent of about:
30 grams of carbohydrates	2 servings of breads, cereals, cooked grains or starchy
17 grams of protein	vegetables
11 grams of fat	2½ ounces of meat or meat substitutes and
235 milligrams of cholesterol	2 servings of fats or oils.
850 milligrams of sodium	

Fish fillet on bun

400 calories	This sandwich is the equivalent of about:
42 grams of carbohydrates	3 servings of breads, cereals, cooked grains or starchy
14 grams of protein	vegetables
18 grams of fat	2 ounces of meat or meat substitutes and
40 milligrams of cholesterol	3½ servings of fats or oils.
640 milligrams of sodium	

Tacos (2 supreme)

330 calories	These tacos are the equivalent of about:
37 milligrams of carbohydrates	3½ servings of breads, cereals, cooked grains or
14 milligrams of protein	starchy vegetables
15 grams of fat	2 ounces of meat or meat substitutes and
30 milligram of cholesterol	3 servings of fats or oils.
740 milligrams of sodium	

Stuffed vegetable pizza (¼ medium)

420 calories	This amount of pizza is the equivalent of about:
48 grams of carbohydrates	3 servings of breads, cereals, cooked grains or
20 grams of protein	starchy vegetables
19 milligrams cholesterol	almost 3 ounces of meat or meat substitutes and
14 grams of fat	almost 3 servings of fats or oils.
1,040 milligrams of sodium	

Source: [42].
aCalories, nutrients and Equivalent Servings are estimated and averaged.

TABLE 11-21 Calories, Fat and Carbohydrates in Snacks

Foods or Beverages	Calories (per serving)	Fat (grams)	Carbohydrates (grams)	Protein (grams)
½ cup vanilla pudding	143 cal	4 g	25 g	2 g
1 bagel	73	0.5	14.5	3
1 tablespoon peanut butter	188	16	7	8
1 cup vegetable soup	178	2	36	6
1 protein bar	180	6	26	9
1 cup low-fat dairy chocolate milk 158	158	3	26	8
1 cup skim milk yogurt	137	0	19	14
1 cup fresh strawberries	49	0	12	1
1 cup cold breakfast cereal with ½ cup dairy skim milk	270	3	48	6
2 fig bars	112	2	22	2
2 graham crackers	60	1	11	1
2 oatmeal cookies	104	6	16	2.25
3 cups popped low-fat microwave popcorn	93	1	19	3

Source: [43].

A diet that is filled with fast foods will likely be high in calories, total fat, saturated fat, cholesterol, sodium and sugar, and too low in fruits, vegetables and whole grains and the nutrients that these foods supply to be healthy long term.

Recipe: Portobello Mushroom Burgers with Basil-Mustard Sauce

*While this **Portobello Mushroom Burger with Basil-Mustard Sauce** in the **Recipe file** which is located within the* Culinary Nutrition *website at www.culinarynutrition.elsevier.com, is not a fast-food burger, the meaty, savory taste of Portobello mushrooms is a good vegetarian substitute. These burgers are lower in calories and fat than traditional beef burgers, with no cholesterol. The tangy basil-mustard sauce adds another layer of flavor—also with little fat. Serve it with lettuce and tomatoes or a micro-green salad on the top to add color, crunch and nutrients. A slice of reduced-fat sharp cheese adds even more taste and nutrients, if calories permit. The finished dish is shown within the centerfold **Photo file** in Plate 11.2.*

513

HEALTHY SNACKS FOR TEENAGERS

Teenager snacks should match their lifestyles and taste preferences: quick to prepare and eat or drink, and tasty with distinct texture, without too many calories, carbohydrates, fats or sodium. Otherwise teenagers may turn to foods and beverages that are not in their best interest. A reasonable guideline is to offer snacks with 30 percent or fewer calories from fat, such as the ones that are shown in Table 11-21.

In addition to these snacks, some of the recipes in this and other chapters that follow can be used for snacks or simple meals, with a few additions. A cup of dairy skim milk or reduced-fat yogurt, some fresh fruit or raw vegetables and dip, or a bowl of hearty bean or vegetable soup can enhance some of these nutritious snacks and transform them into satisfying meals.

Health Snack Recipes	Chapter
Berry Crumble	Chapter 4
Cherry Pistachio Biscotti	Chapter 6
Chocolate Pudding	Chapter 9
Cream of Tomato-Basil Soup with Grilled Cheese Croutons	Chapter 11
Grilled Fruit Skewers with Tropical Yogurt Sauce	Chapter 11
Blueberry-Lemon Muffins	Chapter 11
Mushroom Potato Frittata	Chapter 5

Health Snack Recipes	Chapter
Olive Oil Cake	Chapter 6
Portobello Mushroom Burger with Basil-Mustard Sauce	Chapter 11
Vegetarian Chili	Chapter 4
Healthy Beverages	
Fruit-Flavored Waters	Chapter 8
Green Tea Shake	Chapter 8
Mexican Cocoa	Chapter 8
Papaya Yogurt Smoothie	Chapter 8
Peppermint Chai Tea	Chapter 8
Strawberry Soy Milk Shake	Chapter 8

Other healthy snacks—many that are reduced-fat and whole grain include the following combinations. Fortified soy products can be substituted for dairy products for children and teenagers who are vegetarian or have a milk allergy or lactose sensitivity.

Recipe: Blueberry-Lemon Muffins

*Blueberries contain fiber and manganese and are very high in their antioxidant activity per serving (ORAC value). They have a natural affinity to lemon, which brightens their taste. When added to whole grains, as in these **Blueberry-Lemon Muffins** in the **Recipe file**, which is located within the* Culinary Nutrition *website at www.culinarynutrition.elsevier.com, they are filling, and when teamed with low-fat yogurt, cheese or dairy milk, they have staying power. While perfect for breakfast, these muffins are portable and make an excellent midday snack when other choices may be limited. The finished dish is shown within the centerfold **Photo file** in Plate 6.3.*

Reduced-fat dairy milk or yogurt plus . . .
- Banana, blueberry, bran, carrot, pumpkin or zucchini muffin
- Trail mix made with whole-grain cereal, chopped nuts, roasted soybeans, dried fruit or mini chocolate chips
- Vegetable soup with whole-grain croutons
- Whole-grain bagel with peanut butter and apple, banana or pear slices
- Whole-grain bread with lean meat
- Whole-grain cold or hot breakfast cereal
- Whole-grain waffle with almond, cashew, peanut or soy "nut" butter

Other reduced-fat dairy products plus . . .
- Reduced-fat string cheese *plus* whole-grain crackers
- Reduced-fat cottage cheese *plus* granola, chopped nuts or dried fruit
- Reduced-fat ice cream or frozen yogurt *plus* chopped nuts, dried fruit or 100 percent fruit preserves

100 percent fruit juice or 100 percent calcium-fortified fruit juice or flavored water plus . . .
- Air-popped popcorn with Parmesan cheese
- Cheese and vegetable pizza
- Steamed edamame (immature soybeans) and miso soup
- Fresh raw vegetables with reduced-fat cream cheese or bean dip
- Hard-boiled egg with reduced-fat mayonnaise or mustard
- Hummus with fresh vegetables
- Rice cakes with chocolate hazelnut spread
- Tortilla with refried vegetarian beans

FOOD BYTE

The Centers for Disease Control has reported that in some states four out of five high schools sold candy, and more than three out of four schools sold high-fat, salty snacks—not to mention vending machines and concessions that dispense fruits drinks, regular sodas and sports drinks. Sales from vending machines, canteens and snack bars generally go directly to schools. Due to concerns about childhood and teenage obesity and growing state and federal legislation that regulates the content of food and beverages sold in schools, some schools now substitute healthier food and beverage choices and are still able to bring in revenue. Schools that substitute healthy foods for junk foods may see a drop in revenue at the start, but revenues usually climb back after a year or two [44,45].

TABLE 11-22 Calcium Content of Foods and Beverages

Foods and Beverages	Calcium (milligrams)
4 ounces calcium-set tofu	250–750 mg
4 ounces soft tofu	120–390
1 cup low-fat yogurt	400–450
1 cup fortified soy milk	350
1cup calcium-fortified juice or beverage	350
1 packet calcium-fortified hot cocoa	320
1 cup dairy skim milk	300
1 packet instant breakfast mix	250
1 ounce reduced-fat cheddar or mozzarella cheese	150–200
1 slice calcium-fortified bread	150
1 cup cooked broccoli	180
½ cup cooked greens (such as collards or spinach)	150–250
1 cup low-fat cottage cheese	140
1 cup vanilla ice cream or ice milk	85
1 ounce unblanched almonds	80
1 tablespoon Parmesan cheese	70

Source: [46].

515

SPECIAL NUTRITIONAL NEEDS OF TEENAGERS: CALCIUM, IRON AND FOLATE
Calcium

Calcium is a mineral that is essential during the developmental years of adolescence because it helps to build bones and maintain bone density. Teenage girls and boys aged 14 to 18 years require 1,300 milligrams of calcium daily. Table 11-22 lists some foods and beverages that supply as much as 60 percent of this daily requirement.

By having dairy skim milk instead of fruit juice at breakfast, a yogurt smoothie instead of soda or a sports drink at lunch, a pudding cup or cheese and crackers instead of a candy bar for snacks, and cheese pizza instead of plain pasta for dinner, the level of calcium and other bone-building nutrients can be boosted in a teenager's diet.

By eliminating milk and replacing it with calcium-poor soda, fruit drinks or sports beverages, teenagers may become more susceptible to bone fractures, particularly teenage athletes who engage in contact sports, such as football players, runners or gymnasts. While some calcium-fortified beverages may deliver the same amount of calcium as dairy milk or even more, they may fall short in protein, magnesium, phosphorus, potassium and vitamins A and D.

Some calcium-rich beverages are fortified with vitamin D. The potential benefits of vitamin D include bone strength, immunity, and the potential risk reductions of cancer, diabetes and heart disease. Some dairy products such as yogurt and hard cheese may not be vitamin D–fortified, so make sure to check the nutrition label.

Iron

Iron is a mineral that makes up hemoglobin, the oxygen-carrying component of red blood cells that supplies energy to cells throughout the body. If iron is low in the bloodstream, as in anemia, people may have less energy for normal bodily functions and poor resistance to infection.

TABLE 11-23 Iron Content of Foods and Beverages	
Foods and Beverages	**Iron (milligrams)**
1 cup iron-fortified cold breakfast cereal	18 mg
½ cup roasted soy "nuts"	3.5
3 ounces cooked lean sirloin steak	2.9
½ cup cooked red kidney beans	2.6
3 ounces cooked lean hamburger	1.8
3 ounces skinless chicken breast	0.9
3 ounces roasted lean pork	0.9
3 ounces canned salmon with bones	0.7
⅔ cup raisins	1.8
1 cup cooked oatmeal	1.6
½ cup tofu	1.4
½ cup enriched rice	1.4
1 slice enriched whole grain bread	1
3 ounces cooked pork loin	0.9
½ cup cooked broccoli	0.7
3 dried apricots	0.6
2 tablespoons peanut butter	0.6

Source: [47].

Teenage girls require about 15 milligrams of iron daily for normal needs and to replace menstrual blood loss. Teenage boys require less iron—about 11 milligrams daily for normal needs. Heavy athletic training may contribute to sports anemia, which can be corrected by iron-rich foods and beverages.

Iron is available through foods and beverages in two forms: *heme iron* (the iron-holding portion of hemoglobin) and *nonheme iron*. Meat is an excellent source of heme iron, and foods and beverages from the vegetable kingdom (fruits, grains, nuts and vegetables) are sources of nonheme iron.

A larger proportion of heme iron than nonheme iron is absorbed and available to the body, so vegetarians and vegans are at increased risk of anemia. This is partially due to two substances—*phytates* and *oxylates* in vegetables and grains—that interfere with iron absorption. In particular, meat, fish and poultry contain a factor called MFP that promotes iron absorption. Dried fruit, iron-fortified cereals, green leafy vegetables, legumes and nuts are iron-rich foods in the plant kingdom. Table 11-23 lists some foods and beverages that supply over 100 percent of the daily requirements for iron.

By having iron-rich breakfast cereal instead of a sweet roll for breakfast, a meat or tofu sandwich on iron-fortified whole-grain bread instead of a salad for lunch, mixed peanuts or soy nuts and dried fruit trail mix instead of a bag of chips for an afternoon snack, and a grilled hamburger or vegetarian red bean chili instead of spaghetti for dinner, the level of iron and other blood-building nutrients can be improved in a teenager's diet.

Folate and Folic Acid

In addition to iron, teenage women should have a good source of folate, which is essential for the prevention of neural tube defects in pregnancy. Because teenage pregnancy can be unexpected, it is advisable that daily folate intake of 400 micrograms be consistent throughout childbearing years. If inadequate, a health care provider may recommend a folic acid supplement. The folate content of foods and beverages is shown in Table 11-24.

By having folic acid–fortified breakfast cereal instead of a doughnut at breakfast; bean burritos at lunch instead of a bowl of soup; an orange, some peanuts or some sunflower seeds for a snack instead of a coffee-flavored drink; and a vegetable stir-fry with asparagus and broccoli at dinner instead of an iceberg lettuce salad with diet salad dressing, the level of folate can be raised in a teenage girl's diet. More information about calcium, iron and folate can be found in Chapter 7.

TABLE 11-24 Folate Content of Foods and Beverages	
Foods and Beverages	**Folate (micrograms)**
½ cup cooked lentils	180 mg
½ cup cooked asparagus	146
½ cup chickpeas	141
½ cup black beans	128
2 bean burritos	118
½ cup cooked spinach	113
1 cup cooked broccoli	104
½ cup instant cooked oatmeal	100
1 cup fortified breakfast cereal	100–400
¼ sup sunflower seeds	80
⅓ cup peanuts	71
1 cup tomato juice	48
½ cup cantaloupe	47
1 medium orange	47
½ cup Brussels sprouts	47
1 slice fortified bread	38
2 tablespoons wheat germ	38

Source: [48].

TEENAGE VEGETARIAN DIETS

Teenage years are times to experiment with different diets and lifestyles. Reasons to choose a vegetarian or vegan diet may be ecological, economical, ethical, moral, political or spiritual. Sometimes following a rigid set of dietary guidelines offers control when the rest of a teenager's life seems out of control.

Protein needs are based on body weight and can easily be met or exceeded by a well-planned vegetarian diet. Lacto-ovo vegetarians who include dairy products and eggs may also meet or exceed their other daily nutritional needs. Vegans may require more careful diet planning to ensure adequate amounts of vitamins B12 and D, calcium, iron and zinc.

It may be difficult for teenage vegetarians to obtain enough vitamin B12, since it is only naturally found in animal products. Nonmeat sources of vitamin B12, which include fortified ready-to-eat cereals and soy products, nutritional yeast and B12 supplements, may be an effective means of meeting the teenage DRI for vitamin B12 of 2.4 milligrams per day. A conscious effort to consume this amount of vitamin B12 daily is essential for health and well-being.

Vitamin B12 is essential because a deficiency in this vitamin may cause an anemia that is similar to what is seen in folate deficiency. In this anemia, red blood cells are immature, large and dysfunctional. Undetected vitamin B12 deficiency may lead to nerve paralysis and permanent nerve damage. Vegetarian teenagers should be made aware of these potential consequences and undertake dietary assistance in their food and beverage choices.

Low levels of vitamin D have been linked to high blood pressure and high blood sugar in teenagers, which may foretell other health problems that are associated with aging. The human body makes vitamin D when it is exposed to the sunlight's ultraviolet rays. But dark-colored skin may interfere with optimal vitamin D production. Moreover, African Americans and Hispanics may avoid dairy products due to lactose intolerance or milk allergies.

Vitamin D–fortified foods and beverages, dairy products and fatty fish such as salmon are good sources of vitamin D. The American Academy of Pediatrics (AAP) recommends 400 IU of vitamin D daily for teenagers. This is the equivalent of drinking four cups of vitamin D–fortified dairy milk. The AAP also recommends vitamin D supplementation if intake is insufficient. Vegetarian teenagers who avoid dairy products and vegans—particularly those who reside in cloudy climates—should consider a vitamin D supplement.

The need for calcium, iron and zinc and their food sources have been discussed earlier in this chapter and in Chapter 7. While vegetarians and vegans can obtain enough calcium and iron from fortified plant foods, there may be downsides. By eliminating dairy milk and milk products, good sources of magnesium, protein, phosphorus, potassium and vitamin D may also be jeopardized.

When meat and meat products are eliminated, heme iron and zinc may be at risk. Plus phytates and oxylates in vegetables and grains may interfere with iron and zinc absorption from plant foods [49, 50].

Dietary intake of these minerals can be adequate if a teenage vegetarian or vegan diet is well planned by a registered dietitian or nutritionally informed health care specialist. It is imprudent to follow a restrictive diet just to call oneself a vegetarian or vegan. Furthermore, a poorly executed vegetarian diet—one that is high in fats and sugars—may be less healthy than a meat-based diet.

TEENAGE OVERWEIGHT, OBESITY AND WEIGHT MANAGEMENT

Overweight and obesity are two of the most serious nutritional problems of teenagers today, particularly among low-income Hispanics, African Americans and Native Americans. The association between overweight and obesity and health risks has been documented in adults. Medicare recognized obesity as a disease in 2004. Overweight and obesity in adolescents may be detrimental later in life.

The Harvard Growth Study, which spanned over 50 years, indicated that overweight teenage boys were twice as likely as thin teenagers to die by the age of 70, principally from coronary heart disease. Overweight teenage boys were about five times likelier to develop colon cancer and twice as likely to develop gout (a form of arthritis characterized by sudden, severe attacks of pain, redness and joint tenderness). Overweight teenage girls were 60 percent more likely to develop arthritis and twice as likely to suffer from coronary heart disease in their seventies than teenage girls who were not overweight [51].

When this famous study was conducted and later published, the degree of overweight and obesity in teenagers was not as serious as it is today. This is why the conclusions of this study are still so compelling. To prevent a lifetime of overweight or obesity and the health ramifications that these conditions may bring, it is essential for teenagers to stay at or below their calorie guidelines, which are shown in Table 11-25.

Skipping meals or abstaining from foods and beverages altogether to lose or maintain weight is not a good idea, and it is never a long-term solution to teenage weight problems. For one, skipping meals does not provide the teenage body with the energy that it requires, which can have both physical and mental repercussions. Also, teenagers may overeat or overdrink after skipping meals, which may cause unwanted calories to be stored as fat instead of burned for energy. Longer-term starvation may lead to constipation, decreased immunity, exhaustion, hair loss, poor body temperature regulation, and poor sports performance. Unmonitored, starvation may lead to the dysfunctional organs and body systems, and ultimately death.

There is no magic solution for teenage weight loss. Healthy food and activity habits must be learned and incorporated so they can last a lifetime. Still, teenagers cannot succeed at weight loss alone. They need supportive parents and other role models who create healthy school, home, work and leisure environments.

518

TABLE 11-25 Recommended Calorie Levels for Teenagers	
Age and Gender	**Recommended Daily Calorie Level**[*]
Girls 13 years of age	1,600[*]
Girls 14–18 years of age	1,800
Girls 19–20 years of age	2,000
Boys 13 years of age	2,000
Boys 14–18 years of age	2,400
Boys 19–20 years of age	2,600

Source: [34].
*Based on age, gender and sedentary level of physical activity.

Some commercial weight-control programs, residential programs and weight-loss camps offer specialized diet and activity plans for teenagers. More information can be found in "Hungry for More?" later in this chapter.

TEENAGERS AND ATHLETICS

Teenage athletes require calories and nutrients over and beyond those that are normally needed for teenage growth and development. Some high-energy sports, such as cross-country running, soccer and swimming, may have very high caloric needs. Other sports that are intense but stop and start, such as track and field or gymnastics, may have lower caloric needs.

Fasting, dieting or skipping meals may compromise athletic performance and overall health. Specific food groups, such as dairy products or breads, cereals and grains, should not be eliminated because many of their nutrients are essential for sports training and performance (see Chapter 10).

For some sports, a goal is to carry the least amount of body weight and retain the most energy. Long-distance runners and cyclists fall into this category. "Making weight" may require the help of a qualified health professional, coach or athletic trainer. The ideal percentage of body fat differs among sports, which is why it is important to consult with an exercise, health and/or nutrition professional. Teenage athletes should not try to lose a large amount of weight over a short period of time, especially before a major event; induce sweating to lose excess water; keep calories too low while exercising very hard; use rapid weight-loss aids; or restrict fluids before workouts or important competitions.

Teenage athletes should ensure that they consume enough carbohydrates, protein, fats, vitamins, minerals and fluids to maintain the right percentage of body fat and have the most energy and muscle power according to individual sport requirements. They should only supplement their diet if there are gaps, without exceeding the DRIs, except under the direction of trained health professionals.

COOKING FOR TEENAGERS

519

The diet and nutrition habits of teenagers are mostly the result of a short lifetime of established eating habits combined with a wide range of behavioral, cultural, physical, emotional and environmental issues that affect adolescence. For all these reasons and more, cooking for teenagers at home and in food service operations in community recreation centers, athletic facilities and academic institutions is challenging.

Many of these facilities have become a "home away from home" for fueling our nation's youth. Some teenagers are dependent on these sites for the majority of their daily meals and snacks. Foods and beverages must look very appealing, taste great, be very satisfying, economical and easily consumed on the run. Nutrient-dense foods compete for those that are higher in calories, fats, sugars and sodium. The challenge for nutrition and culinary specialists is how to make healthy food for teenagers good to eat, too—and today's teens can be selective.

FAVORITE TEENAGE FOOD MAKEOVERS

Many US teenagers have a repertoire of foods and beverages that include cheeseburgers and hamburgers, chicken tenders and wings, french fries and cheese fries, hot dogs and other sausages, pasta and macaroni and cheese, pizza and calzones, and tacos and burritos. Many of these favorite teenage foods can undergo healthy makeovers with some food science experimentation, nutritional knowhow and creative cuisine.

Burgers and Fries

Instead of a double cheeseburger and large serving of fries, think lean. Prepare the burger with ground sirloin that contains 13 percent fat (one-half that of regular ground beef). Start with 4 ounces of ground meat and then pound the patties as thin as possible to cook quicker, and grill instead of fry. About ½ ounce of fat should remain and be discarded, which leaves about a 3½-ounce serving.

Toast the bun and bake potato wedges with just enough salt to retain flavor. Besides lettuce and tomatoes, dress the burger with sweet bell peppers, mushrooms, or grilled onions to add more vegetables, and use a little mustard, catsup or salsa instead of mayonnaise-based sauces.

A typical fast-food double cheeseburger contains about 530 calories, with about 30 grams of total fat (51 percent of total calories), about 95 milligrams of cholesterol, and about 1,310 milligrams of sodium. A typical order of large french fries contains about 540 calories, with about 26 grams of total fat (43 percent of total calories) and 1,210 milligrams of sodium. Changing the ingredients and techniques can help cut calories, total fat, cholesterol and sodium without changing protein too much. By using fewer condiments, sodium can be reduced as well.

Hot Dogs

A simple hot dog on a bun contains about 174 calories. Once it is loaded with substantial condiments, such as chili and cheese, it may exceed 500 calories. By choosing lean beef, poultry or soy dogs or sausages; limiting cheese and/or chili to 1 to 2 tablespoons; boiling or grilling instead of frying; adding fresh vegetables such as onions and tomatoes; and toasting the bun for more flavor, this favorite sandwich can be converted into a healthier option.

A typical fast-food hot dog contains about 240 calories, 14 grams of total fat (52.5 percent of total calories), and 730 milligrams of sodium. A typical chili-cheese dog contains about 350 calories, 21 grams of total fat (54 percent of total calories), and 1,070 milligrams of sodium. To reduce calories, substitute a turkey hot dog at about 100 calories (8 grams total fat), a low-fat beef hot dog at about 133 calories (11 grams total fat), or a fat-free beef, pork or turkey hot dog at about 50 calories (0 grams total fat).

Two ounces of cheese sauce contain about 60 calories, 5 grams of total fat (75 percent of total calories), and 360 milligrams of sodium. Two ounces of chili contain about 66 calories, 4 grams of total fat (54.5 percent of total calories), and 348 milligrams of sodium. Other condiments are lower in calories, but the sodium adds up, as shown in Table 11-26.

Macaroni and Cheese

Other than enriched pasta, the basic ingredients in macaroni and cheese are cheese, cream or dairy milk, and butter, which are mostly high in calories, total fat and cholesterol. A typical 1-cup serving of macaroni and cheese contains about 250 calories, 12 grams of total fat (44 percent of total calories), and 470 milligrams of sodium.

A light cheese sauce can be made with a combination of reduced-fat cheese and low-fat or nonfat milk. For each 1 cup of cooked macaroni, add just ¼ cup of light cheese sauce, and once carefully incorporated, add another ¼ cup of light cheese sauce and mix well. Do not top the dish with reduced-fat cheese, since it can toughen.

Cooking with reduced-fat cheese in this manner can be challenging. Here are some tips to maintain both taste and texture:

- Shred, crumble, or finely dice *cold* reduced-fat cheese for quick and consistent melting.
- Blend a small amount of strongly flavored cheese with reduced-fat cheese for more flavor.
- Allow shredded reduced-fat cheese to come to room temperature before adding to hot ingredients.
- Use starch, such as all-purpose flour, cornstarch, or potato flour, to help keep reduced-fat cheese from curdling. All-purpose flour needs a few minutes of cooking to remove its starchy taste.
- Add an acidic ingredient, such as a touch of lemon juice or wine, to help prevent reduced-fat cheese from becoming stringy.
- Heat reduced-fat cheese gradually, since it has different melting characteristics than regular cheese. The less it is heated, the better. Once melted, reduced-fat cheese may be tougher than full-fat cheese.

TABLE 11-26 Calories and Sodium in Common Condiments		
Condiments	**Calories**	**Sodium (milligrams)**
1 tablespoon ketchup	16 cal	175 mg
1 tablespoon yellow mustard	11	190
1 tablespoon brown mustard	14	200
1 tablespoon hot dog relish	14	225
1 tablespoon sweet relish	21	100

Pasta

A fast-food order of spaghetti with meat sauce totals about 2 cups, with about 600 calories, 13 grams of total fat, and 910 milligrams of sodium. This meal contains about one-third of the calories needed daily by some teenagers! Cut the portion in half to 1 cup, substitute whole-grain or high-protein pasta for the enriched white pasta, and use lean ground beef, poultry or texturized soy protein in the meat sauce. Add some ground or roasted vegetables to the sauce for more nutrients. Opt for reduced-fat hard cheese, such as Parmesan, instead of full-fat mozzarella to top the pasta—and watch the amount. By making these simple adjustments, a significant amount of vitamins A, C, and E; thiamin and niacin; and the minerals calcium, iron and zinc can be added—potentially with fewer calories, fat and sodium.

> **Morsel** The Pizza
> Look at itsy-bitsy Mitzi!
> See her figure slim and ritzy!
> She eats a Pizza!
> Greedy Mitzi!
> She is no longer itsy-bitsy!
> —Ogden Nash
> (American humorist
> and poet, 1902–1971)

Pizza

It is possible to make a tasty and wholesome pizza that is lower in calories and fat and higher in nutrients and fiber than a fast-food pizza. The fiber in pizza can be boosted by as much as 50 percent simply by using whole-wheat pizza dough. Two slices of thin crust pizza contain about 2 to 4 grams of fiber. Substitute all-purpose flour with mostly whole wheat flour, and the fiber content may increase to about 8 grams. The addition of garlic, onions, mushrooms, pineapple, sweet bell peppers and tomatoes boosts the fiber content even more.

Select thin pizza before deep-dish pizza; it saves calories, fat and sodium. Two slices of a 12-inch deep-dish cheese pizza made with dairy whole milk cheese contains about 617 calories, 33 grams of total fat (48 percent of total calories), and 1,573 milligrams of sodium. Two slices of a 12-inch thin crust cheese pizza made with dairy whole milk cheese contains about 408 calories, 23 grams of total fat (50 percent of total calories), and 1,285 milligrams of sodium. Change the cheese to a lower-fat option, or use less cheese to save calories, fat, and sodium. One-quarter of a commercial reduced-fat pizza contains about 366 calories and 9 grams of total fat, but the sodium content is still high at 1,460 milligrams per serving.

Tacos

South-of-the-border foods, condiments and beverages are now mainstream in US homes and food service institutions. Salsa, a spicy sauce made with tomatoes and chilies, is one of the most popular condiments in the US next to ketchup. Most tacos in the United States are made with crisp (fried) tortilla shells, but there are also soft versions in both wheat and corn with varying amounts of fiber. Soft tacos are more likely to be found in the Southwest and California.

Two beef tacos with hard shells contain about 442 calories, 28 grams of total fat (57 percent of total calories), and 516 milligrams of sodium. Two beef tacos with soft shells contain about 474 calories, 26 grams of total fat (49 percent of total calories), and about 846 milligrams of sodium.

Tacos with meat and lettuce, tomatoes and onions are a good source of nutrients, with protein; vitamins A, B6, B12, and C; niacin; and the minerals iron and zinc. Bean tacos are a good vegetarian choice, unless they are made with lard. Two typical fast-food bean tacos contain about 278 calories, 5.2 grams of total fat (46.8 percent of total calories), and 772 milligrams of sodium. To decrease the fat, refry the beans in a little vegetable oil or saute in a nonstick pan.

The Middle Years

MOVING INTO ADULTHOOD: AGES 20 TO 65

Most discussion about life cycle food and nutrition glosses over the "in-between" years: ages 20 to 65. This is because it is not a period of growth, but one of stability, where weight, food and nutrition intake and activity should be normal. Other than gender, the DRIs, DVs, MyPlate and other dietary standards are similar for this age group.

After adolescence and before the "older years," the best nutritional advice is to practice modification, moderation, movement and management. Modify old eating and activity habits and integrate new ones; moderate all health behaviors, including food intake, alcohol or drug use, sleep and exercise; move the body at least 30 minutes all days; and manage conditions or diseases as they arise.

The consensus among health professionals for "normal" adults in this age group is to consume *more* of the following:

- Beverages, especially water, antioxidant-rich teas, 100 percent fruit juice, calcium-rich dairy milk or milk substitutes, and wine with the polyphenol resveratrol (if consumed) for fluids, nutrients and protective substances
- Broccoli and other members of the cruciferous family, such as Brussels sprouts, cabbage and cauliflower, with phytonutrients for immunity
- Dairy milk and milk substitutes, calcium-fortified 100 percent fruit juice, green leafy vegetables, and canned salmon and sardines, with calcium for healthy bones and teeth
- Deep leafy green vegetables, such as chard, kale and spinach, with calcium, folate and iron for heart health and cancer protection
- Fatty coldwater fish, such as salmon and mackerel, with omega-3 fatty acids for brain and heart defense
- Fruits and vegetables with edible seeds and skin, such as dried or fresh apricots, berries, grapes and plums, for healthy digestion
- Healthy oils, such as canola and olive, with monounsaturated fatty acids for heart protection
- Lean protein, such as some cuts of beef and pork, fish and shellfish and skinless poultry, for muscle mass and blood sugar stabilization
- Oatmeal, barley and apples, with soluble fiber for healthy digestion
- Whole grains, such as brown rice, quinoa and whole wheat couscous, with B vitamins and fiber for healthy digestion

522

The consensus among health professionals for average adults in this age group is to consume *less* of the following:

- Alcohol
- Animal protein over bodily needs
- Extra sugars
- Fried foods
- Highly processed foods
- Extra fats and oils
- Sodium
- Sweetened beverages

Many people in this age group consume more of the foods and beverages they should be eating less of and less of the foods and beverages they should be eating more of—leading to obesity and nutrition-related diseases. Paying heed to this advice is the best transition to the "older years," when critical nutrients and nutrient requirements change.

Aging

GETTING OLDER: THE GRAYING OF AMERICA AND GLOBAL AGING

When does aging occur? When a person is 50 years of age? 70 years of age? Older? In biological terms, after a person reaches his or her growth potential, they start *aging*: the process of becoming older. Women may stop growing in their late teens, but men may continue to grow until their early twenties. After this point, the body starts to age, or decline. The rate is determined in part by genetics and in part by diet, exercise and healthy or unhealthy lifestyle choices.

> **FOOD BYTE**
>
> Life expectancy and infant mortality rates are used to measure the overall health of a society.
> *Life expectancy* in the United States shows a long-term upward trend, and infant mortality shows
> a long-term downward trend. Overall, death rates in the United States have declined, and the gap in
> life expectancy between African-American and Caucasian populations has narrowed. Between 2000
> and 2007, life expectancy at birth increased more for the US black than white populations. From 1980
> through 2007, life expectancy at birth in the United States increased from 70 years to 75 years for
> men and from 77 years to 80 years for women [52].

AGING: A NATURAL PROCESS

Aging is a predictable, natural process that encompasses all of the changes in an organism over time. In human beings, aging involves physical, psychological and social changes. The chronological age of a person is his age measured in years. Chronological aging is considered to be over 50 years of age. The biological age of a person is her physical state as a result of aging. Antiaging strategies try to prevent the demise of biological systems so people can add years to their lives. As a result, a 70-year-old person who engages in health-enhancing activities may function like a 50-year-old. His or her biological age is 50 years old.

Lifestyle factors that tend to increase life expectancy include a well-balanced and nutritious diet, regular physical activity, a relatively stress-free environment, the abstinence of alcohol and drugs (including nicotine), and the maintenance of normal body weight, blood pressure and cholesterol.

Women tend to outlive men in most cultures, and people in some cultures tend to outlive those in other cultures. For example, people in some Mediterranean and Asian countries have longer life spans that are attributed, in part, to their healthy diets. The average lifespan in the United States is 79 years of age for women and 72 years of age for men. Throughout the twentieth century, the average lifespan in the United States increased by more than 30 years, which is attributed to public health measures, including better food and nutrition [53].

US AND GLOBAL AGING

Due to the baby boom between 1946 and 1964, the number of people who are aging in the United States and worldwide is dramatically increasing. The most rapidly growing segment of the US population is currently aged 65 and older. According to the US Census Bureau, aging Americans are expected to double to about 70 million by 2030, which may be about 20 percent of the US population, or about one in five Americans [54].

The number of people worldwide aged 60 and older is expected to triple to more than 1 billion by 2030. The world's elderly population is increasing by about 800,000 people monthly. In fact, the "oldest old" are the fastest-growing segment of many national populations [55].

Starting in 2010, many baby boomers reached retirement age. Due to improved life expectancy from better disease identification and management, aging baby boomers should enter their senior years healthier than their predecessors. But will they? With increased obesity and related diseases, including cancer, cardiovascular disease, diabetes and hypertension, will life expectancy take a downward turn? A look at "healthy aging" and its relationship to diet may be foretelling.

SHIFTS IN HEALTHY AGING

Improved medical care and preventive efforts have produced a major shift in the leading causes of death in the United States. At the turn of the twentieth century—around the year 1900—people in the United States mostly died from infectious diseases and acute illnesses. At the end of the twentieth century, people mostly died from chronic diseases and degenerative illnesses.

523

It has been estimated that about 80 percent of older Americans live with at least one chronic condition, such as cancer, cardiovascular disease, dementia, diabetes, diverticulosis, hypertension, oral disease or osteoporosis—all of which have food and nutrition connections.

America's aging population is becoming more racially and ethnically diverse. But the health status of minority populations in the United States lags behind nonminorities, especially in blood pressure and vascular diseases, such as cardiovascular disease and hypertension, as well as cancer and diabetes—once again with nutritional roots.

At the crossroad of the twenty-first century—around the year 2000—three lifestyle behaviors—smoking, physical inactivity and poor diet—were the cause of about one-third of the deaths in the United States. These unhealthy behaviors underlie the leading chronic diseases in the United States: heart disease, cancer, diabetes and stroke.

To detect and control chronic diseases, the aging need to improve many aspects of their diet, lose and/or maintain weight, be more active, stop smoking, and seek regular health screenings. The US government and health organizations need to continue to work together to help to decrease health disparities in the aging and to lower health care costs. Many of the opportunities to achieve the most changes are community-based. However, change begins with the individual who still has the potential to alter her own destiny [56].

AGING AND THE USDA HEALTHY EATING INDEX

The Healthy Eating Index (HEI) is a measure of diet quality that assesses food intake compared to US government guidelines. In general, the overall HEI scores for people aged 65 years and older have not changed since 1989, when the first HEI was conducted. Only about 20 percent of people in the United States aged 65 to 74 years and 19 percent of US residents over 75 years of age had good diets.

The lowest HEI scores and the poorest intakes were for fruit and milk, and one of the greatest intakes was for saturated fat. The HEI concluded that most older Americans have poor diets and need improvement in all aspects of their diets, especially in fat reduction. Older Americans need to increase whole grains, dark green and orange or red fruits and vegetables, legumes, and dairy milk, and choose more nutrient-dense foods and less solid fats, added sugars and sodium—much like all Americans. Poor diets in older Americans are equated with food-related diseases and affect health care costs and food systems [57].

DIETARY DECLINE AND AGING

Why do diets decline as people age? The factors that have been suggested are environmental, physiological, psychological and socioeconomic. *Environmental* factors include inadequate transportation, institutional living, isolation, lack of food production facilities, limited food availability, poor housing and restricted services. *Physiological* factors include alcohol or drug abuse, chronic disease, decreased hunger, loss or decline in taste and smell, immobility, inactivity, oral health disorders, physical disabilities and poor dietary intake. *Psychological* factors include cognition disorders, companionship, dementia, depression, emotional isolation, indifference, loneliness, loss of spouse or significant other, and marital status. *Socioeconomic* factors include cultural values, economics, education, health care, religion and society.

This is a golden opportunity for nutrition, food science and culinary professionals to help improve the nutritional quality of foods and beverages for the aging, the accuracy and consistency of their diets, and the sensorial quality of foods and beverages in health care systems [58].

NORMAL PHYSIOLOGICAL CHANGES WITH AGING

Body systems are groups of organs that work together to perform certain tasks. *Senescence* is the decline in organ systems during aging and the increased risks of disease. While all organ systems slow down, they do not decline at the same rate, partially due to differences in health-enhancing efforts. The changes that the body undergoes during the aging process and the diseases that may arise are shown in Table 11-27.

NUTRITIONAL NEEDS, CONSIDERATIONS AND CONCERNS OF AGING

Around age 35, in addition to every organ system, there is a slowdown in every tissue and cell. As a result, there is a decrease in bone mineralization, cardiac output, hand grip flexibility, kidney function, maximum heart rate, maximum oxygen uptake, metabolism, muscle mass, taste and smell, and the vital capacity of the heart, as well as other vital functions. The rate at which this slowdown occurs is determined by the environment, genetics and lifestyle.

TABLE 11-27 Changes in Body Systems and Potential Diseases Associated with Aging

Body System	Disease Potential
Circulatory system	
Heart, blood and blood vessels	Atherosclerosis, decreased cardiac output and increased blood clotting
Digestive system	
Salivary glands, esophagus, stomach, liver, gallbladder, pancreas, intestines, rectum and anus	Decreased gastric acid, intrinsic factor, and saliva and increased constipation, heartburn, ulcers, and other gastrointestinal disorders
Endocrine system	
Hypothalamus, pituitary gland, pineal gland, thyroid, parathyroids and adrenals	Decreased growth, reproductive and thyroid hormone production
Excretory system	
Integumentary, digestive, respiratory and urinary systems	Decreased bladder control, blood filtration rate and kidney function
Lymphatic (immune) system	
Leukocytes, tonsils, adenoids, thymus and spleen	Decreased immune function, increased risk of infections and cancer
Integumentary system	
Skin, hair, nails and sweat and oil glands	Decreased elasticity, pigmentation, and thickness and increased bruising, hair thinning, hair loss and wrinkling
Musculoskeletal system	
Muscles, bones, cartilage, ligaments	Decreased bone formation, muscle mass, strength and stamina, and increased bone loss, fractures, joint stiffness and pain
Nervous system	
Brain, spinal cord and peripheral nervous system	Decreased brain weight, nervous impulses, neurotransmitters, short-term memory and sensory functions
Reproductive system	
Ovaries, fallopian tubes, uterus, vagina, mammary glands, testes, vas deferens, seminal vesicles and prostate	Decreased fertility, male and female hormone production, eggs and sperm count
Respiratory system	
Pharynx, larynx, trachea, bronchi, lungs and diaphragm	Decreased lung capacity and increased susceptibility to infections

525

This slowdown brings decreased needs for certain nutrients and greater needs for other nutrients, including the following. Altered cardiovascular, endocrine, gastrointestinal, musculoskeletal, renal and sensory functions also affect nutritional requirements.

Calories

Caloric needs gradually decline with age. This is because lean body mass decreases, which lowers the basal metabolic rate (BMR). By cutting out extraneous calories and including muscle-building activities to maintain lean body mass, these practices should help normalize weight throughout aging.

Protein

The need for protein declines during aging, parallel to the decrease in lean body mass. But protein intake must still be adequate to sustain body weight. Poor protein intake may decrease immune function and cause the body to be more prone to disease. The DRI for protein ranges from 10 to 35 percent of total daily calories depending on body size and muscular demands. About 46 grams (184 calories) of protein per day are recommended for women over 50 years of age, and about 56 grams (224 calories) of protein per day are recommended for men 50 years of age or over. High-quality lean protein foods such as fish and seafood, lean meats, legumes, reduced-fat dairy products and skinless poultry should be encouraged.

Carbohydrates

About 45 to 65 percent of the total daily caloric intake for people 50 years of age and older should come from carbohydrates, with an emphasis on fruits, vegetables and whole grains for fiber and phytonutrients. Refined and processed carbohydrates should be decreased to allow for these healthier carbohydrates.

The DRI for carbohydrates is about 130 grams (520 calories) daily. Added sugars should be less than 10 percent of total calories. Those who are active and aging may require more carbohydrates; those who are sedentary and aging may require fewer carbohydrates for decreased energy needs.

Fiber

Americans are chronically fiber-poor, but as they age, fiber becomes even more essential. This is because the gastrointestinal tract becomes more sluggish during aging. Other factors that contribute to poor gastrointestinal health include poor fluid intake and decreased activity.

The recommendations for daily fiber intake for people over 50 years of age are 21 grams of fiber for women and 30 grams of fiber for men, or about 14 grams of fiber per 1,000 calories consumed. A variety of fruits, legumes, vegetables and whole grains that the aging gastrointestinal tract can tolerate, with at least 6 to 8 cups of fluid daily, are recommended.

Lipids

While there is no DRI established for lipids, sensible guidelines established by the American Heart Association (AHA) suggest a limit of 30 percent total calories from lipids for people without cardiovascular disease and no more than 20 percent total calories from lipids for people with cardiovascular disease. Healthy fats from monounsaturated vegetable oils and fish are recommended within these guidelines.

Vitamins

Vitamin D may be deficient in the aging due to reduced exposure to sunlight and decreased synthesis of this vitamin in the skin. Vitamin D deficiency may lead to musculoskeletal disorders, such as *osteomalacia*, or bone softening. Fortified dairy products, breads and cereals, and salmon and other fatty fish supply vitamin D.

Levels of antioxidant vitamins A, C and E may be low in the aging from reduced intake of fruits, vegetables and whole grains. This may lead to poor immune function and increased oxidative stress to body tissues. Vitamins A and C are prevalent in brightly colored fruits and vegetables, and vitamin E is rich in nuts, seeds, and fruit and vegetable oils.

Folate may be difficult for the aging to obtain, since it is mostly found in fresh green leafy vegetables, which are expensive and sometimes unavailable. Inadequate folate may lead to anemia and higher risks of cervical and colon cancer. Besides green leafy vegetables, folate is abundant in fortified breakfast cereals, legumes, orange juice and whole grains.

Vitamins B6 and B12 may be substandard in the aging, since they tend to consume less protein, particularly less red meat. This may cause an elevated level of homocysteine in the bloodstream and increased risk of cardiovascular disease. Bananas, figs, low-fat meats, melons and potatoes provide vitamin B6.

Vitamin B12 deficiency is estimated to affect 10 to 15 percent of people over 60 years of age. Compared with younger people, the aging absorb less protein-bound vitamin B12, which results in a high incidence of atrophic gastritis.

Atrophic gastritis is a chronic inflammation of the stomach mucosa that affects the stomach's secretion of hydrochloric acid, pepsin and intrinsic factor—needed in vitamin B12 absorption. Atropic gastritis may lead to digestive disorders, vitamin B12 deficiency and megaloblastic anemia. Stomach acid is not required for the absorption of vitamin B12–fortified foods or vitamin B12 supplements for adequate absorption.

The DRI for vitamin B12 for people 50 years of age and older is 2.4 milligrams daily. If aging people refrain from consuming animal protein, it is essential that they consume vitamin B12–fortified foods or B12 supplements. Foods that are fortified with vitamin B12 include some meat analogs, nutritional yeast, ready-to-eat cereals, and soy- and other plant-based milks.

Minerals

Calcium, iron and zinc may be subnormal in the aging. A lifetime of poor calcium intake, lactose intolerance and decreased gastric acidity may impair calcium absorption and lead to reduced bone mass.

Low levels of iron and zinc may be caused by poor protein intake, particularly red meat, or substances that interfere with their absorption, particularly phytates and oxylates. While anemia is less common after menopause, decreased gastric acidity may impair iron absorption. Chronic blood loss from gastrointestinal disorders may also increase iron needs. Zinc deficiency may affect immune function. Whether or not zinc deficiency affects taste and smell is debatable.

If aging people shun animal products, then calcium, iron and zinc status may suffer. Like vitamin D, calcium is found in dairy products; calcium-fortified foods and beverages, such as juices, breads and cereals; green leafy vegetables, such as broccoli and spinach; and the small bones of fish, such as canned salmon and sardines. If the aging are lactose-intolerant, then nondairy sources of calcium should be favored.

Iron and zinc are mostly found in animal products. Dried fruits, green leafy vegetables, iron-fortified cereals and legumes contain nonheme iron with poorer absorption than heme iron in animal products. Some legumes and enriched cereals contain zinc. Dried fruits and legumes are high in fiber and helpful for sluggish digestion.

Phytonutrients

By consuming an array of plant-based foods and beverages, an aging person should be able to obtain plenty of phytonutrients, disease-protective plantlike substances. Carotenoids in orange and deep yellow fruits and vegetables, especially beta-carotene and lutein, may help to prevent cataracts, decline in vision, and macular degeneration.

Anthocyanins, which lend fruits and vegetables their blue-purple color, and phenolics in such foods as apples, artichokes, berries, cherries, plums and potatoes, may help with memory, urinary tract health and reduced cancer risks. Allicin in onions and garlic and selenium in mushrooms may promote heart health and reduced cancer risks.

Sodium

The recommendation for sodium consumption in people 51 years of age and older is 1,500 milligrams of sodium daily. This is especially critical for people who are African American and those who have high blood pressure, diabetes or chronic kidney disease, who are at higher risk for hypertension and its ramifications: congestive heart failure, heart disease, kidney disease and stroke.

As a whole, the aging should choose and prepare foods with little salt and consume plenty of potassium-rich foods, such as fruits and vegetables, to help reduce the risk of hypertension. People with diagnosed hypertension should also meet the DRI for potassium, which is 4,700 milligrams daily.

Water

Dehydration may be the most important nutritional concern of the elderly. Because aging people have a reduced sense of thirst, they may consume far fewer fluids than their body requires (at least four cups per 1,000 calories). Increased urine output magnifies the need for adequate fluids to prevent dehydration. While coffee and tea supply fluids, they may also increase urination and lead to dehydration and lead to dehydration.

One factor that affects the nutritional requirements of aging is *activity*. To achieve calorie balance and reduce body fat, cardiovascular and muscular activities are necessary throughout aging. Safe and effective cardiovascular activities for the aging include walking and swimming—walking because it stresses the long bone and muscles of the body and swimming because it is buoyant and protects the bones and joints. Other activities, such as biking and running, are still possible during aging as long as a person has good balance

527

and their joints can handle the impact. Muscular activities should include strength training to increase and preserve muscle mass. See Chapter 10 for examples.

CONDITIONS AND DISEASES OF AGING

The following conditions and diseases of aging may alter these nutrient requirements. Recommendations are provided for each.

- *Atherosclerosis:* Carefully monitor calories, sodium and water intake, particularly if congestive heart failure is present. Decrease dietary fats and increase fiber.
- *Cancer:* Increase fruits, legumes, vegetables and whole grains for antioxidants, fiber and phytonutrients. Decrease dietary fats.
- *Depression and dementia:* Serve small, balanced meals that are regularly spaced throughout the day so aging people remember when to eat and are not overwhelmed by large portions.
- *Diabetes:* Serve balanced and moderate meals and snacks to maintain blood sugar, with fewer refined foods and more fiber from fruits, legumes, vegetables and whole grains.
- *Hypertension and stroke:* Reduce sodium, dietary fats and cholesterol and the amount of protein in extreme cases. Increase fruits and vegetables.
- *Oral disease:* Decrease total carbohydrates, especially those that are refined and sticky. Increase foods and beverages with vitamin C, folic acid, calcium and zinc.
- *Osteoarthritis:* Increase foods and beverages with vitamins A and D and calcium.
- *Osteoporosis:* Increase foods and beverages with vitamins A, C, D and K; calcium; phosphorus; and magnesium.
- *Renal disease:* Carefully monitor calories, protein, calcium, phosphorus, potassium and sodium.

DIETARY GUIDELINES FOR THE AGING

The *2010 US Dietary Guidelines* for Americans recommend that healthy, sedentary females aged 51 to 76 years and older consume about 1,600 calories daily. Healthy, sedentary males aged 51 to 60 should consume about 2,200 calories daily. From ages 56 to 76 and older, this amount decreases to about 2,000 calories daily to account for decreased muscle mass and declining energy needs. Table 11-28 shows the recommended average

TABLE 11-28 Recommended Average Daily Intake Amounts for Healthy Aging

1,600 Daily Calories	2,000 Daily Calories	2,200 Daily Calories
5 ounces of breads, cereals, cooked grains or starchy vegetables with one-half (2½ ounces) whole grains (1 ounce serving is about one slice of bread or about ½ cup of cooked rice or pasta)	6 ounces of breads, cereals, cooked grains or starchy vegetables with one-half (3 ounces) whole grains	6 ounces of breads, cereals, cooked grains or starchy vegetables with one-half (3 ounces) whole grains
2 cups of cooked and/or fresh vegetables (1 serving is about ½ cup of cooked vegetables or about 1 cup of fresh vegetables)	2½ cups of cooked and/or fresh vegetables	3 cups of cooked and/or fresh vegetables
1½ cups of fruit (1 serving is about 1 small piece of fruit or about ½ cup of cooked fruit or fruit juice)	2 cups of fruit	2 cups of fruit
3 cups of low or nonfat dairy milk and milk products or substitutes (1 serving is about 1 cup of dairy milk or yogurt)	3 cups of dairy low- or nonfat milk and milk products or substitutes	3 cups of dairy low- or nonfat milk and milk products or substitutes
5 ounces of lean meat or meat substitutes (1 ounce serving is about 1 slice or one 1×1×1-inch cube)	5½ ounces of lean meat or meat substitutes	6 ounces of lean meat or meat substitutes
5 teaspoons of additional healthy oils and fats, such as olive oil, peanut butter, or trans-free margarine (1 serving is about 1 teaspoon regular or 1 tablespoon reduced-fat)	5½ teaspoons of additional healthy fats and fats	6 teaspoons of additional healthy fats and fats

daily intake amounts at calorie levels that range from 1,600 through 2,200 calories. Additional servings at each calorie level are highlighted.

HEALTHY MEAL PLANNING FOR THE AGING

It can be difficult to plan and cook for aging people. Like infants, they can be set in their ways and difficult to please. This list provides some steps to take and ideas for even the most problematic eater.

1. Individualize daily needs for calories, carbohydrates, fiber, protein, fats, vitamins, minerals, sodium and water. Provide:
   a. enough calories to meet daily needs (see "Dietary guidelines for the aging"). Increase about 200 calories if moderately active and another 200 calories if active.
   b. about one-half of total calories from carbohydrates, with at least half of these carbohydrates from whole grains for fiber, vitamins and minerals.
   c. at least two servings (2 to 3 ounces each) of lean protein from lean meats or high-quality vegetable sources.
   d. plenty of fruits and vegetables, prepared as tolerated or as diet permits.
   e. fluids with each meal and in between meals.
2. Adjust calorie level and nutrients for conditions or diseases, or conditions that affect nutritional status (see "Conditions and diseases of aging").
3. Review medications and accommodate for any dietary restrictions.
4. Plan three to six balanced and moderate meals and snacks throughout the day.
5. Control portion sizes. Follow the portion guidelines that are provided in Chapter 1, including plating recommendations. Judgment diminishes as people age. Portion control helps prevent overeating and reminds the aging about the position of food on a plate.
6. Use salt- and sodium-containing foods in moderation. The recommendation for sodium consumption in people 51 years of age and older is 1,500 milligrams of sodium daily. Aging people with hypertension, cardiovascular disease and/or renal disease should be particularly cautious. Check Chapters 7 and 9 for advice on sodium reduction in cooking.
7. Supply enough fiber for gastrointestinal health or GI disease management. A practical guideline is 14 grams of fiber per 1,000 calories consumed. Just 1 cup of cooked oatmeal (5 grams) and 1 cup of fresh raspberries (8 grams) nearly supplies this amount, as does 1 cup of lentil soup (15.6 grams). Check the tips for adding fiber in cooking in Chapter 4.
8. Prepare reduced-sugar foods for prediabetics and those with diabetes. Desserts can be included in diabetic diets as long as they are carbohydrate-controlled. This generally means smaller portions with natural sugars and fiber from fruits, nuts, reduced-fat dairy products and whole grains.
9. Create heart-healthy foods that are reduced in fats and cholesterol. Use lean protein and low-fat cooking methods, including broiling, grilling or roasting. Replace some animal protein with legumes, higher-protein vegetables such as spinach or peas, or whole grains where sensible, such as ground oats or legumes in ground beef recipes.
10. Add calcium to recipes wherever possible. Aging people need calcium for healthy blood, bones, gums, heart, muscles, nerves and teeth. If dairy beverages and foods are not well tolerated, lactose-reduced products can be substituted in recipes. Consider ways to incorporate calcium-rich greens, canned fish with bones, and calcium-fortified breads, cereals and juices in meals.
11. Serve food that is easy to chew and swallow and is not too sticky for denture wearers. Aging people produce less saliva, and they may have trouble moving food around in their mouth. Fruits and vegetables should be torn or cut into mouth-sized pieces; firmer fruits, legumes and vegetables should be fork-tender and diced or minced to promote easy chewing. Recipes should include enough moisture to mix food well and help distribute flavors.
12. Incorporate alcohol sparingly, if at all. Make sure that alcohol is safe to consume with any medications. Alcohol can be used as an appetite stimulant before meals and as a flavor enhancer in some dishes. Wine and beer contain antioxidants, which may have cardiovascular- and cancer-preventive qualities.

529

Morsel "He who eats alone chokes alone."
—Proverb [59]

Bite on This: diet, dementia and Alzheimer's disease

Dementia is a progressive decline in cognitive brain functions that is due to damage or disease. It affects memory, attention, language and problem solving. *Alzheimer's disease* is the most common type of dementia. The relationship of diet, dementia and Alzheimer's disease is complex, debatable and inconclusive to date. Some vitamins and homeopathic remedies have been touted as memory aids. These include vitamin B1 (thiamin), found in legumes, pork, sunflower seeds and whole and enriched grains; vitamin B3 (niacin), found in beef, bran, chicken, mushrooms, peanuts and tuna; vitamin B6, found in bananas, broccoli and spinach; vitamin B12, found mostly in animal products; and folic acid, found in chickpeas, green leafy vegetables, orange juice and sprouts. While the herbs ginkgo and ginseng have been associated with improved memory, research has not fully supported their connections.

Some people with dementia or Alzheimer's disease may develop a constant appetite for food and gain weight from consuming too many foods or beverages or from inactivity. Others may have a poor appetite or lose interest in eating, which may lead to compromised immunity, decreased energy and impaired concentration. People may reject food initially or say they are not hungry. This condition is not to be forced.

Rather, food should be served in a relaxed and unhurried manner. Soft background music may be comforting for some people, but to others, it may be distracting. Carefully test which works best. Some people may prefer to eat in company, while others may prefer to eat alone. By observing and copying others, people with dementia may be prompted to eat on their own.

Offer small, frequent meals and snacks, regularly spaced throughout the day, since people with dementia may forget when to eat or not be able to recall their last meal. Only one course should be served at a time. Without adequate judgment, a person with dementia may be dependent on external regulation. Fluids should be monitored to help prevent dehydration—a common condition among those with memory disorders. Alcohol and caffeinated beverages should be minimized.

Dementia may cause people to reject certain foods that they loved in the past and request new and unusual dishes, or vice versa. They may mix up courses or even start a meal with dessert. Sweetness is comforting; it also encourages people to eat more. Just 1 teaspoon of sugar per pound of vegetables may encourage a person with dementia to consume a serving of vegetables—even if he does not like them. Some people with dementia may eat nonfood items, such as laundry soap, pet-food or potpourri, which may have a sweet taste or smell. Keep anything that is nonedible out of sight.

Tableware should be simple so a person with dementia does not become too distracted. Solid-colored tableware that contrasts with food makes food easier to see. Foods should be clearly plated, or they may be ignored or forgotten.

People with memory loss may lose interest in food if it is the wrong temperature. This can easily happen if people forget to eat, take too long to eat, or have problems with coordination or swallowing. To help solve this problem, insulated plates can be used to keep food warm. Or small portions can be warmed, and, once they are consumed, additional portions can be heated and served. Food that is too cold may be perceived as tasteless. Moderately cool foods and beverages may be better recognized and enjoyed.

If coordination problems persist and become issues, or if managing cutlery is difficult, people with dementia may become agitated. Foods such as peas, sauces and spaghetti may be especially difficult to manage. Some adaptive lightweight cutlery functions as both a spoon and a fork. Nonslip placemats keep plates and cups in place. A cup with two handles permits a steadier grip. Some cups do not spill, and others have spouts—much like child-friendly utensils. Some people with dementia need to relearn these basic eating and drinking skills.

Since the relationship between diet and the brain is still unclear, these guidelines are not fixed. The unconventional food behaviors that may accompany memory loss, Alzheimer's disease and dementia require compassion, diligence and patience. Nutrition, food science and culinary professionals who develop foods and beverages, recipes and meal plans for this unique group of individuals need to be adaptive, creative and resourceful. As the US and global population ages, this will be a growing area of food and nutrition that may offer a number of employment opportunities.

Bite on This: cooking for the aging—foods for one or two

A significant challenge of cooking for aging people is learning how to shop, prepare, cook, and store recipes for just one or two people. Single households are one of the fastest-growing segments of the US population. Typical consumer recipes are still designed to serve a nuclear family—many with six or more portions. After years of cooking for large institutions and families, chefs and care providers need to downsize by making smaller, flavorful portions for tiny appetites. Here are some suggestions:

- Think about convenience and ease. Buy what can be used, and use only what is bought. Purchase foods in single portions or portions that allow thawing only what is needed.
- Downsize recipes. Use recipes that call for small quantities of ingredients, and meticulously measure. The balance of emulsifiers, flavors and leavening agents, and so on must be exact because there is less room for error with such small quantities. Some handy instructions for downsizing recipes are provided in Table 11-29.
- Use cooking times only as guidelines. Appearance, aroma, texture, taste and other sensory elements help to determine whether or not a recipe is "finished." Physical variables such as altitude, type of burner or oven and temperature may also affect a recipe's outcome. Smaller portions for the aging will probably cook or bake faster, so check them often. They may also lose nutrients faster than larger portions, since there is more surface area that is vulnerable to air, light, water and other substances.
- Freeze foods in correct portion sizes. Use the portion guidelines in Chapter 1. They may have to be cut in half or one-third for smaller appetites. Then package foods well for freezing. Almost any food can be frozen in small quantities, except canned foods and eggs in shells. Some foods do not freeze well, such as lettuce and those in mayonnaise or cream sauce. Raw meat and poultry maintain their quality longer when frozen than cooked meats, which lose moisture during cooking.
- Prepare one-dish meals with lean protein, vegetables and whole grains. These include casseroles, chili, soups or stews. Refrigerate and use in one to two days, or freeze in covered, shallow containers within two hours after cooking. Allow air space around the containers for cold air to circulate and to promote rapid and even cooling. Taste and texture may be compromised.

531

TABLE 11-29 How to Downsize Recipes to One-Half or One-Third

To reduce a recipe by one-half, use the measurements on the left, divide by one-half and adjust as needed. Not every recipe will work this precisely. It is best to decrease individual ingredients gradually until the right proportions are reached.

Instead of	Use
¼ cup	2 tablespoons
⅓ cup	2 tablespoons + 2 teaspoons
½ cup	¼ cup
⅔ cup	⅓ cup
¾ cup	6 tablespoons
1 tablespoon	1½ teaspoons
1 teaspoon	½ teaspoon
½ teaspoon	¼ teaspoon
¼ teaspoon	⅛ teaspoon

To reduce a recipe by one-third, use the measurements on the left, divide by one-third and adjust as needed.

Instead of	Use
¼ cup	1 tablespoon + 1 teaspoon
⅓ cup	1 tablespoon + 2⅓ teaspoons
½ cup	2 tablespoons + 2 teaspoons
1 cup	5 tablespoons + 1 teaspoon

- Use the equipment with the correct scale. Use smaller pots and pans for scaled-down recipes, such as a small 1- or 1½-quart saucepan, medium 2- or 2½-quart saucepan, small 6- or 7-inch saute pan, or medium 8- to 10-inch saute pan.
- A mini–food processor or blender and hand mixer are helpful for mixing small quantities. A kitchen scale is useful for measuring tiny amounts of ingredients. Measuring cups and measuring spoons should be calibrated in small increments.
- Reduce cooking and baking times to correspond with scaled-down equipment. Reduce baking time by about 10 minutes if a shallower dish is used than what is called for in a recipe. More exposed surface area increases browning. Increase baking time by about 10 percent if the dish is deeper than what is called for in a recipe. Less exposed surface area may cause a gummier product with little crust.
- Small baked items, such as brownies, cakes and puddings, can be baked in ceramic ramekins, 4-inch springform pans or 4-inch pastry shells. Baking time may have to be increased by 10 to 20 percent. The pastry shells should be placed on insulated baking sheets to promote uniform baking and prevent overbrowning.
- Repurpose leftovers into new dishes, but follow food safety guidelines. Repurposing leftovers is economical and nutritious as long as foods are gently handled or carefully reheated to prevent nutrient loss. Wash your hands before handling foods—especially meats—and use clean utensils and surfaces.
- Change the garnish in vegetable soups or stews; add lean protein, starch (noodles, polenta, potatoes or rice), or cooked legumes, lentils or peas. Before serving, cover and reheat soups, sauces, gravies and other "wet" foods to a rolling boil. More solid foods, such as casseroles, should be reheated to at least 165°F. Cooked vegetables with lean protein and light salad dressing can be combined into entree salads. Do not refrigerate or freeze a second time.
- Use prepackaged single servings to supplement cooked meals. These may include shredded cheese, prechopped vegetables, flash-frozen vegetables in resealable bags, quick-cooking rice, shredded potatoes, and single-serving fruits and vegetables in their own juice or without added sauces.

532

Bite on This: tasty foods when taste and smell decline

Taste and smell begin to decline around 50 years of age, with a more dramatic decline after age 70. Foods and beverages may not be enjoyed with the same appreciation as when people were younger. These sensory enhancement techniques help to make food more appealing when interest in eating diminishes:

- Choose high-quality food at its peak, when it is fresh, brightly colored and full-flavored.
- Make sure that foods have great visual appeal for aging eyes, with bright colors and different textures.
- Select ethnically correct foods that are suitably arranged and garnished.
- Place portions in set layouts on plates with simple patterns and solid colors so people who can no longer smell or taste may still discriminate among foods.
- Arouse hunger by covering or tenting plates or bowls. Remove the covers right before serving, and then encourage an older person to take a big whiff. This causes saliva and gastric juices to flow and helps mastication (chewing) and digestion. It also signals the person that there are more "good tastes" to come.
- Serve aromatic foods, such as baked cookies or chicken soup, to help activate "smell memory." This technique is particularly useful with Alzheimer's patients. However, disagreeable smells from garlic or broccoli may trigger unpleasant memories.
- Encourage people to chew their food well because it helps to break down food, release flavor molecules, and set up air currents for maximum enjoyment.
- Combine familiar tastes with new tastes to broaden the range of foods and nutrients that people consume.
- Contrast textures, sizes, and shapes in a meal to reduce sensory fatigue or boredom.
- Vary temperatures in a meal, but avoid temperature extremes that might overstimulate thermoreceptors. People expect hot food to be at least warm and cold food to be at least cool. Too much variance may be confusing and disturbing.

- Liberalize some diet restrictions, with a few medical exceptions that should be first reviewed by a health care provider. If people have lived this long and are well managed through diet and medications, they should occasionally be able to deviate from rigid diets.

Recipe: Garlic-Enhanced Mashed Potatoes

*Mashed potatoes are a beloved food of many aging people because they often bring memories of home. Usually laden with butter and salt, carbohydrate-filled mashed potatoes no longer fill many plates. These **Garlic-Enhanced Mashed Potatoes** in the **Recipe file** which is located within the Culinary Nutrition website at www.culinarynutrition.elsevier.com, have just enough garlic to perk up aging taste buds without offending them. Because they taste so good, less can be used— which means fewer calories, fat and sodium compared to mashed potatoes of former times. Potatoes contain protein and fiber, vitamins B6 and C, and the minerals copper, manganese and potassium. They are a nutritious side when prepared healthfully, like in this recipe. The finished dish is shown within the centerfold **Photo file** in Plate 10.2.*

SERVE IT FORTH

1a. Alice Waters is the world-renowned celebrated chef and owner of Chez Panisse in Berkeley, California. One of Alice's passions is an edible garden at Berkeley's Martin Luther King Jr. Middle School. This project involves faculty and children in the planting, gardening, harvesting, preparation and consuming of food. It serves to underscore the fundamental relationship of food in children's lives, while it teaches children mutual respect for both one another and the planet. This project is a significant part of the school's curriculum, including its lunch program.

The King Middle School Edible Schoolyard pilot project continues to serve as a model for schools across the country. It has a mission to "transform the health and values of every student by building and sharing a food curriculum for the school system." Check out the Edible Schoolyard Project at http://www.edibleschoolyard.org/.

- If you were hired to recreate an edible schoolyard at a neighborhood school that is based on the Martin Luther King Jr. Middle School Edible Schoolyard, how would you go about doing this?
- Check out the Edible Schoolyard Kitchen at http://edibleschoolyard.org/berkeley/day-kitchen. Based on this model, how would you create a kitchen like this one, and how would it function? What types of recipes and activities would you use and demonstrate?
- For both projects, be specific in your approaches, goals, methods, projected outcomes and evaluations.

2a. Chef Ann Cooper is rightly titled "The Renegade Lunch Lady." Chef Ann served as the executive chef and director of wellness and nutrition at the Ross School in East Hampton, New York, where she developed an integrated school lunch curriculum that was centered on organic, regional, seasonal and sustainable meals. Chef Ann has transformed public school cafeterias in New York City, Harlem, and Bridgehampton in New York; Berkeley, California; and Denver, Colorado, where she has taught students why good food choices matter, using innovative strategies and fresh organic lunches.

Chef Ann wants people to join her on her mission to change the way children are eating. Specifically, she wants to tackle "outdated district spending policies, commodity-based food service organizations, political platforms with no mention of school food or child health—and ultimately the USDA—to ensure that kids everywhere have wholesome, nutritious, delicious food at school."

- Review Chef Ann's mission at http://www.lunchlessons.org and describe what you would do in your neighborhood school district about school lunches based on Chef Ann's work. Be specific in your goals, methods, projected outcomes and evaluations.
- What are the similarities and/or differences in your neighborhood school district compared to Chef Ann's settings in New York and Colorado? (Consider economic, educational, ethnic, religious, rural versus urban, sociological and other factors.) What does this tell you about the ability to recreate programs such as this one?

3a. The number of people who are aged 65 years and older is rapidly growing as baby boomers age. To help meet this market, the Stay-Right-Here hotel chain has moved aggressively into the senior housing arena, called the "life-care industry." The Stay-Right-Here's life-care industry project is a twofold operation. The first operation, called "independent full-service," provides a range of services for people who are totally independent to those that require assistance in day-to-day needs. Meals, transportation services, recreation facilities and some medical services are provided.

The second operation, called "catered living," incorporates a modest level of assistance through skilled nursing for those people who require more advanced care. As people age, they can progress through these various levels of care and services within the Stay-Right-Here facilities.

Residents place a lot of emphasis on food selection and service. Community dining areas and cafes are available; residents also cook and dine in their own apartments if they can and as they choose.

> **Morsel** "The kitchen, reasonably enough, was the scene of my first gastronomic adventure. I was on all fours. I crawled into the vegetable bin, settled on a giant onion and ate it, skin and all. It must have marked me for life, for I have never ceased to love the hearty flavor of raw onions." —James Beard (American chef and food writer, 1903–1985) [60]

○ You have been hired as the executive chef of the Stay-Right-Here hotel chain to plan and supervise the food service for the independent full-service facilities, with recommendations for the catered living facilities.

○ Based on the information you have learned in this chapter about feeding the aging, what recommendations and guidelines would you provide for each of these operations of the Stay-Right-Here hotel chain? Be specific in your responses. Include goals, methods, projected outcomes and evaluations.

Three additional activities can be found within the *Culinary Nutrition* website at www.culinarynutrition.elsevier.com.

WHAT'S COOKING?

1. Interactive food experiments with children: making raisins

Objectives
○ To understand how grapes become raisins
○ To preserve fruit by removing water
○ To compare the sensory characteristics of food
○ To practice food safety

Materials
Large bunch fresh, firm, seedless Thompson grapes; food scale; water; towel; plastic-coated trays; pieces of cheesecloth to cover trays; glass container with airtight lid

Procedure
○ Weigh the grapes and record.
○ Reserve a few fresh grapes for later comparison.
○ Rinse the grapes in water; blot with paper towels.
○ Remove the grapes from their stems; spread the grapes evenly on the trays; cover and secure the trays with cheesecloth.
○ Place the trays outside in direct sunlight to dry where the air can freely circulate but away from any dirt or dust. (The trays can be placed in a 140°F oven until dry.)
○ Test the grapes for dryness. If the grapes spring apart and are leathery and pliable, then they are ready. If not, continue to dry.
○ Remove the grapes from the trays; weigh the grapes again and record.

Evaluation
Compare the weight of the grapes before and after drying. The difference between the two values is the amount of water that is lost during drying. What has happened to this water?

Compare the fresh grapes to the dried grapes in appearance. Describe any changes in color, taste, form and texture or other observations. The color should change from green to brown; the texture should change from smooth to wrinkled; the form should change from round to flattened spheres; and the taste should change from sweet to sweeter. Why should this happen in each instance?

Use a Data Sheet like the one that follows to record these values and observations.

Data Sheet

Fresh Grapes	Dried Grapes
Weight	Weight
Appearance	Appearance
Color	Color
Form	Form
Taste	Taste
Texture	Texture
Other	Other

Culinary applications

Other fruits can be dried in this manner or on a low oven setting (140°F). Add about 2 teaspoons of lemon juice or ⅛ teaspoon of ascorbic acid (Vitamin C) for each 2 cups of light-colored fruit, such as apricots or pineapple, to prevent darkening.

What other culinary applications can you suggest that incorporate your observations?

2. Interactive food experiments with children: making cheese

Objectives

○ To observe the process of cheese production
○ To separate curds from whey
○ To learn about herb and spice combinations and flavor
○ To compare different cheeses that are made from different milks

Materials

1 quart plain, nonfat yogurt; ½ yard doubled cheesecloth; 1 yard strong string or twine; sink; large bowl; any or all of these herbs and seasonings: Italian seasoning, Herbes de Provence, black pepper, garlic or onion granules, dill or parsley and caraway, fennel, or sesame seeds

Procedure

○ Form a bag with the cheesecloth by drawing up the sides.
○ Place the yogurt inside the cheesecloth bag; tie tightly with string or twine.
○ Hang the yogurt-filled bag around a faucet or nozzle over a sink.
○ Let the whey drip from the bag into a large bowl for a few hours or overnight.
○ Note observations on a Data Sheet (see following example).
○ Measure the amount of whey that is produced.
○ When the cheese curds solidify, remove them from the bag.
○ Remove sections of the cheese curds and roll in herbs, spices and/or seeds.
○ Refrigerate the cheese curds and whey separately.

Evaluation: Use a Data Sheet like the one that follows to record your observations.

Data Sheet

Changes in yogurt	Time
Color	
Consistency	
Odor	
Taste with herbs, spices, seeds	
Taste without herbs spices, seeds	

Whey	Amount produced
Color	
Consistency	
Odor	
Taste	

Report any changes in the yogurt and the times these changes occurred. Note the color, consistency, odor, and taste of curds with/without the herbs, spices, and/or seeds.

How much whey was produced? Note the color, consistency, odor and taste on the Data Sheet. Whey can be mixed into smoothies, milk or juice to boost the protein content. It can also be added to hot cereals and casseroles or mixed into cookie or cake batters. Recipes will probably require adjustment for this additional liquid. If the whey is sour, some sweetener may need to be added.

Culinary applications

This exercise can be redone with heated goat, rice, dairy skim milk or soy milk. What do you project will happen to the color, consistency, odor and taste of each of these cheese curds and their whey? How can each of these be used in recipes?

What commercial cheese (if any) is similar to the nonfat cheese curds? Is there any commercial cheese that is similar to the cheese curds that are made from goat, rice, dairy skim or soy milk?

3. Interactive food experiments with children: making bean snacks

Objectives

○ To see how dried legumes absorb water
○ To create a nutritious snack food that is similar to peanuts
○ To understand how soybeans are used in food products

Materials

Dried soybeans, 1 cup measure, large bowl, water, plastic wrap or aluminum foil, refrigerator, baking sheet, oven, vegetable oil, large spoon, herbs and spices (salt and pepper are optional)

Procedure

○ Wash 1 cup of soybeans thoroughly; discard any broken beans.
○ Place soybeans in large bowl; cover with water.
○ Cover bowl with plastic wrap or aluminum foil; refrigerate overnight.
○ Drain beans; spread into single layer on a baking sheet.
○ Bake at 200°F about 2½ hours, or until soybeans are fairly dry.
○ Remove baking sheet from oven.
○ Drizzle the soybeans with vegetable oil, and toss with herbs, spices and salt and pepper, if desired.
○ Place baking sheet back into oven; bake the soybeans another 30 minutes until quite dry.
○ Cool the soybeans thoroughly; store in a covered container in the refrigerator.

Evaluation

Compare the dry soybeans to the soaked and baked soybeans; note any differences in color, hardness, shape and size and other characteristics. Use a Data Sheet like the one that follows to record these observations.

Data Sheet

Dry soybeans	Soaked soybeans	Baked soybeans
Color	Color	Color
Hardness	Hardness	Hardness
Odor	Odor	Odor
Shape	Shape	Shape
Size	Size	Size

How can these differences (if any) be explained?
Commercial dried beans have been dehydrated in large ovens or by the sun. Rehydrated beans, such as those that are canned or frozen, have reabsorbed water. Sodium and other additives and preservatives are often used in canned beans, which can be reduced by rinsing.

Culinary applications

Redo this exercise with raw peanuts or other dried legumes. Compare and contrast the results.
Soybeans and peanuts can be processed into "nut" butters. Which other legumes can be prepared in this manner?
What are other creative culinary uses of soybeans, peanuts and other legumes—aside from adding them to salads, soups and stews?

OVER EASY

Entire volumes have been written about nutrition throughout the life cycle, but not cooking throughout the life cycle. One approach to nutrition for every life cycle group does not fit everyone; neither does one approach to cooking. In this chapter you learned about the essential nutritional needs for pregnancy, lactation, infancy, childhood, preadolescence, adolescence, the middle years, and aging, along with cooking tips and techniques for each of these life cycle periods and groups of people.

The cycle of birth, life, and death is a sequence of building up and slowly tearing down. The nutrients that an expectant woman consumes help determine the longevity and health of her offspring. The lifestyle choices that a person makes, including food intake, drug abstinence or use, emotional and mental well-being, physical activities, weight management—even sleep—affect their health status and future welfare.

Healthy intervention possibilities exist at each stage of the life cycle. Nutrition and culinary specialists can work at or with community centers, long-term care facilities, maternal and child programs, park districts, physicians and health care providers, schools, supported living facilities, and with other organizations to provide healthy and nutritious foods, diets, and menus for people of all ages.

Armed with the information from this chapter, innovative and healthy snacks and beverages can be created for after-school activities, sporting events, and recreational centers; progressive school cafeteria menus can be designed to dually meet nutritional needs and student approval; healthy takeaway meals can be produced for new mothers and their children; and flavorful foods can be formulated to feed the aging.

Now that you know the food and nutrition basics for each of these life cycle stages, think broader. Begin with your extended family, and help improve their diets and health. Work with local groups to ensure that nutritious options are available in your community and in the towns or cities where you reside. The foods and beverages that you create, prepare, and serve today can affect a lifetime.

CHECK PLEASE

1. The _____ is the organ that connects the uterus to the embryo or fetus.
   a. umbilical cord
   b. stomach
   c. placenta
   d. belly button
   e. intestine
2. The average amount of weight that a pregnant woman should gain during her pregnancy is_____ pounds.
   a. 28 to 40
   b. 25 to 35
   c. 15 to 25
   d. less than 15
   e. more than 40
3. The "normal" birth weight of an infant in the United States is about _____ pounds.
   a. under 5
   b. 5 to 6
   c. 6½ to 8
   d. 8½ to 10
   e. There is no normal birth weight.

Essay Question

1. There are two specialized diseases of pregnancy. One involves hypertension, and the other involves diabetes. What are the names of *each* of these diseases? What happens during pregnancy when a woman has *either* of these diseases? What can be done from a nutritional standpoint to help *prevent* each of these diseases?

For additional questions, please see the *Culinary Nutrition* website at www.culinarynutrition.elsevier.com.

HUNGRY FOR MORE?
Pregnancy and Lactation

DHHS. HRSA. Maternal and Child Health Bureau   http://mchb.hrsa.gov
La Leche League International   http://www.llli.org

537

National Center for Education in Maternal and Child Health   http://www.ncemch.org
USDA Daily Food Plans for Pregnancy and Lactation   http://www.choosemyplate.gov/mypyramidmoms

Children and Teenagers

American Academy of Pediatrics   http://www.aap.org
Children Before Birth through Adolescence   http://kidshealth.org
Shanley EL, Thompson CA. *Fueling the Teen Machine*. Palo Alto, CA: Bull Publishing Company, 2001.
Shaping America's Youth   http://www.shapingamericasyouth.org/Default.aspx
Tamborlane WV. *The Yale Guide to Children's Nutrition*. New Haven, CT: Yale University Press, 1997.

Aging

AARP (formerly American Association of Retired Persons)   http://www.aarp.org
Johns Hopkins. *Johns Hopkins Medical Guide to Health after 50*. New York: Leventhal Publishing, 2005.
National Institutes of Health—National Institute on Aging   www.nia.ih.org

TAKE AWAY
Kids in the Kitchen

The kitchen is a laboratory where children can learn about the world of food and nutrition. There are many benefits of cooking with children when they have a readiness to learn, and they can perform a variety of age-appropriate skills. Children enjoy assembling, measuring and chopping tasks that require concentration and execution, and they like projects that have a beginning (preparation), a middle (involvement), and an end (a tasty and successful meal).

Since food appeals to all the senses, and learning is achieved through the senses, food can be a powerful learning tool. A child's physical and social development and his depth of understanding and proficiency in language arts, mathematics, science, social studies and the visual arts can all be fostered by learning about and working with food.

PHYSICAL DEVELOPMENT

Foods can help children expand their sensory development though their physical appearance (sight), the noises they make (sound), and their tastes, smells, textures, touches and other sensations. Small, gradual changes are easier to make than large or sudden ones. When changes in the sensory properties of foods are made too rapidly, some children may refuse to comply. Other children may demonstrate a lifetime of sensory preferences or dislikes.

Food preparation can help in the development of small muscle coordination by using such techniques as chopping, squeezing and stirring, and in the development of large muscle coordination by using such techniques as kneading, mixing and tossing.

SOCIAL DEVELOPMENT

Food experiences may help children to feel confident, cooperative, independent and respectful of themselves and others when these food experiences are age-appropriate and socially acceptable. Early childhood is an excellent time for children to learn about good manners and simple table etiquette, including how to properly set a table and the correct use of serving and eating utensils.

LANGUAGE ARTS

Grocery shopping and purchasing foods can help school-aged children to read labels, follow directions, and differentiate among package and container sizes. Nutrition and health information on food labels can stir up conversation about daily and occasional food choices. Children can learn about food safety, simple recipes, meal and menu planning, and food marketing. Foods can be used for storytelling about families, their differences and similarities, and how they are united in cultures.

MATHEMATICS

Kitchen math helps children make estimations and comparisons and investigates the relationship of parts to wholes. Food is useful in teaching numbers and sizes of servings, understanding fractions in recipes, and translating English into metric units. Food can help children to classify the number and types of ingredients in recipes, the functions these ingredients perform, foods that are similar (such as broccoli, Brussels sprouts, cabbage, collard greens, etc.) and foods that have different sizes and shapes (regularly sized vegetables versus miniature or heirloom).

Food teaches shape, size and space within a dish, pan or pot; area measurements of different-sized plates and place settings; volume measurements of pints, quarts and gallons; and the differences in weights between liquids and solids.

SCIENCE

The kitchen is a living science laboratory where children can investigate and discover the genesis of foods, such as when beans sprout into little plants on sunlight-filled kitchen windows; how flour, sugar and yeast plus heat transform into bread; and why stock that is made with bones, meat and vegetables yields more taste than broth alone.

Children can witness the physical properties of foods, such as how baking powder biscuits rise and how vinegar and oil salad dressing emulsifies. They can experience how foods change states, such as when water turns into ice or steam, or when salt dissolves in water, then reappears as water evaporates.

Children can examine how heat and cold affect fats, such as when oil solidifies when it is chilled and when butter melts when it is warmed. They can see that cooking is food processing, such as when tomatoes are blended into tomato sauce or when corn kernels explode into popped corn.

SOCIAL STUDIES

Kitchen-based food studies help children learn about different people and their cultures. Children can learn about countries by discovering the capture, cultivation, preparation and consumption of local, regional, national and global food. Ethnic recipes can be used to compare and contrast ingredients, techniques, tastes, similarities and differences among world cuisines.

Food helps children see how the world population is interconnected with the food supply, how geography affects food availability, how land is used effectively and efficiently for food production, how different government efforts impact world hunger, and how their food preferences affect how others eat (such as the influx of fast food around the world).

VISUAL ART

Food is an art form, similar to music and painting. It promotes creative expression in balance, color, dimensionality, form, shape and texture. Like artistic expression, food is very hands-on. Give children simple and fun hands-on food tasks such as cracking eggs, sprinkling cheese, spreading icing, and squeezing fruit into juice. Or involve children in rewarding hands-on recipes such as personalized brownies, cookies, simple cakes or pancakes to help further their creativity and broaden their food choices.

FOOD SAFETY

The kitchen is a perfect place to teach food safety. It promotes discussions about safe ingredients, techniques, equipment, food preparation, sanitation and storage. Helpful tools for teaching food safety are these food safety games for children and teenagers at http://www.fda.gov/Food/ResourcesForYou/Consumers/KidsTeens/default.htm.

539

Morsel "The bagel is a lonely roll to eat all by yourself because in order for the true taste to come out, you need your family: one to cut the bagels, one to toast them, one to put on the cream cheese and the lox, one to put them on the table, and one to supervise." —Gertrude Berg (American pioneer of classic radio, 1898–1966)

The Benefits of Breakfast

Breakfast literally means "break the fast." Breakfast is the period of time after dinner or a late-night snack, usually after a full night's sleep. Breakfast helps to refuel the body and prepare it for the rest of the day. When a person skips breakfast, it is similar to starting a car with an empty tank: she will have to refuel, just like a car will need more gasoline.

Eating breakfast raises the metabolic rate and may help the body burn calories the rest of the day. If breakfast is skipped, a person may consume more calories midday and later to accommodate for the calories and nutrients missing earlier in the day.

In general, people who eat breakfast tend to eat healthier overall. They are more likely to participate in physical activities and maintain a healthy body weight. Adults who eat breakfast may eat less at lunch and dinner and may snack less impulsively. People who skip breakfast are more likely to be overweight than those who skip lunch. A change in eating routine may be impactful, because it may make a non–breakfast eater rethink his overall eating habits.

Breakfast foods that are rich in fiber, protein and whole grains and low in sugars help to boost energy and maintain it over time. This promotes increased attention span, concentration, memory and learning. If a person skips breakfast, he may feel irritable, restless and/or tired by midmorning. Starting the day dehydrated may also lead to difficulties in concentration, headaches and irritability.

The best evidence that breakfast matters has been demonstrated in children's breakfast studies. In many of these studies, children were tested within a few hours after eating or skipping breakfast. Children who consumed breakfast demonstrated improved creative thinking, concentration, memory, problem-solving abilities and visual perception.

Similar tests were conducted with adults, and these tests proved differently. Adults managed brain tasks more effectively than children. It may be less important if adults eat breakfast than children. What does matter is *what* adults eat for breakfast. This is because breakfast may impair some functions and enhance other functions in adults. For example, breakfast may help older people perform better on some tests because it supplies the brain with blood sugar [61,62].

It is much easier for a person to meet her nutritional requirements if she eats breakfast. A typical American breakfast of cereal and milk with fruit juice, or bacon, eggs, toast and spread contributes B vitamins, vitamins A and C, calcium, folic acid, vitamin D, fiber, iron, protein, and whole-grain carbohydrates, among other nutrients.

An energy-filled breakfast may contain fortified whole-grain breakfast cereals and/or breads with B vitamins, iron and fiber, and low-fat dairy products or calcium-fortified beverages with calcium and vitamins A and D. Citrus fruits and vitamin C–fortified fruit juices assist with iron absorption from iron-fortified breakfast cereals.

A protein-packed breakfast may feature eggs and lean breakfast meats with protein, B vitamins, iron and zinc, again with low-fat dairy milk or milk products. By consuming carbohydrates, protein and healthy fats at breakfast, this meal will supply and maintain energy and fuel muscles over time. Fiber and healthy fats are filling and satisfying.

Good sources of carbohydrates and fiber, lean protein and healthy fats for breakfast include the following:

- **Carbohydrates and fiber**
  - Cold whole-grain cereals with 5 grams of fiber or more per serving
  - Cooked whole-grain cereals, such as barley grits, multigrain, oatmeal, oat bran or rye
  - Low-fat granola or muesli
  - Quick breads, muffins, scones, pancakes and waffles made with whole-grain flours and dried fruits
  - Fresh fruit, fresh fruit juice with pulp, 100 percent fruit preserves
  - Vegetables, including onions, potatoes, sweet bell peppers, and tomatoes
- **Lean protein**
  - Cheese with 3 to 5 grams of fat or fewer
  - Cooked legumes, such as refried or black beans

- ○ Dairy fat-free (skim) or low-fat milk or yogurt
- ○ Lean meats, such as beef jerky, Canadian bacon or low-fat beef, chicken, pork or turkey sausage
- ○ Meat substitutes (vegetarian bacon or sausage)
- ○ Whole eggs* and egg whites
- **Healthy fats**
  - ○ Nuts, including nut "butters" and seeds
  - ○ Legume "butters," such as peanut or soybean
  - ○ Light butter, cream cheese or margarine

*Whole eggs in moderation, if warranted.

A number of breakfast options exist for time-crunched people, including bagel sandwiches, breakfast and granola bars, individual cereal boxes, nuts and dried fruit mixes, soy or yogurt smoothies, and whole fresh fruit. Bagel sandwiches may be high in carbohydrates and fats from oversized bagels and regular cream cheese. Some breakfast and granola bars may be close to candy bars in calories, sugars and fats, so compare labels. Smoothies can climb in calories with each additional ingredient. Some 22-ounce smoothies contain as much as 375 to 800 calories and 75 to 110 grams of sugar! Healthy and tasteful smoothies and power bar recipes can be found in Chapter 8.

Breakfast does not have to be eggs, toast, bacon or sausage and potatoes. Some unconventional breakfasts may include mini pizzas, soup, tacos or even leftovers. Meals such as these contain various amounts of carbohydrates and fiber, protein and fats to refuel the body and provide satiety. They may be better than some traditional breakfasts—or skipping breakfast altogether.

Many of the following nontraditional breakfasts contain fewer than 500 calories per average serving. This is about one-fourth of the total number of calories required daily, based on a 2,000-calorie diet. Portion sizes are small.

- ○ Bran muffin and yogurt with berries
- ○ Cooked or raw grains (muesli) with dried fruit and reduced-fat yogurt
- ○ Homemade granola with reduced-fat yogurt
- ○ Hot cereal with sweet spices (such as cinnamon or nutmeg) and chopped bananas
- ○ Hummus with whole-grain pita bread, lettuce, tomatoes and cucumbers
- ○ Reduced-fat ricotta or cream cheese with sliced fresh fruit on whole-grain toast or bagel
- ○ Shredded cheese melted inside whole wheat tortilla
- ○ Whole-grain cereal with canned fruit in 100 percent fruit juice
- ○ Whole-grain waffle with 100 percent fruit preserves
- ○ Peanut or nut butter on bagel or whole-grain toast with fresh sliced fruit
- ○ Sliced hard-cooked egg with light mayonnaise in whole-grain roll
- ○ Soy milk or yogurt smoothie blended with fresh or fresh-frozen fruit
- ○ Turkey or chicken breast on whole-grain English muffin
- ○ Vegetable frittata with potatoes and leftover vegetables

References

[1] Institute of Medicine (IOM). Dietary Reference Intakes (DRIs): estimated average requirements, <http://www.iom.edu/Activities/Nutrition/SummaryDRIs/~/media/Files/Activity%20Files/Nutrition/DRIs/5_Summary%20Table%20Tables%201-4.pdf>; [accessed 25.09.08].

[2] Olson CM. Achieving a healthy weight gain during pregnancy. Annu Rev Nutr 2008;28:411–23.

[3] US Department of Agriculture (USDA). Weight gain during pregnancy, <http://www.nal.usda.gov/wicworks/Sharing_Center/MO/Weight_Gain.pdf>; [accessed 25.09.08].

[4] University of Pittsburgh Medical Center (UPMC). Weight gain during pregnancy, <http://www.upmc.com/healthatoz/pages/healthlibrary.aspx?chunkiid = 101071>. [accessed 25.09.08].

[5] American Academy of Pediatrics (AAP). Fetal alcohol syndrome and alcohol-related neurodevelopmental disorders, <http://aappolicy.aappublications.org/cgi/content/full/pediatrics;106/2/358>; [accessed 25.09.08].

[6] March of Dimes. Caffeine in pregnancy, <http://www.marchofdimes.com/pregnancy/nutrition_caffeine.html>; [accessed 25.09.08].

[7] US Environmental Protection Agency (EPA). What you need to know about mercury in fish and shellfish, <http://water.epa.gov/scitech/swguidance/fishshellfish/outreach/advice_index.cfm>; [accessed 25.09.08].

[8] A.D.A.M. Medical Encyclopedia. Sudden infant death syndrome, <http://www.ncbi.nlm.nih.gov/pubmedhealth/PMH0002533/>; [accessed 25.09.08].

[9] US Department of Agriculture (USDA). Health and nutrition for pregnant and breastfeeding women, <http://www.choosemyplate.gov/mypyramidmoms/index.html>; [accessed 25.09.08].

[10] US Food and Drug Administration (FDA). Safe eats—eating out & bringing. In: <http://www.fda.gov/Food/ResourcesForYou/HealthEducators/ucm082539.htm>; [accessed 25.09.08].

[11] Work Group on Breastfeeding. Breastfeeding and the use of human milk. Pediatrics 2005;115:496–506.

[12] Committee on Nutrition American academy of pediatrics. In: Kleinman RE, editor. Pediatric nutrition handbook (5th ed.). Elk Grove, IL: American Academy of Pediatrics; 2004.

[13] Mennella J. Alcohol's effect on lactation, <http://pubs.niaaa.nih.gov/publications/arh25-3/230-234.htm>; [accessed 25.09.08].

[14] Kazal Jr LA. Prevention of iron deficiency in infants and toddlers, <http://www.aafp.org/afp/2002/1001/p1217.html>; [accessed 25.09.08].

[15] Wagner CL, Greer FR. Section on Breastfeeding and Committee on Nutrition: prevention of rickets and vitamin D deficiency in infants, children, and adolescents, <http://aappolicy.aappublications.org/cgi/reprint/pediatrics;122/5/1142.pdf>; [accessed 25.09.08].

[16] SelfNutritionData. Know what you eat, <http://nutritiondata.self.com/facts/baby-foods/477/2>; [accessed 25.09.08].

[17] American Academy of Pediatrics (AAP). Starting solid foods, <http://patiented.aap.org/content.aspx?aid = 5713>; [accessed 25.09.08].

[18] Fiocchi A, Amal A, Sami B. Food allergy and the introduction of solid foods to infants: a consensus document. Ann Allergy Asthma Immunol 2006;97:10–21.

[19] Greer FR, Sicherer SH, Burks AW, et al. Effects of early nutritional interventions on the development of atopic disease in infants and children: the role of maternal dietary restriction, breastfeeding, timing of introduction of complementary foods, and hydrolyzed formulas. Pediatrics 2008;121:183–91.

[20] Sicherer SH. Food for thought on prevention and treatment of atopic disease through diet. J Pediatr 2007;151:331–3.

[21] National Center for Education in Maternal and Child Health. Planning to meet the children's food needs, <http://www.ncemch.org/pubs/PDFs/Nutrition_Stnd/Nutrition_4.pdf>; [accessed 25.09.08].

[22] Florida Department of Health. Nutrition and menu planning for children in the child care food program, <http://www.doh.state.fl.us/ccfp/Nutrition/Children/childnutrmenuplanning.pdf>; [accessed 25.09.08].

[23] Permanente Medical Group. Daily serving sizes for children and adolescents, <http://www.permanente.net/homepage/kaiser/pdf/40863.pdf>; [accessed 25.09.08].

[24] Centers for Disease Control and Prevention (CDC). Childhood obesity facts, <http://www.cdc.gov/healthyyouth/obesity/facts.htm>; [accessed 25.09.08].

[25] Let's Move. Let's Move: America's move to raise a healthier generation of kids, <http://www.letsmove.gov>; [accessed 25.09.08].

[26] Freedman DS, Kettel L, Serdula MK, et al. The relation of childhood BMI to adult adiposity: the Bogalusa heart study. Pediatrics 2005;115:22–7.

[27] Guo SS, Chumlea WC. Tracking of body mass index in children in relation to overweight in adulthood. Am J Clin Nutr 1999;70:S145–148.

[28] Office of the Surgeon General. The Surgeon General's vision for a healthy and fit nation. Rockville, MD: US Department of Health and Human Services; 2010.

[29] US Department of Agriculture. Dietary guidance: DRI tables, <http://fnic.nal.usda.gov/nal_display/index.php?info_center=4&tax_level = 3&tax_subject = 256&topic_id = 1342&level3_id = 5140>; [accessed 25.09.08].

[30] Sherry B, McDivitt J, Birch LL, et al. Attitudes, practices, and concerns about child feeding and child weight status among socioeconomically diverse white, Hispanic, and African-American mothers. J Am Diet Assoc 2004;104(2):215–21.

[31] US Department of Agriculture. Food groups, <http://www.choosemyplate.gov/food-groups/>; [accessed 25.09.08].

[32] Academy of Nutrition and Dietetics. Juice Products Association: nutrition fact sheet: the role of 100 percent juice in a healthy diet, <http://www.wellnessproposals.com/nutrition/nutrition_fact_sheets/role_of_100_percent_juice_in_a_healthy_diet.pdf>; [accessed 25.09.08].

[33] Juice Products Association. Health benefits, fruit juice facts, <http://www.fruitjuicefacts.org/healthbenefits.html>; [accessed 25.09.08].

[34] US Department of Agriculture (USDA). Dietary guidelines for Americans, <http://www.cnpp.usda.gov/dietaryguidelines.htm>; [accessed 25.09.08].

[35] Eisenberg ME, Olson RE, Neumark-Sztainer D, et al. Correlations between family meals and psychosocial well-being among adolescents. Arch Pediatr Adolesc Med 2004;158:792–6.

[36] Gillman MW, Rifas-Shiman SL, Frazier AL, et al. Family dinner and diet quality among older children and adolescents. Arch Fam Med 2000;9:235–40.

[37] Larson NI, Neumark-Sztainer D, Hannan PJ, et al. Trends in adolescent fruit and vegetable consumption, 1999–2004: Project EAT. Am J Prev Med 2007;32:147–50. [accessed 25.09.08]

[38] Irish Universities Nutrition Alliance (IUNA). National Teen's Food Survey—preliminary results 2008, <http://www.iuna.net/>; [accessed 25.09.08].

[39] Growth and your 13 to 18 year old. Kid's Health. 2011. Nemours Foundation. Retr. 25 Sept. 2008, <http://kidshealth.org/parent/growth/growth/growth_13_to_18.html>.

[40] Smith RN, Mann NJ, Braue A, et al. A low-glycemic-load diet improves symptoms in acne vulgaris patients: a randomized controlled trial. Am J Clin Nutr 2007;86:107–15.

[41] Smith RN, Mann NJ, Braue A, et al. The effect of a high-protein, low glycemic-load diet versus a conventional, high glycemic-load diet on biochemical parameters associated with acne vulgaris: a randomized, investigator-masked, controlled trial. J Am Acad Dermatol 2007;57:247–56.

[42] FastFoodNutrition.org. Fast food nutrition facts, <http://www.fastfoodnutrition.org/index.php>; [accessed 25.09.08].

[43] SelfNutritionData. Know what you eat, <http://nutritiondata.self.com/>; [accessed 25.09.08].

[44] Centers for Disease Control and Prevention (CDC). Competitive foods and beverages available for purchase in secondary schools—selected sites, United States, 2006, <http://www.cdc.gov/mmwr/preview/mmwrhtml/mm5734a2.htm>; [accessed 25.09.08].

[45] Aptos Middle School PTSA. Schools and school districts that have improved school food and beverages and not lost revenue, <http://www.cspinet.org/nutritionpolicy/improved_school_foods_without_losing_revenue2.pdf>; [accessed 25.09.08].

[46] University of California San Francisco. Calcium content of foods, <http://www.ucsfhealth.org/education/calcium_content_of_selected_foods/index.html>; [accessed 25.09.08].

[47] Harvard University Health Services. Iron content of common foods, <http://huhs.harvard.edu/assets/File/OurServices/Service_Nutrition_Iron.pdf>; [accessed 25.09.08].

[48] Ohio State University. Folate (folacin, folic acid), <http://ohioline.osu.edu/hyg-fact/5000/5553.html>; [accessed 25.09.08].

[49] DeNoon DJ. The truth about vitamin D: how much vitamin D do you need?, <http://www.webmd.com/osteoporosis/features/the-truth-about-vitamin-d-how-much-vitamin-d-do-you-need>; [accessed 25.09.08].

[50] Associated Press. Lack of vitamin D tied to teen health problems, <http://www.msnbc.msn.com/id/29642547/ns/health-childrens_health/t/lack-vitamin-d-tied-teen-health-problems/>; [accessed 25.09.08].

[51] Must A, Jacques PF, Dallal GE, et al. Long-term morbidity and mortality of overweight adolescents—a follow-up of the Harvard Growth Study of 1922 to 1935. N Engl J Med 1992;327:1350–5.

[52] Centers for Disease Control and Prevention (CDC). Health, United States, 2010: with special feature on death and dying, <http://www.cdc.gov/nchs/data/hus/hus10.pdf>; [accessed 25.09.08].

[53] Centers for Disease Control and Prevention (CDC) Ten great public health achievements—United States, 1900–1999. JAMA 1999;281:1481.

[54] National Institutes of Health (NIH). Dramatic changes in US aging highlighted in new census, <http://www.nih.gov/news/pr/mar2006/nia-09.htm>; [accessed 25.09.08].

[55] Kinsella K, Velkoff VA. An aging world: 2001, <http://www.census.gov/prod/2001pubs/p95-01-1.pdf>; [accessed 25.09.08].

[56] Centers for Disease Control and Prevention (CDC). The state of aging and health in America, 2007, <http://www.cdc.gov/aging/pdf/saha_exec_summary_2007.pdf>; [accessed 25.09.08].

[57] US Department of Agriculture (USDA). Diet quality of older Americans in 1994–1996 and 2001–2002 as measured by healthy eating index—2005, <http://www.cnpp.usda.gov/Publications/NutritionInsights/Insight41.pdf>; [accessed 25.09.08].

[58] US Department of Agriculture (USDA). Quality of diets of older Americans: nutrition insight 29, <http://www.cnpp.usda.gov/Publications/NutritionInsights/Insight29.pdf>; [accessed 25.09.08].

[59] Quote Garden. Quotations about food, <www.quotegarden.com/food.html>; [accessed 25.09.08].

[60] Robbins MP.. In: The cook's quotation book: a literary feast. New York: Pushcart Press; 1983.

[61] Pollitt E, Cueto S, Jacoby ER. Fasting and cognition in well and undernourished schoolchildren: a review of three experimental studies. Am J Clin Nutr 1998;67(Suppl):779S–84S.

[62] Pollitt E, Mathews R. Breakfast and cognition: an integrative summary. Am J Clin Nutr 1998;67(Suppl):804S–13S.

543

CHAPTER 12

Global Food and Nutrition: World Food, Health and the Environment

Practical Applications for Nutrition, Food Science and Culinary Professionals

OBJECTIVES

1. Define *globalization* and explain its effects on world food, diets and health

2. Recognize the differences and similarities among world cuisines

3. Note the economic, political, sociocultural and technological issues that encompass globalization

4. Distinguish among inclusive cuisines and cultures:

   a. African American

   b. Hispanic

   c. Asian

   d. Mediterranean

Culinary Nutrition. DOI: http://dx.doi.org/10.1016/B978-0-12-391882-6.00012-1

5. Differentiate among regional cuisines and cultures:
   a. Cuban, Mexican and Puerto Rican
   b. Chinese, Japanese, Korean and Taiwanese
   c. Cambodian, Laotian, Malaysian, Filipino, Thai and Vietnamese
6. Define fusion cooking and highlight healthful combinations
7. Identify specialized cooking equipment used by global cuisines
8. Apply healthy cooking principles when recreating ethnic recipes
9. Incorporate ethnic recipe ideas when preparing US recipes
10. Respect how religious beliefs affect some world cuisines
11. Recognize difficulties in changing customary food habits
12. Identify countries with environmentally active measures in food and nutrition and compare/contrast to US measures
13. Apply environmentally active global measures in food and nutrition to US efforts

INTRODUCTION: BENEFITS AND CONCERNS OF GLOBAL FOOD AND NUTRITION

Morsel "Food is our common ground, a universal experience."
—James Beard (American chef and food writer, 1903–1985) [1]

Globalization and the US Food Supply

Globalization is the process of transforming local, regional or national foods, beverages, concepts and perspectives into global ones. Foods and beverages help to unify the world, along with the economic, political, sociocultural and technological issues that surround them.

When countries were more defined and contained than they were in the twenty-first century, food systems were more specialized. Hispanic cuisine defined the hot climate and lush vegetation of Central and South America, with chilies, corn and legumes. Asian cuisine symbolized the ancient cultures of China, Japan, Korea, Vietnam and Thailand, with soy products, vegetables and flavorful sauces. Mediterranean cuisine portrayed the sun-filled countries that flank the Mediterranean Sea, with their fresh fruit and vegetables, fish, olive oil and red wine.

Thanks to globalization, the distinction among these world cuisines and others is less clearcut. Global cuisines now embrace Tex-Mex, Pan-Asian, French-Asian and a host of other fusions. Some ingredients and techniques are harmonious and others are discordant; some enhance diets and others diminish diet quality. As a result of "cuisines without borders," issues such as food safety, labeling, regulations and health—especially food allergies and sensitivities—have come to the forefront.

This chapter examines the main cuisines that have permeated the US melting pot: African American, Asian, Hispanic and Mediterranean, with an overview of other cuisines that have an influence on the US diet: Cajun, Caribbean, Eastern Indian, European, Native American and others. Each of these cuisines is discussed in terms of its history, culture, diet, nutrition, culinary characteristics, health and its place in the US diet. They provide an important glimpse of the rapidly changing world of nutrition, food science and the culinary arts for future nutrition, food science and culinary professionals.

MAIN COURSES

AFRICAN-AMERICAN CUISINE

African-American cooking is not exclusively from the southern United States, nor is it entirely African. Rather, African-American cuisine has evolved from both countries and cultures. It is a combination of passed-down recipes, techniques and tales that have crossed boundaries and modernized.

The first English colony in America was settled in 1607 in Jamestown, Virginia, where Native Americans already resided. The local foods, which included corn, legumes, peas, pumpkins and squash, were introduced to and integrated with the cattle, chickens, goats, horses, pigs, and sheep that the settlers brought from England. These settlers also brought or introduced the Native Americans to apples, barley, root vegetables and wheat. With local and borrowed ingredients, Native Americans prepared dishes such as hominy, hot-water cornbread and strawberry bread (which Europeans reinvented as strawberry shortcake).

Around 1619, the first group of African slaves was brought to work the colony fields and kitchens. Colonists transitioned from farmers to plantation owners. Cotton, rice and tobacco plantations yielded large profits and required even more African slaves to handle the growing demands. Some southern plantations became so wealthy that they were able to import foods, wines and spirits from Spain and France. African cooks became adept at integrating these foreign foods and beverages into their southern cuisine.

Typical English food of this time period included sweet and savory English breads, cakes, pies, trifles and *syllabub* (made from rich dairy milk or cream, seasoned with sugar and lightly curdled with wine or cider). Traditional African foods included black-eyed peas, *benne* (sesame seeds), coconut, *jollof rice* (West African risotto), okra, peanuts and peanut oil.

SOUL FOOD

African-American cuisine embodies *soul food*, a blend of traditional African and southern US cooking. "Soul" is a term that historically described African-American culture, including food. In general, soul food is more intensely flavored than the southern US or European cuisines that originally dominated US cooking.

Soul food was the first cuisine to crop up, along with Creole cuisine, in the French Louisiana territory. In the 1870s, Czech, German and Irish immigrants brought their own traditions and cuisines to the southern US, which further influenced soul food.

Soul food cooking incorporates a simple and thrifty use of foodstuffs that are either grown or raised, such as collard and turnip greens, peanuts, peppers, and pig carcasses, including backbones, *chitterlings* (fried slices of small or large intestine), ears, fat, feet, hocks, pork ribs and salt pork.

547

Fish, meats, poultry and vegetables are traditionally fried in pig fat until crisp and then highly seasoned with hot and peppery sauces. Corn and rice are the carbohydrate foundations of soul food. Corn is a multipurpose vegetable, both fresh and processed; it is featured in such dishes as cornbread, grits and hominy. Rice is a versatile grain; it is integral in some casseroles, soups and stews, such as gumbo.

Besides corn, the vegetables that African Americans cooked on plantations included the tops of beets, dandelions and turnips, which later included collards, cress, mustard, kale and pokeweed. They were flavored with bay, garlic, onions and thyme, among other local herbs and spices. Wild meat was hunted and incorporated into hearty dishes, which included opossum, rabbit, raccoon, squirrel, turtle and sometimes waterfowl.

Leftovers were reused—even in small quantities. Leftover fish was combined with breadstuffs to form *croquettes*, small deep-fried and breaded fritters. Stale bread was converted into *bread pudding*, with dried fruit, eggs, sugar, spices and suet. *Potlikker*, the leftover liquid from cooked greens, was used in gravies.

Many of these soul food dishes are still popular today: candied yams, cornbread, collards and smoked pork, fruit cobbler, gumbo, *Hoppin' John* (black-eyed peas and rice), macaroni and cheese, okra, one-pot pork chops (also common in Cajun cooking), pecan and sweet potato pies, southern fried chicken and spoon bread.

Hoppin' John is also known as *Whippoorwill peas and rice* and *crowder peas and rice*. Okra, a vegetable that exudes a sticky substance with thickening properties when cut, is used in *gumbo*, a hearty meat and/or shellfish stew. Cobblers have their roots in English dishes, but African Americans have created their own versions with apples, berries and peaches. A typical African-American southern-style menu may include such dishes as:

- Baked or cured ham
- Barbecued or fried chicken
- Cheese grits
- Collard greens with smoked meat
- Corn pudding

- Country-style ribs
- Fruit cobbler or pudding
- Hoppin' John
- Macaroni and cheese
- Pimento cheese
- Smoked pulled pork
- Smothered chicken with gravy
- White cornbread

In comparison, a typical *West African–style* menu may include the following dishes, some of which are highly flavored with chilies, onions and other pungent spices:

- Beef kabobs with peanut butter marinade
- Black-eyed peas
- Cassava
- Croquettes with fish or meat
- Goat
- Greens
- Joulouf rice with beef or chicken
- Lamb
- Meat pies
- Okra
- Peanuts
- Pepper chicken or fish
- Plaintains
- Rice bread
- Sweet potatoes
- Tomatoes
- Yams

A typical blended **American South and Mississippi Delta–style** menu may include such dishes such as:

- Banana pudding
- Chicken and sausage jambalaya
- Collard and mustard greens
- Coleslaw
- Cured ham
- Onions and ham hocks
- Smoked pulled pork
- Tomato and pimento cheese sandwiches
- White cornmeal cornbread

Caribbean and South American immigrants have since influenced African-American and southern US cuisines. Typical dishes that reflect these influences include:

- Brazilian *feijoada* (beans with beef and pork)
- Fried plantains
- Jamaican jerk chicken
- Puerto Rican **habichuelas** (beans with rice, potatoes or other vegetables and ham)

CAJUN AND CREOLE COOKING

Cajun and Creole cooking originated from French and Spanish influences and then blended with African-American cooking. The items that African-American cooks lent to traditional French and Spanish cuisines were indigenous spices, okra and Native American foodstuffs, including crab, crawfish, oysters, pecans and shrimp.

At first, Cajun cooking meant the country cooking of the Acadian people of French origin who had settled in the French colony of Nova Scotia around 1632. The term *Cajun* may have been a mispronunciation of the word *Canadian* from its French roots. In fact, the French **roux** (a one-to-one mixture of flour and fat) is still central to Cajun cooking.

Cajun meals were initially bland, the result of boiled, one-pot recipes. Rice stretched out Cajun meals to feed many people. Today, Cajun cooking tends to be spicier and more full-bodied than some Creole cooking. A traditional Cajun menu may have included such dishes as:

- *Andouille* (smoked pork) and **boudin** (French) sausages
- Catfish
- **Coush-coush** (creamed corn)
- Crawfish
- Dirty rice
- Gumbo
- Jambalaya
- *Sauce piquant* (hot peppers, spices and tomatoes)

An updated Cajun menu with variations on traditional dishes may include such dishes as:

- Alligator piquant
- Blackened fish (catfish or other white fish)
- Cajun seafood salad
- Champignons (mushrooms)
- Chicken and andouille
- Corn and crab bisque
- Crawfish boil
- Gumbo
- *Hush puppies* (cornbread fritters)
- *Pain perdu* ("lost bread" or savory French toast)
- Seafood jambalaya
- *Shrimp boulettes* (little fried balls of stuffing)
- Spiced coffee

Creole cooking reflected "city cooking," along with homegrown, local ingredients. Traditional Creole dishes tended to be more refined than Cajun dishes. They included such classic recipes as *Bananas Foster, Oysters Rockefeller* and *Shrimp Remoulade*.

Tomatoes most often show up in Creole dishes before they do in Cajun recipes, but they are sometimes used both in gumbo and jambalaya. Both Cajun and Creole recipes rely upon celery, green peppers, onions and roux (flour cooked in fat—generally pork fat or butter).

AFRICAN-AMERICAN FOOD AND CELEBRATION

Kwanzaa is a holiday that originated from African harvest festivals. It is celebrated annually from December 26 to January 1. Kwanzaa is dedicated to the celebration of African-American culture and community. It is also a cultural and culinary festival.

Kwanzaa recipes use dominant flavors from aromatic spices, such as cumin, cardamom, cinnamon and nutmeg; flavorful herbs; and seasonal fruits and vegetables, including lentils, okra and sweet potatoes. These robust flavors help to decrease dependence on fat and salt in some recipes.

AFRICAN-AMERICAN FOOD, NUTRITION AND HEALTH

The ten leading causes of death of African Americans are heart disease, cancer, stroke, unintentional injuries, diabetes, homicide, chronic lower respiratory disease, nephritis, HIV/AIDS, and septicemia (life-threatening infection). Furthermore, African Americans have a disproportionately higher prevalence of hypertension, infant mortality and tuberculosis. Hypertension increases the risks for cardiovascular disease, kidney disease and stroke. Calcium helps to maintain normal blood pressure through its role in vascular contraction and vasodilation. The calcium intake of African Americans does not meet the DRI, which is related to their increased hypertension, obesity and osteoporosis [2].

As a whole, African Americans show evidence of more overweight and obesity. At the beginning of the year 2000, about one-half of African-American women were overweight, according to the Centers for Disease Control and Prevention (CDC). Among African-American men, the prevalence of obesity had increased significantly from earlier years.

By 2008, 72 percent of African-American men, 78 percent of African-American women, and 22 to 24 percent of African-American children were considered to be overweight or obese. African-American women now have the highest rates of overweight or obesity compared to other US population groups [3–5].

While African-American women tend to have higher bone mineral density (BMD) than white American women throughout their lifespan, they are still at risk of developing osteoporosis. This may be because osteoporosis is underrecognized and undertreated in African-American women. Diseases that are more prevalent in African Americans, such as sickle-cell anemia and lupus, can increase the risk of developing osteoporosis [6].

African Americans are genetically more prone to lactose intolerance than other US population groups. Lactose intolerance is a food sensitivity to lactose, the milk sugar in dairy products, which can hinder optimal calcium intake. Lactose intolerance is highly individualized; some foods and beverages with less or no lactose may be tolerated. These include yogurt with active cultures, cottage or Swiss cheese, and lactose-reduced or lactose-free dairy milk and dairy products.

Certain ingredients that are common to African-American cuisine have health benefits. Collards and other greens are excellent sources of the vitamins A, B6, C and folic acid; the minerals calcium, iron and manganese; fiber; omega-3 fatty acids; and phytonutrients. Legumes, peas and lentils combined with rice or corn are good sources of inexpensive plant protein. Sweet potatoes and yams are excellent sources of beta-carotene, a precursor to vitamin A.

AFRICAN-AMERICAN HEALTH DISPARITIES

According to the 2000 US census, there are major diet-related health disparities between African Americans and Caucasians in rates of cancer, diabetes, heart disease and stroke. The age-adjusted death rate for cancer was 25.4 percent higher in African Americans than in Caucasian Americans; for heart disease it was 30.1 percent higher; for stroke it was 41.2 percent higher, and for diabetes it was more than twice as high as Caucasian Americans.

Eliminating these disparities requires a collaboration of culturally appropriate public health initiatives (including ones that are food and nutrition focused), community support and equal access to quality health care [7].

AFRICAN-AMERICAN FOOD CHOICES AND DIET PLANNING

The Oldways Preservation Trust created the African Heritage Diet Pyramid in 2011 (Figure 12-1) as a healthy eating model for African Americans. It portrays the traditional healthy eating patterns of African Heritage that optimize health, which are rooted in America, Africa, the Caribbean and Central and South America. It is shaped like a pyramid to show how to "base" food consumption in *decreasing* order.

A healthy lifestyle forms the foundation of the African Heritage Diet Pyramid. It is followed by a diet that is filled with an abundance of fruits, greens, legumes, nuts and seeds, tubers and other vegetables and whole grains at every meal; fish and seafood at least two times weekly; moderate portions of dairy products or calcium-rich foods; eggs; healthy oils; meats and poultry daily or weekly; sweets occasionally; water daily; and alcohol in moderation, if consumed.

Another tool for healthy meal planning for African Americans is provided at USDA MyPlate.gov. Traditional African-American foods choices can be "exchanged" for typical US foods and beverages in the amounts that are shown in Table 12-1. The higher-fat choices should be selected less frequently.

550

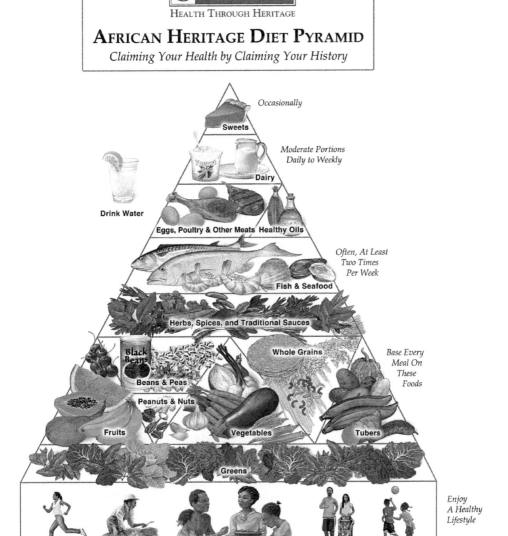

FIGURE 12-1
African Heritage Diet Pyramid.

CHARACTERISTIC FOODS AND BEVERAGES IN AFRICAN-AMERICAN DIETS AND HEALTHIER CHOICES

Most diets can use some improvements, African-American diets included. Emphasis should be placed on purchasing healthier food and beverages, consuming foods and beverages from all of the major food groups, choosing healthier food preparations, practicing food safety, and preserving maximum nutrients. Table 12-2 shows characteristic foods and beverages in African-American diets and healthier choices.

AFRICAN-AMERICAN RECIPE MODIFICATIONS
Lard and Fats in Cooking

Many African-American dishes are traditionally cooked and seasoned with pork and often fried in lard. Lard, or pig fat, is commonly used in many global cuisines as a cooking fat or shortening, or as a spread that is similar to butter.

TABLE 12-1 Common African-American Foods and Beverages and Equivalents

Foods and Beverages	One Serving Equals
Bread, cereal, rice, pasta and starchy vegetables	½ cup cooked grits ½ cup cooked hominy ½ cup cooked macaroni ½ cup cooked rice 1-ounce piece cornbread 1-ounce piece pound cake 1 small hush puppy 1 medium biscuit 1 small sweet potato
Vegetables	½ cup coleslaw (*plus 1 teaspoon of fat*) ½ cup cooked greens ½ cup cooked okra ½ cup cooked succotash ½ cup cooked turnips
Fruit	½ cup blackberries ½ cup muscadines (*grapes*) ½ cup watermelon 1 medium orange 1 medium peach 2 small plums
Dairy milk, yogurt and cheese	1 ounce reduced-fat cheddar-type cheese ½ cup reduced- or low-fat ice cream 1 cup reduced- or low-fat dairy milk 1 cup reduced-fat buttermilk
Meat, poultry, fish, dry beans, eggs and nuts	2 to 3 ounces *lean* chicken, fish, pork or turkey, or reduced-fat sausage (*Limit sausage with 8 grams of fat or more per ounce to 3 servings per week*) ½ cup cooked red beans or black-eyed peas (*equals 1 ounce of meat*) ¼ cup egg whites (limit whole eggs to 3 per week) 1 tablespoon peanut butter (*equals 1 ounce of meat plus 1 teaspoon of fat*)
Fats, oils and sweets (*use sparingly*)	1 teaspoon reduced-fat or light butter 1 teaspoon lard (*use sparingly*) 1 teaspoon reduced-fat or light margarine 1 teaspoon vegetable oil 1 teaspoon nonhydrogenated vegetable shortening 1 tablespoon reduced-fat or light mayonnaise 1 to 2 tablespoons reduced-fat or light salad dressing 2 tablespoons chitterlings (*boiled, fried or stewed pig intestines*) (*use sparingly*)

In comparison to butter, lard has less saturated fatty acids and more monounsaturated fatty acids. The culinary qualities of lard vary, depending on the part of the pig where the fat was obtained and how the lard was processed (see Chapter 6). Pork is raised leaner today than it was during the time of southern plantations.

Traditionally lard was reused because early African-American cooks were thrifty. Used cooking lard was considered as a "repurposed" ingredient. The problem with heating lard to the temperature required for frying, and then cooling and reheating it, is that fatty acids can break down and form potentially dangerous substances. Plus, frequent consumption of lard and fried foods may lead to cardiovascular disease, diabetes, hypertension and obesity.

Healthful alternatives to lard and other fatty foods in the African-American diet include substituting vegetable oil for lard, substituting smoked poultry for fattier cuts of pork, and pan-frying foods instead of deep-frying them.

TABLE 12-2 Characteristic Foods and Beverages in African-American Diets and Healthier Choices

Characteristic African-American Foods and Beverages	Healthier Choices
Dairy products	
Limited dairy milk consumption; buttermilk often preferred	Lactose-free milk for drinking; dry and evaporated skim milk for cooking
Cheese sandwiches and macaroni and cheese	Reduced-fat cheese
Protein foods	
Beef: hash and stew; cured beef tongue	Leaner and skinless protein cuts
Eggs: fried and scrambled	Lower-fat preparations: broiling, grilling, roasting or steaming
Fish and shellfish: fresh catfish, crawfish and white buffalo; boiled and stewed shrimp and oysters; fried scallops, shrimp and oysters	
Game: opossum, rabbit and squirrel	
Legumes: black-eyed peas, beans with salt pork, peanuts and peanut butter	
Poultry: fried chicken and turkey legs	
Pork: cured ham, hog jowls, ham hocks and pig's feet	
Variety meats: brains, chitterlings, heart, kidneys and lungs	
Vegetables	
Beans: green and wax with pork	Remove baking soda from cooking water
Corn, corn products: grits, hominy	Reduce or remove pork products
Leafy greens: cabbage, collards, mustard or turnip with bacon, ham hocks or salt pork	Quick cooking to preserve vitamins and minerals
Pot liquor (vegetable cooking liquid)	Lower-fat preparations: reduce or eliminate
Potatoes: sweet (baked, candied or fried) and white	
Tomatoes: breaded or fried and stewed	
Fruits	
Limited citrus fruits	Fortified fruit juices
Seasonal berries, peaches, plums and watermelon	Frozen or canned fruit in 100% fruit juice
Breads, cereals and grains	
Biscuits with molasses, cornbread	Enriched and whole-grain breads and cereals, including oatmeal
Dumplings (corn pancakes)	Combinations of refined grains
Hominy grits with gravy	
Limited whole-grain breads, cereals	
Pancakes	
White or polished rice (with ham hocks, onions, okra or tomatoes)	
Fats and oils	
Bacon	Decrease fats and oils
Butter	Reduced-fat or fat-free cooking methods
Gravy	Replace solid fats with liquid oils where possible
Salt pork	
Vegetable oil (for frying)	
Sweets	
Cakes, cookies, pastries, pies and sweet breads	Lower-fat and reduced-fat baked goods
Ice cream	Reduced- and low-fat frozen desserts
Cane syrup	Fruit-based desserts
Molasses	Reduced sweeteners, jams and jellies
Lemonade	Lower-calorie and lower-sugar beverages
Soft drinks	

553

Although deep-fat frying is associated with too much fat, if foods are fried quickly at high temperature and with a minimum of healthy oil, deep-fat frying may be better than once thought. If foods are fried under these conditions, the water in the food should boil out as steam. This outward force of steam should be greater than the inward force of oil entering the food, so the food should absorb little oil. But heavy breading retains oil, so it may make deep-fat fried foods too fatty and unhealthy to consume.

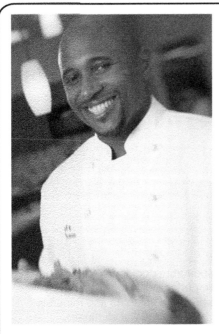

THE COOK'S CORNER: JEFFERY E. MCGOWAN, CHEF AND FOOD SPECIALIST

After completing his undergraduate studies at Southern University in Baton Rouge, Louisiana, Jeffery McGowan spent four years in retail management and nine years as a sales representative for Kraft Foods in Northfield, Illinois. Jeff pursued his passion for cooking, and in 2004 he attended the School of Culinary Arts at Kendall College in Chicago. After completing his culinary training, Jeff decided to make a change. He became a food specialist in the Kraft kitchens and supported the Kraft Macaroni and Cheese, Stove Top Stuffing, and A1 Steak Sauce brands. Jeff is now employed at another food and beverage company.

Chef McGowan has modified traditional African-American Simmered Collard Greens and created Vegetarian Greens with similar appeal, but meatless and lower in calories and fat.

FIGURE 12-2
Jeffery E. McGowan.

SIMMERED COLLARD GREENS—TRADITIONAL RECIPE

Ingredients

2 pounds ham hocks or turkey necks
Water
1 large onion (about 1 cup), chopped
1 large green pepper (about 1 cup), chopped
2 cloves garlic, minced
¼ cup vinegar
½ teaspoon crushed red pepper
2 large bags (about 10 cups) collard greens or mixed turnip and mustard greens, rinsed

Instructions

1. Place ham hocks in a large pot with enough water to cover. Bring to a boil; simmer 45 minutes to 1 hour, or until tender.
2. Add onions, green pepper, garlic, vinegar and crushed red pepper to pot with meat. Place greens on top of meat; cook until greens begin to wilt.
3. Cover and continue cooking for 45 minutes to 1 hour.

Serving size: 8 to 10 servings

Nutrients per serving: 320 calories, 21.2 grams total fat, 7.7 grams saturated fat, 4.5 grams carbohydrates, 1.9 grams fiber, 26.5 grams protein, 235.3 milligrams sodium

VEGETARIAN GREENS—MODIFIED AND HEALTHIER RECIPE

Ingredients

2 tablespoons olive oil
½ cup onion, chopped
½ cup green pepper, chopped
2 cloves garlic, minced
¼ teaspoon seasoning salt
¼ teaspoon red pepper, crushed
4 cups collard greens or mixed turnip and mustard greens, rinsed
1 cup water

Instructions

1. Chop greens and set aside.
2. Heat olive oil in large skillet on medium-high heat. Add onion, green peppers, garlic, salt, and crush red pepper to skillet and stir.
3. Add greens and water to skillet and stir.
4. Cover and reduce heat to low; cook 15 to 20 minutes, or until tender.

Serving size: 4 servings

Nutrients per serving: 85 calories, 7.5 grams total fat, 1 gram saturated fat, 5.3 grams carbohydrates, 2 grams fiber, 1.4 grams protein, 156 milligrams sodium

For more African-American cooking idea substitutions, check out "Hungry for More?" in this chapter.

Mediterranean Cuisine

The Mediterranean is loosely defined as the area around the Mediterranean Sea. In fact, 21 nation-states have a coastline on the Mediterranean Sea. These include those in Europe, including Albania, Bosnia and Herzegovina, Croatia, France, Greece, Italy, Malta, Monaco, Montenegro, Slovenia and Spain; Asia, including Cyprus, Israel, Lebanon, Syria and Turkey; and Africa, including Algeria, Egypt, Libya, Morocco and Tunisia.

Territories that border the Mediterranean Sea include the British territory of Gibraltar; the Spanish enclaves of Ceuta, Melilla and nearby islands; the British sovereign base area of Akrotiri and Dhekelia; and the Palestinian National Authority.

THE MEDITERRANEAN DIET

The "Mediterranean diet" is a modern concept with nutritional recommendations that are based on the traditional dietary patterns of countries that flank the Mediterranean Sea. The idea of the Mediterranean diet began in 1958 by physiologist Ancel Keys at the University of Minnesota, who conducted his now famous Seven Countries Study. Keys examined the diet and disease rates of men in rural areas of Finland, Italy, Greece, Japan, the Netherlands, the United States and Yugoslavia. Of 12,000 men studied, those least likely to develop heart disease lived on the island of Crete.

Those who consumed the most saturated fat had the highest blood cholesterol levels and the greatest incidence of heart attack. While the almost-vegetarian diet and active Cretan lifestyle have significantly changed since 1970, this island retains the distinction of embracing a diet and lifestyle that many other countries have tried to follow. The original Cretan diet was not low in fat. In fact, more than 35 percent of calories came from fat, but primarily from olive oil with monounsaturated fatty acids—the hallmark of the Mediterranean diet, both then and now.

The Mediterranean diet also consists of wine with resveratrol and quercetin, two phytonutrients with heart protective properties; an abundance of fruits and vegetables; legumes and nuts; cheese and yogurt; poultry and eggs a few times weekly; meats; and sweets (just a few times monthly). This dietary protocol is the direct opposite of many Western diets, including those in the United States.

The Lyon Diet Heart Study, published in 1999, followed 600 men in Lyon, France, who had previously suffered a heart attack. The men who followed a traditional Mediterranean diet showed a major reduction in heart attacks and complications compared to those who ate a prudent low-fat, heart-healthy diet. This study showed that the Mediterranean diet group had consumed more olive oil with its heart-protective monounsaturated fatty acids [8,9].

A 2008 review of the relationship among the Mediterranean diet, mortality, and the incidence of chronic diseases in nearly 600,000 participants concluded that greater adherence to the Mediterranean diet resulted in significant improvement in health status.

Those who strongly adhered to the Mediterranean diet had significant reduction in overall mortality (9 percent); mortality from cardiovascular diseases (9 percent); incidence of or mortality from cancer (6 percent); and incidence of Parkinson's disease and Alzheimer's disease (13 percent). These results were clinically relevant to encourage a Mediterranean diet for chronic disease prevention [10].

> **FOOD BYTE**
>
> Squid (calamari) is commonly used in Mediterranean and Asian cuisines. Japan is the world's biggest consumer. Squid meat provides just 85 calories per 100 grams. Although it is low in fat, squid is high in cholesterol, with good amounts of copper, manganese and zinc. Squid can be stuffed whole, cut into flat pieces, or sliced into rings. Its arms, tentacles and ink are also edible. Cook squid very quickly over high heat to prevent toughening, or cook it slowly in a liquid such as tomato broth to break down its muscle fibers. Squid can be barbecued, braised, grilled or pan-fried.

556

FOODS IN THE MEDITERRANEAN DIET

The Mediterranean diet is characterized by a range of fresh ingredients that are indigenous to the Mediterranean countries, with many local and regional varieties. Given the close geographical proximities of all of these nation-states and territories, it is not surprising that the foods are so fresh and readily available and that the cuisines have greatly influenced one another over time.

The Mediterranean diet is not just one approach but an interpretation and translation of many different dietary patterns. The Mediterranean landscape favors goats and sheep, and fish is abundant from the vast coastal sources of the Mediterranean Sea. Olive oil is produced throughout Greece, Italy, Portugal, Spain, Turkey and other Mediterranean nation-states. The terrain is ripe with grapes for eating and wine production.

Southern Italian cuisine emphasizes grains, herbs such as basil and oregano, and garlic. Traditional Greek cuisine features dairy products, such as cheese and yogurt; fruits; spices such as cinnamon and cloves; and unleavened flatbreads, similar to those that are found in the Middle East. Spanish cuisine relies on garlic and olive oil and adds ground almonds, onions, peppers and tomatoes to some of the neighboring cuisines. Southern French cuisine has more meat and fewer grains, but it still relies on garlic and olive oil, with Herbes de Provence, a mixture of marjoram, rosemary, sage and thyme, predominant. Pita bread, hummus and falafel are popular in eastern Mediterranean cuisine, scented with cardamom, coriander and cumin.

The *Mediterranean triad* refers to three foods that comprise the Mediterranean diet: grapes (and wine), olives (and olive oil), and wheat and wheat products. Mediterranean inhabitants have consumed these foods since biblical times.

Today, wheat is stored as raw grain, processed into flour, or transformed into a number of wheat products, including breadstuffs, cracked wheat and pasta. Olives are eaten raw as fruit or preserved and stored. Olive oil is used while still young or indefinitely if properly stored. Grapes are consumed raw, dried or fermented as wine.

These three foodstuffs provide carbohydrates, some protein, healthy fats and phytonutrients. Small portions of cheese, fish, fowl, legumes, nuts, seasonal fruits and vegetables and yogurt supplement these Mediterranean staples and form what is known as the *Mediterranean Food Guide Pyramid*.

THE MEDITERRANEAN FOOD GUIDE PYRAMID

Oldways, a nonprofit "food issues think tank," is perhaps best known for developing the well-known Mediterranean Diet Pyramid, shown in Figure 12-3. The Oldways Traditional Healthy Mediterranean Diet Pyramid was the first in a series of food guide pyramids that illustrated the healthy traditional food and dietary patterns of various cultures and regions worldwide. Other food guide pyramids included the Asian, Latin American and Native American pyramids.

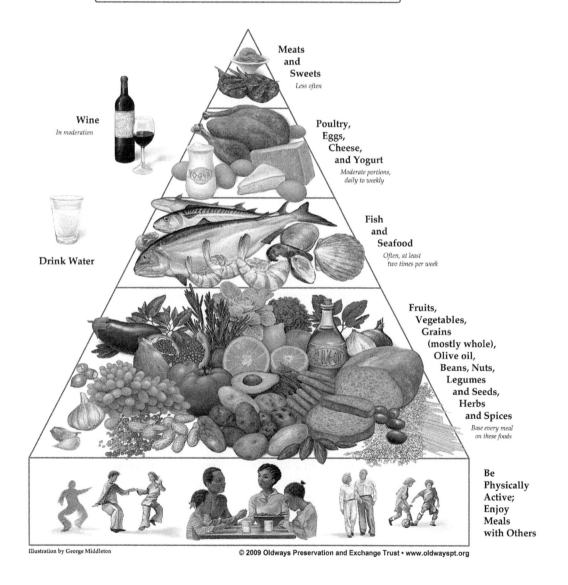

557

FIGURE 12-3

The Mediterranean Diet Pyramid.

These food guide pyramids were an outgrowth of the USDA Food Guide Pyramid of 1992 that reflect clinical and epidemiological research about what constitutes optimal human nutrition. The design of the Traditional Healthy Mediterranean Diet Pyramid and the others in the series shows the proportion of foods in each of these diets, with the number and frequency of servings.

Regular physical activity is the foundation of the Oldways Traditional Healthy Mediterranean Diet Pyramid. An abundance of plant foods, including breads and grains, fruits and vegetables, legumes, nuts and seeds, and potatoes are recommended daily, along with moderate amounts of cheese and yogurt.

Seasonally fresh and locally grown foods are encouraged. Olive oil is promoted as the principal fat. Low to moderate amounts of fish and poultry, zero to four eggs, and a moderate amount of sweets are limited to weekly consumption. Lean red meat consumption is restricted to just a few times monthly. Wine is advocated in moderation with meals, but it is optional. A variety of minimally processed foods are incorporated where necessary.

MEDITERRANEAN FOODS

While there is a commonality of foods in Mediterranean cuisines, some countries are noted for their local ingredients. This is just a sampling of the countless products that are representative of some of the nation-states of the Mediterranean.

Cow, Goat, and Sheep Milk and Milk Products

The traditional Mediterranean diet does not focus on dairy milk. When dairy products are used in recipes, they are usually yogurt or cheese. Yogurt plays a very important role in Greek, Eastern Indian, Middle Eastern and Turkish cuisines as a tangy ingredient, marinade and tenderizer. Yogurt-inspired dips, dressings, salads, sauces and soups are plentiful, including Eastern Indian *lassi* (a yogurt-based drink) and *raita* (a seasoned yogurt condiment) and Greek *tzatziki* (a yogurt and cucumber dip or salad).

558

Mediterranean cheese is widely diverse in appearance, aroma, taste, texture and versatility. Some French, Greek, Italian, Middle Eastern and Spanish cheeses include the following:

French Cheese

- *Brousse* is a soft goat's or sheep's milk cheese. It is the Provençal equivalent of Italian ricotta cheese in both taste and texture. Brousse is excellent paired with grapes or pears.
- *Chèvre* is a tart and slightly salty semisoft goat's milk cheese with a characteristic odor. It is stark white because goat's milk lacks carotene, the yellow pigment that is found in cow's milk.

Chèvre contains about the same amount of fat as cow's milk cheese, but it has a higher amount of medium-chain fatty acids, which creates its unusual odor. It can be paired with chutney, cured meats, dried fruits, and olives, but not citrus fruits.

- *Roquefort* is an aged blue-veined sheep's milk cheese with a characteristic odor and flavor. Roquefort is aged in caves and carries a French-protected designation of origin. Pair Roquefort with figs, pears, raisins or fruit, and nut breads.

Greek Cheese

- *Feta* is one of the oldest cheeses in the world. In 2002, Greece won the rights to own the name "feta." Feta is made from sheep's milk or a combination of sheep's and goat's milk, in both full-fat and reduced-fat varieties. Its flavor ranges from mild to tangy and salty. Feta is used in salads, and it blends nicely with eggplant, onions, shrimp and tomatoes.
- *Kasseri* is a semihard and slightly crumbly ewe's and goat's milk cheese. It has a sweet-tart, olive-like flavor. Kasseri is used to make saganaki (flaming cheese).
- *Kefalotiri* is made from ewe's or goat's milk. It has a salty, piquant flavor and rich aroma. Because kefalotiri is so hard, it is ideal for grating. Kefalotiri is used to make spanakopita (spinach and phyllo pie).

Italian Cheese

- *Fontina* is a semisoft cow's milk cheese with a sweet, buttery flavor. It is the primary ingredient in Italian fonduta (cheese fondue) and is also used as a table or dessert cheese.
- *Gorgonzola* is a blue-veined cow's milk cheese with a full, earthy flavor. It is commonly used in pasta dishes and salads, or paired with dried fruit.
- *Mascarpone* is a naturally light and sweet, soft cow's milk cheese, frequently used in tiramisu (a dessert that integrates Italian biscuits, brandy and coffee).
- *Mozzarella* is both a stringy-textured buffalo milk cheese and a fresh pasteurized or unpasteurized cow's milk cheese. Whole or part-skim and smoked mozzarella are widely used in the food service industry in Italian-influenced dishes.
- *Parmesan* is a hard cheese. As Parmesan ages, it becomes more pungent and flavorful. Parmigiano-Reggiano is made from cow's milk that has aged a minimum of 24 months. Parmesan is used in pastas and pizzas and as an essential ingredient in some sauces, such as pesto.
- *Ricotta* is a sheep's milk whey-based cheese. Like mascarpone, ricotta is a flavorful ingredient in Italian desserts, such as cheesecake and cannoli (a Sicilian pastry).

Middle Eastern Cheese

- *Aackawi* is a soft white cow's milk cheese that is native to Lebanon and Syria. It is primarily used as a table cheese.
- *Kenafa* is an unsalted fresh soft sheep's milk cheese that is used in cheesecake-type desserts.
- *Jibneh arabieh* is a fresh white cow's milk cheese that is popular in Egypt. It is similar to feta but less salty, so it can be used in similar dishes.

Spanish Cheese

- *Manchego* is made from pasteurized sheep's milk. It pairs with salmon or lamb and is often eaten with *dulce de membrillo* (quince paste).
- *Picos de Europa* is a blue cheese also known as Valdeon. It is eaten with honey for breakfast and with cured and smoked meats. Picos de Europa is a combination of cow's, sheep's and goat's milk.
- *Queso Iberico* is an aged semicured ewe's milk cheese that is slightly piquant and nutty. Queso Iberico is a table cheese, but it is also used for grating and grilling.

559

Fish and Seafood

The Mediterranean Sea is filled with anchovies, clams, **cuttlefish** (sepia or inkfish), eel, *langoustes* (saltwater crayfish), lobster, mackerel, mussels, octopus, oysters, *pilchards* (sardines), prawns, salt cod, scallops, shrimp, snapper, squid, swordfish and tuna, among others. The traditional Mediterranean methods of cooking fish include boiled in hearty soups and stews; grilled with olive oil and herbs; poached in flavorful liquid or wine; and wrapped in parchment and baked.

Recipe: Gazpacho with Bay Scallops (Spain)

*Traditional gazpacho soup is a cold tomato-based raw vegetable soup. It originated in the southern region of Andalucía and is popular in Spanish/Portuguese cuisines, where fish-laden soups are common. This version of **Gazpacho with Bay Scallops** in the **Recipe file** which is located within the Culinary Nutrition website at www.culinarynutrition.elsevier.com, adds low-calorie and lean bay scallops to the tomato-vegetable mixture. A small cup can be paired with a simple pasta entree, or a larger serving can be paired with a cheese course similar to the cheese pairings above. The finished dish is shown within the centerfold **Photo file** in Plate 12.1.*

Fruits and Vegetables

Traditional fruits in Mediterranean cuisine include apricots, figs, grapes, lemons, melons, oranges and plums. Fruit is often the sign of the end of a meal. Dessert is often simply an assortment of seasonal fruits.

Traditional vegetables in Mediterranean cuisine include beets, broccoli, cabbage, carrots, cauliflower, dandelion and other greens, eggplant, kale, okra, onions, peppers, spinach and turnips. Vegetable-inspired dishes are often the center of the meal, such as Middle Eastern *baba ghanoush* (roasted, mashed and seasoned eggplant), Indian carrot curry or *mutah paneer* (pea and cheese curry).

> **Morsel** "It is not really an exaggeration to say that peace and happiness begin, geographically, where garlic is used in cooking," —Marcel Boulestin (French author, chef and restaurateur, 1878–1943) [11]

Garlic and Onions

Garlic is predominant in many Mediterranean recipes. A number of the Mediterranean nation-states have versions of garlic sauces that accompany meats, poultry and fish, such as Greek skordalia, French aioli, Italian pesto, Lebanese garlic sauce, and Spanish aigo bouido (a soup that is made with an entire head of garlic). Parsley is often added to Mediterranean dishes to freshen the strong taste and odor of garlic.

Onions are the foundation of many Mediterranean dishes. They create a solid, nonassertive flavor base that melts into a dish over time. French *confit d'oignon* (onion jam) and Italian *cipolline arrostite* (roasted onions, often in olive oil) are prime examples of the versatility of onions.

Like garlic, onions have cardiovascular health benefits. A study of the effects of onion-infused olive oil on arterial blood pressure showed that the onion–olive oil mixture helped dilate blood vessels and reduce blood platelet stickiness [12].

Legumes

The Mediterranean diet includes a daily serving of (⅓ to 1 cup cooked) legumes. The Mediterranean's most famous legumes are chickpeas (garbanzos), fava beans (broad beans) and lentils. Other Mediterranean legumes and their location of origin include the following:

Type of Legume	Locality
Carob or St. John's bread	Syria
Cowpea or asparagus beans	West Africa
Cultivated field and sweet peas	Near Eastern Mediterranean
Flageolets	France
Hyacinth	East Africa
Lupines	Southern Mediterranean and northern Africa

Mediterranean legume-based dishes include southwestern French *cassoulet* (a stew with white flageolets beans and haricots or green beans), Italian *fagioli all'uccelletto* (white bean ragout) and *lenticchie con pancetta* (lentils with pancetta), and Middle Eastern *hummus* (garbanzo puree).

Meats

Meats traditionally make up only a small portion of the Mediterranean diet. When the Mediterranean diet was first studied in 1952, only about 13 ounces of meat were consumed weekly; some people consume this amount today in one meal! In the 1950s, meat was used in the Mediterranean diet as a condiment, not as an entree as it is used today.

In the Mediterranean regions, meats are generally cooked by low, slow cooking methods, such as simmering or stewing, or by quick methods that sear the meat and retain nutrients, such as grilling or sauteing. Beef, kid, lamb, pork, poultry and veal are common in Mediterranean recipes. The following are some typical Mediterranean meat dishes:

- **Beef:** Italian *bistecca* (beef steak) and Middle Eastern *kefta* (hamburger)
- **Kid (Young Goat):** Italian *capretto alla cacciatora* (kid with garlic, rosemary and vinegar) and Greek *chevon souvlaki* (skewered goat)
- **Lamb:** Moroccan *lamb tangine* (a stew with lemons and olives) and Greek *souvlaki* (lamb brochette)
- **Pork:** Florentine *costata de maiale* (grilled pork chop) and Portuguese *lomo de porco* (pork fillet)
- **Poultry:** Moroccan *bastilla* (pigeon pie) and Turkish *tavuk izgara* (grilled chicken with yogurt)
- **Veal:** Milanese *ossobuco* (veal shank) and Sicilian *scaloppine* (pounded veal)

Nuts and Seeds

Almonds are a common nut throughout the Mediterranean. Almonds are high in protein and fiber and relatively low in fat—especially saturated fat. They are also a good source of vitamin E, copper, magnesium, manganese and phosphorus.

Whole and ground almonds are used in Spanish *ajo blanco* (white garlicky gazpacho) and *turrón* (almond candy); Greek *amygdalota biscuits* (cookies); French *financiers, macaroons, marzipan* and *nougats* (pastries and sweets); and Indian *pasanda-style* (curries) and *badam halva* and *sohan burfy* (sweets).

Pine nuts, also called *pignoli*, are small, oval, sweet nuts that have been associated with the Mediterranean region, particularly Italy, for over 2,000 years. Pine nuts are also popular in Greek, Lebanese, Spanish and Turkish cuisines.

Italian cooks stuff escarole with pine nuts, anchovies and capers; add pine nuts to fresh sardine sauce for pasta; and blend pine nuts, bread crumbs, broth, chives, garlic, lemon juice and olive oil into a sauce that accompanies grilled or baked chicken or fish. Spanish cooks use pine nuts with braised rabbit and over fried sole. Greek and Turkish cooks stuff fresh mussels with pine nuts, herbs and rice.

Sesame seeds are used in Greek cakes and *pastel* (roasted sesame honey candy); Middle Eastern *tahini* (sesame seed paste); Middle Eastern, East Asian and Indian *halvah* (honey confection); Punjabi and Indian *pinni* (sweet balls); Sicilian and French *ficelle sesame* (baguettes topped with sesame seeds); and in Togo West African (soup).

Olives and Olive Oil

Olive oil, produced from the fruit of the olive trees throughout Greece, Italy, Portugal, Spain, Turkey and other Mediterranean countries is indispensable in the Mediterranean food pantry and diet. Products packed in olive oil, such as artichoke hearts, pimentos and tuna, while higher in total fat, are a good source of monounsaturated fatty acids. Because of olive oil's higher smoke point, it can be used for quick deep-frying, such as in Spanish *boquerones britos* (anchovies).

Olive oil is common in Catalan *pa amb tomaquet* (bread with garlic, tomatoes and olive oil); French Provencal *tapenade* (puree of anchovies, capers, olives and olive oil); Greek *moussaka* (eggplant casserole); Italian *pesto* (pasta sauce); Lebanese *tabouli* (cracked wheat salad with parsley and tomatoes); Middle Eastern *tahini* or *tartor* (sauce); and Sicilian *caponata* (a celery, eggplant and sweetened vinegar appetizer or salad).

Wheat and Other Grains

Wheat and other grains, such as bulgur from Turkey, couscous from North Africa, cornmeal from Northern Italy, and rice from Spain, Greece and Turkey, provide the backbone of the Mediterranean diet.

- **Bulgur (bulghur or burghul)**, is coarse or fine cracked wheat that has been partially cooked. Bulgur is a staple in Lebanon, Palestine, Syria and Turkey, where it is used in traditional dishes such as Lebanese *kibbeh* (a mixture of ground meat and spices), or Turkish *tabouleh* (a salad with olive oil, parsley and tomatoes).
- **Couscous** is a quick-cooking grain that is produced from crushed semolina wheat, and sometimes corn or pearl millet. It absorbs flavors easily like rice. Couscous comes in both refined and whole grain varieties. It is used in traditional North African Moroccan and Middle Eastern cuisines with fish, lamb, or poultry and vegetables with broth or spicy sauce, such as Moroccan *charmoula* (a spicy marinade).

> **Recipe: Tabbouleh with Pickled Vegetables (Lebanon)**
> *There are many different versions of tabbouleh, a salad that is based on cracked bulgur wheat, tomatoes, cucumbers, parsley, mint, olive oil and lemon juice. It is popular in Armenia, Cyprus, Israel, Jordan, Lebanon, Syria and Turkey and growing in popularity in the United States.*
> ***Tabbouleh with Pickled Vegetables*** *pairs this Mediterranean staple with lightly marinated vegetables for more color, texture, taste and phytonutrients. The recipe can be found in the **Recipe file** which is located within the Culinary Nutrition website at www.culinarynutrition.elsevier.com. The finished dish is shown within the centerfold **Photo file** in Plate 12.2.*

- **Cornmeal** is commonly cooked into Northern Italian *polenta* (gruel or porridge) with flavorful herbs and spices and bits of protein. Typical combinations include *polenta e gorgonzola* (gorgonzola cheese), *missultin e polenta* (fish) and *polenta e osei* (small song birds).
- **Rice** is a versatile staple grain in the Mediterranean region, particularly in Greek, Northern Italian, Spanish and Turkish cuisines. Three types of rice commonly used are:
  - ○ **Short-grain rice** (such as *bomba*) is used in Catalan and Valencian *paella* (a dish made with rice, legumes, meat, seafood and vegetables) and Arabic and Greek *rice pudding*.
  - ○ **Medium-grain rice** (such as *arborio*) is the foundation of Northern Italian recipes. Arborio rice easily absorbs liquids without turning soggy. It transforms into smooth and creamy dishes such as *risotto* (a dish made with fish, legumes, meat, seafood or vegetables—often with cheese or wine). Arborio rice is also used in *pilaf* (sauteed and seasoned rice) and salads.
  - ○ **Long-grain rice** (such as *basmati or patna*) is used in eastern Mediterranean, Greek and Turkish *pilaf*; Greek *avgolemono* (a sauce and soup made with lemon and egg); Turkish *dolma* (stuffing for vine leaves and sweet bell peppers); and Egyptian, Arabic eastern Mediterranean and North African *kushary*, *mjadarah* and *mudardara* (variations of dishes made with rice with lentils).
- **Wheat and wheat products** that are minimally processed are characteristic of the Mediterranean diet. *Hard durum or semolina wheat* is higher in protein by about one-third and slightly lower in carbohydrates than all-purpose wheat flour. It is best for Southern Italian and Sicilian pasta. Hard durum or semolina wheat will not lose its shape or become too sticky when cooked.

  Semolina and whole wheat are used in breads that include among others Catalan *coques* (pizza-like); Egyptian *fiteer* (flatbread); French hard-wheat baguette (long loaves); Middle Eastern pita (flat pocket bread); Italian pizza and focaccia (flatbread related to pizza); Lebanese *manoushe* (breakfast pizza) and *tabouneh* (sourdough pita); and Middle Eastern *lavash*.
- *Phyllo (filo)* are sheets of paper-thin unleavened dough that are mostly used in sweet and savory Greek, Middle Eastern and Turkish pastries and pies. Phyllo dough is available in both white flour and whole-grain varieties. Phyllo recipes are typically made with butter or oil to help tenderize the pastry sheets.

562

Wine and Vinegar

Moderate consumption of wine with meals is an integral feature of the Mediterranean diet. The skin and seeds of grapes contain powerful substances called *oligomeric proantho cyannidins (OPCs)*, which may block cancer-causing free radicals in the environment.

Drinking grape juice may have the same beneficial effects as drinking wine. About 1 to 2 (4-ounce) glasses of wine per day for men, and 1(4-ounce) glass of wine per day for women is considered as moderate if alcoholic beverages are consumed.

Wine vinegar, made from red or white wine, is a common ingredient in some Mediterranean cuisines. Wine vinegar tends to have lower acidity than cider or white vinegars. Common wine vinegars include French *champagne* vinegar, Spanish *sherry* vinegar and Italian *balsamic* vinegar, which is full-bodied, slightly sweet, and somewhat syrupy. Balsamic vinegar is excellent in salads, sauces and fruit desserts.

> ## Recipe: Stuffed Figs in Port Wine Sauce (Portugal and Spain)
>
> *Sometimes the simplest of desserts are the most satisfying. This recipe for **Stuffed Figs in Port Wine Sauce** in the **Recipe file** which is located within the Culinary Nutrition website at www.culinarynutrition.elsevier.com, is a perfect finale for a meat-filled or vegetarian Mediterranean meal. Figs are native to the Mediterranean and Middle East, where they were one of the first plants that was cultivated. Figs are high in calcium and fiber from their chewy skin and countless seeds. They are also rich in copper, magnesium, manganese, potassium, vitamin K, flavonoids and poplyphenols. The finished dish is shown within the centerfold **Photo file** in 12.3.*

MEDITERRANEAN MEAL PLANS

The typical US "meat and potatoes" diet, with an emphasis on protein, fat and refined carbohydrates, can benefit from a Mediterranean-type diet makeover with less protein, healthier fats and whole grains. The wholesome Mediterranean foods and ingredients just described are available from many US food suppliers, supermarkets and specialty stores. They can easily be integrated into typical US meals as shown following. Here is a sample Mediterranean menu that incorporates these ingredients:

Breakfast

- Foccacia with feta cheese and grapes
- Fruit and nut bread with goat cheese and fresh orange slices
- Whole-grain baguette with melted cheese
- Whole-grain muffin with yogurt and fresh melon
- Whole-grain phyllo pastry filled with ground walnuts and honey
- Whole-grain toast with almond butter and date or fig jam

Lunch

- Arborio rice salad with mixed seafood and vegetables
- Arugula salad with shaved Parmesan cheese and garbanzo beans (both salads with lemon juice and olive oil dressing)
- Falafel in whole-grain pita bread with lettuce, tomatoes and tahini dressing
- Mashed white bean spread with sesame seed crackers, cucumbers and tomatoes
- Tapenade with whole-grain flatbread, sweet bell peppers and onions
- Vegetable and bean soup with fresh fruit and goat's or sheep's milk cheese

Dinner

- Braised chicken with asparagus, garlic and lemon
- Grilled chicken and zucchini with olive oil, basil and wine
- Grilled leg of lamb with artichokes, bay leaves, olives and tomatoes
- Mixed bean soup with whole-grain croutons and grated cheese
- Penne pasta with prosciutto, ricotta and spinach
- Polenta with oregano, porcini mushrooms and steamed kale
- Red peppers filled with parsley, pine nuts, Parmesan cheese and cooked long-grain rice
- Pilaf with couscous, garbanzos, mint, onions and sweet bell peppers
- Seafood paella with grilled whole-grain garlic bread
- Tomatoes filled with white bean puree and topped with toasted almonds
- Veal shank with gremolata (garlic, lemon zest and parsley)
- Zucchini boats filled with caramelized onions and topped with Romano cheese

563

Accompaniments

- Baba ghanoush with chunky eggplant
- Flavored olives, plain and stuffed
- Fresh herb salad with balsamic vinaigrette
- Grilled seasonal vegetables or salad
- Marinated feta or other semifirm cheese
- Pickled beets, carrots, cabbage, cauliflower, sweet bell peppers or turnips
- Pita triangles with garlic and herbs
- Roasted pears with quince paste
- Vegetable pesto pizza
- Yogurt with honey and almonds
- White bean hummus with pomegranate seeds

Desserts

- Apricots, berries, grapes, clementines (variety of Mandarin orange), melons, oranges or plums
- Bread pudding
- Compote (cooked fruit in sweetened liquid)
- Flan (caramel custard)
- Ground almond tart
- Olive oil cake

- Rice pudding
- Ricotta cheesecake
- Sponge cake with wine
- Walnut and honey tart

Beverages

- Coffee, fruit juice, tea, yogurt-based drinks, water and/or wine

SAMPLE MEDITERRANEAN MENU

A sample Mediterranean menu can be created by selecting one dish from each of the above categories. Balance ingredients, flavors and textures when making choices to add interest to these simple, flavorsome ingredients. If consumed in moderation, a Mediterranean menu such as the one in Table 12-3 should provide many of the benefits of the traditional Mediterranean diet. The abundance of fresh, local, minimally processed ingredients are difficult to match year-round in the United States—especially in climates far north of the equator.

TABLE 12-3 A Sample Mediterranean Diet Menu

	Breakfast	Lunch	Dinner
Meal Components	Bread, fruit, nuts and yogurt with specialty coffee	Legumes, herbs, olives and salad with mint tea	Chicken, pizza, vegetables and nut tart with red wine
Main course	Fruit and nut bread with goat cheese and fresh orange slices	Falafel in whole-grain pita bread with lettuce, tomatoes and tahini dressing	Grilled chicken and zucchini with olive oil, basil and wine
Accompaniments	Roasted pears with quince paste	Flavored olives, plain and stuffed	Grilled seasonal vegetable salad
	Yogurt with honey and almonds	Fresh herb salad with balsamic vinaigrette	Vegetable pesto pizza
Beverage	French or Turkish Coffee	Mint tea	Red wine
Dessert	Dried fruit	Fresh Fruit	Walnut and honey tart

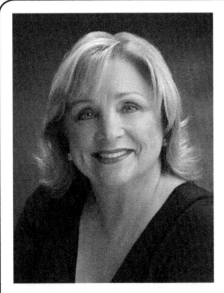

FIGURE 12-4
Maria Battaglia.

THE COOK'S CORNER: MARIA BATTAGLIA, ITALIAN FOOD AUTHORITY

Maria Battaglia, founder and president of La Cucina Italiana, Inc., is a leading bilingual English/Italian authority on Italian food, wine and tourism. Maria has developed, directed, and taught culinary courses across Italy and the United States. She is an accomplished food writer, syndicated restaurant reviewer and correspondent. Her work has appeared in *Food & Wine*, *Santé* and *Vinotizi*, among other publications. Maria has been a consultant and spokesperson in the United States for Barilla America, Contadina Foods, the Italian Cultural Institute and Italian Trade Commission, and Paterno Imports, and in Italy for MASI, Serègo Alighieri Winery and *Vialone Nano* Rice. Maria was voted "one of the five best cooking teachers" by *The Chicago Tribune* and is a recipient of Italy's prestigious *Diploma di Merito* (Diploma of Achievement) from the Federation of Italian Chefs in Italy. Maria believes that good food and wine should do more than merely fill the void; they should be enjoyed, savored and respected as works of culinary art. Maria presents this traditional **Lasagna with Artichokes and Asparagus** recipe and a healthier adaptation that follows with fewer calories and fat.

LASAGNA WITH ARTICHOKES AND ASPARAGUS—TRADITIONAL RECIPE

Ingredients

1 (8-ounce) package frozen artichoke hearts, thawed and coarsely chopped

1 (8-ounce) package frozen asparagus, thawed and coarsely chopped

Unsalted butter

1½ cups heavy cream, divided

¼ cup (packed) fresh basil leaves, chopped

1 (15-ounce) container whole-milk ricotta cheese

½ cup freshly grated Parmigiano-Reggiano cheese

1 large egg

1 teaspoon salt

2 tablespoons fresh flat-leaf parsley, chopped

1 (9-ounce) box (about 12 noodles) no-boil lasagna noodles

4 cups (about 1 pound) shredded mozzarella cheese, divided

Instructions

1. Preheat oven to 400 °F.
2. Brush 13×9×3-inch glass baking dish with unsalted butter.
3. Mix artichokes, asparagus, ½ cup heavy cream and basil in medium bowl.
4. Puree remaining 1 cup cream, ricotta cheese and next four ingredients in food processor; blend.
5. Spread 1 cup ricotta mixture over bottom of prepared baking dish.
6. Arrange four noodles in single layer over ricotta mixture; break noodles as needed to cover.
7. Spread ½ artichoke/asparagus mixture over noodles.
8. Spread 2½ cups ricotta mixture over artichokes/asparagus mixture.
9. Sprinkle 1 cup mozzarella cheese over artichoke/asparagus mixture.
10. Repeat with four noodles, artichoke/asparagus mixture, 2½ cups ricotta mixture, and 1 cup mozzarella cheese; top with four noodles.
11. Spread remaining ricotta mixture over noodles; sprinkle remaining 2 cups mozzarella over ricotta mixture. (Up to this point, lasagna can be prepared ahead of time.)*
12. Tent lasagna with foil; seal edges.
13. Bake lasagna about 30 minutes.
14. Remove foil; continue to bake until bubbles form at edges and top is browned, about 25 minutes.
15. Let stand about 15 minutes before serving.

Serving size: 8 to 10 servings

Nutrients per serving: 461 calories, 30 grams total fat, 18 grams saturated fat, 25 grams carbohydrates, 3 grams fiber, 24 grams protein, 679 milligrams sodium

*Prepare ahead: before baking, cover and refrigerate up to two days, or freeze up to three months. Thaw before baking 30 minutes at 400 °F.

LASAGNA WITH ARTICHOKES AND ASPARAGUS—MODIFIED AND HEALTHIER RECIPE

Ingredients

1 (8-ounce) packages frozen artichoke hearts, thawed and coarsely chopped

1 (8-ounce) package frozen asparagus, thawed and coarsely chopped

Nonfat cooking spray

¾ cup 2% dairy milk, divided

¼ cup (packed) fresh basil leaves, chopped

1 (15-ounce) container nonfat ricotta cheese

1 large egg

1 teaspoon salt

2 tablespoons fresh flat-leaf parsley, chopped

1 (9-ounce) box (12 noodles) no-boil lasagna noodles
4 cups (about 1 pound) shredded part-skim mozzarella cheese, divided

Instructions
1. Preheat oven to 400 °F.
2. Prepare 13×9×3-inch glass baking dish with nonfat cooking spray.
3. Mix artichokes, asparagus, ½ cup 2% milk, and chopped basil in medium bowl.
4. Puree remaining ¼ cup milk, ricotta and next four ingredients in food processor; blend.
5. Spread 1 cup ricotta mixture over bottom of prepared baking dish.
6. Arrange four noodles in single layer over ricotta mixture; break noodles as needed to cover.
7. Spread ½ artichoke/asparagus mixture over noodles.
8. Spread 2½ cups ricotta mixture over artichokes/asparagus mixture.
9. Sprinkle 1 cup mozzarella cheese over artichoke/asparagus mixture.
10. Repeat with four noodles, artichoke/asparagus mixture, 2½ cups ricotta mixture and 1 cup mozzarella cheese; top with four noodles.
11. Spread remaining ricotta mixture over noodles; sprinkle remaining 2 cups mozzarella over ricotta mixture. (Up to this point, lasagna can be prepared ahead of time.)*
12. Tent lasagna with foil, seal edges.
13. Bake lasagna about 30 minutes.
14. Remove foil; continue to bake until bubbles form at edges and top is browned, about 25 minutes.
15. Let stand about 15 minutes before serving.

Serving size: 8 to 10 servings

Nutrients per serving: 330 calories, 13 grams total fat, 7.8 grams saturated fat, 25.9 grams carbohydrates, 3 grams fiber, 26.1 grams protein, 864.8 milligrams sodium

*Prepare ahead: before baking, cover and refrigerate up to two2 days, or freeze up to three months. Thaw before baking 30 minutes at 400 °F.

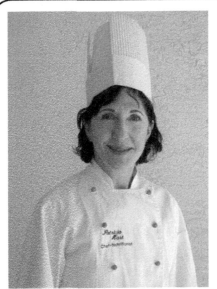

FIGURE 12-5
Patricia Hart.

THE COOK'S CORNER: CHEF PATRICIA HART, REGISTERED DIETITIAN AND MEDICAL TECHNOLOGIST

Chef Patricia Hart has 25 years of experience in the fields of food preparation, human nutrition, food chemistry, sanitation and medicine. Patricia holds a bachelor's degree in medical technology, an AOS degree in culinary arts from the Culinary Institute of America, and a master's degree in food science and human nutrition. Patricia also studied cooking and flavor balancing with renowned chef Madeleine Kamman in France.

Chef Hart teaches culinary skills and nutritional concepts to a variety of professional audiences and writes about these topics in many consumer and trade magazines. For the last 20 years, she has developed food products for many of the major food companies. She is often called upon by her peers for her expertise in culinary development, research, training and writing.

Chef Hart has created a healthier version of baba ghanoush, a Middle Eastern eggplant dip, with less calories and fat. According to Chef Hart, "Baba ghanoush is a Middle Eastern dish that is eaten with vegetables or as a spread with bread. It is a creamy dish. In this modified version, the creaminess comes mostly from using yogurt, which also adds a tart taste. The small amount of tahini is used to highlight the familiar fatty taste that is found in many Middle Eastern appetizers."

BABA GHANOUSH—TRADITIONAL RECIPE

Ingredients

1 globe eggplant (approximately 1 to 2 pounds)*
2 cloves garlic
3 tablespoons tahini (sesame seed paste)
3 tablespoons lemon juice
½ teaspoon salt

Instructions

1. Preheat oven to 350 °F.
2. Prick eggplant several times with fork.
3. Bake eggplant until soft, about 45 minutes.
4. Allow eggplant to cool; scoop out flesh and discard skin.
5. Combine eggplant and remaining ingredients in blender or food processor; process until smooth.

*Note: Most globe eggplants are about 1 to 2 pounds.

Nutrients per entire recipe: 388 calories, 22.7 grams total fat, 3.2 grams saturated fat, 43.8 grams carbohydrates, 20.1 grams fiber, 13.3 grams protein, 1,219 milligrams sodium

BABA GHANOUSH—MODIFIED HEALTHIER RECIPE

Ingredients

Nonfat cooking spray
1 globe eggplant (approximately 1 to 2 pounds)*
Olive oil
3 tablespoons nonfat plain yogurt
1½ tablespoons tahini (sesame seed paste)
2 teaspoons lemon juice
2 teaspoons cumin powder
1½ teaspoons chopped fresh garlic
¼ teaspoon salt
4 drops hot sauce (optional)

*Note: Most globe eggplants are about 1 to 2 pounds.

Instructions

1. Preheat broiler.
2. Prepare sheet pan with nonfat cooking spray.
3. Place whole eggplant over medium-high heat over gas stovetop burner. (The eggplant can be placed under a broiler and turned frequently to char.)
4. Rotate eggplant with tongs to burn eggplant skin all over (eggplant flesh should be soft).
5. Remove eggplant from heat; slice lengthwise down center,
6. Brush cut sides with olive oil; place cut sides down on prepared sheet pan.
7. Place eggplant under broiler to burn skin all over (eggplant flesh should be soft).
8. Scoop out flesh with large spoon; place in blender or food processor; blend. Discard skin or compost.
9. Add remaining ingredients; process about 45 seconds, until smooth.

Nutrients per entire recipe: 301 calories, 12.4 grams total fat, 1.8 grams saturated fat, 42.3 grams carbohydrates, 18.1 grams fiber, 13.6 grams protein, 672.4 milligrams sodium

> ### FOOD BYTE
>
> Organ meats commonly appear in some Hispanic (and Asian) recipes. Organ meats (offal) are the entrails (intestines) and internal organs of butchered animals. They include the brain, chitterlings (pig's small or large intestine), heart, head (pig, calf, lamb and sheep), kidney, liver, lights (lungs), scrotum, snout (nose), sweetbreads (thymus), tongue, tripe (stomach), and trotters (feet). Many of these organ meats are high in fat and cholesterol.

Hispanic Cuisine

Hispanics are people who originated from Central or South America, Cuba, Mexico, Puerto Rico and other Spanish-speaking areas of Latin America. After Latin American immigration into the United States substantially increased during the late 1900s, Hispanics became the largest minority subpopulation in the United States. Most Hispanics settled in the southwestern United States, particularly in California and New Mexico.

The three major Hispanic groups that comprise the US Hispanic population today are Cubans, Mexican Americans, and Puerto Ricans. Mexican Americans represent the majority of Hispanics in the United States.

The present US Hispanic diet is a mixture of the traditional dietary patterns of these immigrants with modern, time-saving influences. Many regional differences still exist, particularly within diet composition and food preparation. Common to the various Hispanic cultures is family life, with its emphasis on home-prepared family meals.

THE HISPANIC DIET, NUTRITION AND HEALTH

Overall, Hispanics tend to consume more beef, eggs, legumes and rice and drink more dairy whole milk than Caucasians. They also tend to consume fewer vegetables and slightly more fruits.

Hispanics, especially Mexican Americans, have a higher intake of dietary fiber compared to Caucasians, with much of this dietary fiber from legumes. In general, Hispanics have low intakes of calcium, vitamin E and zinc compared to the Dietary Reference Intakes (DRIs).

The US culture, including foods and beverages, has significantly influenced the traditional Hispanic diet. Today, Hispanic Americans who still use Spanish as a primary language at home tend to consume healthier diets than those who use English as a primary language. They also tend to eat less fat, saturated fat and cholesterol.

Acculturation and the changing Hispanic diet have serious health implications. Type II diabetes is two to three times higher in Hispanics than in Caucasians, and it is especially high in Mexican Americans. Hispanics with diabetes have two to four times the risk of developing cardiovascular disease. This increased risk of diabetes is accompanied by an increased risk of obesity [16–18].

THE CUBAN DIET AND CUISINE

Cuban cuisine is influenced by Arabic, African, Chinese, French, Portuguese and Spanish cultures that were brought by explorers to this Caribbean island. Traditional Cuban cooking is chiefly peasant cuisine, with little concern for measurements and orderly procedures—like many other ethnic cuisines. It relies on *sofrito* as a base for legumes, rice and stews. In Cuban cuisine, sofrito consists of garlic, green pepper, ground pepper, onions and tomatoes sauteed in oil. Other flavorful ingredients in Cuban cuisine include *cilantro* (the leaves of the coriander plant, also known as Chinese parsley), *culantro* or *recao* (a stronger version of cilantro that is used in legumes, soups and stews), cumin, *laurel* (bay), and oregano.

Cuban root vegetables include *boniato* (sweet potato), *malanga* (similar to taro root), *plantain* (similar to banana, used for cooking), sweet and white potatoes, and *yuca* (similar to cassava, used for tapioca). Vegetables are often flavored with *mojo* (a marinade that is also used with black beans, meat dishes, stews and tomato-based sauces). Traditional Cuban mojo contains juice from sour oranges, but equal parts of freshly squeezed orange and lime juice can be used. Other Cuban sauces include *mojo criollo* (garlic sauce) and *alcaparrado* (a sauce that is made with capers, olives and pimiento).

Meats and poultry are usually marinated in citrus juices, especially lime and sour orange, and then sauteed or slow-roasted over low heat until very tender. Pork products are commonly used. These include *chorizo* (sausage), *jamón* ham, *torcino* (bacon) and lard. Very few foods are deep-fried or served with creamy sauces.

TYPICAL CUBAN MEALS
Breakfast

A typical Cuban breakfast consists of a grilled *tostada* (corn pancake) and *café con leche* (strong espresso coffee with warm milk) or *café cubano* (Cuban coffee). The tostada is often torn into pieces and then dunked into the coffee. *Croquetas* (lightly breaded and fried finger rolls with smoky creamed ham) may also be served at breakfast.

Lunch

A typical Cuban lunch consists of *empanadas* (chicken or meat turnovers) or Cuban sandwiches that are lightly toasted in a *plancha sandwich press*, which is similar to an Italian *panini press*. Cuban sandwiches are often accompanied by thinly sliced plantain chips.

Cuban sandwiches include the *mixto* that is made with glazed ham, roast pork, Swiss cheese, pickles and mustard on sweetened egg bread; *media noche or midnight* (named for its popularity in Havana's night clubs), which is similar to the mixto sandwich, but without the glazed ham; and *pan con bistec* that is made with thinly sliced *palomilla steak* on Cuban bread and garnished with lettuce, tomatoes and fried potato sticks.

Dinner

A typical Cuban dinner consists of fish, meat or poultry often accompanied by some starchy combination, such as *congrí* (red beans and white rice), *Moors and Christians* (black beans and white rice), *maduros* (sweet fried plantains), or *yuca con mojo* (yucca with garlic sauce).

Meat dishes include *ajiaco* (chunky meat and vegetable stew), *boliche* (chorizo-stuffed roast), *lechon asado* (roast pork from the whole pig), *pavo rellano* (stuffed turkey), *picadillo* (ground beef, spices and vegetables), and *ropa vieja* (sauteed shredded beef, onions and peppers). A small salad of avocadoes, onions, and/or tomatoes is often served with meat dishes.

A special Cuban holiday meal may include a small pig that is first marinated with garlic, salt and sour orange juice, and then slowly roasted for several hours over an open fire.

Desserts

Sweet desserts and *cafe cubano* often follow the dinner meal. Desserts include *flan* (caramel-flavored custard); *natilla* (chocolate or coconut pudding); or coconut, guava or papaya marmalade with cheese.

Snacks

Cuban snacks include bakery items, fruits and sweetened beverages. Baked and fried snacks include *bocaditos* (bite-sized sandwiches layered with ham spread), *croquetas* (small rolls filled with mashed potatoes, minced meat, shellfish or vegetables, covered in breadcrumbs and fried), *empanadas* (baked or fried pastries stuffed with seasoned mincemeat), and *pastelitos* (small flaky turnovers filled with cheese, guava or meat).

Beverages

Cuban beverages include freshly squeezed citrus juices, *guarapo* (sweet "juice" of freshly pressed sugar cane) and *baditos* (icy fruit-based alcoholic drinks including *daiquiris* and *mojitos*) that are made with lime juice and pure cane rum.

THE CUBAN DIET, NUTRITION AND HEALTH

The Cuban diet has a rich history that is tied into its economics. The traditional Cuban diet is filled with starchy root vegetables, grains and legumes that create the foundation of Cuban casseroles, side dishes and soups. This heavy emphasis on starches sometimes comes at the expense of other vitamin- and mineral-filled vegetables. While Cubans do use some avocado, lettuce, onions, peppers and tomatoes in salads and to garnish dishes, these foods are typically not featured in meals. This dietary imbalance may be the consequence of Cuba's economic history.

The Cuban economy thrived until the 1990s. As in other thriving economies, food was abundant. A collapse in industrialized farming due to lack of fuel and equipment caused food shortages, malnutrition and suffering. Within five years, the prevalence of obesity and rates of death from coronary artery disease, diabetes and stroke in Cubans *decreased*.

The average daily caloric intake in Cubans fell from about 2,900 calories per person to about 1,800 calories per person. The proportion of physically active adults increased because fuel shortages forced people to walk or ride bicycles. Many Cubans became organic and sustainable farmers, instead of relying on chemicals, food and oil from other countries. Rice from Vietnam and some apples and beef from the United States were imported. Today, Cubans face similar diet and health concerns like the rest of the world [13].

THE MEXICAN-AMERICAN DIET AND CUISINE

When Mexicans migrated to the American Southwest, they brought their native ingredients: beans, chilies, legumes and squash. Native Americans were already living on berries, corn, fish, game, squash and wild greens. The Spanish Indians of northern Mexico brought goat, pig, sheep, and steer. Fruit, rice and wheat were introduced by the Spaniards.

While foodstuffs were varied, the core of the traditional Mexican diet in the American Southwest in the 1820s was chilies, grains (particularly corn) and legumes. Corn was ground and made into *tortillas* (flat, thin cakes). Tortillas were filled with mixtures of chilies, legumes and meats, crisply fried into *tacos*, softened into *enchiladas*, and steamed into *tamales*.

Recipe: Grilled Tilapia Fish Tacos with Corn Salsa (Mexico)

*Tilapia is a delicate-tasting white fish that is low in calories, total fat and saturated fat and a good source of protein; the vitamins niacin and B12; and the minerals phosphorus, potassium and selenium. Tilapia is commonly breaded and fried for fish tacos. The tilapia in **Grilled Tilapia Fish Tacos with Corn Salsa** in the **Recipe file** which is located within the Culinary Nutrition website at www.culinarynutrition.elsevier.com, is lower in calories and fat because it is grilled. Sliced cabbage and radishes, traditional fish taco accompaniments, often complete this popular Mexican dish that is eaten any time of day. The finished dish is shown in within the centerfold **Photo file** in Plate 12.4.*

570

TYPICAL MEXICAN-AMERICAN MEALS

In the American Southwest of 1820s, breakfast included tortillas, beans and chilies, coffee and brown sugar. Trail lunches included bean tacos rolled in cornhusks. Dinner was similar to lunch, with bits of meat added to the beans. Chocolate and tea were consumed or traded.

Today, Mexican foods are still based on these traditional ingredients but with contemporary influences. Corn is used both fresh and ground in chilaquiles, enchiladas, tacos, tamales and tortillas. Other vegetables consist of squash, sweet potatoes and tomatoes.

Popular legumes include black, fava, kidney, pinto, and red beans, and lentils. Favored fruits include avocado, coconut, lemon, lime, mango, papaya, pineapple and Seville oranges. Herbs and spices add heat and zest and include allspice, cilantro, cloves, cumin, marjoram, oregano and thyme. Some specialized ingredients, preparations and techniques that are popular in Mexican recipes are shown in Table 12-4.

THE MEXICAN DIET, NUTRITION AND HEALTH

Clinical studies consistently show a high occurrence of cardiovascular disease, dental caries, obesity and overnutrition and undernutrition in the US Mexican population. As Mexicans migrate and assimilate in the United States, they often acquire unhealthy dietary changes. These include the increased consumption of fats, such as butter, margarine and salad dressings; high-sugar drinks in place of traditional fruit-based beverages and meats with saturated fats; and the decrease in inexpensive yet healthy sources of complex carbohydrates like beans and rice and in low-fat dairy products.

These dietary changes may be significantly economically based. The desire for cheaper foods and beverages may have increased some of these unhealthy diet changes. In 2010, US Mexicans comprised 12 percent of individuals below the poverty line [19].

TABLE 12-4 Specialized Ingredients, Preparations and Techniques in Mexican Recipes

Achiote	Coloring and seasoning
Adobo	Chili sauce
Albondiga	Ground meat and egg ball
Arroz	Rice
Cabrito al asador	Broiled young kid
Cajeta	Caramelized goat's or sheep's milk
Calabazade tacha	Pumpkin baked with brown sugar
Caldo	Broth
Canela	Cinnamon
Ceviche	Marinated fish
Chayote	Pear-shaped squash-like vegetable
Chilaquiles	Fried tortillas in chili and tomato sauce
Chilies:	Mild to hot chili peppers
ancho, cascabel, chipotle, guajillo, habanero,	
jalapeno, mulato, pasilla, pobalano and serrano	
Chiles rellenos	Stuffed chili peppers
Churros	Fried pastries
Cocada	Coconut candy
Cochinita	Roasted suckling pig
Cocotero	Coconut
Coctel de camarones	Shrimp cocktail
Crema	Crème fraiche
Crepas de huitlacoche	Huitlacoche[a] crepes in cheese sauce
De la olla	Boiled and served in light broth (generally bean stew)
Dulce de nuez	Walnut candy
Epazote	Strong-tasting herb
Flor de calabaza	Squash blossoms
Frijol:	Legumes (beans)
frijol negro (black)	
frijol bayo (red)	
frijol canario (yellow)	
Guacamole	Avocado sauce or dip
Huitlacoche[a]	Corn stalk fungus
Jicama	Large root vegetable with sweet taste
Masa	Fresh dough of processed dried corn
Mole poblano	Chili sauce
Nopales	Prickly pear cactus paddles
Pepitas	Pumpkin seeds
Piloncillo	Unrefined sugar
Platano macho (plantains)	Starchy fruit used as vegetable, often fried
Refrito	Refried in lard (generally beans)
Romerito	Strongly flavored rosemary-like herb
Salsa	Spicy sauce, often tomato
Seviche	Pickled raw fish
Sopa de tortillas	Tortilla soup
Tamarindo	Brown pods of tamarind tree
Tomatillos	Small tart green tomatoes
Zapotes	Avocado-like creamy fruit

Source: [14,15]
[a]*Mexican corn fungus*

571

THE PUERTO RICAN DIET AND CUISINE

The cuisine of Puerto Rico is an exotic blend of African, American, Spanish and Taíno (Bahamian) influences. Its roots can be can be traced to the original inhabitants of Puerto Rico, the *Arawaks* and *Tainos*, who thrived on a diet of corn, seafood and tropical fruit.

In 1493, when Ponce de León arrived with Columbus, they brought beef, olive oil, pork, rice and wheat. Then Spanish settlers planted sugarcane and imported slaves from Africa, who brought okra and *yautia* (taro root) and integrated these ingredients into the island's already blended cuisines. Traditional Puerto Rican cuisine, *cocina criolla*, has its roots in all of these ingredient fusions.

Seasonings

Herbs and spices have played a central role in traditional Puerto Rican cuisine. Adobo and sofrito, two blends of herbs and spices with distinctive taste and color, are characteristic of many Puerto Rican dishes. *Adobo* is a mixture of crushed garlic, oregano, peppercorns and salt with olive oil and lime juice or vinegar. It is used as a rub for meats before roasting. *Sofrito* is a mixture of coriander, garlic, onions, and peppers that are browned in olive oil or lard and colored with *achiote* (annato seeds). Sofrito provides flavor and color for rice, soups and stews.

Meats, Poultry and Fish

Typical Puerto Rican meat dishes include *carne frita con cebolla* (fried beefsteak with onions), *lengua rellena* (stuffed beef tongue), *pastelón de carne* (ham and salt pork meat pies), roasted leg of pork or lamb *a la criolla* (Creole-style), *riñones guisados* (calf's kidneys), *sesos empanados* (breaded calf's brains), *ternera a la parmesana* (veal with Parmesan cheese), and *veal a la criolla* (veal shoulder with Creole sauce).

Common Puerto Rican chicken dishes include *arroz con pollo* (chicken with rice), *pollo agridulce* (sweet and sour chicken), *pollo al jerez* (chicken in sherry wine), and *pollitos asados a la parrilla* (broiled chicken).

Fresh fish is often marinated with garlic, lime juice, and olive oil and then grilled or fried, as in *mojo isleño* (fried fish with tomato-olive sauce) and *pescado dorado* (golden fish). Caribbean shellfish dishes include *camarones en cerveza* (shrimp in beer), *jueyes hervidos* (boiled crab), *paella*, and *pescado en escabeche* (citrus marinated seafood).

Soups, Gumbos, and Stews

Soups, gumbos, and stews are popular starters to Puerto Rican meals. They include *caldo gallego* (Galician sausage and greens soup), mondongo (tripe soup), *sopón de garbanzos con patas de cerdo* (chickpea soup with pig's feet), *sopón de pescado* (fish soup), and *sopón de pollo con arroz* (chicken soup with rice).

Asopao is a traditional Puerto Rican stew that includes *asopao de pollo* (chicken stew) and *asopao de gandules* (rice and pigeon pea stew). Other stews include *carne guisada puertorriqueña* (beef stew), *habichuelas rosadas secas* (red bean stew), and *sancocho* (root vegetable stew).

Typical soup and stew ingredients are asparagus, capers, chili peppers, chorizo sausages, cilantro, cured ham, garlic, green peas, green peppers, olives, onions, oregano, paprika, pimientos, potatoes, raisins, salt pork and/ or tomatoes.

Fruits and Vegetables

Fresh tropical fruits are fundamental to the traditional Puerto Rican diet. Common and unusual tropical fruits include the *acerola* cherry, avocado, banana, bitter orange, breadfruit, *carambola* (starfruit), *chironja* (orangelo—a combination of orange and pomelo), coconut, cucumber, *frambuesa* (raspberries), grapefruit, *guanábana* (soursop), guava, *guineos niño* (ladyfinger bananas), *jobo* (yellow mombin), key lime, lemon, lime, *mamey* (apple-like), *quenepa* (lychee-like), Mandarin orange, mango, *nance* (wild cherry), okra, orange, papaya, passion fruit, pineapple, *pomarosa* (tropical apple), pomegranate, sea grape, tamarind, tomato and watermelon.

Plantains (coarsely textured, starchy bananas) are served baked, boiled or fried, such as in *mofongo* (mashed plantains and pork cracklings) and *tostones* (fried green plantain or breadfruit).

Other starchy and green vegetable dishes include *batatas en almíbar* (candied sweet potatoes), *berzas and grelos* (collard and turnip greens), *chayotes rellenos* (stuffed baked chayote squash), *frijoles negros* (black beans), *quimbombo guisado* (stewed okra), *papas empanada al horno* (potato pudding), and *papas y zanahorias* (roasted potatoes and carrots).

Desserts and Beverages

Besides *arroz con dulce* (rice pudding), many Puerto Rican desserts and sweets make creative uses of fruits and vegetables. These include banana cupcakes, *boudin de pasas con coco* (coconut bread pudding), *buñuelos de name* (yam buns), *bizcocho de chinas frescas* (orange cake), *flan de piña* (pineapple custard), *nisperos de batata* (sweet potato balls), *pastel de coco* (coconut pie), pastel de limón verde (lime pie), *polvo de amor* or *love powder* (crisp, browned coconut sugar), *tembleque* (coconut pudding), and *dulce de lechosa rallado* (papaya pudding).

Rum, which is made from sugarcane, is the national drink of Puerto Rico. Wine is not produced on Puerto Rico, but *cerveza* (beer) is common. Other popular Puerto Rican beverages include *batidos* (fruit shakes), *coquito* (coconut eggnog), *maví* (a fermented bark beverage), limeade, and alcoholic and nonalcoholic *piña coladas* (pineapple-coconut beverages). A Puerto Rican meal is often completed with strong, black, aromatic Puerto Rican coffee. Coffee beans were once imported from the Dominican Republic.

TYPICAL PUERTO RICAN MEALS

Three meals a day are generally consumed in a traditional Puerto Rican diet: *desayuno* (breakfast) *por la manana* (in the morning); *almuerzo, comida* or *lonche* (lunch) *por la tarde* (in the afternoon); and *cena* (dinner) *por la noche* (at night). Supper is sometimes served.

Breakfast may include sweetened breads and café con leche, fruit juices or hot chocolate. Sometimes there is a second breakfast when eggs are served. *Tortilla espanola* (Spanish potato omelet with olive oil, onions and potatoes) is a favored dish at this meal. Other breakfast options include cooked grains and starches dishes, including *arroz con leche* (rice with milk), *batatas asadas* (baked sweet potatoes), *avena* (oats and milk), *farina* (wheat and milk), and *funche* (cornmeal and milk).

Lunches and dinners generally start with hot appetizers including *bacalaitos* (cod fritters), *empanadillas* (turnovers with beef, conch, crab or lobster), and *surullitos* (sweet fried cornmeal fingers). Many of the traditional Puerto Rican foods and ingredients just described are then combined into flavorsome and hearty meals. Supper, if consumed, is generally lighter.

Large, extended Puerto Rican families often gather for birthdays, holidays and weddings—often planned around festive meals. *Lechón asad* (barbecued pig) is a festival dish that is traditionally served at picnics. The pig is basted with *jugo de naranjas agría* (sour orange juice) and *achiote* for coloring. It is often served with a traditional dressing, *ali-li-monjili* (sour garlic sauce), and green plantains as a side dish.

THE PUERTO RICAN DIET, NUTRITION AND HEALTH

Puerto Ricans are more inclined to develop arthritis, cancer, diabetes (three to five times higher than the general US population), gastrointestinal disorders, heart disease, high blood pressure and obesity.

Almost three-quarters of the foods and beverages in Puerto Rico are imported from the United States. As a result, the Puerto Rican diet—particularly that of Puerto Rican youth—has become quite Americanized. Favorite foods include fast foods such as hot dogs and pizza, plus canned soups, cold cereals and spaghetti. Carbonated beverages have replaced traditional unsugared fruit juices.

The typical Puerto Rican diet has many positive features. It is high in a variety of complex carbohydrates from breadstuffs, corn and rice. Incomplete proteins, such as those found in legumes, rice and beans, are often eaten in combinations that are both economical and healthy.

A typical Puerto Rican diet includes some calcium through dairy milk and milk products and greens. Milk is consumed in café con leche (coffee with milk) and flan (custard). However, increased low-fat dairy products and a variety of vegetables would improve the intake of calcium, fiber and other vitamins and minerals.

Puerto Ricans should be discouraged from consuming too much sugar from refined carbohydrates and using excessive cooking fats by learning a greater variety of preparation styles. Bilingual children can play a major role in promoting the best traditional dietary practices with healthier modifications [20].

THE LATIN AMERICAN DIET PYRAMID

The Latin American Diet Pyramid is shown in Figure 12-6. It is a blend of the traditional diets of three cultures: indigenous Aztecs, Incas, Maya and Native Americans; Spanish settlers who arrived in the 1500s; and Africans who came to Latin America as slaves.

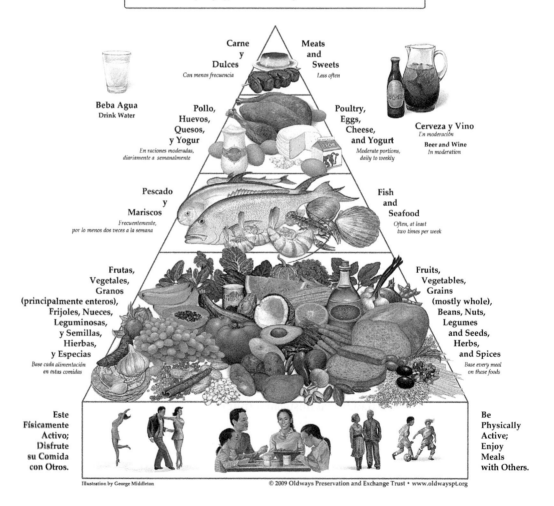

FIGURE 12-6
The Latin American Diet Pyramid.

The pyramid contains a base of physical activity, followed by an abundance of fruits, vegetables, grains (especially whole), beans, nuts, other legumes, seeds, herbs and spices; then fish and shellfish; followed by cheese, eggs, poultry, yogurt, with limited meats and sweets at the pinnacle. Water and alcohol in moderation are also included. This healthy Latin American Diet Pyramid was devised in 1996 and still serves as a model diet for these populations.

THE COOK'S CORNER: SYLVIA KLINGER, CROSS-CULTURAL SPANISH CUISINE, NUTRITION AND HEALTH EXPERT

Cooking lighter Hispanic foods is a specialty of Sylvia Klinger, a registered dietitian, certified personal trainer, and founder of Hispanic Food Communications, a food communications and culinary consulting company in Hinsdale, Illinois. A bilingual Hispanic native and leading expert in cross-cultural Hispanic cuisine as it relates to nutrition and health, Ms. Klinger has appeared on *CNN Spanish*, *Univision*, *Telemundo*, *America Teve*, *TV Azteca*, *Telefutura*, *Despierta America*, *Hispanics Today*, and *4 San Antonio Living*, among others and is published in *Latina Magazine* and *Hispanic Business South Florida*.

Ms. Klinger addresses specific health issues that are increasingly important to the escalating US Hispanic population. She leverages the tasteful Latin cuisine and the health-conscious Hispanic lifestyle with increasing health problems that are fast overcoming the US Hispanic population. Here is an example of how she modifies a traditional enchilada recipe into a healthier version with fewer calories and fat.

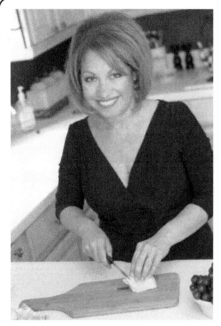

FIGURE 12-7
Sylvia Klinger.

575

ENCHILADAS VERDES (GREEN SAUCE)—TRADITIONAL RECIPE

Prep time: 40 minutes
Cook time: 15 minutes
Preheat oven to 350 °F.

Ingredients
1 to 2 pounds chicken thighs (about 6 to 8 per package), or 1 whole chicken breast
6 cups water
½ teaspoon coriander seeds
1 medium onion, chopped
1 medium carrot or red bell pepper, chopped
Cumin
Salt
1 whole garlic clove, divided into ½ chopped and ½ roasted
2 Serrano chilies (handle with gloves)
Olive oil
1 green bell pepper, chopped
2 pounds tomatillos (green husk tomatoes), husks removed, rinsed and diced (or canned if fresh unavailable)
½ to 1 cup table cream (Mexican crème)
Nonfat cooking spray
2 cups grated Monterrey Jack, cheddar cheese or crumbled queso fresco (queso fresco is traditional)

1 cup cilantro, coarsely chopped
12 corn tortillas
3 to 4 cups lard or shortening (to fill 8-inch skillet ½-inch high)
Guacamole and crumbled cheese to garnish (optional)

Instructions

Step 1: Prepare the chicken.

1. Remove skin from chicken; place chicken in pot and cover with water.
2. Add ½ teaspoon coriander seeds.
3. Add ½ of chopped onion, ½ of chopped carrot or red bell pepper, and cumin and salt to taste.
4. Bring to boil; simmer until chicken falls off bones, about 20 minutes.
5. Roast ½ of the garlic clove over flame or in skillet; add to chicken broth.
6. Remove chicken from broth; reserve stock.
7. Shred chicken; set aside.

Step 2: Prepare the green sauce.

1. Roast Serrano chilies over flame or in skillet; put into baggie and seal until skin loosens.
2. Add olive oil to large skillet; when hot, saute chopped green bell pepper and ¼ of the chopped onion and ½ of the chopped garlic until translucent.
3. Using gloves, slice chilies in half lengthwise; remove seeds. Chop and add to skillet.
4. Add chopped tomatillos and tomatillo liquid (if canned).
5. Lower heat; simmer, stirring often, until tomatillos start to break up. (If sauce becomes thick, add some chicken stock.)
6. Adjust spices; add slight amount of cream if sauce is tart.
7. In a blender, puree tomatillos, garlic, chilies and remaining ¼ chopped onion.
8. Add cilantro; process briefly so cilantro is not processed too fine.
9. Add 1 cup reserved chicken stock.

576

Step 3: Prepare the enchiladas.

1. Prepare 13×9×2-inch baking pan with nonfat cooking spray.
2. Shred cheese; place to side of stove.
3. Place shredded chicken to side of stove.
4. Heat lard or shortening in 8-inch skillet on medium-high heat to ½-inch level.
5. Using tongs, carefully immerse tortilla into hot lard or shortening, about 5 to 10 seconds on each side to soften for rolling. Let drip onto paper towels; place on platter.
6. Apply thin row of shredded chicken down center of tortilla; cover with thin row of shredded cheese.
7. Spoon about 1 teaspoon to 1 tablespoon green sauce over cheese.
8. Spoon about 1 teaspoon heavy cream over cheese.
9. Roll up tortilla and place in prepared baking pan; repeat process until baking pan is filled with enchiladas, side-by-side.
10. Spoon any remaining sauce over enchiladas; pour cream over top and cover with cheese.
11. Tightly cover baking pan with foil.

Step 4: Bake the enchiladas.

1. Bake enchiladas at 350°F until cheese melts and sauce bubbles (about 15 to 20 minutes).
2. Remove foil to brown, if desired.
3. Serve with additional cream, guacamole and crumbled cheese, if desired.

Servings: 12 servings (1 enchilada per serving)

Nutrients: 757 calories, 68.5 grams total fat, 21.2 grams saturated fat, 20.8 grams carbohydrates, 3 grams fiber, 17.4 grams protein, 529.2 milligrams sodium

CHICKEN ENCHILADAS WITH GREEN SALSA—MODIFIED HEALTHIER VERSION

Prep time: 40 minutes
Cook time: 15 minutes
Preheat oven to 350°F.

Ingredients

1 to 2 pounds chicken thighs (about 6 to 8 per package) or 1 whole chicken breast
6 cups water
½ teaspoon coriander seeds
1 medium onion, chopped (divided)
1 carrot or red bell pepper, chopped
1 teaspoon cumin
1 whole garlic clove, ½ diced and ½ roasted
2 Serrano chilies
2 pounds tomatillos (green husk tomatoes), husks removed, rinsed and diced (or canned if fresh unavailable)
1 green bell pepper, chopped
1 cup fresh cilantro, coarsely chopped
Nonfat cooking spray
12 corn or whole wheat tortillas
2 cups low-fat Monterrey Jack or cheddar cheese, shredded (crumbled queso fresco is traditional, but may not be available in low-fat version)
½ to 1 cup nonfat half & half cream or low-fat cream (Mexican crème)

Instructions

Step 1: Prepare the chicken.

1. Remove skin and visible fat from chicken.
2. In a large saucepan, boil water and chicken with coriander seeds, ½ of the chopped onion, chopped carrot or red bell pepper, and cumin.
3. Bring to boil; simmer until chicken falls off bones, about 20 minutes.
4. Roast ½ of the garlic over flame or in skillet; add to chicken broth.
5. Remove chicken from broth; reserve stock
6. Shred meat; set aside by shredded cheese.

Step 2: Prepare the green sauce.

1. On a baking sheet, place Serrano chilies, chopped tomatillos, chopped green pepper, and the remaining onion and garlic.
2. Bake at 350°F for 5 to 10 minutes, or until translucent. Let cool 10 to 15 minutes.
3. Using gloves, slice chilies in half lengthwise; remove seeds.
4. In a blender, add roasted vegetables and cilantro; puree about 1 to 2 minutes or until cilantro is pureed. Add 1 cup reserved chicken stock until sauce-like consistency. (If sauce becomes thick, add more chicken stock.)

Step 3: Prepare the enchiladas.

1. Prepare 13×9×2-inch baking pan with nonfat cooking spray.
2. Heat about 1 cup tomatillo sauce in 8-inch skillet on medium-high heat
3. Using tongs, quickly immerse tortilla into sauce, enough to soften for rolling. Let drip; place onto plate.
4. Apply thin row of shredded chicken down center of tortilla. Cover with thin row of shredded cheese.
5. Spoon 1 teaspoon to 1 tablespoon green sauce over cheese.
6. Spoon about 1 teaspoon cream over cheese.
7. Roll up tortilla and place in prepared baking pan; repeat process until baking pan is filled with enchiladas side-by-side.

577

8. Spoon any remaining sauce over enchiladas.
9. Sprinkle about ½ cup cream over top; cover with remaining cheese (about 1 cup) and aluminum foil.

Step 4: Bake the enchiladas.

1. Bake enchiladas at 350 °F about 10 to 15 minutes, or until cheese melts and sauce bubbles. Remove foil to brown, if desired.

Yield: 6 servings (about 1 enchilada per serving)

Nutrients: 255.8 calories, 10.8 grams total fat, 4.4 grams saturated fat, 22.44 grams carbohydrates, 3 grams fiber, 18 grams protein, 307.5 milligrams sodium

Morsel "A nation, though uncultured, may, all of a sudden or at times, produce a genius, whether in art or in literature, but only a people of culture can have a good cuisine, because the former is particular and transient, whereas the latter is general and permanent." —F. T. Cheng (Chinese author, gourmet and judge, 1884–1970) [1]

Asian Cuisine

Like the Hispanic and Mediterranean diets, the Asian diet is not representative of just one country, culture, menu or set of ingredients. Rather, the Asian diet represents three major regions: *East Asia* (China, Japan, Korea and Taiwan), *Southeast Asia* (Malaysia, the Philippines and Singapore), and *South Asia* (India and Sri Lanka). There are about 47 countries throughout Asia, with countless tribes and other geographic groups, hundreds of dialects, and a multitude of cuisines.

The geography and climate of Asia create great diversity in these countries—from the rice paddies in the Philippines, throughout the metropolitan areas of Hanoi, Shanghai and Tokyo, and to the Indonesian rainforest in between. This geographical diversity provides a wealth of fruits, vegetables, herbs and spices, many of which are unfamiliar to Western consumers, but others that are rapidly assimilating into Western diets.

Around 1840, during the gold rush, many foreigners were attracted to the United States, including Asians. Not only did they come to discover gold, but they came for "golden" employment opportunities, including work on the Central Pacific Railroad.

At this time, Asian immigrants consumed a traditional diet of mostly rice, vegetables and tea. Wherever they settled, they established vegetable gardens for fresh produce. They helped advance the fish industry in the northwestern United States and worked as cooks, domestics, farmers, gardeners, laundry workers and small-time merchants.

Asian Americans are now a large and growing segment of the US population. At the turn of the twenty-first century, Chinese Americans (not including Taiwanese Americans) were the leading Asian subpopulation group, followed by Filipinos and Asian Indians. Other Asian Americans include Cambodian, Hmong, Japanese and Vietnamese.

Asians Americans display great diversity in age, country of origin, education, language, length of time in the United States, location, socioeconomic status, religion, social class—and food and nutrition. The US Asian population is expected to triple by 2050 [21,22].

THE TRADITIONAL ASIAN DIET

The traditional Asian diet, like the Mediterranean diet, has been a model diet for the Westernized world. This is because many diet-related diseases, such as obesity, coronary heart disease, diabetes, hypertension and certain cancers, are not as common in Asia as they are in Westernized countries.

The nutrient composition of the traditional Asian diet is very similar to the Mediterranean diet. Both diets are largely plant-based, and meat is just occasionally consumed in very small amounts. Like the Mediterranean diet, the Asian diet is thought to contribute to long life spans, which are common throughout Asia. Physical activity also contributes to Asian health and longevity.

The traditional Asian diet is rich in fish, fruits, grains (corn, rice and wheat), nuts, soy foods, vegetables, vegetable oils and tea. These foods and beverages provide generous amounts of antioxidants, fiber, phytonutrients, and vitamins and minerals for health protection and maintenance. Among these foods, the three foods that best depict the traditional Asian diet are rice, vegetables and tea.

The lack of functional pastures has had a strong influence on traditional Asian dietary habits, since it restricted the amount and variety of dairy foods and limited meats to mostly pork, some poultry and fish. As a result, dairy foods are not a traditional part of the Asian diet; eggs and poultry are not the mainstay of every meal like they are in the United States, and meat is mainly used as a condiment.

Since Asian food industries were historically less developed than in Westernized countries, minimal amounts of processed meats were and are consumed. Instead of richer cuts of meat, a substantial amount of protein in the Asian diet is from plant-based sources, such as legumes—especially soy, including miso, soy milk, tempeh and tofu.

Steaming and stir-frying are frequently used cooking techniques in the Asian diet. These techniques reduce the amount of fat in food preparation and promote nutrient retention.

The beverages Asians consume have diet and health significance. As mentioned, dairy milk and dairy products have little history in Eastern and Southeast Asia. A variety of beers and some wines are consumed in moderation to enhance meals.

Teas are an integral part of the Asian diet for nutrition, taste and medicinal benefits. In China, tea is the most common beverage, though soda is also popular. In Japan, Japanese green tea is especially popular, and rice wine (mirin or sake) is served both cold and warm. In Korea, green tea, herbal teas, scorched rice tea and coffee are popular drinks. Other well-enjoyed beverages in various Asian cuisines are made from barley, cinnamon, citron, corn, ginger, ginseng, rice and sesame seeds. Vietnamese coffee is made with condensed milk and served over ice.

UNIFYING FEATURES OF THE ASIAN DIET

Two unifying features of the Asian diet are meals that emphasize fish, fruits, nuts, legumes, rice and vegetables and the cooking techniques that are used to produce these meals.

Fish

The Asian diet has a wide variation in fish and seafood. These are associated with its large land mass, including the interiors of China, India and Korea, where fish may seldom be consumed, compared to its many and varied seacoasts and islands, where fish is a dietary staple. Traditional Asian fish and seafood include abalone, clams, cockles, crab, eel, king fish, mussels, octopus, oysters, roe, scallops, salmon, sea bass, shrimp, squid, tuna, whelk and yellowtail, among others.

Fruits

Due to the tropical Asian climate in the south and southeast, and the milder climate in Eastern Asia, the conditions are perfect for some tropical fruits to thrive. In southern and Southeast Asia, sweet mangoes (originally from India) are eaten out-of-hand or made into ice cream and other confections, and green mangoes are widely used as chutneys or curries in India, the Philippines and Vietnam.

In East Asia, cherries, dates, grapefruit, oranges, pears, quince, peaches, strawberries and watermelon are widely consumed. Other tropical fruits include *carambola* (starfruit), *durian* (the odorous "King of Fruits"), guava, jackfruit, *longan* (with a nutlike flavor), lychee, mangosteen, pineapple, papaya, pawpaw, *rambutan* (lychee-like) and *soursop* (a cross between pineapple and strawberry).

Nuts and Legumes

Significant amounts of nuts and legumes are added to grain and vegetable dishes, reduced to pulpy sauces, such as Malaysian and Indonesian *satays* (peanut-based sauces), and consumed as snacks. Coconuts and coconut milk are popular in Thailand, Malaysia, Indonesia, South India, Myanmar and the Philippines and are used in curries, desserts, entrees and salads. Chinese use almonds, hazelnuts, and macadamia nuts in cookies, ice cream and steamed cakes. Asian Indians use almonds, hazelnuts, sesame seeds and walnuts with raisins and other fruit in rice pudding and in *halwah* (a ground sesame seed confection).

Rice

Rice is the mainstay of the Asian diet, since is it a staple food that is essential to survival and so versatile. Rice is central to each meal as a main ingredient or side dish. It appears in beverages, cakes, candies and cookies, and it is fermented to make beer and wine (sake).

Rice is considered to be sacred in some Asian cultures and cuisines. It is sometimes presented to deities in order to ensure a good harvest.

Vegetables

Fresh vegetables are fundamental to the Asian diet, used in entrees, side dishes and as ingredients. Vegetables provide aroma, color, taste, texture and balance to Asian meals. They are mostly consumed raw, barely cooked or pickled to preserve their nutrients, maximize their flavors, and balance rice, noodles and other grains. Common vegetables to many Asian cuisines include bamboo shoots, bok choy, broccoli, cabbage, carrots, chilies, bean sprouts, leafy greens, mushrooms, scallions and sweet bell peppers.

Cooking Techniques

Food preparation in the Asian diet is purposeful and ceremonial. Asian cooking techniques mostly include barbecuing, boiling, deep-frying, steaming and stir-frying, many of which are healthy cooking techniques.

Ingredients are meticulously prepared before cooking, much like the *mise en place* (everything in its place) of Western cooking. Most Asians prefer fresh food for cooking. They select live seafood, fresh meats and seasonal fruits and vegetables from local markets to ensure freshness.

> **FOOD BYTE**
>
> **Chinese tea culture** refers to all of the elements that are involved in Chinese tea preparation, including the equipment, type of tea brewed, occasions in which tea is consumed, and means of the people who prepare the tea. Some of the special circumstances in which tea is prepared and consumed in Chinese tea culture include offering apology and appreciation, connecting large families and passing on traditions. In addition to being a hot beverage, Chinese tea has a very prominent place in traditional Chinese medicine (TCM), as discussed in Chapter 9, and in Chinese cuisine.

THE TRADITIONAL CHINESE DIET

The traditional Chinese diet has been advocated as a means to reduce the risks of coronary heart disease and certain cancers. Chinese cuisine and cooking techniques are influenced by the *yin-yang* philosophy of balancing *fan* (grains and rice) with *ts'ai* (vegetables and meat) and cold temperatures with those that are hot. Tea drinking is symbolic and an integral part of the Chinese approach to diet and health.

The traditional Chinese diet mainly consists of four food groups: fruits, grains, meats and vegetables. Common Chinese fruits, herbs and vegetables include bamboo shoots, bean sprouts, bok choy, cabbage, coriander, cucumbers, daikon (giant white radish), eggplant, grapes, maize, melons, mushrooms, mustard greens, onions, peanuts, peas, pomegranates, sesame, snow peas, sweet potatoes, tomatoes, water chestnuts, winter radishes, yard-long beans and others.

Rice is the universal grain, except in northern China, where wheat flour is more prevalent (much like in the northern and southern Mediterranean countries). Starchy vegetables, including potatoes, taro and yams, are consumed when rice and wheat are not available.

Chicken, duck and pork are more widely consumed than beef. Many Chinese people use soy products, such as soy milk and tofu for protein, calcium and phytonutrients. Soy products are more widely used in China than they are in the United States.

Preserved foods are common in Chinese cuisine. They are treated by pickling, salting, smoking and other techniques to halt or hinder spoilage, be it loss of edibility, nutritional value or quality. Preserved foods include fermented and pickled vegetables and smoked and salted meats. Chinese seasonings include black fungus, chilies, *douche* (salted black beans), garlic, ginger, hoisin and oyster sauce, scallions, sesame seeds, sesame oil, and different varieties of soy sauce.

The Chinese first carefully prep the ingredients, and then the majority of the food is cooked by stir-frying or steaming in a *wok* (a deep pan with sloping sides). Very little peanut, soy, or other vegetable oil is used for stir-frying. Chinese specialties vary according to different regions. Some common Chinese regional specialties include:

- Beijing, Mandarin and Shandong: steamed bread and noodles
- Cantonese and Chaozhao: *egg foo yung* (egg patties), eel, egg roll, snails, snakes and sparrows
- Chekiang and Kiangsu: minced chicken, mullet, perch, shad, shrimp and tofu
- Fujian: bamboo shoots, glutinous rice dumplings with meat stuffing, mushrooms and seafood
- Peking: *chiaotse* (cabbage), *paotse* (pork buns) and *Peking duck* (duck with pancakes, spring onions and hoisin (sweet noodle sauce)
- Shanghai: spicy chili flavoring and red-colored meats
- Szechwan: hot, fiery pepper recipes with *fagara* (Szechuan pepper)

THE TRADITIONAL TAIWANESE DIET

Many Asian cuisines are embodied in Taiwanese cuisine (especially Chinese and Japanese) due to waves of immigration to this island that began in 1949. Taiwanese cuisine is similar to the food of China's Fujian Province (see Chinese specialties above). Much of Taiwan's population emigrated from Fujian to Taiwan beginning in the seventeenth century.

Taiwanese cuisine is filled with pork, seafood and vegetables. It features the umami taste and emphasizes texture. Soups tend to be extra thick, and **Q** (similar to the Italian *al dente*, or "to the tooth") is important in noodles, fish balls, tapioca and other chewy dishes.

581

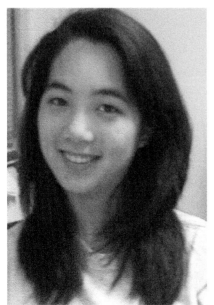

FIGURE 12-8
Annie W. Lin.

THE COOK'S CORNER: ANNIE W. LIN, REGISTERED DIETITIAN

Annie W. Lin graduated from the University of Illinois at Urbana-Champaign with high honors and received her master's degree in clinical nutrition from Rush University Medical Center in Chicago, Illinois. Her future goals include pursuing a PhD degree in nutritional sciences at Cornell University in Ithaca, New York. When not studying, Annie enjoys watching competitive cooking shows and dining at new restaurants around Chicago. These are traditional and modified versions of pan stick dumplings. The traditional recipe is from the Lin family. According to Annie, "The ingredients from the traditional recipe were changed; however, the cooking process has not been altered."

PAN STICK DUMPLINGS—TRADITIONAL RECIPE

Ingredients

5 cups all-purpose flour, plus extra for dusting dough
1 cup water
1¼ cups ground pork
4 tablespoons chives, chopped
¼ cup corn oil
Water to seal dumplings

Seasoning A

½ teaspoon salt
½ teaspoon black pepper
1½ teaspoons ground ginger
1½ teaspoons sesame oil

Seasoning B (optional)

⅓ cup vinegar
½ teaspoon chili oil

Instructions

To make the outer wrapping:

1. Combine flour and water; knead until smooth
2. Roll dough into a sausage-like shape (approximately 1 inch in diameter); cut into 1-inch lengths.
3. Using your palms, slightly flatten each piece of dough.
4. Roll each piece of dough into a round shape; make dough slightly thicker in the center than the edges.
5. Dust each piece of dough lightly with flour.

To make the filling:

1. Mix pork and chives with Seasoning A ingredients.
2. Place 2 teaspoons (or as desired) of mixture in center of each rounded piece of dough.
3. Brush edges of dough with water.
4. Fold edges together; make pleats; make sure edges are completely sealed.
5. Lightly press bottom of dumplings to flatten.

To cook:

1. Heat corn oil in frying pan over medium heat.
2. Place 8 to 10 dumplings in frying pan.
3. Cook 1 minute; raise heat; add about 2 tablespoons water to frying pan.
4. Cover; cook until water evaporates.
5. Remove lid; continue cooking until dumplings are lightly browned on bottom.

Optional:

1. Blend together ingredients in Seasoning B.
2. Sprinkle over dumplings and serve.

Servings: 4

Nutrients per serving: 449.3 calories, 16.95 grams total fat, 3.9 grams saturated fat, 60.1 grams carbohydrates, 1 gram fiber, 14.15 grams protein, 374.6 milligrams sodium

PAN STICK DUMPLINGS—MODIFIED HEALTHIER VERSION

Ingredients

3 cups all-purpose flour
2 cups whole wheat flour
1 cup water
1¼ cups lean ground pork
¼ cup scallions, chopped
1½ cups minced Napa cabbage
3 tablespoons olive oil
Water to seal dumplings

Seasoning A

½ teaspoon salt
½ teaspoon black pepper
1½ teaspoons ground ginger
1½ teaspoons sesame oil

Optional:

⅓ cup vinegar (for dipping dumplings)

To make the outer wrapping:

1. Combine all-purpose and whole wheat flour; knead until smooth
2. Roll dough into a sausage-like shape (approximately 1 inch in diameter); cut into 1-inch lengths.
3. Using your palms, slightly flatten each piece of dough.
4. Roll each piece of dough into a round shape; make dough slightly thicker in the center than the edges.
5. Dust each piece of dough lightly with flour.

To make the filling:

1. Mix pork, scallions and Napa cabbage with Seasoning A ingredients.
2. Place 2 teaspoons (or as desired) of mixture in center of each rounded piece of dough.
3. Brush edges of dough with water.
4. Fold edges together; make pleats; make sure edges are completely sealed.
5. Lightly press bottom of dumplings to flatten.

To cook:

1. Heat olive oil in skillet over medium heat.
2. Place 8 to 10 dumplings in frying pan.
3. Cook 1 minute; raise heat; add about 2 tablespoons water to frying pan.
4. Cover; cook until water evaporates.
5. Remove lid; continue cooking until dumplings are lightly browned on bottom.

Optional:

1. Blend together ingredients in Seasoning B.
2. Sprinkle over dumplings and serve.

Servings: 4

Nutrients per serving: 421.5 calories, 14.21 grams total fat, 3.9 grams saturated fat, 58.49 grams carbohydrates, 5.21 grams fiber, 15.2 grams protein, 170.6 milligrams sodium

THE TRADITIONAL JAPANESE DIET

Some Japanese-American families span four generations: a vanishing first generation of grandparents, an aging second generation of parents, a growing third generation of children, and a beginning fourth generation of grandchildren. Contrary to Japan, where generations live together and share family meals, Japanese Americans may be spread across the country, making Japanese family meals less common.

The traditional Japanese diet is largely established by its geography. Although Japan is a small island nation, it has temperature extremes that produce a variety of foodstuffs. There is little available land mass for cattle and dairy grazing. As a result, significant amounts of fish and sea vegetables are part of the traditional Japanese diet.

Fish is usually fresh; prepared as *sashimi* (raw), *shioyaki* (broiled) and *tempura* (fried in deep fat). It is also served dried, pickled and salted. There are generally two fish courses served at each meal: one cold and one hot. Fish soups are considered to be strengthening. Carp soup is traditionally given to women after childbirth.

Like the traditional Chinese diet, the foundation of the traditional Japanese diet is rice. Noodles that are made with wheat flour, egg yolks and salt are also featured. Japanese noodles are also made with buckwheat, rice and sweet potatoes. Noodles are often consumed with chicken or duck, and sometimes with lobster and frequently in broth.

The traditional Japanese diet also includes more soy protein and less red meat than Westernized diets. Meats include beef, chicken, duck, eel and pork, usually grilled and served with a mixture of soy sauce, *mirin* (sweet wine), *sake* (rice wine), vinegar and sugar. Japanese Kobe beef is very tender but high in fat. Beef liver, tripe and other organ meats are common. Like the Chinese people, the Japanese tend to avoid dairy products.

About one-quarter of the dishes in Japanese cuisine contain some variety of seaweed, such as *kombu*, *nori* and **wakame** (see Chapter 5). Instead of salads, boiled spinach or watercress is often served cold with soy sauce. Common vegetables include *azuki* (small red beans), bamboo shoots, beets, burdock, carrots, daikon, eggplant, green beans, green peppers, lettuce, lotus root, onions, red bell peppers, shiitake mushrooms, spinach, sweet potatoes, tomatoes, turnips and zucchini.

A typical Japanese meal may include *miso* (fermented soy-based soup), steamed rice or noodles, seaweed and other vegetables and beef, fish, poultry, pork or seafood. Western-type desserts are uncommon. An assortment of seasonal fruits or fruit in light syrup, breaded chestnuts, mashed sweet potatoes, or *mochi* (pounded sticky rice) with sweet bean paste may complete a meal. Rice wine (sake) is served throughout meals. Japanese tea (often green) concludes meals.

Japanese food is predicated on meticulous preparation, distinctive presentation and visual appeal that signifies balance, delicacy and proportion. Many separate dishes convey a sense of harmony among foods and tastes. Meals are often served within elaborate ceremony. Even *bento* (Japanese lunch boxes filled with compartments of foods and condiments) are also nutritionally balanced art forms.

THE TRADITIONAL KOREAN DIET

The traditional Korean diet can be traced to ancient myths and legends. It has been highly influenced by Chinese and Japanese cultures and cuisines, yet it has evolved with its own distinctive dishes and flavors.

The foundation of Korean cuisine is *kimchi* or *gimchi* (pickled and fermented vegetables, such as cabbage or carrots, with chili, garlic, ginger and salt). Kimchi is used both as a condiment and as a side dish. Other seasonings in Korean cuisine include *doenjang* (fermented soybean paste), *gochujang* (red chili paste), sesame oil and soy sauce,

The Korean national dish is *bulgogi* (fire beef), which is beef strips that are marinated in chili, garlic, sesame oil and soy sauce. *Gogi gui* (Korean barbecue) is a method that is used to grill beef, chicken, pork and other meats, often tableside. Fish and seafood are major dietary staples in Korea. Deer, hen, pigs and wild boar are also consumed.

Rice is the staple grain in Korean cuisine; it is made into dumpling or rice-cake soup, five-grain rice and rice gruel, among other preparations. Korean noodles are ever-present and made from buckwheat, legumes, rice, soy and wheat. Common vegetables used in Korean cuisine include bamboo shoots, ferns, leeks, lettuce, lotus roots, mushrooms, taro and turnips.

Korean desserts typically include fresh fruit or *sweetmeats* (candy), made from chestnuts, cinnamon, honey and ginger. Popular Korean beverages include coffee, green tea, herbal teas, scorched rice tea, sweet rice drinks and beverages that are made from local ingredients such as barley, cinnamon, citron, corn rice, ginger, ginseng and sesame seeds.

Like Japanese meals, traditional Korean meals are carefully prepared and presented with many dishes. Traditional Korean meals are noted for their number of *banchan* (side dishes). A *hanjeongsik* (full-course Korean meal) contains an array of banchan.

> **Morsel** Do not dismiss the dish by saying that it is just simple food. The blessed thing is an entire civilization in itself." —Abdulhak Sinasi (Turkish novelist, 1887–1963) [1]

FOOD BYTE

Curry powder, also known as *masala* (spice) powder, is actually a mixture of spices. It is used in a variety of dishes in Bangladeshi, Indian, Indonesian, Malaysian, Nepali, Sri Lankan and Thai cuisines. Most commercial curry powders use ground turmeric, which lends a yellow color. Other ingredients may include allspice, bay, black pepper, cardamom, chili powder, cinnamon, cloves, coriander, cumin, fenugreek, ginger, mace, mustard, nutmeg, white pepper and/or salt. The spices are gently fried or toasted to bring out their flavor and to avoid pungency and bitterness.

TRADITIONAL SOUTH ASIAN DIETS: BANGLADESH, INDIA, PAKISTAN AND SRI LANKA

Like other Asian cuisines, the South Asian Indian diet is centered on cereals, chilies, rice, legumes and vegetables. Indian Hindus from these regions consider the cow sacred and refrain from consuming beef. As a result, they have developed some of the world's finest vegetarian cuisine. Still, India is not predominantly vegetarian.

Bangladesh, India, Pakistan and Sri Lanka cuisines depend on *chutneys* (sweet and spicy relishes) and spices for their complex flavors. Aromatic and hot spices include aniseed, cardamom, celery seed, cinnamon, cloves, coriander, cumin, curry leaf, fenugreek, garlic, ginger, mustard, nutmeg, saffron, tamarind and turmeric.

Indian Hindu specialties include *biriyani* (rice with spices and vegetables), *idlis* (steamed rice and lentil cakes), *pakoras* (fried vegetables in chickpea batter), *raita* (yogurt with fruits or vegetables), and *samosa* (fried pastries with vegetables). Almonds, cashews, coconut and coconut milk and pistachios are often found within, these dishes or used for garnish.

Indian Hindu breadstuffs are baked, fried or roasted; they include *chapatti*, *naan*, *pappadam* and *paratha*. Vegetables consist of banana flowers, cucumbers, lotus root, onions, potatoes, pumpkin, radishes, tomatoes and yams. Sweets include *halwah* (ground almonds, and sugar or honey) and *keer* (creamy rice pudding).

In comparison, Eastern Indian cuisine includes dairy products in the form of cheese, cream, dairy milk and yogurt. Northern Indian cuisine contains meats dishes, such as chicken, goat or sheep. Western Indian cuisine is the most diverse. It ranges from spicy and largely vegetarian to slightly sweet (a pinch of sugar is added to most dishes). It also includes fresh coconut-based hot and sour curries with fish and seafood and rich, piquant dishes that are strongly flavored with red chilies and vinegar.

The influence of the South Asian Indian diet can also be seen in Afghanistan and Bali Indonesia, where hot curries with rice and *hoppers* (fried pancakes) are accompanied by honey-sweetened yogurt. Meat and seafood are staples in these countries, as are teas.

FOOD BYTE

The *Filipino-American diet* is higher in fat and cholesterol than other Asian-American diets. Organ meats, including pork blood, pork and chicken intestines, poultry liver, and tripe, are favored. In Italy, the consumption of entrails is quite widespread, including fried or stewed brain and boiled stomach (trippa). In some Hispanic countries, such as Mexico, almost all organ meats are consumed, including boiled or fried chicken hearts, gizzards and livers [23,24].

585

THE ASIAN FOOD BOWL

Southeast Asia encompasses 11 countries: Brunei, Cambodia, East Timor, Indonesia, Laos, Malaysia, Myanmar, the Philippines, Singapore Thailand and Vietnam, and Northeast India. In mass, these countries are considered the "food bowl" of Asia. This is because the cooking styles are strongly influenced by a combination of Chinese, Eastern Indian and Malaysian cuisines. Foods range from the rich and spicy dishes of the Muslims and the Eastern Indians that reside in Brunei, East Timor, Indonesia, Malaysia and Singapore, to the fairly plain Chinese dishes from bordering Chinese regions and communities.

The most distinctive features of Southeast Asian cuisines are the abundance of seafood and the liberal use of herbs and spices. The Southeastern Asia diet consists mostly of rice or noodles as the foundation of meals. Fish is the main source of protein, accompanied by an abundance of fruits and vegetables that are highly flavored by herbs and spices. Heavy rains and lush vegetation contribute to this wealth of fresh fruits and vegetables.

TRADITIONAL SOUTHEAST ASIAN DIETS

The Cambodian Diet

A typical Cambodian meal consists of soup, salad, fish, vegetables, rice and dessert. As in other Asian cuisines, fish and rice are staples. Seafood is abundant in coastal areas, especially crab and shrimp. Fermented fish sauce and fish paste add protein and flavor to Cambodian dishes, which are intensified by coconut milk, garlic, ginger, hot peppers, kaffir lime juice, lemongrass, mint, ginger, tamarind and turmeric. Beef, eggs, pork and poultry may be consumed on special occasions.

Rice is less milled than in other rice-dependent Asian countries. Several kinds of noodles are also consumed. Typical Cambodian fruits and vegetables include bananas, *galangal* (a ginger-like fruit), kaffir limes, mangoes, palm fruit, papayas and *rambutan* (a lychee-like fruit). Similar to other Asian delicacies, dessert is based on fresh fruit and grains, such as bananas and sticky rice.

Cambodian specialties include *amok* (fish cooked in coconut milk), *num treap* (sticky rice with toasted sesame seeds) and *prahok* (fiery fish paste).

The Laotian Diet

Laotian food is influenced by its Southeast Asian neighbors and its colonial French legacy. Traditional Laotian food is dry and spicy, and, like other Southeast Asian cuisines, it revolves around rice.

Traditional Laotian rice is *khao niaw* (glutinous sticky rice) that is rolled into a ball and eaten by hand. Sticky rice is often accompanied by *naam paa* (fish sauce), parboiled vegetables, salad, soup and various curries that include beef, chicken, duck, fish, pork, prawns and water buffalo. Laotians eat family style, sharing dishes.

Laoian food is quite similar to Thai food—likely due to its proximity. Popular Laotian dishes include *pho* (noodle soup), *laap* (spicy minced meats and seasoned grains), *kaeng jeut* (minced pork and bitter gourd soup), *khao laat kaeng* (curry with long-grain rice), *ping kai* (grilled chicken), *som moo* (raw or cooked fermented pork sausage), *naem nuang* (barbecued som moo), *tam mak houng* (spicy papaya salad), and *tom khaa kai* (chicken soup with ginger and coconut milk).

A wide variety of exotic and familiar Laotian fruits include bananas, coconut, custard apple, durian, guava, jackfruit, mango, mangosteen, papaya, pineapple, rambutan, starfruit and watermelon. Vegetables readily grown in fertile Laotian fields include cabbages, chilies, cucumbers, eggplants, mushrooms, onions, salad leaves, snake beans, tomatoes, winged beans and yams.

Pho is popular for breakfast or snacks, as are *yaw jeun* (deep-fried spring rolls) and *pah thawng ko* (deep-fried Chinese dough sticks). *Khao jii* (French baguettes) are freshly baked daily and may accompany *moo yor* (pork pate) for breakfast. Khao jii are also dunked into thick, strong Laotian coffee. Chinese tea is often a free accompaniment for meals. Soft drinks and lemonade are common, as are canned and bottled beer.

The Malaysia and Singapore Diets

Malaysia and Singapore incorporate Indian, Muslim and Chinese traditions that are reflected in their spicy cuisines. Rice is a staple food as in other Asian cuisines. The most commonly consumed rice is from Thailand, but Indian basmati rice is used in *biryani* dishes, and Japanese short-grain rice appears in the Malaysian diet.

Noodles such as *bi hoon* (rice vermicelli), *kuay teow* (fettuccine-shaped rice noodles), *mee* (yellow noodles), *mee suah* (fine wheat vermicelli), *tang hoon* (transparent noodles made from green beans) and *yee meen* (prefried noodles) are an option to rice or are consumed with rice. Indian-style breads such as *canai, idli, naan, poori, roti* and *thosai* are regularly consumed—especially at breakfast.

Kampung chicken (village or free-range) is used for soup or steamed dishes. Duck and goose are also popular poultry. Beef is used in curries, roasts and stews and with noodles. Pork is largely consumed by the Chinese Malaysian community. Mutton is used in curries, soups and stews. Fresh fish, such as cod and salmon, are popular, along with clams, cockles, crabs, cuttlefish, octopus, prawns or shrimp, snails and squid. Some Hindis and Buddhists refrain from consuming meats and seafood.

Malaysian dishes are based upon *rempah* (spice paste). Typical Malaysian dishes include *laksa* (creamy chicken or seafood curry) and *tahu goreng* (fried tofu in peanut sauce). *Satay* (meat kebab in spicy peanut sauce) is a Malaysian creation and the national dish.

Vegetables are usually available year-round, since Malaysia does not have much seasonal weather variations. They include bamboo shoots, chilies, ferns, greens and wild vegetables. Typical Malyasian fruits include durian, longan, lychee, mango, mangosteen and rambutan.

Popular Malaysian desserts include *endol* (sugar syrup, coconut milk and green noodles) and *is kacang* (beans and jellies with condensed milk). The cuisine of Singapore resembles the cuisine of Malaysia due to their historical and cultural ties. While a number of dishes are common, most differences lie in food preparation.

The Filipino Diet

Philippine cuisine is a mixture of American, Chinese, Malaysian, Japanese and Spanish influences. Unlike other Asian cuisines that use hot chilies, Philippine cuisine is often mild. Four daily meals are served in the traditional Phillipine household: breakfast, lunch, *merienda* (snack) and dinner. Popular merienda include *pancit* (noodles with *puto* or spongecake) and *cuchinta* (glutinous rice cake).

As with other Asian cuisines, rice is the staple food in most meals. Lunch is the heaviest meal of the day, consisting of rice, vegetables, meat and sometimes fish. In general, vegetables are not as important to the Philippine diet as in Eastern Asian diets, but meat is more significant, especially pork. Beef and chicken are also consumed, and water buffalo is enjoyed in the provinces. Seafood, such as crab and shrimp, may be prepared uncooked with *kilawin* (vinaigrette), *ihaw* (grilled), or stuffed with onions and wrapped in banana leaves.

Vegetables include bean sprouts, broccoli, Chinese broccoli, bitter melon, corn, eggplant, *kangkung* (local spinach), mung beans and okra. Common fruits and nuts include bananas, coconuts, mangoes and pineapple.

Coffee and sugarcane are common in the Philippine diet, as are coconuts. Coconuts are used in desserts such as *bibingka* (coconut milk and ground rice pudding topped with fresh, salted duck eggs). Other desserts include *buchi* (filled doughnuts), *crema de fruita* (fruit and custard cake) and *macapuno* (thick dessert jam).

The Thai Diet

The cuisine of Thailand is both spicy and rich from hot peppers, coconut oil and lard. Thai curries and soups are made from chicken or fish broth and whole coconut milk, with a variety of herbs and spices. These include anise, basil, chilies, coriander, cumin, garlic, ginger, lemongrass, lime, mint nutmeg, and turmeric. Fish sauce and shrimp paste are common condiments and create a unified umami taste.

Thai dishes are always served with rice. Long-grain polished rice is used in central and southern Thailand, while glutinous rice is the mainstay in northern and northeastern Thailand. A significant public health problem in rural Thailand has been *beriberi*, a vitamin B deficiency disease from overreliance on polished or milled white rice.

Seafood is plentiful in the Thai diet, including eels, crab, mackerel, salted and dried fish, and shrimp. Raw or pickled pork and beef are available at restaurants. Chicken, duck, eggs and water buffalo are commonly consumed, as are caterpillars, frogs, lizards, rats, snakes, snails and squirrels.

Vegetables include baby corn, cabbage, celery, cucumber, eggplant, gourds, kale, lettuce, mushrooms, mustard greens, onions, radishes, swamp cabbage, water chestnuts, and winged and yard-long beans. Fruits include bananas, plums and tamarinds. *Citrus hysteric* (Kaffir lime) and *momordica chiantria* (bitter melon) are distinctive to the Thai cuisine.

Soy foods assume a minor role in Thai cuisine, as opposed to Chinese or Japanese. Bean curd is used in soups, and fermented soybeans, soybean paste and soy sauce are used as condiments. Black beans and mung beans are sprouted or used in sweets.

Thai desserts are made from bean paste, coconut and/or fermented glutinous rice and are sweetened with palm sugar or unrefined cane sugar. In general, sweeteners are sparingly used.

Recipe: Thai Lettuce Rolls (Thailand)

Thai lettuce rolls are delicate appetizers filled with a mixture of fresh vegetables and steamed instead of fried like Chinese egg rolls. They make a light starter to a multicourse Asian dinner. **Thai Lettuce Rolls** *can be prepared in advance and dressed with reduced-sodium soy sauce and a sprinkle of toasted sesame seeds, if desired. Or serve them with cooked brown rice for a flavorful and nourishing vegetarian entree. The recipe can be found in the* **Recipe file**, *which is located within the* Culinary Nutrition *website at www.culinarynutrition.elsevier.com.*

The Vietnamese Diet

Vietnamese cuisine is primarily based on rice, eggs and vegetables. It also incorporates dishes from other Asian cuisines. What distinguishes Vietnamese cuisine is its generous use of dipping sauces, which are combinations of garlic, green and red chilies, lime juice, sugar and vinegar. *Nuoc mam* (fish sauce) is the main condiment used in almost every dish except sweets. Very little fat or oil is used in Vietnamese cuisine.

The national dish of Vietnam is *pho* (broth), made with *banh* (round rice noodles), beef, chicken or pork, and garnished with basil, bean sprouts and seasonings. The most popular Vietnamese vegetables include *gia* (germinated bean sprouts) and *rau muong* (bindweed). Vietnamese salads contain flavorful herbs and *rau song* (scented leaves), including cilantro, *perilla* (like lemon balm), mint and *rau rum* (coriander). Fruits such as bananas, coconuts, mangoes, mangosteens, oranges, papayas, pineapple, tangerines and watermelon are an integral part of Vietnamese meals.

An urban Vietnamese meal may consist of fish or vegetable soup with gia, rau song and fried shrimp, or fish stewed in nuoc mam, shredded banana stalks with scented leaves and cucumbers, and a rice dish. Delicacies such as abalone, fox fangs, half-hatched eggs, octopus, shark's fin and swallow's nests are sometimes added. Vietnamese coffee made with sweetened condensed milk or hot green tea often completes a meal such as this one.

A rural Vietnamese meal is much less elaborate; it may include bindweed, hard-boiled duck eggs with nuoc mam, pork fat, shrimp and a rice dish. Vietnamese street foods feature *duramam* (preserved cucumber), fried omelets, fish, shrimp, rice and tea. "Hot Shoppe" meals are balanced on vendors' shoulders. They include rice soup with hog intestines, liver or stomach, or rice noodles with clear meat consommé.

MICRONUTRIENT DEFICIENCIES IN ASIAN DIETS

As healthy as the Asian diet is, dietary insufficiencies are still widespread in Asia, especially in rural areas. Vitamin A, iodine and iron deficiencies are of particular concern. Some of the greatest vitamin A deficiencies occur in South and Southeastern Asia, where roughly three-quarters of children under 5 years of age are affected. Vitamin A deficiency in children under age 5 may compromise their immune system, cause blindness and retard growth. Rice is the staple food of these regions. Milled white rice contains almost no pro–vitamin A. Unmilled brown rice contains very little. Vitamin A deficiency (VAD) also occurs when vitamin A–rich foods, such as carrots, egg yolks, mango, squash, sweet potatoes, tomatoes and watermelon, are unavailable, as they are in these rural areas.

Iodine deficiency disorder (IDD) can lead to brain damage, stunted growth and goiter in children and affect their ability to hear, move or speak. Iodine is found in iodized salt and refined breadstuffs in Western countries and in seafood, which is expensive and in limited supply in some inland Asian countries.

Iron deficiency is the most common micronutrient deficiency worldwide. Inadequate iron intake causes anemia and impairs cognitive development in children. Adolescent girls and young adult women are the most severely affected. Southeast Asia has the most iron deficiency and anemia worldwide. Heme iron from meats is better absorbed than nonheme iron from plant foods, which are so common in Asian diets. Whole grains and tea, also common in Asian diets, interfere with iron absorption.

Dairy milk and dairy products are not traditionally used in East and Southeast Asia. This is because these populations are not able to digest the milk sugar lactose. Since milk and dairy products are a significant source of calcium and vitamins A and D, responsible for healthy bones and teeth, the inability to tolerate lactose may compromise bone mineralization and bone strength in these populations.

FOOD BYTE

Fish sauce, a condiment made from fermented fish, salt and sometimes herbs and spices, has ascended traditional Vietnamese, Thai, Lao, Cambodian and Filipino cuisines. Fish sauce is now used in modern-day cooking. It is added during cooking to casseroles, soups and stews and served with meats, poultry, fish and seafood to create a full-bodied umami taste. Asian chefs select a fish sauce like Western chefs select wine or balsamic vinegar. If a fish sauce is overused, a dish can be ruined. Straight fish sauce tends to be overpoweringly strong, sharp and salty, which makes it challenging as a versatile ingredient, like soy sauce. Usually fish sauce is cut with citrus juice and sugar for Western tastes [25,26].

THE MODERNIZATION OF TRADITIONAL ASIAN DIETS

589

As Asians adopt Western diets, there has been a general shift from vegetarian to nonvegetarian diets, and traditional foods are often replaced by nontraditional foods and ingredients. These dietary changes, coupled with decreased physical activity and other lifestyle changes, have led to more cardiovascular disease, certain cancers, diabetes, hypertension and obesity among indigenous Asians and Asian Americans.

Indigenous Asians have high rates of cervical, liver and lung cancers, hepatitis B and tuberculosis. Asian Indian US immigrants have increased rates of coronary artery disease, and Southeast Asian immigrants have increased rates of parasitic infections.

The United Nations Food and Agricultural Organization (UN/FAO) and Oxfam International (OI) are two organizations that monitor Asian diets and health and help to foster food security and sustainable agriculture to improve food accessibility, nutrition and well-being [26,27].

THE ASIAN FOOD GUIDE PYRAMID

The Asian Food Guide Pyramid was created in 2000 by Oldways Preservation & Exchange Trust. It depicts foods and beverages that replicate the traditional Asian diet for good health and longevity. It is shaped like a pyramid to show the recommended proportions of foods and beverages—heavier consumption at the bottom of the pyramid and lighter consumption at the peak.

While the USDA replaced MyPyramid with MyPlate in 2010, the Asian Food Guide Pyramid still reinforces the choices that are the foundation of a healthy Asian diet. The Asian Food Guide Pyramid is shown in Figure 12-9.

The Asian food pyramid portrays a mostly plant-based low-fat Asian diet, with a strong foundation that is built on daily physical activity. Rice, rice products, noodles, breads, millet, corn and other whole grains comprise the next layer, topped by a substantial layer of fruits, legumes, nuts and seeds and a sizeable amount of vegetables. This layer is topped by a smaller layer of vegetable oils, followed by fairly equal layers of fish and shellfish, eggs and poultry, sweets and meat, with meat at the pinnacle of the pyramid.

590

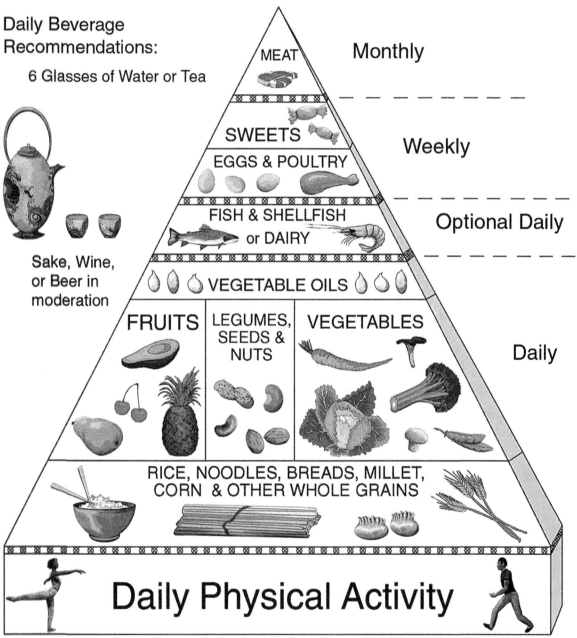

The Traditional Healthy Asian Diet Pyramid

Daily Beverage Recommendations:

6 Glasses of Water or Tea

Sake, Wine, or Beer in moderation

MEAT — Monthly

SWEETS

EGGS & POULTRY — Weekly

FISH & SHELLFISH or DAIRY — Optional Daily

VEGETABLE OILS

FRUITS | LEGUMES, SEEDS & NUTS | VEGETABLES — Daily

RICE, NOODLES, BREADS, MILLET, CORN & OTHER WHOLE GRAINS

Daily Physical Activity

© 2000 Oldways Preservation & Exchange Trust   www.oldwayspt.org

FIGURE 12-9
The Asian Food Guide Pyramid.

Daily servings of grains, fruits, legumes, nuts, seeds, vegetables, and vegetable oils are recommended, with optional daily servings of dairy, fish and shellfish. Eggs, poultry and fish are recommended weekly, and meat is recommended monthly. Eight glasses of water or tea are recommended daily, and sake, wine and beer are recommended in moderation [28].

THE FUTURE OF ASIAN DIETS

What can both Asian nationals and immigrants do to reverse the diet and nutrition trends that are seen in Westernized Asian diets?

1. *Retro-acculturate*, which is a process that integrates cultural customs and traditions back into daily life. Follow the traditional Asian diets in customary proportions. Many Asian ingredients are now available in Western markets.
2. *Replicate* traditional meal plans with available Asian ingredients, such as the following. Substitute or add traditional foods and beverages as desired.
   a. *Breakfast:* Clear soup; converted white or brown rice; egg and tea
   b. *Lunch:* Vegetable salad with Asian dressing; fish or tofu; enriched white or brown rice or whole-grain noodles; and fresh fruit or pure fruit juice
   c. *Snack:* Fruit, nuts and grain- or legume-based snacks (such as fortified rice milk or edamame)
   d. *Dinner:* Clear soup with fish, meat, poultry or tofu; vegetable salad with Asian dressing; steamed, baked or broiled fish; converted white or brown rice or whole-grain noodles; stir-fried vegetables; fresh fruit and tea
3. *Incorporate* fortified soy milk or grain-based milks that supply the nutrients that are found in dairy foods.
4. *Integrate* more fresh fruits, nuts, legumes, vegetables and whole grains in the diet.
5. *Implement* healthy cooking techniques. Steam, bake, broil or grill meats, poultry, fish, and shellfish instead of frying them.
6. *Decrease* red meat and organ meats.
7. *Reduce* the amount of salt, soy sauce, and sodium in sauces and pickled items. Make greater use of fresh and dried herbs and spices.
8. Drink *more* green and black tea for antioxidants and protective health values.
9. Drink *less* beer, wine and spirits.
10. *Activate* lifestyle. Walk or bike for transportation, which is reminiscent of home countries.

Bite on This: ethnic cooking equipment and tools

A well-stocked ethnic kitchen depends on many pieces of essential equipment and tools that are described in Chapter 3. Some global cuisines depend on very little equipment or tools to create healthy and flavorsome beverages and foods. However, specialized equipment and tools can make certain tasks easier, and sometimes with better results.

African-American Cooking Equipment and Tools

The simplicity of African-American cooking is one pot, and the pot is often cast iron.
Cast-iron cookware is heavy, nontoxic iron cookware with excellent heat retention and diffusion capabilities. It is available either bare or enameled. Bare cast-iron cooking pots and pans have been used for hundreds of years.

Different types of bare cast-iron cookware include Dutch ovens, flattop grills, fry pans, deep fryers, griddles, **tetsubin** (Japanese cast-iron pots with pouring spouts and handles), potjies (African three-legged pots) and woks. Bare cast-iron cookware that is useful in the preparation of African-American recipes includes a 12-inch cast-iron skillet, flattop grill or griddle, and a four-quart Dutch oven with lid.

Because cast iron withstands and maintains high temperatures, it is excellent for searing or frying. Since cast iron diffuses and retains heat well, it is also excellent for lengthy cooking of stews or braises. As cast iron develops a nonstick patina from seasoning and use, it creates an exceptional cooking surface for sauteing with less fat and helps produce golden crusts on cornbread and cakes. A small amount of iron may leach into foods that are cooked with cast iron. Since African Americans tend to have iron deficiency and anemia, this could be beneficial.

Other useful equipment and tools for healthier African-American cooking include the following items with their functions. Control higher-fat ingredients and char-grilled and heavily smoked foods.

Equipment and Tools	Functions
Barbecue or wood-burning grill	Grilling meats and vegetables
Corn muffin tins	Baking whole-grain muffins
Crock pot or slow cooker	Slow cooking hearty vegetables, legumes and meats
Pressure cooker	Fast cooking hearty vegetables, legumes and meats
Smoker	Smoking meats, poultry, fish and vegetables

Mediterranean Cooking Equipment and Tools

Mediterranean cooking creates fresh flavors and maintains deep, intense flavors that are reflected in its choice of equipment and tools. Dispensers, graters, grinders, mortar and pestles and presses help produce bright finishing flavors, illustrative of modern Mediterranean cooking. Slow cookers and pressure cookers help generate long and slowly developed flavors, which are reminiscent of traditional Mediterranean cooking. Useful equipment and tools intended for Mediterranean cooking include the following items with their functions:

Equipment and Tools	Functions
Barbecue wood-burning grill	Grilling meats and vegetables
Box cheese grater	Grating hard cheese
Couscoussiere	Cooking couscous
Crock pot or slow cooker	Slow cooking fish, hearty vegetables, legumes, poultry and meats
Flan pan	Baking egg custard
Garlic press	Finely mincing garlic
Gnocchi board	Preparing flour or potato dumplings
Hand-crank or electric pasta machine or pasta attachment for food processor	Making fresh pasta
Olive oil dispenser	Pouring olive and other oils
Mortar and pestle	Crushing herbs, spices, nuts and seeds
Panini press or contact grill	Pressing sandwiches
Pasta drying rack	Drying freshly made pasta
Pasta pot with colander	Cooking and draining pasta
Pepper grinder	Grinding pepper varieties
Pizza stone	Crisping pizza crust
Pressure cooker	Fast cooking hearty vegetables, legumes and meats
Rice cooker	Cooking different varieties of rice
Spice grater	Grating garlic, ginger, nutmeg and other larger spices

592

FOOD BYTE

The **mortar and pestle** are tools for crushing, grinding and mixing. The pestle is a heavy baton, and the mortar is a bowl. The Mexican version of the mortar and pestle is the **molcajete (mortar)** and **tejolote (pestle)**. The word *molcajete* is derived from the Aztecs who were early Mexican inhabitants. The Mexican molcajete and tejolote are made of volcanic rock called basalt. Foods that are traditionally prepared with a molcajete and tejolote include guacamole, mole and salsas. They are also used for grinding chilies, garlic, herbs and spices.

Hispanic (Latina) Cooking Equipment and Tools

Traditional Hispanic cooking is **scratch cooking** (from the beginning), with homemade herb and spice blends for meats, soups, stews and vegetables. More preparation equipment and tools may be required than last-minute utensils. Some unique items that are listed following can be interchanged with nonreactive heavy-gauge or cast-iron cookware.

Since highly acidic chili peppers, garlic, onions and sweet peppers are common ingredients in Hispanic cuisines, it is important that equipment and tools are nonreactive. Otherwise, a metallic taste may affect the final flavors. Functional cooking equipment and tools that are designed for Hispanic cooking include the following:

Equipment and Tools	Functions
Bamboo skewers	Grilling fish, meats, poultry and vegetables
Barbacoa Mexicana (Mexican barbecue pit)	Barbecuing fish, meats, poultry and vegetables
Caldero (heavy kettle)	Boiling soups and stews
Chili pepper grill	Grilling chili peppers
Chili pepper stove-top smoker	Smoking chili peppers
Flan pan	Baking egg custard
Comal (griddle)	Grilling meats, spices and tortillas
Huarachera or huarache press	Pressing masa (corn) cakes
6-2/5 quart pressure cooker	Fast cooking hearty vegetables, legumes and meats
7½-inch traditional cast-iron hand or electric tortilla press	Preparing fresh tortillas or electric tortilla press
10-inch round cast-iron griddle	Grilling meats, spices and tortillas
Lime press and juicer	Pressing and juicing limes and lemons
Masa grinder	Grinding corn into paste
Masa spreader	Spreading corn husks or banana leaves
Metate y mano (corn grinding stone)	Grinding corn
Molcajete y tejolote (stone mortar and pestle)	Crushing and grinding spices; blending guacamole and salsa
Stainless-steel grater	Grating hard cheese and vegetables
Tamale steamer	Steaming tamales
Tostonera for tostones	Frying plantains
Wooden molinillo	Frothing hot chocolate

593

Asian Cooking Equipment and Tools

Asian cooking embodies form and function. Some equipment and tools are especially designed for distinctive Asian ingredients and recipes. These include the following with their functions:

- **Bamboo steamer baskets** to set over boiling liquid in a wok or large pot. Bamboo steamer baskets can be used for steaming dumplings, poultry, seafood or vegetables and for serving.
- **Cast-iron noodle pot** to cook noodles and soups with nonreactive ingredients.
- **Cleaver** to chop almost everything, except for butchering. A cleaver should be made from high-carbon steel and medium weight, with a large, heavy rectangular blade that is easy to sharpen.
- **Heavy spun-steel 16-inch wok** to steam whole fish, cook a considerable amount of vegetables, or shallow- or deep-fry (in moderation). The wok should have a round bottom and curved sides to help diffuse heat and facilitate easy stir-frying. It should be properly "seasoned" (treated to withstand high heat) in order to develop a nonstick surface that can easily be maintained.
- **Hibachi barbecue grill** to grill foods with less heat variation across the cooking surfaces due to its small size.
- **Rice cooker** to cook all types of rice to perfection and free up burners for other cooking. A rice cooker can also be used for steaming vegetables. A large rice cooker with a tight lid is most practical.
- **Sushi tools** to prepare fresh sushi. These consist of a bamboo rolling mat, paddle and rice cooker.
- **Small spice grinder or coffee grinder** to pulverize spices for custom-made spice blends.
- **Slow cooker** for making curries, dal and other long-cooking, sauce-based dishes.
- **Sticky rice steaming pot and basket** to cook this specialty Asian rice that is used in Burmese, Chinese, Filipino, Japanese, Korean, Laotian, Malaysian, Thai and Vietnamese cooking.
- **Wok tools** to stir-fry, remove and skim food. These consist of a **shovel** for stir-frying; a **skimmer** with a flat, perforated disk for removing food and skimming stock; a **mesh strainer or spider** for retrieving food from hot fat; **cooking chopsticks** that are longer than chopsticks used for eating; and a **cleaning whisk** for scrubbing the wok (washing is generally discouraged).

Bite on This: Pan-Asian, Tex-Mex and California cuisines

Fusion cooking is a contemporary cooking term that has traditional roots. Fusion cooking is the synthesis of ingredients and techniques from different cuisines, much like how cuisines evolved since antiquity. When Columbus arrived in the New World, he brought Spanish and Portuguese influences to Native American cuisine, with the addition of ingredients such as black-eyed peas, cattle, goats, horses, okra, pigs, sheep, spices and watermelon. Similarly, Native Americans traded chilies, citrus fruits, cocoa, corn, grapes, legumes, peanuts, potatoes, sweet potatoes and tomatoes with the Spanish and Portuguese settlers, who brought these foods back to Europe to fuse into European cuisines. Before this time, tomatoes did not appear in Mediterranean cooking, and chilies did not create fiery Thailand and Szechwan dishes.

Chocolate, indigenous to the Central America rainforests, played an important role in Maya and Aztec royal and religious events. When Columbus and other explorers brought chocolate back to Europe, it was enhanced with refined sugar and dairy milk—two previously unknown ingredients in Mexico. It was not until the nineteenth century that this beverage of the gods was emulsified into the solid chocolate bar that we know today.

Due in part to globalization, there is a new wave of fusion among traditional cuisines. Open borders have brought ingredients from around the world to regional and local markets, food emporiums and malls, complete with salad bars, sushi counters, wok stations, and cold and hot international buffets. Year-round farmers markets with a wide variety of ethnic breads, cheeses, herbs, meats and vegetables are now the norm. The popularity of these venues mirrors the influx of Africans, Asians, Central Americans, Caribbeans, Mediterraneans, Mexicans and other ethnicities in the United States [29]. Pan-Asian, Tex-Mex and California cuisines help to illustrate the concepts behind fusion cuisine.

Pan-Asian Cuisine

Pan-Asian is roughly defined as all of Asia. In *Pan-Asian cuisine*, traditional Asian cuisines are deconstructed and recombined, borrowing elements and styles from neighboring Asian cuisines into new fused dishes. Many early Pan-Asian dishes were fused from Chinese, Eastern Indian, Thai and Vietnamese cuisines, along with French influences. Pan-Asian ingredients provide stimulating taste counterpoints of hot and sour, salty and sweet, bitter and sweet, and others. Here are some Pan-Asian cuisine combinations:

- Eastern Indian eggplant curry with Japanese rice noodles, topped with chopped peanuts and cilantro
- Japanese ahi tuna with Vietnamese fish sauce and Korean kimchi
- New England stir-fried scallops with Chinese fermented black bean curry sauce and Thai chili crostini
- New York strip steak with fresh lime, Japanese wasabi-mashed potatoes, sauteed shiitake mushrooms and Chinese broccoli
- Shanghai noodles with Szechuan green beans, Vietnamese chilies and Thai peanut dressing
- Spicy Korean barbecued rabbit with rosemary, chilies and Japanese hoisin sauce
- Stir-fried Eastern Indian coconut chicken curry with Chinese bok choy and basil
- Thai grilled squab with Eastern Indian banana salsa

Tex-Mex Cuisine

Tex-Mex cuisine exemplifies a regional American cuisine that blends the foods and beverages of the southwest Native Americans with those of Mexico. The term Tex-Mex likely originated with the *Tejanos* (Texans of Hispanic descent). It was a hybrid of Spanish and native Mexican cuisines when Texas was part of New Spain and later Mexico.

Tex-Mex cuisine is characterized by avocado, cheese, cilantro, chipotle and other chilies, corn, meat (particularly beef), legumes (especially pinto and red beans), Mexican-style tortillas, tomatoes and spices. It incorporates flavors from other spicy cuisines, such as cumin, which is common in Middle Eastern dishes. The following are some typical Tex-Mex combinations:

- Chili con carne (chili beans with meat)
- Chili con queso (chili beans with cheese)

- Chili gravy
- Fajitas (grilled meats on flour tortillas)
- Mexican pizza
- Nachos (corn chips with cheese and garnishes)
- Salsas
- Taco salad
- Tortilla chips with hot sauce or salsa
- "Combination plate" with several of these dishes on one platter

California Cuisine

California cuisine was created as a result of some bold culinary movements along the California coastline during the last several decades. It is noted for its fusion of dissimilar cooking styles and ingredients and its use of freshly gathered and simply prepared local ingredients. California cuisine is produced with significant attention to the sensory qualities of food, including presentation and flavor.

Chef Alice Waters of the renowned restaurant Chez Panisse in Berkeley, California, is often credited with creating California cuisine in 1971. Chez Panisse is recognized for serving dishes that are created with fresh ingredients from local farmers and ranchers. Chef Wolfgang Puck is also renowned for creating and promoting California cuisine. Chef Puck is known for fusing local California ingredients with French culinary techniques.

California represents a melting-pot of cultures, from the Mexican and Spanish influence in the south, the Asian influence (particularly Chinese and Japanese) in the north, and the international influence of western Europe throughout the rest of the state.

Due to its large agricultural industry and close proximity to the Pacific Ocean, California cuisine incorporates a large variety of fresh fruits, herbs and spices, meats, fish, and seafood. Some of the trademark ingredients of California cuisine include abalone, almonds, artichokes, avocadoes, chicken, citrus fruits, dates, Dungeness crab, garlic, goat cheese, grapes, lamb, olive oil, salmon, sourdough breads, sun-dried tomatoes and wine.

595

Most dishes in California cuisine are cooked quickly in order for the ingredients to retain their nutritional values. Blanching, grilling, steaming and stir-frying are popular cooking techniques. Today, California cuisine is synonymous with healthful eating, just like California is identified with a healthy lifestyle. The following are some examples of California fusion cuisine:

- Brick-oven taco pizza with cheddar and pepper jack cheese, refried beans, fresh vegetables and salsa (Mexican and western Europe/Italian cuisines)
- Chinese snow pea and Napa cabbage slaw with Dungeness crab (Chinese and Californian cuisines)
- Crab and shiitake tortellini with lemongrass sauce (Californian, Japanese and Thai cuisines)
- Gingered peach cobbler (Chinese and Californian cuisines)
- Roasted garlic and bean puree with Thai basil shrimp salad (Californian, western European and Thai cuisines)
- Tamarind glazed duck breast with fresh corn salsa (Eastern Indian and Californian cuisines)
- Tuna and avocado tartare with California caviar and sesame wonton crackers (western European, Californian and Chinese cuisines)

SERVE IT FORTH

1a. The Cruz family has relocated to a midwestern US city from the Virgin Islands in the Caribbean. They have never been to the United States before, and they wonder how they can recreate their favorite Virgin Islands recipes, such as *kallaloo (callaloo) soup*, with Midwestern ingredients.

A typical recipe for *Caribbean Kallaloo Soup* follows. Kallaloo soup uses high-sodium meats and conch to create the distinctive flavor of this native recipe. Conch is a large, edible snail. Its meat is used in burgers, chowders, fritters, gumbos and salads.

The ingredients in this kallaloo soup recipe are hard to find in typical US grocery stores. They are also high in sodium and fat. Midwestern ingredients that can be substituted include Canadian bacon, scallops and shrimp for the conch; beet greens, spinach and Swiss chard for the dasheen leaves; and dried mushrooms.

How would you adapt this traditional Caribbean recipe for the Cruz family? What would you substitute and why? Would you need to reduce or increase the amounts of each of these ingredients? What would you do to make sure that you maintain the traditional Caribbean flavors and textures?

Analyze the original and revised recipes, and then compare and contrast the nutrients to especially see if the amounts of fat and sodium have decreased in the revised recipe. You can use *SuperTracker* at https://www.choosemyplate.gov/SuperTracker/default.aspx, or a cooking and recipe analysis program from the Nutrition and Food Web Archive (NAFWA) at http://www.nafwa.org/the-library/free-nutrition-software/free-cooking-and-recipe-software.html.

2a. The Chins are planning to relocate from a mostly rural Chinese village to the southwestern United States to join their extended family. The Chins follow a traditional Chinese diet and are not well educated about Westernized diets. They are lactose intolerant, so they do not drink dairy milk or consume milk-based products.

CARIBBEAN KALLALOO SOUP

Ingredients
½ pound salt beef
½ pound pig's tail or pig's feet
1 ham bone
10 cups cold water, plus additional water if needed
1 pound mixed red snapper, goatfish and/or grouper, cleaned
2 crabs, backs removed, cleaned and cooked
Vegetable oil
3 pounds dasheen leaves, chopped
½ pound okra, chopped
1 medium onion, chopped
1 tablespoon fresh thyme, finely chopped
½ teaspoon allspice
2 hot chilies, seeded and minced
2 teaspoons vinegar

Instructions
1. Soak meat overnight in large bowl covered with 5 cups cold water.
2. Drain meat; fill large heavy-gauge stockpot with 5 cups fresh cold water; boil meat until tender.
3. Remove meat from stockpot with slotted spoon; cut meat away from bones; finely chop and reserve.
4. Add fish to stock; boil until tender.
5. Carefully lift out fish with slotted spoon; remove bones; finely chop and reserve.
6. Add vegetable oil to large saute pan; heat to medium hot.
7. Saute dasheen, okra, onion, thyme, allspice and chilies until tender.
8. Add vegetables to stock along with meat, fish, crab and vinegar.*
9. Boil over medium heat about 20 minutes.

*Note: Vinegar prevents slime that rises to the surface of the soup. It also adds a tangy taste.

The Chins are accustomed to eating a limited amount of meat. Their diet includes mostly eggs, fish and pork. They consume chicken and shellfish much less frequently. They only eat Chinese vegetables, which include the Chinese varieties of bamboo shoots, bok choy, broccoli, Brussels sprouts, carrots, corn, eggplant, greens, kohlrabi, leeks, mushrooms, radishes, snow peas, soybeans, spinach, sweet potatoes, turnips and watercress.

Fruits are a delicacy in the Chins' diet, but sometimes they eat seasonal apples, bananas, dates, figs, lichee nuts, mango, oranges, papaya, pears, persimmon, pineapple, plums, tangerines and winter melon. They mostly consume wheat noodles and steamed breads, millet and both long-grain and sticky rice. They use peanut and soybean oil and lard for cooking; sugar, molasses, brown sugar and occasionally preserves for sweetening; and chilies, ginger, garlic, pepper, salt and vinegar for seasoning. They boil, steam and stir-fry food. The Chins rarely use an oven to bake foods. How can the Chins retain their traditional Chinese diet in the southwestern United States?

Use the diet planning guidelines in Chapter 1 to create a daily meal plan (breakfast, lunch, dinner and snacks) for the Chins that respects their traditional Chinese diet, yet integrates the southwestern foods and ingredients of their new locale. Which traditional Chinese foods should the Chins consume to meet the nutrients normally found in dairy products?

3a. Sari Patel is planning to become a US Registered Dietitian. Once Sari is credentialed, she hopes to return to her homeland in North India and improve the traditional diet, which is mostly vegetarian but high in fat and calories.

North Indian cuisine is well-known for its abundant use of dairy products, which include whole milk *paneer* (cheese), *ghee* (clarified butter) and whole milk yogurt. Gravies are often dairy-based. Breads such as *puri* (fried, puffy whole wheat bread) and *bhatoora* (fried bread with chickpeas) often accompany meals. *Samosas* (deep fried pastry snacks with savory fillings) and *chaat* (snacks and fast food dishes) are often made from refined white flour and oil). Coconuts and coconut oil (high in saturated fatty acids) are often used as condiments. *Masala chai tea* (brewed spiced tea) is often made with whole milk.

This is an example of a North Indian daily meal plan:

Morning: *Lentil dal, puri, yogurt, banana, Masala chai tea*

Afternoon: Chickpea curry, basmati rice, barfi (ice cream-type confection), coconut water

Snack: Chaat and samosas

Evening: Vegetable *tikka* (tandori-cooked vegetables with yogurt), basmati rice, *aloo mattar* (potato and pea curry), bhatoora, *halwa* (semolina pudding), Masala chai tea

1. What do you think that Ms. Patel will learn about these traditional North Indian foods in her diet and nutrition training? Support your comments.
2. What is your evaluation of the North Indian daily meal plan in comparison to current diet and nutrition recommendations? Support your comments.
3. How do you think that Ms. Patel can adjust these traditional North Indian foods to decrease fat and calories? (See **Chapter 6** for ideas for reducing fat in cooking.)
4. Revise this North Indian daily meal plan by incorporating your suggestions in #3 above.
5. Since fat is a carrier of flavor, what do you propose to retain the complex and full-bodied flavors of North Indian cuisine?
6. How do you think these ideas will be perceived by traditional North Indian residents?
7. What would you recommend to improve their diet adherence?
8. What effect(s) do you anticipate as a result of these dietary changes?

Three additional activities can be found within the *Culinary Nutrition* website at www.culinarynutrition.elsevier.com.

WHAT'S COOKING?

1. Introduction to Leavening Agents in Ethnic Cuisines: Baking Soda

While European cuisines are noted for leavened breads, Mediterranean cuisines are distinguished by unleavened breads, and Asian cuisines are known for consuming little to no breads. Ethnic cuisines often rely on natural fermentation for leavening.

Objectives
- To introduce the properties of baking soda
- To apply this information to ethnic cuisines

597

Materials

2 glasses, 1 cup water, 2 teaspoons baking soda, measuring cup, measuring spoons, spoon, 1 cup of apple, grapefruit or lemon juice

Procedure

1. Fill the first glass ⅔ full of water; add 1 teaspoon baking soda, and stir; observe and note reactions on a Data Sheet similar to the one that follows.
2. Fill the second glass ⅔ full with one fruit juice; add 1 teaspoon baking soda, and stir; observe and note reactions on Data Sheet.
3. What happens with the application of heat?

Data Sheet

Liquid	Liquid *plus* baking soda	Observations	Reactions
Water			
Fruit Juice			

Evaluation

Baking soda is *sodium bicarbonate* (also known as bicarbonate of soda). Bicarbonate of soda is a weak alkaline or base. In cooking, baking soda acts to neutralize acidic ingredients, such as dairy products or fruit juices, and break down proteins. This quality of baking soda accounts for its usefulness as a tenderizer and leavening agent—particularly for making baked goods rise.

There should be no reaction between the baking soda and the water. However, when the baking soda mixes with the fruit juice, bubbles should form. These bubbles are carbon dioxide. The final product is a fruit juice–based soda water that contains carbon dioxide gas, salt and water.

Many recipes that use baking soda as a leavening agent also contain an acidic ingredient, such as brown sugar, fruit juice (as in this experiment), honey or milk.

Culinary applications

Repeat this experiment with other fruit or vegetable juices, especially those that are native to African, Asian, Hispanic and Mediterranean countries. Buttermilk, molasses, sour cream and yogurt (common in many ethnic cuisines) can also be used, since they are all acidic and should also bubble. Once baking soda is added to batter or dough that is made with any of these acidic ingredients, after the bubbles form, then the dough should rise.

This reaction should occur immediately once the batter or dough is mixed. The gas bubbles expand with heat and rise to the top of the batter or dough, and yield fluffy griddle cakes, light quick breads and airy cookies.

2. Introduction to Leavening Agents in Ethnic Cuisines: Baking Powders

This experiment can be repeated with baking powder, which is a combination of baking soda (a base) and an acid. Both baking soda and baking powder contain sodium bicarbonate. Baking powder also contains cream of tartar (an acid), which should affect the results.

When baking powder is added to water or dairy milk, carbon dioxide bubbles should form in both liquids. When a recipe contains baking powder and baking soda, the baking powder does most of the leavening.

Baking soda tends to be unstable at higher temperatures and with longer baking times. The cream of tartar in baking powder acts as a second leavening agent, and it reacts when baking soda becomes inactivated from long exposure to heat. This is why baking powder is often required in biscuits, muffins, cakes and nonyeast breads.

Objectives

- To introduce the properties of baking powder
- To apply this information to ethnic cuisines

Materials

There are three types of baking powder, all of which contain baking soda and an acid: *tartrate baking powder* (cream of tartar), *phosphate baking powder* (monocalcium phosphate), and *double-acting baking powder* (combination of calcium acid phosphate and sodium aluminum sulfate).

2 glasses, 1 cup water, 2 teaspoons baking powder, measuring cup, measuring spoons, spoon, 1 cup dairy milk

598

Procedure

1. Fill the first glass ⅔ full of water; add 1 teaspoon of one of the baking powders and stir; observe and note reactions on a Data Sheet similar to the one that follows.
2. Fill the second glass ⅔ full with milk; add 1 teaspoon of one of the baking powders and stir; observe and note reactions on Data Sheet.
3. Repeat this experiment with each of the other baking powders with both water and milk.
4. What happens with the application of heat?

Data Sheet

Liquid	*plus* Tartrate Baking Powders	*plus* Phosphate Baking Powders	*plus* Double-acting Baking Powders	Observations	Reactions
Milk					
Water					

Culinary applications

Which of these baking powders should be used in ethnic bread and breadstuff recipes that require a leavening agent? Which ethnic bread and breadstuff recipes would perform better with baking soda? Be specific according to cuisine. (Hint: Look for quicker baking versus longer baking recipes, and those that require acidic ingredients, such as fruit juice, versus milk or water.)

3. Candy Making with a Leavening Agent

Several ethnic cuisines depend on honey with its distinctive flavor, high fructose content and sweetening power. Honeycomb candy is a Mediterranean sweet with an unusual texture created by a leavening agent. It serves to make a lighter sweet because of its airiness.

Objectives
- To make an ethnic-inspired sweet by utilizing a combination of sweeteners
- To incorporate baking soda, a leavening agent, in a sugar solution

Materials

Baking sheet, nonfat cooking spray, 3/4 cup white granulated sugar, 2 tablespoons honey, 2 tablespoons water, saucepan, spatula, stovetop, candy thermometer, 1½ teaspoons baking soda, wire whisk, airtight container with lid

Procedure

1. Prepare baking sheet with nonfat cooking spray.
2. Add sugar, honey and water to saucepan; stir with spatula.
3. Cook over high heat without stirring until mixture reaches 300 °F on candy thermometer.
4. Remove saucepan from heat; whisk baking soda into sugar syrup, just to mix ingredients.
5. Spoon mixture onto prepared baking sheet; do not spread.
6. Cool candy mixture until brittle; break or cut it into pieces.
7. Store candy mixture in airtight container.

Evaluation

Sugar will start to melt and caramelize when heated to an amber color. When baking soda is added, this will cause the sugar syrup to foam. Small bubbles will form and become larger, caused by carbon dioxide bubbles trapped in the sugar syrup.

Culinary applications

Carbon dioxide is produced when baking soda (sodium bicarbonate) is added to hot sugar syrup. This is a similar process that causes some baked goods to rise. Instead of being trapped in a butter-flour-sugar matrix, the bubbles are trapped in sugar syrup. When this sugar syrup dries, it forms a crisp candy. The holes in the candy make it light in weight and produce a honeycomb-like appearance. Spreading the mixture will cause the bubbles to pop and produce a denser candy. A few chopped nuts or seeds can be added for texture and nutrients. Flavor extracts and spices add different dimensions.

This is how classic peanut brittle is made. For peanut brittle, light corn syrup, salt, butter or vanilla are often added. Swap the peanuts for sesame seeds, and it becomes a sweet that is popular in both Mediterranean and

599

Asian cuisines. Experiment with different nuts, seeds, extracts, and spices. Record your observations and taste preferences. Conduct a taste test to determine which combination is the most popular.

OVER EASY

Throughout the course of history, geographic barriers among countries have been broken, and different food cultures have spread and blended into others. Even in Greek and Roman times, Greek slaves brought their own cooking methods to the Romans, much like Africans brought their ingredients and customs to America. In modern times, with the creation of the European Union (EU), independent countries are now a unification of cultures and cuisines, fusing their indigenous ingredients in new, creative and futuristic ways.

Globalization has and continues to make the world smaller. Unusual dishes and ingredients in foreign cookbooks now regularly appear on grocers' shelves and in specialty markets. From cosmopolitan cities to tiny towns, ethnically inspired dishes crop up on a variety of menus and in a multitude of consumer products.

With seemingly shrinking distances among countries and more affordable widespread travel, people now journey to exotic places with out-of-the-ordinary cuisines. They experience new foods and beverages in traditional settings and then return to the United States to attempt to recreate their culinary experiences. In turn, foreigners immigrate to the United States to establish new lives, and try to retain the traditional dishes of their homelands. In this manner, both US travelers and foreign immigrants are global messengers of food, nutrition and the culinary arts.

The fascinating diversity of the world's food and beverages is presented in this chapter though four blended US cuisines: African American, Asian, Hispanic and Mediterranean. Each cuisine has very significant characteristics that are strongly reflective upon their unique traditional ingredients and recipes. Fusion cuisine merges some of their most striking qualities into Pan-Asian, Tex-Mex, California cuisine and others, often by utilizing fresh local ingredients and healthy-cooking techniques.

Traditional and modern-day ingredients and foods are highlighted for each of these four blended US cuisines, with attention to the dietary, nutritional and health issues of each of these populations.

Asian and Mediterranean diets have been touted for their mostly plant-based cuisines, while African-American and Hispanic diets have been noted for their robust and succulent dishes. The Cook's Corner features expert chefs and registered dietitians who modified traditional recipes to make them healthier without sacrificing flavor.

Although globalization continues to bring a broad range of foods and beverages into the US diet, it also has some drawbacks. For example, first-time exposure to new foods and beverages can provoke food sensitivities and/or allergies in sensitive individuals. Foreign foods can challenge US food safety with resistant and dangerous bacteria and viruses. Foreign food imports can squeeze out small US food producers and manufacturers. And foreign foods and beverages are disallowed unless they contain permissible US ingredients or are reformulated and carry FDA-compliant food labels. This is just the tip of the iceberg as globalization broadens and deepens.

As you review the chapter, note that many of the dishes that are described can be found in the Word Pantry at the end of the book. The most representative ingredients, foods and beverages are featured. Add your favorites—or create new ones as you explore the fascinating diversity of global food.

CHECK PLEASE

1. A US cuisine that blends traditional African-American and southern US cooking is called:
   a. Creole
   b. Caribbean
   c. Southern
   d. Soul food
   e. Tex-Mex

2. Kwanzaa is an:
   a. African tool for crushing herbs and spices
   b. African vegetable brought to the United States by slaves
   c. African-American ground peanut dish
   d. African-American translation for salt pork
   e. African-American holiday that originated from African harvest festivals
3. The Mediterranean diet is:
   a. one dietary pattern
   b. an interpretation and translation of many different dietary patterns
   c. a marketing idea created by Mediterranean people
   d. a guarantee for good health and longevity
   e. a high-protein diet for weight loss

Essay Question

1. Name and describe five dishes that illustrate African-American cuisine. Suggest how these dishes can be prepared using healthy cooking and/or baking methods and techniques. Support your choices.

For additional questions, please see the *Culinary Nutrition* website at www.culinarynutrition.elsevier.com.

HUNGRY FOR MORE?
General

Food and Agriculture Organization of the United States—Food Guidelines by Country
   http://www.fao.org/ag/humannutrition/nutritioneducation/fbdg/en/
Oldways Preservation Trust   http://www.oldwayspt.org/
Achtterberg CL. *Multicultural Pyramid Packet*. University Park, PA: Penn State Nutrition Center 1996.
Hafner D. *United Tastes of America—Recipes and the Cultural Origins of Your Favorite Dishes*. New York: Ballantine Books 1997.
Gabaccia DR. *We Are What We Eat—Ethnic Food and the Making of Americans*. Cambridge, MA: Harvard University Press, 1998.

African-American Diet

Heart-Healthy Home Cooking African American Style
http://www.nhlbi.nih.gov/health/public/heart/other/chdblack/cooking.pdf
Oldways Preservation Trust   http://www.oldwayspt.org/AHH-pyramid
Gates Jr HL, Appiah KA, eds. *Africana: The Encyclopedia of the African and African American Experience*, 2nd ed. Oxford University, Oxford, UK 2005.
Harris JB. *Iron Pots and Wooden Spoons: Africa's Gifts to New World Cooking*. New York: Atheneum, 1989.
Ferguson S. *Soul Food: Classic Cuisine from the Deep South*. New York: Weidenfeld & Nicolson, 1989.
Hultman T, ed. *The Africa News Cookbook—African Cooking for Western Kitchens*. New York: Penguin Books, 1985.

Asian Diet

Asian Nation—Asian American History, Demographics and Issues
http://www.asian-nation.org/asian-food.shtml
The China Study   http://www.thechinastudy.com/about.html
Oldways Preservation Trust   http://www.oldwayspt.org/asian-diet-pyramid
Campbell TC, Campbell TM. *The China Study: The Most Comprehensive Study of Nutrition Ever Conducted and the Startling Implications for Diet, Weight Loss and Long-Term Health*: BenBella Books, Dallas, TX 2006.
Trang C. *Essentials of Asian Cuisine: Fundamentals and Favorite Recipes*. New York: Simon & Schuster, 2003.

Hispanic Diet

Oldways Preservation Trust   http://www.oldwayspt.org/latino-nutrition
Food, Recipes and Nutrition in Latin America   http://lanic.utexas.edu/la/region/food/

Tausend M, Ravago M. *Cocina de la Familia: More than 200 Authentic Recipes from Mexican-American Home Kitchens*. New York: Simon & Schuster, 1997.

Bayless R. *Rick Bayless's Mexican Kitchen: Recipes and Techniques of a World-Class Cuisine*. New York: Scribner, 1996.

Sanjur D. *Hispanic Foodways, Nutrition and Health*. Boston: Allyn and Bacon, 1995.

Mediterranean Diet

Oldways Preservation Trust   http://www.oldwayspt.org/traditional-mediterranean-diet

Watson R, Thelander T. *The MediterrAsian Way: A Cookbook and Guide to Health, Weight Loss, and Longevity, Combining the Best Features of Mediterranean and Asian Diets and Lifestyles*. New Jersey: John Wiley, 2007.

Jenkins NH. *Mediterranean Diet Cookbook: A Delicious Alternative for Lifelong Health*. New York: Bantam Books, 1994.

Goldstein J. *The Mediterranean Kitchen*. New York: William Morrow, 1989.

TAKE AWAY

The China Project: Then and Now

The China Project was a diet and mortality study that began in 1983 and lasted for over 20 years. It surveyed the death rates of 6,500 Chinese adults in more than 130 villages and 65 rural counties. Specifically, it examined the relationship between the consumption of animal foods and diseases, including autoimmune diseases; cancers of the breast, large bowel and prostate; coronary heart disease; degenerative brain disease; diabetes; macular degeneration; obesity; and osteoporosis. The China Project was conducted by T. Colin Campbell, a professor of nutritional biochemistry at Cornell University in Ithaca, New York, and his colleagues at Oxford University and the Chinese Academy of Preventive Medicine.

602

The study concluded that diets high in protein, particularly meat and cow's milk, were strongly linked to diseases, especially coronary heart disease, cancer and Type II diabetes. The researchers recommended that people consume a plant-based diet and avoid beef, poultry, dairy milk and their by-products to decrease and/or reverse the incidence and development of chronic diseases [30].

In 2006, Campbell and his son Thomas released *The China Study*. In this acclaimed book, they outlined eight principles of food and health. These principles were based on the idea that genes do not solely determine diseases. Instead, the Campbell's asserted that genes must be activated or expressed and that nutrition plays a critical role in their activation or expression. The Campbells advocated good nutrition starting early in life for disease prevention, combined with a plant-based diet throughout life [31].

According to the Campbells, one of the strongest predictors of chronic disease is serum (blood) cholesterol. As serum cholesterol levels decreased in rural Chinese, cancers of the brain, breast, colon, esophagus (throat), liver, lungs, rectum, stomach and childhood and adult leukemia decreased. As serum cholesterol levels in rural Chinese rose, the incidence of Western diseases such as these also rose.

At the time of the China Study, Western diseases were relatively rare in China. Animal protein in the rural Chinese diet averaged only 7.1 grams daily, whereas animal protein in the American diet at that time averaged about 70 grams daily. The authors concluded that the lower the percentage of animal protein, the greater the health benefits.

Today, like the rest of the world, China is struggling with a serious obesity epidemic. In 2008, about one-quarter of Chinese adults were considered overweight or obese. The rate of overweight adults in China is predicted to double by 2028 without health interventions. The adoption of a Westernized diet, China's newly gained affluence and urban lifestyle, and decreased activity have all been implicated with their overweight and obesity. Even low-income Chinese in rural areas are susceptible to these conditions [32].

While there have been many critics of the scientific thoroughness of the China Project, it is evident that a Western-style diet with higher protein has affected the nutrition and health of this country. It may be valuable to revisit the dietary patterns of the traditional Chinese diet and restore some of its principles to help curtail nutrition-related diseases, improve health, and increase longevity.

Food Security and Insecurity

Food security is the availability of food and a person's access to food. A person is considered "food secure" when they do not live in hunger or fear of starvation. Two common definitions of food security have been established by the United Nation's Food and Agriculture Organization (FAO) and the US Department of Agriculture (USDA). These definitions state the following:

- Food security exists when *all people*, at *all times*, have access to *sufficient, safe and nutritious* food to *meet* their dietary needs and food preferences for an *active* and *healthy* life. (FAO)
- Food security for a household means access by *all members at all times* to *enough* food for an *active, healthy* life. Food security includes at a minimum (1) the ready availability of nutritionally adequate and safe foods, and (2) an assured ability to acquire acceptable foods in socially acceptable ways (that is, without resorting to emergency food supplies, scavenging, stealing, or other coping strategies). (USDA) [33]

Food is not always readily available or accessible across Africa, Asia, Central and South America, the Mediterranean countries, and some "food deserts" in the United States due to complex geographic, social and political factors. Food deserts are areas in industrialized societies where affordable and healthful foods are difficult to obtain. Food deserts are also in rural low-socioeconomic minority communities without access to grocery stores with affordable and healthful foods.

The complex geographic social, political factors that may affect food availability or accessibility include climatic changes that cause natural catastrophes, such as droughts, earthquakes, floods, hurricanes and typhoons; economics; land loss to industrial and residential development; population growth; and other factors.

About half of the world's population live in urban environments but are dependent on rural food production. If there are major problems that affect the growing, harvesting and transportation of food, then urbanites will no longer have availability or accessibility of food. People who should normally be food secure would then face food insecurity. For example, when Hurricane Katrina destroyed the city of New Orleans, Louisiana, in 2005, food distribution to this major US city was perilous.

In developing countries, such as some that were featured in this chapter, the reverse is true: considerably fewer people live in urban areas than rural areas. By investing in the preservation of small farms, residents may be inspired to stay on their land, continue to provide food for their communities, and help feed urbanites. The complex social and political factors of globalization may interfere with this natural cycle and course of action. Once again, people who could be food secure would face food insecurity; in this example, the rural farmers are particularly vulnerable.

Morsel "All people are made alike. They are made of bones, flesh and dinners. Only the dinners are different." —Gertrude Louise Cheney (American poet, 1918–) [1]

From time to time, countries worldwide experience natural disasters that cause food distribution problems and food shortages. If these events multiply, chronic hunger and malnutrition may follow. A look at some of the natural disasters over the last decade—earthquakes, hurricanes, tornadoes and tsunamis—have proven this to be true.

There is a direct relationship between lack of food and poverty. Poorer families tend to suffer the most chronic hunger and malnutrition during food shortages. Wealthier families may have the means to stockpile foods and beverages during times of crises; poorer families must rely on public aid, like the impoverished residents of New Orleans in 2005.

Chronic hunger and malnutrition can stunt infant and child growth and development and cause a host of nutrition-related health problems, such as severe anemia, compromised immunities, defective cognitive development, infections, failure to thrive, and infant and childhood mortalities. These conditions can also have long-term effects. For example, healthy organs and body systems should decline slowly with aging, but

603

early malnourishment can accelerate premature organ failure. A poor 50-year-old person may have the body of an 80-year-old and die earlier than normal life expectancy.

Food insecurity is a persistent problem in the United States due to population inequalities, especially among minorities such as those discussed in this chapter. There is a lack of healthy food alternatives, a disproportionate amount of fast food, and an increasing gap between food availability and accessibility among racial and ethnic groups. It is time to look at our own food insecurities, equalize food availability, eradicate hunger and starvation, and improve the nutrition and health of all Americans.

References

[1] Coriander Leaf. Food quotes. <http://www.corianderleaf.com/foodquotes.html/>; [accessed 08.07.08].

[2] 3aday.org. <http://www.3aday.org/SiteCollectionDocuments/PDFs/africanAmericanHealthRolePDF.pdf/>; [accessed 08.07.08].

[3] Ogden CL, Carroll MD, Curtin LR, et al. Prevalence of overweight and obesity in the United States, 1999–2004. JAMA 2006;295:1549–55.

[4] Centers for Disease Control and Prevention (CDC). Health, United States, <http://www.cdc.gov/nchs/data/hus/hus09.pdf/> 2009; [accessed 08.07.08].

[5] Office of Minority Health (OMH). Obesity and African Americans. <http://minorityhealth.hhs.gov/templates/content. aspx?ID=6456/>; [accessed 08.07.08].

[6] National Institute of Arthritis and Musculoskeletal and Skin Disease. Osteoporosis and African American women. <http://www.niams.nih.gov/Health_Info/Bone/Osteoporosis/Background/default.asp/>; [accessed 08.07.08].

[7] Centers for Disease Control and Prevention (CDC). Health disparities affecting minorities—African Americans. <http://www.cdc.gov/omhd/Brochures/PDFs/1PBAA.pdf/>; [accessed 08.07.08].

[8] De Lorgeril M, Salen P, Martin JL, et al. Mediterranean diet, traditional risk factors, and the rate of cardiovascular complications after myocardial infarction—final report of the Lyon Diet Heart Study. Circulation 1999;99:779–85.

[9] Explorations Fonctionnelles Cardiorespiratoires et Métaboliques. CHU de Saint-Etienne (M.d.L., P.S., I.M.), Saint-Etienne; and INRETS Epidemiology Unit (J.L.M.). Hôpital Cardiovasculaire (J.D.) and INSERM Unit 265 (N.M.), Lyon, France.

[10] Sofi F, Cesari F, Abbate R, et al. Adherence to Mediterranean diet and health status: meta-analysis. BMJ 2008;337:a1344.

[11] Rowinski K, editor. The quotable cook. New York: The Lyons Press; 2000.

[12] Kalus U, Pindur G, Jung F, et al. Influence of onion as an essential ingredient of Mediterranean diet on arterial blood pressure and blood fluidity. Arzneimittelforschung 2000;50:795–801.

[13] Franco M, Orduñez P, Caballero B, et al. Obesity reduction and its possible consequences: What can we learn from Cuba's Special Period?. CMAJ 2008;178:1032–4.

[14] Kenyon C. Mexican ingredients and terms at a glance. <http://mexicanfood.about.com/od/introtomexicanfood/a/mexcookglossary. htm/>; [accessed 08.07.08].

[15] MyMexicanRecipe. The Mexican pantry. <http://www.mymexicanrecipes.com/ingredients/>; [accessed 08.07.08].

[16] Hobbs F, Stoops N.. In: Demographic trends in the 20th century. Washington DC: US Government Printing Office; 2000.

[17] Romero-Gwynn E, Gwynn DL, Grivetti R, et al. Dietary acculturation among Latinos of Mexican descent. Nutrition Today 1993;28:6–11.

[18] Therrien M, Ramirez RR.. In: The Hispanic population in the United States: population characteristics. Washington DC: US Government Printing Office; 2000.

[19] Ohio State University. Cultural diversity: eating in America Mexican-American. <http://ohioline.osu.edu/hyg-fact/5000/pdf/5255. pdf/>; [accessed 08.07.08].

[20] Ohio State University. Cultural diversity: eating in America Puerto Rican. <http://ohioline.osu.edu/hyg-fact/5000/pdf/5257.pdf/>; [accessed 08.07.08].

[21] US Census Bureau. <http://www.census.gov/Press-Release/www/releases/archives/population/012496.html/>.

[22] US Department of Agriculture (USDA). Food security in the United States: measuring household food security. <http://www.ers. usda.gov/Briefing/FoodSecurity/measurement.htm/>; [accessed 08.07.08].

[23] Lee MM, Shen JM. Dietary patterns using traditional Chinese medicine principles in epidemiological studies. Asia Pac J Cin Nutr 2008;17:79–81.

[24] McLagan J.. In: Odd bits: how to cook the rest of the animal. Berkeley, CA: Ten Speed Press; 2011.

[25] Faqs.org. Diet of Asians. <http://www.faqs.org/nutrition/Ar-Bu/Asians-Diet-of.html/>; [accessed 08.07.08].

[26] Popkin BM, Horton S, Kim S. The nutritional transition and diet-related chronic diseases in Asia: implications for prevention, International Food Policy Research Institute. <http://www.unescap.org/65/documents/Theme-Study/st-escap-2535.pdf/>; [accessed 08.07.08].

[27] US Department of Commerce. The emerging minority marketplace: minority population growth: 1995–2050, Washington, DC: US Department of Commerce; September, 1999.

[28] California Pacific Medical Center. Asian food guide for meal planning. <http://www.cpmc.org/learning/documents/asianfd-guide.pdf/>; [accessed 08.07.08].

[29] Powis TG, Hurst WJ, Carmen-Rodríguez M, et al. Oldest chocolate in the New World, Antiquity. <http://antiquity.ac.uk/projgall/powis/index.html/>; [accessed 15.02.11].

[30] Campbell TC, Chen J.. In: Diet and chronic degenerative diseases: a summary of results from an ecologic study in rural China. N. Totowa: Humana Press; 1994.

[31] Campbell TC, Campbell TM.. In: The China Study: the most comprehensive study of nutrition ever conducted and the startling implications for diet, weight loss and long-term health. : Benbella Books; Dallas, TX, 2006.

[32] China and India: reform goes global. Health Aff (Millwood) 2008;27:1064–1076.

[33] World Health Organization. South-East Asia progress towards health for all (1977–2000). <http://www.searo.who.int/LinkFiles/Health_Situation_SEA_Progress_Towards_Health_For_All_1977-2000.pdf/>; [accessed 08.07.08].

605

Absorption: movement of nutrients and other substances into cells or tissues

Acesulfame-A: all-purpose sweetener; 200 times sweeter than table sugar or sucrose; stable at high temperatures and soluble in water; used in baked goods, candies, chewing gum, desserts, diet drinks, gelatins and puddings

Acetaldehyde: intermediate product of ethanol breakdown into acetate, then into carbon dioxide and water

Acetate: intermediate product of ethanol breakdown into carbon dioxide and water

Achiote: annatto seeds; used to color butter, cheese, rice and smoked fish

Acid and base balance: equilibrium between acid and bases within body fluids; partially maintained by proteins

Acidophilus milk: milk fermented by acidophilus bacteria; potential gastrointestinal benefits

Acidosis: condition that occurs when blood becomes acidic; pH of arterial blood falls below 7.35

Acids: chemical compounds with pH measure of less than 7 when dissolved in water

Acidulated water: water with added acid such as lemon juice, vinegar or wine

Actual body weight: current body weight

Acupuncture: technique of inserting and manipulating fine needles into specific body points; used for pain relief and therapy

Added sugars: sugars and caloric sweeteners added to foods during processing or preparation

Addiction: condition where body relies on addictive substances to function; develops physical dependence

Additive: substance added to food or becomes part of food during processing

Adenosine triphosphate: high-energy molecule that stores and supplies the energy for life

Adipose cells: connective tissue cells that synthesize and contain fat globules

Adiposity: state of being overly fat

Adobo: mixture of crushed garlic, oregano, peppercorns and salt with olive oil and lime juice or vinegar

Adolescence: transitional stage of development from childhood to adulthood; between the ages of 13 and 19 years

Adult-onset (Type II) diabetes: blood sugar disorder characterized by insulin resistance, reduced insulin sensitivity and/or reduced insulin secretion; usually occurs in adulthood

Adverse reaction: unfavorable response to food; includes both food allergies and intolerances or sensitivities

Aerobic bacteria: bacteria that require oxygen to derive energy

Aerobic metabolism: metabolism (the breakdown of nutrients to create energy) in the presence of oxygen

Aflatoxins: poisons produced by molds in grains, legumes and meals for livestock

Agar-agar: gelatinous substance in cell membranes of red algae or seaweed; used as clarifying agent in brewing; thickener in soups, jellies and ice cream and vegetarian gelatin; common in Japanese cuisine

Agave syrup and nectar: concentrated sweeteners; produced from Mexican agave plant; can be substituted for honey or sugar in some recipes

Aging: physical, psychological and social changes over time

Aioli: French garlic mayonnaise

Alcohol (ethanol): colorless, unstable liquid with mild odor; produced by fermentation of sugars

Alcohol dehydrogenase: enzyme in liver that helps break down ethanol into acetaldehyde and water

Alcohol dependency: addiction to ethanol; unstoppable consumption coupled with harmful physical, emotional and/or social effects

Alcoholism: disease that causes continual use of alcohol despite negative consequences

Aldosterone: hormone that causes kidneys to retain sodium and water

Alkalis (bases): chemical compounds with pH measure greater than 7 when dissolved in water

Allergens: substances (usually protein) that body recognizes as foreign; may cause allergic reactions

Allergic reaction: acquired and abnormal immune response to otherwise harmless substances that involves the human body's immune system

Allergy: negative response to ordinary substances (usually proteins) that involve the immune system; may cause broad range of inflammatory reactions

All-purpose (AP) flour: blend of hard and soft flours; designed for wide range of foods

Almuerzo: lunch in Spanish-speaking countries

Alpha-lactoalbumin: protein in human breast milk

Alzheimer's disease: most common form of dementia; symptoms may include aggression, confusion, irritability, language breakdown, long-term memory loss, mood swings and/or withdrawal

Amaranth: ancient "pseudograin" still grown in Central America and India; suitable for people with celiac disease and gluten intolerance since gluten-free

Amenorrhea: cessation of menstruation; often associated with the "female triad" and heavy exercise

Amino acids: building blocks of protein

Amniotic sac: sac in which fetus develops

Anabolic steroids: synthetic male hormones often used to build muscles

Anabolism: chemical reactions that cause molecules to form larger and more complex cells, cell membranes, enzymes, proteins, tissues, and organs; necessary for growth, maintenance and repair

Anaerobic bacteria: bacteria that do not require oxygen to derive energy

Anaerobic metabolism: metabolism (the breakdown of nutrients to create energy) in the absence of oxygen

Anaphylaxis: sometimes fatal reaction to an allergen; characterized by decreased oxygen to lungs and heart

Anardana: spice made from wild pomegranate seeds; notable in Indian and Pakistani cuisines

Anemia: condition where human body has insufficient healthy red blood cells with diminished oxygen transport to body tissues

Anencephaly: neural tube defect; occurs when head end of neural tube fails to close, usually between 23rd and 26th day of pregnancy; may be outcome of folate deficiency pre- or during pregnancy

Aneurysm: blood-filled dilation of blood vessel; most common in arteries at base of brain and aorta

Angiogenesis: growth of new blood vessels from pre-existing vessels

Anorexia nervosa: eating disorder of acute self-starvation from extreme fear of fatness

Anthocyanins: water-soluble plant pigments; color fruits and vegetables in shades from red to blue

Antibodies: large proteins produced by immune system in response to allergens

Antidiuretic hormone (ADH): hormone that functions to increase water reabsorption in kidneys

Antioxidants: protective compounds that defend human body from potentially damaging effects of oxygen; includes vitamins A, C, E and selenium

Aojiru: Japanese vegetable juice made from carrot, kale, tomato, turnip and V8 juices

Appearance: state, condition, manner or style in which objects appear; determines whether or not foods are desired or consumed

Appetite: psychological desire to obtain and consume food

Arabica coffee beans: species of coffee native to Ethiopia and Yemen; known as "mountain coffee"

Arawaks and Tainos: original inhabitants of Puerto Rico

Arborio: medium grain rice; foundation of Northern Italian dishes

Arrowroot: root of common West Indies plant; produces silky-smooth powdery starch that gelatinizes (thickens) at high temperatures when mixed with liquid; does not thin out or get stringy like other root starches, and sets clear

Arroz con leche: Puerto Rican rice with dairy milk

Arroz con pollo: Spanish and Hispanic chicken and rice

Artisan water: water drawn from well in isolated water-bearing rock or formation

Ascorbic acid: water-soluble acid with antioxidant properties; also called ascorbate and vitamin C; primarily found in citrus fruits, leafy green vegetables and tomatoes

Asopao: traditional Puerto Rican stew; often made with chicken or pigeon and rice

Aspartame (Nutra-Sweet and Equal): general, all-purpose sweetener 160 to 220 times sweeter than table sugar (sucrose); loses sweetness at high temperatures over time; used in beverages, chewing gum and as tabletop sweetener; should not be used by people with **phenylketonuria** (genetic disorder of metabolism)

Atherosclerosis: form of cardiovascular disease; characterized by fatty deposits accumulated as plaque within walls of arteries

Atropic gastritis: chronic inflammation of stomach mucosa; reduces gastric cells and impairs hydrochloric acid, pepsin and intrinsic factor; may lead to poor vitamin B12 absorption, vitamin B12 deficiency and pernicious anemia

Au jus: French for "with (its own) juice"; light sauce for beef recipes

Autism Spectrum Disorders (ASD): range of disorders displayed by autism, a neural development disease

Ayurveda: therapeutic and complementary system of Eastern medicine; stresses moderation and plant-based treatments for therapeutic purposes

Azuki: small, red Japanese beans

B-complex vitamins: eight water-soluble vitamins; play important roles in cellular metabolism; include vitamin B1 (thiamine), B2 (riboflavin), B3 (niacin), B6, B12, folate, pantothenic acid and biotin

Baba ghanoush: roasted, mashed and seasoned eggplant

Baby bottle caries: syndrome characterized by severe tooth decay in infants, due to prolonged contact of liquids with fermentable carbohydrates and cariogenic bacteria

Bacteria: harmful or beneficial microscopic organisms

Baking: dry-heat method of cooking food without direct exposure to flames; typically in oven or enclosed compartment

Baking powder: leavening agent primarily used in baking, mostly double *acting* (helps dough or batter rise when first prepared and later at higher temperature)

Baking soda (sodium bicarbonate): leavening agent primarily used in baking; reacts with other substances to release carbon dioxide and help dough rise

Balsamic vinegar: Italian condiment made from sweet wine grape reduction

Bamboo steamer basket: wooden basket for steaming and serving Asian foods

Banchan: Korean side dishes

Bariatric medicine: medical treatment of overweight and obesity

Bariatric surgery: treatment option for obesity; especially suitable for people who have not experienced and sustained long-term weight loss

Barley: cereal grain cultivated around Dead Sea 9,500 years ago; contains soluble fibers as gluten-free; used for animal feed, beer production and human consumption

Basal metabolic rate (BMR): rate body uses energy to support and sustain metabolism

Basal metabolism: all chemical activities inside cells that sustain body at rest

Bastilla: Moroccan pigeon pie

Basting: technique that adds moisture, flavor and color via flavorful liquid applied to foods, such as pork loin, standing rib roast, whole chicken or turkey

Bean curd (tofu): white, cheese-like food made by coagulating soy milk; then pressing curds into blocks

Beer: alcoholic beverage produced by brewing and fermentation of starches; derived from cereals

Beet sugar: type of sugar extracted from beets with hot water and alkaline solution to remove impurities; then evaporated and concentrated into crystallized sugar

Behavior modification: psychological protocol for changing behavior; used in combination with diet and exercise programs for weight loss and weight management

Bento: Japanese lunch boxes filled with compartments of food and condiments

Beriberi: central nervous system disorder characteristic of vitamin B1 (thiamine) deficiency; common in diets based on polished rice

Beta-carotene: vitamin A precursor; antioxidant primarily found in brightly colored green, orange, red and yellow fruits and vegetables

Betalains: plant-based substances; responsible for red and yellow pigments in plants, such as beets

Bifidobacteria: bacteria that comprise gut flora and reside in colon; aid in digestion; used as probiotics

Bifidus factor: compound that enhances growth of bifidobacteria in human intestines; associated with lower incidence of allergies

Bile: bitter, alkaline, yellow or green liquid secreted by liver; assists in digestion and absorption of lipids

Bilirubin: product of red blood cell breakdown excreted in bile; elevated in certain diseases; responsible for bruises and jaundice

Bingeing: uncontrolled, chronic overeating with or without vomiting or laxatives

Bioavailability: efficiency of gastrointestinal tract in absorbing and using nutrients

Biodiversity: variation of life forms within an ecosystem

Bioelectrical impedance (BI): method of estimating body fat based on passage of electrical current through body

Biological age: age of organism; reflects health of organs and systems due to aging

Biotechnology: field of applied biology; includes biology, cellular biology, chemical engineering, chemistry, embryology, genetics, information technology, molecular biology and robotics

Biriyani: Indian Hindu rice dish with basmati rice, spices and vegetables

Bistecca: Italian beefsteak

Bitter orange: diet aid and ephedra substitute; increases calories burned; long-term effects unknown

Blackstrap molasses: thick syrup with bitter-tart taste; remains after sugar beets or sugarcane processed to make white sugar; contains lowest amount of sugar within molasses group of sweeteners

Black tea: variety of tea more oxidized than green, oolong or white tea

Blanching: steaming or boiling to destroy enzymes that destruct flavor and nutritional value

Blood clot: clump of blood cells and fibrin strands; called *thrombus* when blocks blood flow

Blood sugar: glucose; simple or single sugar in bloodstream

Body mass index (BMI): figure that represents body weight in relation to height; corresponds with body fat and health risks

Boiling: moist-heat method of cooking; cooks food in liquid at boiling point (just until evaporation)

Bouquet garni: herbal mixture of bay, parsley and thyme

Bovine growth hormone (BGH): hormone used to increase milk production in cows

Bragg's Liquid Aminos: unfermented soy sauce alternative with meatlike flavor; can be used to flavor hearty dishes such as braises, chilis, soups and stews

Brainstem: lower part of brain that joins to spinal cord; provides main motor and sensory nerves to face and neck through cranial nerves

Braising: moist-heat method of cooking; cooks food slowly by simmering in moderate amount of liquid

Bread pudding: dessert often made with egg, dried fruit, milk, spices (such as cinnamon, mace, nutmeg or vanilla), stale bread, suet (or other fat) and sugar (or golden syrup)

Breathalyzer: device for estimating blood alcohol content (BAC) from breath sample

Broiling: dry-heat method of cooking; cooks food beneath high heat source

Broth: commercial stock made with protein base, vegetables, herbs and seasonings

Brown adipose tissue (BAT): brown fat; mainly functions to generate body heat

Brown rice syrup: syrup made by cooking brown rice with enzymes to convert starches into about 50 percent sugars; about half as sweet as white sugar, with mild butterscotch flavor

Brown sugar: sugar produced during sugar refining process when sugar crystals are mixed with molasses

Buckwheat: technically herb in buckwheat family; originated in Asia where made into buckwheat noodles; found in breads, cookies, crackers, muffins and waffles; toasted buckwheat **groats** (hulled, crushed buckwheat kernels) known as **kasha**

Bulgogi: national dish of Korea; also called "fire beef"

Bulgur (bulghur or burghul): Middle Eastern partially cooked coarse or finely cracked wheat

Bulimia nervosa: eating disorder of self-induced vomiting and/or laxatives; connected to extreme fear of fatness

Butter: dairy product made by churning fresh or fermented cream or milk; separates into a soft, white or yellow semisolid of tiny water droplets and milk proteins encased by butterfat

Buttermilk: cultured or fermented dairy product; made by adding bacteria to dairy milk; characteristically sour taste with thick and creamy texture

Butyric acid: type of fatty acid found in animal fats and plant oils; noticeable in rancid butter and Parmesan cheese due to unpleasant smell, pungent taste and sweet aftertaste

Cacao: dried, partially-fermented fatty seeds of South American evergreen tree (Theobroma cacao); used in cocoa, cocoa butter and chocolate production; also called cacao bean, cocoa bean

Café con leche: strong espresso coffee with warm milk

Caffeine: substance that acts as psychoactive stimulant drug and mild diuretic

Caffeine Dependency Syndrome: addiction to caffeine characterized by physical symptoms of addiction and continual consumption despite symptoms

Calamari or squid: common seafood in Asian and Mediterranean cuisines

Calcium: major mineral in earth's crust and seawater; assists muscular contractions, regulates metabolism, builds bones and teeth and transmits nerves; primarily found in dairy products, fish with small bones, and leafy green vegetables

Caldero: heavy kettle for soups and stews used in Hispanic cooking

California cuisine: fusion of dissimilar cooking styles and ingredients using fresh and local ingredients

Calorie: amount of heat (energy) needed to raise temperature of 1 gram of water by 1 °C; unit that measures food energy

Calorie balance: calories consumed through food and beverages in equilibrium with calories expended through basal metabolism, physical activities and thermic effect of food

Calories: quantity of food or drink capable of producing specific amount of energy

Camellia sinensis (tea oil): volatile oil extracted by distilling dried camellia branches and leaves; light color and fragrance and consistency of olive oil

Cancer: group of diseases characterized by uncontrolled cell growth, invasion and metastases

Cane sugar: sugar produced from sugarcane; filtered, treated to remove impurities; neutralized, cooled and centrifuged; *caster* and *superfine* cane sugars (also called *baker's* or *bar sugar*) dissolve quickly; useful in meringues and flavoring beverages

Caponata: Sicilian appetizer made with celery, eggplant and sweetened vinegar

Carambola: Asian star fruit

Caramelization: cooking process that oxidizes sugar; results in nutty flavor and brown color

Carbohydrate counting: process that clarifies how each type of carbohydrate (dairy, fruit, starch, vegetable and sweets) affects blood glucose

Carbohydrates: one of six major nutrients found in both animals and plants; compounds made of single or multiple sugars linked together; include sugars, starches and fibers; one gram equals four calories

Carbon footprints: greenhouse gas (GHG) emissions from events, organizations, people and/or products; released through production and consumption of foods and activities and construction, fuel production, manufacturing and transportation

Carbonated soft drinks: commonly known as soda, in contrast to carbonated "hard drink"

Carbon monoxide: colorless, odorless, tasteless and highly toxic gas; produced from incomplete burning of carbon-containing fuels

Carcinogen: substance that may cause cancer

Cardiovascular disease: class of diseases that involve heart and blood vessels; related to atherosclerosis

Cardiovascular endurance: efficiency of heart, lungs and vascular system in delivering oxygen to working muscles to prolong physical work over time

Cardiovascular fitness: efficiency of heart, lungs and vascular system in delivering oxygen to working muscles to prolong physical work

Carnitine: compound needed for fatty acid transport to generate energy

Carob or St. John's bread: Syrian legume; edible seed pod that can replace chocolate in some recipes

Carotenoid: vitamin A precursor (beta-carotene); acts as antioxidant; essential for vision

Carotenoids: plant-based substances; responsible for bright orange and red color in carrots, pumpkins, sweet potatoes, tomatoes and other orangey fruits and vegetables

Carrageen: species of red algae; used as thickener and stabilizer in milk products, such as ice cream, and in processed foods, such as luncheon meats; source of carrageenan

Carrageenan: starch-like substance from red seaweed; used to increase viscosity (thickness) and stability of desserts, dressings, ice cream, milkshakes, sauces and processed foods

Casein: predominant protein in dairy milk and cheese

Cassoulet: Southwestern French stew of white flageolet and haricot legumes and meats; often contains pork and sausages

Cast-iron cookware: heavy nontoxic iron cookware with excellent heat retention and diffusion capabilities

Catabolism: process by which molecules break down into smaller units and energy

Catalysts: substances that accelerate rates of chemical reactions; stay intact so can be reused

Celiac disease: autoimmune disorder of small intestine; symptoms include chronic diarrhea, fatigue and failure to thrive in children; lifelong disability that requires strict avoidance of gluten-containing foods and food products

Cellulite: dimpled condition of abdomen, lower limbs and pelvic region after puberty

Cellulose: component of cell walls in green plants; often called dietary fiber or roughage; indigestible by humans

Cena: dinner in Spanish-speaking countries

Cerebellum: region of brain; plays important role in integration of coordination, motor control and sensory perception

Cerebral cortex: structure within brain; plays key role in attention, consciousness, language, memory, perceptual awareness and thought

Cerebral vascular disease: group of brain dysfunctions; related to blood vessel supply to brain; hypertension significant cause

Chai tea: brewed spiced South Indian tea; often served with cream or dairy milk

Chapatti, naan, pappadam, and paratha: baked, fried or roasted Eastern Indian breads

Chaso (FenPhen): appetite suppressant; FefPhen substitute; may lead to coronary heart disease

Chèvre: French tart and slightly salty semisoft goat's milk cheese

The China Project: Chinese diet and mortality study during 1983 to 2003

Chinese five-spice powder: seasoning used in Chinese cuisine; incorporates five basic flavors of Chinese cooking: bitter, salty, savory, sour and sweet; contains cinnamon, cloves, fagara, fennel and star anise

Chinese tea culture: elements of Chinese tea preparation, equipment and occasions

Chitosan: diet aid; blocks fat absorption

Chitterlings: fried slices of small intestine

Chloride: mineral required for metabolism; maintains acid-base balance; component of sodium chloride (table salt)

Chlorophyll: colorful green pigment in most green plants and algae; essential in photosynthesis whereby plants obtain energy from light

Chocolate: raw or processed seeds of tropical cacao tree; food that contains cocoa solids, fats (primarily cocoa butter), flavor ingredients and sugar

Cholecalciferol: form of vitamin D normally added during fortification

Cholesterol: sterol (type of lipid); occurs in all animal tissues, especially in brain, spinal cord and fat tissues; serves as protective agent in skin and nerve cells; detoxifier in bloodstream and precursor of steroids; blood cholesterol contributing factor in cardiovascular disease

Cholesterol controversy (lipid hypothesis): hypothesis developed in 1950s to explain atherosclerosis, or "hardening" of the arteries; proposed connection between blood cholesterol and coronary heart disease (CHD)

Choline: water-soluble essential nutrient usually grouped with B vitamins; functions in metabolism and nerve transmission; primarily found in egg yolks, lecithin, liver (beef, turkey, veal) and soy

Chorizo: Mexican and Caribbean pork sausage

Chronological age: age of organism in years

Chutney: condiment made of raw or cooked mixtures of ingredients, such as chilies, fruits, herbs, sugar, spices, vegetables and vinegar

Chylomicrons: lipoproteins that transport lipids from intestine through blood and lymph; mostly carry triglycerides

Cilantro: leaves of coriander plant; also known as Chinese parsley

Cirrhosis: chronic degenerative liver disease; caused by chronic ethanol abuse; marked by liver obstruction; can lead to coma and death

Cis bond: chemical bond used in hydrogenation of fatty acids; safer than trans bond; implicated in increased blood cholesterol and risk of cardiovascular disease

Clarified butter (ghee): type of butter used in Indian cuisine; made by simmering unsalted butter until liquid has boiled off and milk solids have settled, leaving only butterfat; higher smoke point and longer shelf life than standard butter

Clean: condition whereby visible dirt and residue have been removed; used as guideline in food safety

Clementine: variety of Mandarin orange

Clenbuterol: diet aid similar to ephedrine; increases metabolism; impairs heart and lung functions

Clostridium: bacteria present in soil and intestines of humans and animals

Club soda: artificially carbonated water; some types have added salts and/or minerals

Coagulation: to congeal; irreversible change in proteins from liquid to semisolid state by heat

Cocoa: dried and partially fermented fatty seeds of cacao tree made into powder; beverage commonly known as hot chocolate

Coconut: fruit noted for high saturated fat content; filled with flesh, coconut milk and coconut water; used in cooking and baking for flavor and texture; reduced-fat coconut products available

Coffee: stimulating beverage produced by roasting, grinding and brewing coffee seeds; high in antioxidants

Cola: sweet, carbonated drink that contains caramel coloring; with or without caffeine

Cola nuts: tree nuts native to African tropical rainforests; used to make cola; contains bitter flavor and caffeine

Colonoscopy: procedure that examines large colon and small bowel with specialized camera

Colon polyp: fleshy growth on colon or rectum lining; may lead to colorectal cancer if untreated

Color: hue as opposed to black, white or gray

Collagen: main protein found in connective tissue in animals; requires vitamin C for synthesis and maintenance

Colloid: substance evenly dispersed throughout another substance

Colostrum: form of "first" breast milk; produced by mammary glands in late pregnancy and first days after birth

Community/municipality sourced water: water from community/municipality source; origin must appear on water bottle labels

Community Supported Agriculture (CSA): memberships with farms by which shares are purchased in exchange for seasonal fruits and vegetables; builds relationships with farmers and supports local agriculture

Complementary proteins: process that balances incomplete proteins, such as peanut butter and bread, or beans and rice

Complete protein: protein with all essential amino acids, such as eggs or meat

Compote: cooked fruit in sweetened syrup

Computed tomography (CT): medical imaging method for measuring body fat; supplements x-rays and ultrasound

Conch: large edible snail; meat used in burgers, chowders, fritters, gumbos and salads

Condensed milk or sweetened condensed milk: dairy milk with water removed and sugar added; yields thick, sweet liquid

Conditionally essential nutrients: nutrients that must be supplied to human body under special conditions, such as aging, illness or stress

Conduction: direct transfer of heat (energy); heat moved from flame or coil to food; when pot or pan with food is placed on flame or burner

Congri (Moors and Christians): Cuban black beans and rice

Conjugated linoleic acid (CLA): beneficial trans fatty acid found in meat and dairy products with antioxidant and anticancer properties; dietary aid; used to reduce body fat, build muscle, decrease appetite

Contaminated iron: iron that leaches into food; may lead to toxicity

Contamination: infection by pathogenic bacteria, viruses, prions or parasites; usually arises from improper food handling, preparation or storage

Convection: transfer of heat in fluid or gas by circulation

Cooking: process of preparing foods for consumption; includes wide variety of ingredients, methods and tools that affect sensory qualities and/or digestibility of foods

Corn syrup: liquid starch (syrup) made from corn; mainly glucose (sometimes called glucose syrup); used for maintaining freshness, moistening, sweetening, thickening

Cornstarch: starch derived from corn; used as thickener and binder in food products, where more effective than wheat starch; best dissolved in cold water; useful in gluten-free recipes

Coronary arteries: network of arteries that supply blood to heart

Cortisol: "stress" hormone produced by adrenal gland; increases blood pressure and blood sugar; reduces immune responses

Cosmetic surgery: medical procedure that enhances appearance through surgical and medical techniques

Costridium botulinum: bacteria that produces botulin toxin; causes botulism, a rare but serious paralytic illness

Coulis: thickened hot or cold sauce; made with pureed fruits or vegetables

611

Couscous: quick-cooking grain produced from semolina wheat or sometimes corn or pearl millet

Couscoussiere: double boiler used for couscous and stews

Coush-coush: Cajun creamed corn dish

Couverture chocolate: very high-quality chocolate; contains extra cocoa butter (32 to 39 percent); more sheen, firmer "snap" and creamier mellow flavor than regular chocolate; used for coating, dipping, garnishing and molding

Cream: dairy product with high butterfat layer skimmed from dairy milk surface before homogenization

Cream of tartar: potassium hydrogen tartarate; white, powdery substance frequently combined with baking soda in baking powder; used to stabilize egg whites, prevent sugar syrup from crystallizing and reduce discoloration of vegetables

Creams: light, fluffy, thickened mixtures made with whipped egg whites; serve as basis of desserts; includes crème anglaise (custard sauce), crème au beurre (buttercream frosting), crème pâtissière (pastry cream) and frangipane (almond-flavored cream)

Crème fraiche: soured heavy European cream; butterfat content about 28 percent; counterpart to soured cream

Crohn's disease: autoimmune disease that affects gastrointestinal tract; characterized by areas of inflammation, abdominal pain, constipation, vomiting and weight gain or loss

Croquettes: small deep-fried and breaded fritters

Cross contamination: indirect bacterial contamination of food from one substance to another; caused by contact with other food or nonfood sources, such as clothes, cutting boards, knives or machinery

Crytosporidium: organism that causes gastrointestinal illness with diarrhea

Culinary: related to or connected with cooking

Culinary arts: art of cooking

Culinary herb: fragrant leaves and stems of plants used for culinary purposes rather than medicinal purposes

Culinology®: registered trademark of Research Chefs Association (RCA); approach to food that blends culinary arts and food technology

Cultured soy yogurt: yogurt made with cultured or fermented soy milk; replicates consistency and taste of cultured dairy yogurt

Curcumin: antioxidant and anti-inflammatory; found in turmeric

Curdle/curdling: separation of dairy milk or egg mixtures into liquid and solid states by acid, high heat or overcooking

Curry powder or masala powder: South Asian spice blend

Custards: liquids thickened by coagulated egg proteins; includes cheesecake, crème brulee, crème caramel, pots de crème, quiche, sweet flans and timbales

Cyanocobalamin: another name for vitamin B12

Cysteine: nonessential amino acid found in foods of both animal and vegetable origin

Cystic fibrosis: genetic disease; affects mucus glands of intestines, liver, lungs, and pancreas; causes progressive disability

Daikon: giant white Japanese radish

DASH diet (Dietary Approaches to Stop Hypertension): diet created by National Heart, Lung and Blood Institute (National Institutes of Health of US Department of Agriculture); limits sodium, red meat and refined carbohydrates; promotes fish, fruits, lean poultry, nuts, vegetables and whole grains

Date sugar: intense sweetener made from pulverized dates; slightly more granular than white sugar; contains fiber and some minerals

Decompose: to rot or reduce into simple forms of matter

Dehydrated milk: powdered milk; made from dried or dehydrated milk solids; longer shelf life than liquid milk; does not need refrigeration

Dehydration: removal of water; deficiency of water molecules in relation to dissolved solutes

Deionized water: purified water from any source; physically processed to remove impurities; most common form of purified water along with distilled water

Dementia: progressive decline in cognitive function due to brain damage or disease; accompanied by decline in attention, language and problem solving

Demineralized water: water with all minerals removed; also called **purified water**

Denaturation: undoing natural structures through chemical or physical processes; often proteins by acids, agitation, bases, heat or salts

Denatured protein: protein that has lost shape and functionality from acids, bases, heat, high salt concentration or whipping

Dental caries (cavities): formation of cavities (pitted areas) or decay in teeth; caused by oral bacteria

Dental plaque: film made from bacteria, by-products and saliva that adheres to teeth

Desayuno: breakfast in Spanish-speaking countries

Dessicated coconut: shredded or flaked and dried coconut "meat"

Destination spas: wellness facility where environment fosters diet, fitness, healthy eating, relaxation and renewal

Deteriorate: diminished or impaired character, quality or value

Dextrose: form of glucose derived from starch

Diabetes (also known as diabetes mellitus and hyperglycemia): disease characterized by inadequate or ineffective insulin; results in poor blood sugar regulation; differentiated as Type I and Type II

Diastolic blood pressure: blood pressure reading represented by "bottom" number (when heart is resting)

Diet: all foods and beverages routinely consumed; quality, composition and effects of foods and beverages on health; plan for eating and/or weight loss

Diet aids: dietary, herbal and pharmacological aids to weight loss

Dietary fiber: nondigestible substance; mostly polysaccharides (long chains of sugars) from leaves, seeds and stems of plants

Dietary Guidelines: scientifically-based guidelines for health promotion and disease prevention; achieved through diet and physical activities

Dietary Reference Intakes (DRIs): group of values for calories and nutrients established by USDA; used for assessing and planning diets

Dietary supplement: oral product that contains "dietary ingredient(s)" intended to supplement diet

Dieting: process of ingesting foods and beverages in prescribed manner to achieve or maintain controlled weight

Digestion: process of breaking down foods and beverages chemically and physically, then converting into substances for absorption, use and storage

Digestive diseases: disorders of digestive system; includes stomach, small and large intestine, organs and glands

Digestive system: body system responsible for ingestion, digestion, absorption, metabolism and excretion of food and beverages

Direct contamination: direct infection by pathogenic bacteria, viruses, prions, or parasites

Disordered eating: general term for eating disorders, including anorexia nervosa, bulimia nervosa and binge eating disorder; arises from excessive and distorted preoccupation with body weight

Distilled water: water with impurities removed through distillation (process of purifying liquid by boiling and condensing vapors, leaving solid contaminants)

Distilling: physical process of separating mixtures; based on volatile differences in boiling liquid

Dissolving agent: liquid substance able to dissolve other substances

Diuretics: substances that cause increased fluid excretion

Diverticulitis: digestive disease in large intestine; develops from diverticulosis (outpouching of intestinal wall)

Diverticulosis: condition of outpouching of intestinal wall; outpouches or sacs protrude, rupture and become infected

Docosahexaenoic acid (DHA): omega-3 essential fatty acid found in fish oil; may reduce risk of coronary heart disease by reducing level of triglycerides

Doneness: degree meat is cooked: rare, medium rare, medium, medium well or well done; other foods that have completed different stages of cooking

Dopamine: brain neurotransmitter; affects processes that control ability to experience emotional responses, movements, pleasure and pain

Double-acting baking powder: leavening agent; mixture of acidic ingredient as cream of tartar, baking soda and starch; releases carbon dioxide when mixed with liquid for early and secondary rises

Double sugars: two single sugars bonded together; include sucrose (white table sugar), lactose (milk sugar) and maltose (malt sugar)

Doufu: Japanese term for tofu

Duodenal ulcer: raw area in lining of upper part of small intestine (duodenum) that connects to stomach

Duration: amount of time; length of time one participates in exercise

Durian: odorous Asian "King of Fruits"

Eating behavior: consumption of foods and beverages in relation to environment

Eco-consciousness: awareness of environment and ecological (biological) systems

Edamame: immature pods of soybeans

Edema: condition whereby fluids leak from blood vessels into tissues and cause swelling; due to protein deficiency

Egg foams: airy protein structures; created when egg whites are incorporated with air; includes meringues, mousses, sabayon, soufflés and zabaglione

Egg foo yung: Cantonese egg patties

613

Eicosapentaenoic acid (EPA): omega-3 essential fatty acid; found in fish, some plants and algae; reduces inflammation (associated with cardiovascular disease)

Einkorn: tough grain grown in Europe since 11,000 years BC; precursor of durum wheat; may be safe for gluten-free diets

Electrolyte: free ions including chloride, magnesium, potassium and sodium; conduct electricity when dissolved in solution; help regulate water balance

Embryo: organism from time of implantation until end of eighth week of pregnancy, when called a *fetus*

Emmer (faro): original staple grain of ancient Egypt and Turkey; precursor of durum wheat; earthy taste and gritty texture

Empanadas: turnovers; often made with chicken or meat

Emulsifier: substance that stabilizes emulsions by increasing stability; includes egg yolk, honey, mustard, protein, soy lecithin

Emulsify: process by which ingredients are combined into an emulsion (suspension of tiny droplets of liquid in another liquid that ordinarily do not mix)

Emulsions: uniform mixture of immiscible ingredients, made with liquid, emulsifier and mechanical action; includes butter, margarine, mayonnaise and vinaigrette salad dressing

Enchiladas: filled corn tortillas; covered with chili sauce or **verdes** (green sauce)

Endorphins: morphine-like chemicals mainly produced in brain and spinal cord; released in response to neurotransmitters; act as analgesics and sedatives

Energy drinks: soft drinks with physiological and psychological effects, especially energy promoting

English system: classification of measurement primarily used in United States; also called United States Customary System

Enriched grains: refined grains enriched with B-vitamins (folic acid, niacin, riboflavin and thiamin) and iron; restores vitamins and minerals affected during processing

Enzymes: protein catalysts; help chemical reactions catalyze or speed up reactions; remain intact after use

Ephedra (Ma Huang): diet aid; decreases appetite; side effects include high blood pressure, irregular heartbeat, heart attack, seizure, stroke and death; banned for safety issues

Ergocalciferol: form of vitamin D; also known as vitamin D2

Ergogenic: the capacity to exercise or work

Ergogenic aids: mechanical, nutritional, pharmacological, physiological, and psychological aids that help increase capacity to exercise or work

Escherichia coli (E. coli): bacteria normally found in human gastrointestinal tract; may cause different types of diarrhea and gastrointestinal disease

Essential amino acids: amino acids that must be consumed in food, drink or supplements; cannot be made by human body

Essential fat: fat necessary for maintenance of life and reproductive functions

Essential fatty acids: fatty acids that must be consumed in food, drink or supplements; cannot be made by human body in needed amounts; much like essential amino acids

Essential (primary) hypertension: hypertension with no specific medical causes

Ethanol (ethyl alcohol, grain or drinking alcohol): volatile, flammable, colorless liquid in alcoholic beverages

Evaporated milk (dehydrated milk): shelf-stable canned dairy milk with 60 percent water removed

Exchange lists: food lists with similar calories and nutrients; specifies portion sizes

Exercise: body activities that enhance or maintain physical fitness and overall health

Extracellular water: water outside of cells

Extract: concentrated mixtures of alcohol and flavored oils, such as almond or vanilla

Extrusion reflex: reflex that causes infant to thrust tongue forward and extrude food

Fan: balance of grains and rice in Chinese cooking

Fasting: willingly abstaining from food or drink for prescribed time

Fat cell theory: overweight and obesity theory; suggests certain fat cells created during growth; enlarge or decrease with weight gain or loss

Fat-free mass: lean body mass

Fats: lipids that are solid at room temperature

Fat separator (degreasing pitcher or gravy separator): separates heavy gravy or liquid from fat or oil for discarding

Fat soluble: ability of substance or solute to dissolve in fat (solvent)

Fat-soluble vitamins: vitamins A, D, E and K; primarily found in dietary fats; stored in body fat

Fat substitutes: synthetic and natural chemical compounds made from carbohydrates, protein and lipids; resemble lipids in structure and function

Fatty acids: building blocks of lipids; can be saturated, unsaturated or polyunsaturated

Feta: sheep's milk, or sheep's and goat's milk cheese; Greece owns rights to "feta" name

Fetal Alcohol Effect (FAE): effects of alcohol consumption by women during pregnancy; may not cause permanent birth defects

Fetal alcohol syndrome (FAS): group of symptoms in infants or children of mothers who consume excess alcohol during pregnancy; characterized by growth retardation, impaired central nervous system and distorted facial features

Fetus: developing mammal after embryonic stage and before birth

Fines herbes: herbal mixture of chervil, chives, parsley and tarragon

Fitness: general state of good health; usually result of nutrition and exercise

F.I.T. Principle: principle of frequency, intensity and time to achieve fitness

Five basic tastes: bitter, salty, sour, sweet and umami (Japanese for deliciousness)

Five senses: hearing, sight, smell, taste and touch

Flageolets: French legumes

Flan: caramel custard

Flavonoid phenolics: category of antioxidant compounds that include flavonoids; found in almost all fruits, grains and vegetables

Flavonoids: phyto- (plant) nutrients that are water-soluble pigments; thought to have antioxidant and anti-inflammatory properties; also called bioflavonoids

Flavor: distinctive qualities of appearance, mouth feel, smell, sound, taste, temperature and texture of foods or beverages as perceived by senses

Flavored oils and vinegars: oils and vinegars flavored by fruits, herbs, spices, vegetables and other ingredients

Flavr Savr™ tomato: first genetically-engineered food licensed for human consumption; modified to prevent rotting and increase flavor and shelf life

Flaxseed oil (linseed oil): used in cooking or added to finished dishes; contains omega-3 and omega-6 essential fatty acids, B vitamins, fiber, lecithin, magnesium, potassium, protein and zinc

Flaxseeds: seeds from flax plant; used as egg replacer in baking for binding; rich in omega-3 and omega-6 essential fatty acids

Flexibility: ease in movement of joints and/or muscles

Fluorosis: damage during tooth development from overexposure to fluoride; characterized by pitting or mottling of enamel, yellowing of teeth and white spots

Foam: substance formed by trapping gas bubbles in liquid or solid

Focaccia: flat Italian bread; often topped with herbs and spices

Folate acid (folic acid, folacin): B vitamin vital to new cell production and maintenance, especially during growth (as in pregnancy and infancy); primarily found in fortified grain products, leafy green vegetables and legumes; folic acid found in supplements

Food allergy: adverse reaction by immune system to otherwise harmless substances

Food aversion: dislike of certain foods

Foodborne infection: harmful microorganisms transferred by foods or beverages to host; uncontrolled growth of harmful microorganisms in body parts or tissues of host

Food chemistry: field of study that examines food molecules in chemical reactions

Food cooperatives: grocery stores commonly supported and community owned with local, organic foods and beverages; appeal to eco-conscious consumers

Food cravings: strong desires for food or drink

Food deserts: areas without access to healthy foods in industrialized societies and rural communities; affordable and healthful foods are difficult to obtain

Food engineering: field of study that examines development and manufacturing of new food products

Food intolerance: nonallergic food or beverage hypersensitivity; does not involve immune system

Food jags: periods of time of erratic food behaviors; associated with children and teenagers

Food microbiology: field of study that examines interactions among microorganisms and foods

Food packaging: process by which food is packaged to preserve maximum nutrients after processing

Food preservation: field of study that examines causes and prevention of food degradation (breakdown)

Food rituals: practices that demonstrate faith, disciplined behavior and respect for higher being; fundamental to some religions

Food safety: field of study that examines causes, prevention and communication of foodborne illnesses

Food science: study of technical aspects of food from growing, harvesting, slaughtering, cooking and consumption through digestion, absorption and metabolism; includes food engineering, food safety, food technology, molecular gastronomy and sensory analysis

Food security: availability of food; person's access to food

Food technology: field of study that examines physical aspects of foods, as flavor and texture

Fortified foods: foods and food products that contain 10 percent or more of the Daily Value (DV) for certain nutrients; foods are fortified to help prevent nutrient deficiencies or chronic diseases

Free radicals: highly reactive substances associated with oxidative and cellular damage

Freezer "burn": condition whereby frozen food is damaged by dehydration and oxidation

Freezing: process where liquids change into solids at freezing temperatures (32 °F or 0 °C)

French Paradox: phenomenon first noted in 1819; contradiction is that French people have low incidence of coronary heart disease despite diet rich in saturated fats

Frequency: rate of recurrence; how often exercise is repeated

Fructose (fruit sugar): sweetest of all single sugars (monosaccharide); also found in honey

Fruit-based water: water with predominant fruit flavor; does not contain fruit juice

Frying/pan-frying: dry-heat method of cooking foods in hot fat or oil; food fried in pan as opposed to wok or other cooking equipment

Functional foods: fresh or processed foods with reputed health-promoting or disease-preventing properties beyond nutritional functions

Functional tolerance: alteration in sensitivity to alcohol—that is, nerve cells become heightened to counteract inhibitory effects of alcohol

Fusion cooking: contemporary cooking term; combination of ingredients and techniques from different cuisines

Gag reflex: reflex contraction in back of throat; prevents substances from entering throat and choking

Galactose: single sugar (monosaccharide); found in milk and other dairy products

Gallbladder: pear-shaped, muscular sac attached to undersurface of liver where bile is stored

Gallbladder disease: slows or obstructs flow of bile out of gallbladder; causes bloating, heartburn and pain

Garnish: food or nonfood used to decorate plate or platters; also used to indicate ingredients contained in dish

Gastric banding: procedure that restricts stomach's content; designed for obese people with body mass index (BMI) of 40 or greater, or between 35 and 40 with other conditions

Gastric bypass: medical procedure that divides stomach into pouches and rearranges small intestine; reduces stomach volume; alters physiological and psychological responses to food

Gastritis: inflammation of gastric mucosa in stomach

Gastroplasty: most common restrictive medical procedure for managing obesity; known as stomach stapling

Gelatin: colorless, nearly tasteless and translucent substance; extracted from collagen inside connective tissues; commonly used as emulsifier

Gelatinization: cooking process by which starch absorbs fluid, softens, swells and clarifies upon exposure to heat

General fitness: body's overall ability to meet physical demands

Genetic engineering: purposeful manipulation of genetic material of organisms

Genetically engineered foods (GM foods): made from genetically-modified organisms with changes to their DNA by genetic engineering

Genetically modified starch: starch made from genetically-engineered plants

Genistein: isoflavone found in soybeans with reported health benefits

Gestational diabetes: type of diabetes that starts or diagnosed during pregnancy; condition whereby women without previous diabetes exhibit high blood glucose during pregnancy; marked by mild diabetic symptoms, including abnormal blood sugar

Ghee: clarified butter with the milk solids removed; common in Indian cuisine

Gliaden: gluten-type protein found in barley, rye and wheat

Globalization: transformation of local, regional or national foods, beverages, concepts and perspectives into global equivalents

Glucose: single sugar (monosaccharide) found in both plants and animals; building block of complex carbohydrates (starches)

Glucuronolactone: naturally occurring chemical compound produced by glucose metabolism; important structural component in connective tissues; found in plant gums

Glutamic acid: amino acid abundant in animal protein and some vegetable protein; responsible for umami taste

Glutathione: antioxidant; protects cells from toxins as free radicals

Gluten intolerance (celiac disease): extreme sensitivity to gluten protein; found primarily in barley, rye and wheat

Gluten sensitivity or intolerance (celiac disease): disorder of immune system that affects small intestine; inability to tolerate gluten (protein in grains including barley, rye and wheat); symptoms include anemia, diarrhea, fatigue and/or weight loss

Glycemic Index: ranking of foods; based upon ability to raise blood sugar levels in comparison to glucose as standard

Glycerol: organic compound; backbone of triglycerides, along with three fatty acids

Glycogen: storage form of carbohydrate in humans; primarily made/stored by liver and muscles

Gogi gui: Korean barbecue

Golden rice™: rice produced by genetic engineering to biosynthesize beta-carotene (vitamin A precursor)

Gorgonzola: Italian blue-veined cheese

Gout (metabolic arthritis): disease caused by buildup of uric acid in cartilage of joints, tendons and surrounding tissues; causes inflammation

Granulated or white refined sugar (sucrose): double sugar composed of glucose and fructose; made by dissolving and purifying raw sugar or by filtration

"Green" movement: organized effort for addressing environmental issues; affects ecology, health and human rights through individual actions and public policies

615

Green tea: tea originated from China; made with leaves of *Camellia sinensis*; undergoes minimal oxidation during processing

Green tea extract: diet aid; increases calorie, fat metabolism; decreases appetite

Gremolata: Italian chopped herb condiment; made from anchovies, garlic, lemon zest and parsley; traditional accompaniment to Ossobuco alla Milanese (Milanese braised veal shank)

Grilling: dry-heat cooking method; food cooked on grate directly over dry heat, as charcoal or gas grill or stovetop grill pan

Groundwater: water sourced from underground body; does not contact surface water

Growth spurts: periods of rapid growth; generally during childhood and adolescence

Guaranine: caffeine chemical in guarana (South American plant); used in energy drinks, herbal teas and sweetened or carbonated soft drinks

Guar gum: gum found in baked goods; thickener in dairy products, as yogurt

Gum Arabic: gum found in hard, gummy candies, soft drinks and syrups

Gumbo: hearty meat and/or shellfish stew

Gums: carbohydrates that create viscosity in solutions; used as emulsifiers, gelling agents, stabilizers and thickening agents

Gums: guar, locust-bean and xanthan: complex carbohydrates chiefly derived from plants; used as gel-forming agents, stabilizing agents and thickeners; increase viscosity (thickness of liquids)

Half-and-half: very light cream, typically used in coffee; butterfat content about 12.5 percent

Halwah: Eastern Indian honey or sugar confection made with ground almonds and milk

Hangover: physiological effects from heavy ethanol consumption; includes depression, headache, lethargy, nausea, sensitivity to light and noise and thirst

Hanjeongsik: full-course Korean meal

Hard water: type of water with high mineral content, as calcium or magnesium

Hazard Analysis Critical Control Points (HACCP): system of self-inspection; used to manage and maintain sanitation in food service operations

Health: state of complete mental, physical and social well-being, as opposed to absence of disease

Health claims: statements made by food manufacturers about association of food and disease or condition; regulated by US FDA

Healthy baking: sum of all processes and techniques used to bake foods with maximum nutrients and minimal excesses

Healthy cooking: sum of all processes and techniques used to cook foods with maximum nutrients and minimal excesses

Healthy Eating Index (HEI): measure of diet quality; assesses conformance of US population and low-income subpopulations to federal dietary guidelines

Heart attack: sudden interruption or insufficiency of blood to heart; due to occlusion or obstruction of blood flow to heart muscle

Heartburn: painful or burning sensation in esophagus below breastbone; associated with regurgitated gastric acid

Heart Leaf (Country Mallow): diet aid that contains ephedra; decreases appetite and increases calorie expenditure

Heat exhaustion: heat-related illness; includes dizziness, fainting, headache, heavy sweating, muscle cramps, nausea or vomiting, paleness, tiredness, weakness

Heatstroke: perilous condition when heat builds in body; causes series of reactions, including cessation of sweating, confusion, convulsions, fast pulse rate, high body temperature and loss of consciousness

Height: focal point in food plating; distance from base of dining plate to top

Height-weight tables: tables that determine body weight using height, weight, frame and gender classifications

Helicobacter pylori (H. pylori) bacteria: bacteria that inhabit stomach and duodenum; cause chronic inflammation of stomach lining; leads to duodenal and gastric ulcers and stomach cancer

Heme iron: form of iron in hemoglobin and myoglobin; found in animal foods

Hemochromatosis: iron overload

Hemoglobin: iron-containing oxygen-transport protein; found in red blood cells

Herbal teas: beverages made from steeping or boiling herbs, unlike teas

Herbes (Herbs) de Provence: dried herb mixture from Provence region of France; contains basil, fennel, lavender, savory and thyme; used in longer-cooking dishes or infused in oil

Heterocyclic amines (HCAs): carcinogenic chemicals formed from muscle meats cooked at high temperatures

Hibachi barbecue grill: small grill with less heat variations than larger grill

High-carbohydrate diet: diet with higher proportion of carbohydrates than protein or lipids

High-density lipoproteins (HDL): small, dense lipid and protein particles; enable lipid transport in bloodstream; protect against cardiovascular disease

High fructose corn syrup (HFCS): group of corn syrups; undergo enzymatic processing to increase fructose content, then mixed with pure corn syrup (100 percent glucose); very intense economical sweetener

Hippocampus: part of brain; important for formation of new memories

Hispanics: people who originate from Central or South American, Cuba, Mexico, Puerto Rico and other Spanish-speaking areas of Latin America

Histamine: substance released in allergic reaction by immune system; causes inflammation and other symptoms throughout body

Hollandaise sauce: buttery, rich-tasting emulsion; made with butter, egg yolk and lemon juice

Homeostasis: stable, constant environment in living organisms

Homocysteine: substance produced when protein broken down by human body; may damage lining of arteries, increase blood clots and lead to coronary heart disease; linked to higher-protein diets

Homogenized milk: dairy milk broken into smaller-sized particles by homogenization to prevent separation; accomplished by forcing milk through small holes at high pressure

Honey: viscous food and sweetener; mainly fructose and glucose with maltose, sucrose, other complex carbohydrates, trace vitamins and minerals; produced by honeybees from flower nectar

Hoodia: diet aid; decreases appetite; not for children, pregnant women

Hoppin' John (Whippoorwill Peas and Rice and Crowder Peas and Rice): black-eyed peas and rice

Hormones: protein messengers, such as insulin or testosterone; secreted by gland to targeted tissues

Huarache press: corn cake press

Hummus: Middle Eastern garbanzo puree

Hunger: physiological drive to locate and consume foods and/or beverages to decrease physical sensations

Hush puppies: cornbread fritters

Husk: dry outside covering of certain fruits and seeds

Hydrochloric acid: powerful acid secreted in stomach to help digest protein

Hydrogenation: chemical process that converts unsaturated fatty acids to saturated fatty acids by adding hydrogen; partially or fully hydrogenates vegetable oils

Hyperglycemia: high blood sugar; characteristic of diabetes

Hypertension (high blood pressure): medical condition in which blood pressure is chronically elevated

Hypertonic: higher concentration of solutes inside cell

Hypoglycemia: low blood sugar; symptoms include cold, shaky, tired or weak; if undetected may cause unconsciousness or death

Hyponatremia: electrolyte disturbance; sodium concentration in blood plasma low

Hypothalamus: part of brain that senses bodily conditions; links nervous system to endocrine system via pituitary gland to initiate changes

Ice: crystalline solid phase of water

Ideal body weight: weight believed ideal; based on age, build, gender and height

Immiscible: unmixable

Immunoglobulin E (IgE): antibody that plays important role in allergic responses

Incomplete protein: protein that lacks one or more essential amino acids; often found in plant foods

Indigestion: feeling of discomfort and pain in upper abdomen and chest; symptoms may include belching, bloating, fullness and/or nausea

Infant formula: alternative complete nourishment for infants other than human breast milk

Infection: invasion by and uncontrolled growth of harmful microorganisms in body parts or tissues; foodborne infection transferred by food or beverages to host

Infusion: extract prepared by soaking plant leaves in liquid

Initiators (cancer): substances that initiate cancer progression

Inositol: once considered vitamin B8; can be synthesized by body; primarily found in cereals with high bran content, fruits (especially cantaloupe melons and oranges), legumes and nuts

Intensity: strength or power; how hard exercise is executed

Intestinal obstruction: obstruction of bowel due to disease or infection

Intracellular water: water inside cells

Intramuscular fat: fat lined within muscle fibers

Intrinsic factor: glycoprotein produced by cells in stomach lining; necessary for vitamin B12 absorption in ileum

Inulin: fermentable, subtly sweet fiber; promotes mass health of intestinal bacteria; used to replace sugar, fat and flour, or improve flow and mixing qualities of ingredients in product development

Invert sugar: sucrose-based syrup treated with enzymes to split into glucose and fructose; sweeter than sucrose and less prone to crystallization; contributes long-lasting moistness

Involuntary muscles: smooth muscles not directly or willingly controlled; found in digestive system, internal organs, iris muscles, major blood vessels, reproductive system and skin; controlled by autonomic nervous system

Iodine: trace mineral necessary for thyroid hormone production; primarily found in iodized salt and seafood

Iron-deficiency anemia: most common type of anemia; occurs when dietary intake or iron absorption insufficient and hemoglobin cannot be formed

Iron overload: condition caused by accumulation of iron; affects endocrine glands, heart and liver

Irradiation: process of using radiation to destroy harmful microorganisms

Irritable bowel syndrome (IBS): disorder characterized by abdominal pain, bloating, constipation, cramping and/or diarrhea

Isoflavones: chemical compounds in soy-based foods, vegetables and fruits; may be protective against certain cancers

Isopropanol: type of alcohol known as rubbing alcohol

Isotonic: state of equilibrium with surroundings; balance of water exiting and entering cells

Jamón: Spanish or Mexican ham

Jaundice: yellow color in skin and whites of eyes; caused by excessive bilirubin in blood (yellow chemical in hemoglobin)

Juice cocktail: blend of fruit juice with other beverages

Juice drink: any drink with juice, even if 1 percent total volume

Juvenile (Type I) diabetes: autoimmune disease where immune system destroys pancreatic insulin-producing cells; generally occurs in children under 12 years of age

Kallaloo or callaloo soup: Caribbean soup with conch, greens and meats

Kamut: large "ancient" grain, similar to durum wheat; probable roots in Egyptian history; requires long simmering time to soften

Kanten: flavorless dried seaweed, also known as agar-agar; high in fiber; useful as a thickening agent

Kefta: Middle Eastern hamburger

Keratinization: condition of fibrous structural protein; causes skin to harden

Ketones: substances produced when body burns fat for energy

Ketosis: condition of abnormal ketones in blood and urine (ketones used for energy when glucose not available); produced from incomplete fat breakdown in absence of glucose

Kibbeh: Lebanese mixture of ground meat and spices

617

Kidneys: organs that maintain body fluid balance; filter and secrete end-products of metabolism and minerals with water as urine

Kidney stones: solid crystal fragments of dissolved minerals in urine; typically form inside kidneys or bladder

Kilocalories: 1,000 calories; designated by "K" or "kilo"

Kimchi or gimchi: pickled and fermented Korean vegetables

Kola: genus of trees; related to South American cacao

Kombu: type of seaweed used to flavor hearty dishes as braised tempeh

Kosher salt: also called **koshering salt;** used in process of koshering meats by removing blood

Kudzu: starchy powder, like arrowroot or cornstarch; used to thicken gravies, sauces and stews

Lactation: period of time when milk secreted from mammary glands to feed infants

Lactic acid: product of carbohydrate metabolism with low oxygen; higher production with strenuous exercise

Lactobacillus acidophilus: probiotic; "friendly bacteria" used in production of acidophilus-type yogurt

Lactobacillus bifidus: property of breast milk; interferes with growth of pathogenic bacteria in infant's gastrointestinal tract; reduces incidence of diarrhea

Lactococcus lactis bacteria: bacteria used in production of buttermilk and cheese

Lactoferrin: protein found in milk with antimicrobial functions

Lactose: double sugar composed of glucose and galactose; naturally found in dairy milk and dairy products

Lactose intolerance: inability to digest milk sugar (lactose), due to deficiency of enzyme lactase; lactose collects in intestine where metabolized by bacteria, which cause fermentation; produce range of symptoms, including bloating, cramps, diarrhea and/or gas; not true food allergy

Lactose-reduced and lactose-free dairy milk: reduced or free of milk sugar lactose; produces few to no ill effects from lactose

Lard: rendered pork fat

Lassi: Eastern Indian yogurt-based drink

Lavash: Armenian cracker bread

Lean body mass: all body components except storage fat

Lecithin: type of lipid (phospholipid); naturally occurs in animals, plants (soybeans) and eggs; used by body and food industry as emulsifier

Leptin: hormone that keeps appetite in control; produced in fat cells; communicates with brain

Letdown reflex: stimulation that causes hormonal release, muscular contraction and movement of human breast milk into milk ducts to feed infants

Limbic system: set of brain structures; includes hippocampus and amygdala; supports variety of functions, including emotion, behavior, long-term memory and olfaction

Linoleic acid: omega-6 essential polyunsaturated fatty acid; forms lipid component of all cell membranes

Linolenic acid: omega-3 essential polyunsaturated fatty acid; roles in bone health, brain function, growth and development, metabolism, reproduction, skin and hair growth

Lipidemia: presence of excess lipids in blood

Lipids: components of cells that supply energy; include cholesterol, fats, oils and phospholipids, among others

Lipolysis: breakdown of stored fat into free fatty acids released into bloodstream; produces ketones which are used by body for energy

Lipoprotein lipase: enzyme on surface of fat cells; converts triglycerides into fatty acids; transports fatty acids into storage; may malfunction in obesity

Lipoprotein profile: blood test after fasting; indicates total cholesterol, LDL, HDL and VLDL cholesterol, triglycerides and lipid ratios

Lipoproteins: packages of lipids and proteins; help transport lipids through bloodstream and lymph

Liposuction: medical procedure for vacuuming fat cells from body sites

Liqueur: sweet alcoholic beverage; often flavored with bark, cream, flowers, fruits, herbs, roots, seeds or spices

Listeria: bacterium commonly found in food, plants, sewage, soil and stream water; able to infect fetus and newborns

Liver: large, red-brown, glandular organ located in upper right side of abdomen; secretes bile; functions in digestion and metabolism of lipids

Locavore movement: collaborative movement; emphasizes people eat locally, buy from farmers markets and local farms, join CSAs, and/or grow their own food

Locust bean gum: gum found in cream cheese, cultured dairy products and frozen desserts

Long-chain fatty acid: lipid structure containing long chain of carbon units; difficult for body to digest or break down

Low-calorie diet: under 1,200 calories; may not meet nutrient needs

Low-carbohydrate diets: diets that restrict total carbohydrates in diet; typically replace carbohydrate calories with proteins and fats

Low-density lipoproteins (LDL): major carrier proteins of cholesterol in bloodstream; high levels of LDL cholesterol associated with cardiovascular disease

Lower-body obesity: overfatness in lower extremities; not associated with coronary heart disease or obesity; more commonly seen in women

Lymph: clear fluid; transports substances throughout body; lymphatic system major component of immune system

Macerating: soaking fruits or vegetables in liquid to soften and absorb flavor; makes food more flavorful, easier to digest

Macronutrients: nutrients required by human body in large quantities; include carbohydrates, lipids and proteins

Magnesium: major mineral that strengthens bone; component of enzymes; responsible for heart and nerve function; found in chlorophyll in leafy green vegetables

Magnetic resonance imaging (MRI): medical imaging technique; commonly used to visualize structure and function of body; provides detailed images of body fat in any plane

Maillard reaction: chemical reactions among amino acids, reducing sugars and heat; creates browning

Malnutrition: medical condition caused by improper or insufficient diet; also result of disease, infection or starvation

Malted barley: barley germinated by soaking in water and drying with hot air; used for brewing beer

Maltose: double sugar composed of two glucose sugars; primarily used in beer production

Manchego: Spanish pasteurized sheep's milk cheese

Manganese: trace mineral; cofactor for enzymes in carbohydrate reactions; primarily found in legumes, nuts, oats and tea

Maple syrup: liquid sweetener with distinctive maple flavor; made by boiling down maple sap; contains calcium, manganese, potassium and zinc and trace amounts of amino acids

Margarine: butter-like product made from refined vegetable oils; sometimes blended with animal fat and emulsified with water or milk; commercially available in both hardened and softened varieties

Marinating: process of soaking foods in seasoned, often acidic, liquid before cooking

Mascarpone: Italian light and sweet soft cheese

Mast cells: cells that contain histamine; released during allergic reactions, which causes inflammation

Mateine: stimulant similar to caffeine; found in dried leaves of yerba mate

Maximum heart rate: highest number heart can contract in one minute; achieved during maximal physical exertion

Mayonnaise: thick sauce made from emulsified vegetable oil and egg yolk; white to yellow in color; may be flavored with variety of herbs, spices, juices, vinegars and other ingredients

Media noche: Cuban midnight sandwich; similar to *mixto* without glazed ham

Medical nutrition therapy (MNT): medical and nutritional services that help prevent diabetes, manage existing diabetes and slow development of diabetes complications

Medical spas: facility that provides comprehensive medical and wellness care; integrates spa services and alternative therapies under trained personnel

Medicinal foods: fresh or processed foods; claims of health-promoting or disease-preventing properties beyond nutritional functions

Medicinal herbs: leaves or stems of plants with suspected medical-like effects

Mediterranean diet: set of nutritional recommendations based on traditional dietary patterns of countries that flank Mediterranean Sea

Mediterranean triad: three foods that comprise Mediterranean diet: grapes (and wine), olives (and olive oil), and wheat (and wheat products)

Medulla: lower portion of brainstem; controls autonomic functions, such as breathing, blood pressure and heart rate

Megaloblastic anemia: anemia characterized by larger than normal red blood cells; caused by inhibited DNA synthesis; due to vitamin B12 and/or folic acid deficiencies or lack of intrinsic factor

Melanin: pigment that gives skin color

Melt: process of slowly softening, then liquefying fats

Melting/melting point: temperature at which solid and liquid phases of substances are equal; causes solid substance to "melt" or fuse

Menaquinone: vitamin K2; normally produced by bacteria in intestines

Mercury: heavy metal; may accumulate in highly toxic forms in food chain of aquatic ecosystems

Merienda: snack in Spanish-speaking countries

Metabolic syndrome: condition characterized by three or more disease risk factors, including abdominal obesity, high blood pressure, high triglycerides, insulin resistance and/or low HDL cholesterol; linked to increased risk of cardiovascular disease and Type II diabetes

Metabolic tolerance: condition where alcohol (ethanol) metabolized faster than normal; increased amounts needed to experience alcohol's effects

Metabolic water: water produced by metabolism

Metabolism: all physical and chemical processes by which energy is created and made available for life

Metastasis: spread of disease from one organ or tissue to another

Methanol: also called methyl alcohol, carbinol, wood alcohol, wood naphtha, or wood spirits; simplest alcohol

Methionine: essential amino acid; found mostly in animal proteins and some vegetable proteins, including Brazil nuts, corn, spinach and potatoes

Methylcellulose: diet aid and appetite suppressant

Methylxanthines: group of alkaloids; used as mild stimulants and bronchodilators; notable for treating asthma

Metric system: classification of measurement; used internationally by most countries other than United States; also called **International System of Units**

Micronutrients: nutrients needed by human body in small quantities, such as trace minerals; include chromium, cobalt, copper, iodine, iron, manganese, molybdenum, selenium and zinc

Microorganisms: tiny-celled organisms in plants and animals; only seen through microscope

Microwave cooking: method of cooking; relies on radiation to penetrate foods, then conduction and convection to cook foods

Milk allergy: one of most common food allergies; caused by allergic reaction to protein in dairy milk and dairy products

Millet: principal grain and food source in desert regions of world; used in fermented drinks and porridges; millet flour used for chapatti (dense, whole-grain bread) and roti (flat, thin cake)

Mill white sugar, plantation white sugar, crystal sugar and superior sugar: types of raw sugar without colored impurities; bleached white by sulfur dioxide

Minerals: small, naturally occurring, essential chemical substances; needed by human body for structure and vital processes

Mineral water: water from underground source; at least 250 parts per million (PPM) dissolved solids

Mirepoix: mixture of chopped carrots, celery and onions; fundamental to aroma and flavor of sauces, soups, stocks and stews

Mirin: Japanese sweet wine

Mise en place: French term for preparation and assembly of all necessary ingredients and equipment before cooking

Miso: Japanese fermented soy-based soup; also condiment

Mixto sandwich: Cuban pressed sandwich of mixed meats, cheese and condiments on sweetened egg bread

Mochi: Japanese pounded rice

Moderate fat, protein, and carbohydrate diet: diet about 50 percent carbohydrates, 30 percent fat and 20 percent protein

619

Modern wheat: type of wheat deeply rooted in three grain varieties: einkorn, emmer and spelt; harvested in Europe and Near East for over 9,000 years

Modified food starches: starches modified for stability against acids, excessive heat and freezing; used as thickeners, stabilizers and emulsifiers

Molasses (treacle or sorghum): thick syrup with slight bitter taste; by-product of sugarcane or sugar beet processing into sugar; used primarily in baking and baked beans

Molcajete and tejolote: Mexican version of mortar and pestle

Molecular gastronomy: study of molecules linking chemical and physical processes of cooking

Molinillo: kitchen tool for frothing Mexican hot chocolate

Monosaccharide: single sugar, such as fructose, galactose or glucose

Monounsaturated fatty acids: fatty acids with one point of unsaturation; mostly found in avocados, nuts, olives and vegetable oils

Morning sickness: nausea of pregnancy; usually experienced in morning when blood sugar level is low

Mother Sauces: sauce base for other sauces: **bechamel** (white), **espagnole** (brown), **tomat** (red), **veloute** (roux or liasion, as egg yolk or cream) and **hollandaise** (butter)

Mottling: irregular white spots on teeth; usually due to excess fluoride during enamel formation in budding teeth

Moussaka: Greek eggplant casserole

Mozzarella: Italian stringy-textured buffalo milk cheese; also fresh pasteurized or unpasteurized cow's milk cheese; moisture content provides soft texture and mouthfeel

Muscular endurance: ability of muscles to sustain repeated contractions against resistance for extended time

Muscular fitness: includes muscular strength and endurance; allows performance of tasks with less physiological stress; helps maintain functional independence throughout life

Mushrooms: fungi produced above ground on soil or food source

Mutation: changes in genetic material during cell division; caused by chemical mutagens, ultraviolet or ionizing radiation or viruses

Myoglobin: protein that contains heme iron; found in muscle tissue

Myristic acid: saturated fatty acid; found in butterfat, nutmeg and palm oil

Naam paa: Laotian fish sauce

Naphthoquinone: organic compound found in vitamin K

Natural sugar: sugar that naturally occurs; includes fructose, found in fruit; lactose, found in dairy milk and dairy products and honey, produced by bees from nectar of flowers

Negative nitrogen balance: condition where more nitrogen excreted by body than consumed in foods

Neotame: general, all-purpose sweetener, stable at high temperatures; 7,000 times sweeter than table sugar (sucrose); found in baked goods, beverages, dairy products, frozen desserts and gums

Neural tube defects: interference with neural tube closure related to maternal folate intake; causes abnormality of brain and spinal cord; leads to spina bifida and anencephaly

Niacin (or nicotinic acid): B vitamin responsible for metabolism and healthy skin; precursor of tryptophan; deficiency causes pellagra, decreased tolerance to cold and lowered metabolism

Nicotine: colorless, poisonous substance in tobacco; increases dopamine leading to euphoria and relaxation; constricts blood vessels and burdens the heart

Nightblindness: condition that causes difficulty or impossibility to see in low light; related to vitamin A intake

Night eating: pseudo eating disorder; late-night overeating

Nitrogen balance or equilibrium: when nitrogen consumed in foods equals nitrogen excreted by body

Nonessential amino acids: amino acids that can be made in human body; do not require food source

Nonheme iron: form of iron mainly found in plant foods and supplements

Nonpurging bulimia: bulimia without purging; episodes of binge eating followed by excessive exercise, fasting, or strict dieting

Nonreactive: substances or materials that do not react with other substances or materials

Nonvitamins: substances with vitamin-like effects on human body; absence does not create vitamin deficiencies

Normal nutrition: nutrients most people need under normal circumstances

Nuoc man: Vietnamese fish sauce

Nutraceuticals: food extracts with reputed pharmaceutical benefits

Nutrient density: measure that compares amount of calories in food or drink with amount of nutrients

Nutrients: substances in food and drink used for growth, repair and maintenance of human body

Nutrigenomics ("personalized nutrition"): emerging field that applies human **genome** (entirety of organism's hereditary information) to nutrition and health for individual dietary recommendations

Nutrition: science of how organisms take in and utilize food material for nourishment

Nutritional yeast: nutty, cheese-like powder; source of protein and vitamins, especially B- complex

Oats: gluten-free cereal grain; dates back to 2000 BC in Middle East; types include oat groats, rolled oats and oat flour; used in breads, cold and hot cereal, cakes, cookies, granola, muesli, beer and stout

Obesity: 20 percent or more over desirable weight for height; BMI of 30 or greater

Offal or organ meats: entrails (intestines) and internal organs of butchered animals

Oils: category of lipids; derived mostly from plants; liquids at room temperature

Oligomeric proantho cyannidins (OPCs): substances in skin and seeds of grapes; block cancer-causing free radicals

Omega-3 fatty acids: polyunsaturated fatty acids associated with heart health and disease prevention; may help decrease cholesterol and triglyceride levels, platelet clotting and inflammatory and immune reactions; primarily found in fatty fish, flaxseeds and flax oil, nuts and some fruits and vegetables

Omega-6 fatty acids: polyunsaturated fatty acids found in eggs, fortified cereals, nuts, poultry, whole-grain breads and vegetable oils; more omega-6 fatty acids consumed in US diet than omega-3 fatty acids; best to have 1:1 ratio

Oolong tea: traditional Chinese tea; between green and black in oxidation; ranges from 10 to 70 percent oxidation

Organic: contains carbon; refers to USDA standards of growing and processing crop and livestock without additional chemicals

Organic foods: produced without food additives, genetically modified organisms, industrial solvents, irradiation or synthetic fertilizers and pesticides

Osmosis: diffusion of solvent (frequently water) through semipermeable membranes; moves from solution with low solutes to high solutes

Ossobuco: veal shank; often Milanese

Osteoarthritis (degenerative arthritis): syndrome of low-grade inflammation and joint pain; obesity factors in development

Osteomalacia: disease in adults related to vitamin D deficiency; characterized by bone softening from defective mineralization

Osteoporosis: disease in adults related to calcium deficiency; characterized by brittle bones and bone loss

Overnutrition: excessive intake or overconsumption of calories and certain nutrients

Overweight: between 10 and 20 percent above desirable weight for height; a BMI of 25 to 29.9

Oxalic acid (oxylate): binder found in leafy green vegetables; forms precipitates with metals, such as iron; makes nutrients less bioavailable

Oxidation: interaction of compounds with reactive and unstable oxygen; often produces damaging effects

Oxytoxin: female hormone; released in large amounts during labor; facilitates birth and breastfeeding

Paella: Catalan entree or side dish of rice, legumes, meat, seafood and vegetables

Pakoras: Indian Hindu fried vegetables in chickpea batter

Palmer grasp: infant grasp where palm supports objects and fingers used to scoop food

Palmitic acid: saturated fatty acid; major component of oil (palm and palm kernel) from palm trees

Pan-Asian cuisine: fusion cooking; combines different Asian cuisines

Pancreas: gland located near stomach; secretes digestive fluid into intestine and hormone insulin

Pancreatic amylase: enzyme produced in pancreas that assists lipid digestion

Pancreatitis: inflammation of pancreas; can result from alcohol overconsumption

Panini press: Italian sandwich press

Pantry: storeroom for nonperishable items, such as bottled, canned or packaged goods

Parmesan: hard Italian cheese; often used for grating

Pasteurization: heating liquids to destroy bacteria, molds, protozoa and yeasts

Pathogens: organisms as bacteria, fungi or viruses; capable of causing diseases

Pectin: gelatin-type carbohydrate; stabilizes fillings and sweets; thickens jams and jellies; "shortens" or tenderizes baked goods; source of dietary fiber

Peking duck: duck with pancakes, spring onions and hoisin or sweet noodle sauce

Pellagra: vitamin deficiency disease; caused by lack of vitamin B3 (niacin) and protein, especially essential amino acid tryptophan

Pepsin: digestive enzyme found in stomach; breaks down protein molecules into smaller segments

Peptic ulcers: sores in gastrointestinal tract

Peptides: short protein fragments formed when protein broken down

Periodontal disease: inflammatory disease; may affect tissues surrounding and supporting teeth; if untreated may lead to bone and teeth loss

Peritonitis: inflammation of peritoneum (lining) of abdomen

Pernicious anemia: form of megaloblastic anemia; caused by poor absorption of vitamin B12 due to lack of intrinsic factor

Pesco-vegetarian: vegetarian who consumes fish and fish products

Pesto: Italian garlic sauce with basil, olive oil, Parmesan cheese and pine nuts

Phenylketonuria (PKU): genetic disease characterized by enzyme deficiency necessary for metabolism; affects brain development; leads to progressive mental retardation and seizures

Phenylpropanolamine (PPA): diet aid; diuretic and appetite suppressant; increases blood pressure, stroke

Pho: Laotian and Vietnamese noodle soup

Phospholipids: lipids similar to triglycerides; contain phosphorus; emulsify lipids

Phosphoric acid: mineral acid; used to acidify foods and beverages as colas

Phosphorus: major mineral; part of structural component of bones and teeth; component of DNA and other organic compounds; maintains acid-base balance; found in dairy products, fish and meat

pH scale (measure): measure of acidity or alkalinity of solutions; numbered 1 to 14 with 1 most acidic, 14 most basic and 7 neutral

Phyllo (filo): paper-thin Greek pastry dough

Phylloquinone: fat-soluble substance; often called vitamin K1

Physical activities: bodily movements; result of skeletal muscle contractions

Physical digestion: mechanical motion, such as chewing and churning in stomach

Physical fitness: general fitness; state of health and well-being; based on ability to perform certain sports or activities

Physiological anemia: changes in plasma volume and red cell mass during pregnancy

Phytic acid (phytate): principle storage form of phosphorus in plant tissues, especially bran and seeds; binds calcium, iron, magnesium and zinc

Phytoestrogens: substances in plants that act like hormone estrogen

Phytosterols: plant sterols with structures similar to cholesterol; potential protective and disease-fighting benefits

Pica: abnormal appetite for nonfoods, including dirt

Pilaf: entree or side dish of sauteed and seasoned rice

Pincer grasp: ability of infant to grasp small objects between tip of thumb and index finger

Pine nuts (pignoli): Mediterranean small, oval and sweet nuts

Pituitary gland: gland that secretes hormones and regulated homeostasis

621

Placenta: structure attached to wall of uterus; nourishes fetus during pregnancy

Plancha sandwich press: Cuban sandwich press

Plantain: starchy root vegetable; similar to banana

Plaque: accumulation of cells, cell debris, lipids (cholesterol and fatty acids), calcium and fibrous connective tissue; may block arteries and lead to cardiovascular disease

Plasma: liquid component of blood where blood cells suspended; makes up 55 percent total blood volume; composed of carbon dioxide, clotting factors, glucose, hormones, ions, minerals, proteins and water

Poaching: moist-heat cooking method; transfers heat by convection from hot liquids to foods contained within liquids

Polenta: Northern Italian gruel or porridge

Polycyclic aromatic hydrocarbons: potentially toxic chemicals found in grilled meat

Polysaccharide: long chain of sugar molecules bonded together, as starch

Polyunsaturated fatty acids: fatty acids with two or more points of unsaturation; mainly found in fatty fish, nuts and vegetable oils

Port: fortified wine; dry, semidry, or sweet varieties; often served as dessert wine

Portion sizes: amounts of foods chosen versus amounts of foods recommended (serving sizes)

Positive nitrogen balance: occurs when more nitrogen taken into body than excreted

Potassium: major mineral and electrolyte; responsible for maintaining fluid balance, acid-base balance and transmitting nerve impulses; found in dairy products, fruits, legumes, vegetables and whole grains

Potato starch: gluten-free starch; used to thicken soups and gravies

Potentially hazardous foods: foods that carry microorganisms; can be hazardous and sometime fatal

Potjies: African three-legged pots

Potlikker: liquid from cooked greens; used for gravy

Powdered milk (dry milk): substance made from dried (dehydrated) milk solids

Powdered sugar, confectioner's sugar or icing sugar: sugar made by grinding table sugar (sucrose) into fine powder

Prebiotics: category of functional foods; nondigestible food ingredients; selectively stimulate growth or activity of bacteria in colon

Precursor: compound that participates in chemical reactions; produces other compounds, such as beta-carotene and vitamin A

Preeclampsia: condition of pregnancy; characterized by abrupt hypertension, protein in urine, and edema in face, feet and hands

Prefrontal cortex: anterior frontal lobe of brain; responsible for planning complex cognitive behaviors, expressing personality and moderating social behavior

Pregnancy: period of time women carry one or more offspring inside their uterus; typically 38 weeks

Pregnancy-induced hypertension (PIH): development of new arterial hypertension in pregnant women after 20 weeks' gestation

Prehypertension: systolic pressure of 120 to 139 mm Hg, or diastolic pressure of 80 to 89 mm Hg

Prenatal: before birth

Prepubescence: before puberty

Preservatives: chemicals added to foods or beverages; help prevent spoilage from microbes or chemical changes

Probiotics: dietary supplements; contain potentially beneficial bacteria or yeast

Processed cheese: dairy-based cheese; made with emulsifiers, food colorings, regular dairy cheese, salt, unfermented dairy ingredients and whey

Processed foods: foods altered from raw states by chemical or physical methods; practices include aseptic processing, canning, dehydration, freezing, refrigeration and others

Processed soy foods: soy foods that have been processed, usually to resemble animal foods, such as soy bacon or sausage

Prolactin: hormone secreted by pituitary gland; stimulates and maintains milk secretion

Promoters (cancer): substances that promote cancer progression

Prostaglandins: substances that play essential roles in blood, cell membranes, muscles and nerves

Protein: essential nutrient for human body; made from plant and animal tissues; supplies amino acids for growth, maintenance and repair

Protein-Calorie (Energy) Malnutrition (PEM): condition whereby insufficient amounts of protein and calories (energy) are consumed; causes malnutrition

Prothrombin: protein involved in coagulation and vitamin K activity

Pro-vitamins: substances that convert into vitamins; include antioxidant beta-carotene, which converts into vitamin A, and amino acid tryptophan, which converts into niacin

Psyllium: soluble fiber from seeds; FDA allows foods that contain 1.7 g of psyllium to claim there may be reduced risk of heart disease from regular consumption

Puberty: complex biologic and psychological process involving accelerated growth and sexual development

Puree: mixture of food processed to smooth pulp by mashing, straining or very fine chopping

Purging bulimia: eating disorder with purging from laxatives or self-induced vomiting

Purified water (demineralized, distilled or deionized water, or reverse osmosis): water without minerals

Pyrodoxine (vitamin B6): assists sodium and potassium balance; promotes red blood cell production and cardiovascular health; found in lean meats and other protein foods

Q: "to the tooth" in Chinese; like *al dente* in Italian

Quatre épices: French term for "four spices"; spice blend of cloves, ginger, ground pepper (black, white or both), ginger and nutmeg; used in sausages, soups, stews and vegetables

Queso fresco: fresh soft white Mexican cheese

Quinoa: technically fruit, since contains a seed; grown in South America for more than 5,000 years; one of few plant foods that provides complete protein; also gluten-free

Radiation: cooking method where energy transferred by heat or light; does not depend on physical contact between heat source and food; two types of radiant heat are infrared (broilers, toasters) and microwave

Radura logo: symbol for irradiation; must be placed on food labels of irradiated foods

Raita: Indian Hindu yogurt dish with fruits or vegetables

Rancidity: spoiled condition caused by decomposition of fats or oils; results in unpleasant taste and smell; could predict unsafe food or beverage

Raw milk: milk without pasteurization to destroy microorganisms

Raw sugar: made by clarifying sugar at syrup stage; done by boiling and drying syrup until crystalline solid; minimal chemical processing; demerara, muscovado and turbinado raw sugars

Recommended Dietary Allowance (RDA): average daily amounts of nutrients adequate to meet needs of most (97 to 98 percent) healthy people; based on age and gender

Reduced-fat (2%) milk: milk with less total fat than whole milk (3.2 to 4%)

Reducing sugars: sugars with specific shapes and reactive aldehyde (CHO) group; donate ions to other molecules; assist in browning

Relish: savory or sweet condiment; made of chopped, cooked or pickled fruits or vegetables

Research Chefs Association (RCA): foremost association that advocates principles of Culinology®; merges culinary arts with food science

Resveratrol: plant substance naturally found in skin of red grapes, mulberries, peanuts and red wine; produces anticancer, anti-inflammatory, beneficial blood sugar and cardiovascular effects

Retina: light sensitive part of inner eye

Retinoids: chemical compounds related to vitamin A; regulate epithelial cell growth; play roles in vision and immune function

Retro-acculturation: process that integrates cultural customs and traditions into daily life

Retrograde/retrogradation: chemical and physical process whereby grains cook and cool, starch molecules bond and grains harden

Retrograded starch: starch that returns to its cooked state; reformed and firmed

Reverse osmosis: solvent forced by pressure from high-solute concentration through membrane to low-solute concentration

Rhodopsin: pigment in retina; responsible for photoreceptor cells and light perception

Rice cooker: gas or electrical device for cooking rice and steaming vegetables

Rice starch: finely textured starch from rice; not often used in Western countries

Rickets: vitamin D deficiency disease in children; characterized by abnormal growth and bowed legs

Ricotta: Italian sheep's milk whey-based cheese

Risotto: entree or side dish of fish, legumes, meat, seafood or vegetables; often made with cheese or wine

Roasting: dry-heat cooking method; uses uncovered pan in contained environment as oven; commonly used for protein foods and vegetables

Robusta beans: species of coffee; originates in western Africa; limited to lower-grade coffee blends as filler; included in instant coffee and espresso blends; twice caffeine as Arabica

Roquefort: aged blue-veined sheep's milk cheese; French-protected designation of origin

Roux: classically cooked combination of fat (generally pork fat or butter) and flour in equal parts by weight

Saccharide: general term for sugars (monosaccharides) and starches (polysaccharides)

Saccharine (Sweet 'N Low, Sweet Twin): sugar substitute used in baked goods, candy, chewing gum, jams, soft drinks and tabletop sweeteners; 200 to 700 times sweeter than table sugar (sucrose); stable at high temperatures

Saganaki: flaming Greek kasseri cheese

Sake: Japanese rice wine

Salmonella: type of bacteria; causes foodborne illness, especially in chicken and eggs

Salsa: chunky mixture of fruits, herbs, spices and vegetables; sauce for protein or dip for vegetables and snack foods

Samosa: Indian Hindu fried pastries with vegetables

Sanding sugar, decorating sugar or sugar nibs: large, irregular sugar crystals that reflect light; can add "sparkle" to baked goods, candies and cookies

Sanitary: clean and safe environment; protected from food contamination and/or foodborne illnesses

Sashimi: Japanese raw fish

Satay (sate): Malaysian and Indonesian marinated, skewered and grilled meat, often served with peanut-based sauce

Satiety: feeling of satisfaction after consuming foods or beverages

Saturated fatty acids: fatty acids with completely filled hydrogen bonds to "saturation"; mostly found in animal foods and some plant-based foods, including tropical oils; associated with elevated blood cholesterol levels and cardiovascular disease

Sauce: liquid of various thicknesses; used to moisten and flavor foods

Sauce piquant: sauce mixture of hot peppers, spices and tomatoes

Sauteing/dry-sauteing: dry-heat cooking method; transfers heat by conduction from burner or flame to hot pan and food, usually in small amount of fat or oil

Scaloppine: Sicilian pounded meat dredged in flour and sauteed; often veal or chicken

Schmaltz: rich and flavorful cooking fat; made from rendered chicken, goose or pig fat; used in quick sauteing, to enrich savory dishes and spread on bread

Scratch cooking: from the beginning; feature of traditional Hispanic cuisine

Scurvy: vitamin deficiency disease from inadequate vitamin C; needed for collagen synthesis; leads to bleeding from mucous membranes, spongy gums and spotty skin

Seasonal affective disorder (SAD): mood disorder; symptoms range from depression, little energy and/or too much sleep

Seasoning: process by which cookware is prepared before using; closes pores and prevents oxidation, rusting and/or pitting

Seaweeds: single-celled marine plants notable for protein, vitamin and mineral content; include alaria, arame, carrageenan, dulse, egregia, focus, hijiki, Irish moss, kelp, nori, sea lettuce, wakame and others

Selenosis: selenium toxicity; may lead to cirrhosis, fatigue, garlic odor on breathe, gastrointestinal disorders, hair loss, irritability, neurological damage, pulmonary edema, sloughing of nails and/or fatality

623

Seltzer: tap water with injected carbon dioxide bubbles; no added salts

Senescence: process of aging, decline and death

Senses: faculties by which body perceives five senses: sight, smell, sound, taste and touch; affect how foods and beverages are distinguished

Sensory analysis: process that investigates how food is perceived by senses

Sensory science: science that investigates preferences for foods and beverages

Serotonin: neurotransmitter found in gastrointestinal tract and brain; helps regulate appetite, mood and sleep

Serving sizes: amounts of foods recommended versus amounts of foods chosen (portion sizes)

Set point: theory that maintains human body seeks certain predestined weight despite physiological, psychological and environmental influences

Shape: two-dimensional appearance, configuration or outline of object as food

Sherry: fortified wine with brandy after fermentation, unlike other wines

Shioyaki: Japanese broiled fish

Shocking: plunging just blanched vegetables into ice water to halt cooking process

Short-chain fatty acids: short units of lipids; more easily digested than longer-chain fatty acids

Shortening: semisolid fat; used in baked goods to create "short" or crumbly textures

Shoyu or soya sauce: salty, fermented condiment made from soy

Silken tofu: light version of tofu; can be used for sauces and dressings

Simmering: moist-heat cooking method; uses convection heat to cook food in hot liquid

Simple goiter: enlargement of thyroid gland from inadequate thyroid hormone; may result from iodine deficiency

Single-action baking powder: sodium bicarbonate; produces carbon dioxide when combined with moisture and acidic ingredients; expands with heat; causes baked goods to rise

Single sugars (simple sugars): contain one sugar molecule, such as glucose, fructose or galactose

Skim, 1%, 2%, part-skim and whole dairy milk: types of dairy milk according to butterfat content; 0.5 to 0 percent butterfat in skim milk, 1 and 2 percent butterfat, and 5 percent butterfat in whole milk

Skinfold thickness: measurement of subcutaneous fat directly under skin; done by grasping skin and subcutaneous fat away from underlying muscle tissue

Skordalia: Greek garlic and bread sauce

Sleep apnea: sleep disorder characterized by pauses in breathing during sleep; potential side effect of obesity

Slow cookers: electrical appliance for cooking foods unattended at low temperatures for lengthy times; useful for pot roasts and stews

Slow cooking: cooking method where foods cook at relatively low temperatures for long cooking times

Slow Food Movement: movement founded by Carlo Petrini to resist and combat fast food; purpose to preserve culture of cuisine in ecological regions; also domestic animals, farming methods, foods, plants and seeds representative of regions

Smen: traditional cooking oil common in North African and Middle Eastern cuisines; made by using butter from sheep's or goat's milk

Smoke point: temperature at which fats or oils break down, smoke or burn, and create unpleasant taste and/or smell

Sodium: trace mineral and electrolyte; responsible for fluid balance, acid-base balance and nerve impulse transmission; found in processed foods, seafood and table salt

Sodium aluminum sulfate: substance used in manufacturing baking powder

Sodium chloride: table salt (NaCl)

Sofrito: base for legumes, rice and stews; consists of garlic, green pepper, ground pepper, onions and tomatoes sauteed in oil

Soft water: type of water; contains few or no calcium or magnesium ions

Soluble fibers: dietary fibers that dissolve or swell in fluid; may increase bulk and soften stool; include algae (such as carrageenan), gums, hemicellulose, mucilages and pectin; may be beneficial in prevention of digestive diseases, including colon cancer, diverticulosis and hemorrhoids

Solute: dissolved substance in solvent (solution)

Solution: homogeneous mixture; composed of two or more substances (solute dissolved in solvent)

Solvent: liquid or gas that dissolves solid, liquid or gaseous solute; forms solution

Sorghum syrup: by-product of sugar-making process; sometimes mistaken for blackstrap molasses; contains iron, calcium and potassium; can be substituted in equal quantities for corn syrup, honey, maple syrup and molasses

Soul food: American cuisine; blends traditional African-American and southern US cooking

Sour cream: rich dairy product made by fermenting cream with lactic acid bacteria; reduced-fat sour cream optional

Soursop: Asian fruit; cross between pineapple and strawberry

Soy-based infant formulas: soy-based, dairy-like milk beverages used for feeding infants

Soybeans: legumes with complete protein, similar to meat, isoflavones and other phytonutrients; formulated into variety of products, including butter, flour, lecithin, meal, dairy milk, oil, sauce, texturized protein, yogurt and others

Soy protein: protein from soybeans; used to increase protein and other nutrients in breads, breakfast cereals, beverage powders, cheeses, frozen desserts, imitation meats, infant formulas, nondairy creamers, pastas, salad dressings, soups and whipped toppings; also used for emulsifying and texturing

Spa: medical or destination facility for cosmetic and wellness services

Spanakopita: Greek spinach and phyllo (filo) pie

Sparkling water: water with natural carbonation

Specific heat: measure of heat energy required to increase temperature of specific quantity of substance a certain temperature

Spelt (faro in Italy and dinkle in Germany): ancient grain with distinctive nutty flavor; precursor to durum wheat; originated in Mesopotamia about 9000 BC

Spina bifida: developmental birth defect from folate deficiency; partial closure of neural tube; results in incompletely formed spinal cord and permanent damage to infant

Spirits: alcoholic beverages; typically contain 37.5 percent alcohol or greater; some modern spirits infused with flavors after distilling

Sports drinks: beverages that help people who exercise rehydrate, replenish carbohydrates, electrolytes and other nutrients

Spring water: water from underground source; flows naturally to surface

Stabilizers: substances that prevent unwanted changes in other substances; includes agar-agar, carrageenan, lecithin and pectin

Starch blockers: diet aids; substances that inhibit starch digestion

Starches: storage forms of carbohydrates in plants; complex carbohydrates made from repeated sugar units; found in bulbs, grains, leaves, rhisomes, roots and tubers

Starters: grains, liquids or seeds colonized by microorganisms for fermentation; used in beer, bread and yogurt production

Starvation: severe reduction of calorie and nutrient intake; most extreme form of malnutrition

Steam: vaporized water; invisible gas

Steaming: method of cooking by steam to quickly cook food

Stearic acid: saturated fatty acid; derived from both animals and plants; can be made by hydrogenation of vegetable oils; may elevate blood lipids, contribute to cardiovascular disease

Sterols: lipids that resemble cholesterol; found in both animal and plant tissues

Stevia: sweetener 300 times as sweet as white sugar (sucrose); negligible effect on blood sugar; acceptable sugar substitute for carbohydrate-controlled diets; stable at most temperatures; can be used for both cooking and baking

Stewing: moist-heat cooking method; small pieces of food first browned by conduction, then cooked in moderate amount of liquid

Stir-frying: dry-heat cooking method; foods quickly cooked by conduction over high heat, usually in wok or fry pan with sloped sides

Stock: clear, thin liquid; flavored with herbs, protein, spices and vegetables

Strength: muscular ability to perform work against resistance

Stroke: loss of brain functions due to blood vessel disturbances in brain

Subcutaneous fat: fat found just beneath skin

Sucralose or Splenda: general, all-purpose sweetener; 600 times sweeter than table sugar (sucrose); used in baked goods, chewing gum, dairy products, frozen desserts, jams, salad dressings, soft drinks, syrups and tabletop sweeteners; marketed as "no-calorie sweetener," since nondigested

Sucrose: white sugar or table sugar; double sugar made of glucose and fructose

Sugar alcohols: sugars with alcohol groups attached in chemical structures; absorbed slower and metabolized differently than other sugars; may be advantageous in carbohydrate-controlled diets; do not promote dental cavities

Sugars: types of carbohydrates primarily from sugarcane and sugar beets; provide energy for human body; supply sweet taste to foods and beverages

Sulfur: major mineral found in protein-rich foods; component of vitamins and amino acids

Sustainability: ability to persist; maintenance of diverse, productive biological systems for human well-being

Sweating: dry-heat method of cooking vegetables with little to no fat; vegetables release liquid; flavors extracted and concentrated

Sweetened condensed milk: dairy milk with water removed and sugar added; very thick shelf-stable canned beverage and ingredient

Systolic blood pressure: blood pressure reading represented by "upper" number; when heart is beating

Table food: age-appropriate foods; not pureed

Tabouli (tabouleh): Lebanese cracked wheat salad with parsley and tomatoes

Taco: soft or hard tortilla with filling

Tahini: Middle Eastern sesame seed paste

Tallow: rendered beef or mutton fat processed from suet; stored for extended periods without refrigeration

Tangine: Moroccan slow-cooked stew with broth, meat and vegetables

Tapenade: French Provencal puree of anchovies, capers, olives and olive oil

Tapioca: starch from cassava or manioc root; mainly grown in South America; commonly used in puddings due to neutral flavor

Target heart rate: safe rate at which person should exercise for cardiovascular fitness

Taro: starchy Asian root vegetable

Taste: one of the five senses; experienced all over oral cavity, not only on tongue

Taurine: organic acid; major constituent of bile; found in lower intestine and tissues

Tea: infusion made by steeping processed tea buds, leaves, or twigs in hot water; high in antioxidants

Teff: staple grain of Ethiopian cooking for thousands of years; main ingredient in traditional flat bread, injera; gluten-free; higher in protein than barley or wheat

Tejanos: Texans of Hispanic descent

Tempeh: fermented soybean "cake" made from whole soybeans and grains

Temperature danger zone (TDZ): range of temperatures between 40 °F and 140 °F that promote bacteria multiplication

Tempura: battered seafood or vegetables fried in deep fat or oil

Tetsubin: Japanese cast-iron pots with pouring spouts and handles

Tex-Mex cuisine: Southwest Native American and Mexican blend of regional cuisines

Texturized soy or vegetable protein (TVP): made from texturized soy flour; once rehydrated, replicates meat

Theaflavin: polyphenols formed from catechins in tea leaves during oxidation

Theine: form of caffeine

Theobromine: xanthine in cacao plants; found in chocolate; structure and effects similar to caffeine

Theophylline: xanthine in tea plants; structure and effects similar to caffeine

Thermic effect of food: energy spent to digest foods and beverages after consumption

Thermogenesis: process of heat production in organisms

Thirst: craving for liquids; basic instinct of humans or animals

Thrombin: protein involved in coagulation and vitamin K activity; converts into prothrombin

Time-and-temperature principle: rule for keeping hot food hot and cold food cold

Tinnitus: perception of sound in absence of sound

Tocopherol: class of several closely related chemical compounds in egg yolk, leafy green vegetables and wheat germ oil; jointly comprise vitamin E

Toddler: young child learning to walk or "toddle"

Tofu: cheese-like substance made from soy milk and coagulant; available in firm and silken forms

Tolerance: decreased response to functional effects of ethanol in alcoholic beverages

Tonic water: artificially carbonated water; added sugar or sugar substitute, salt and quinine

Tooth decay or cavities: result of dental caries, infectious disease that damages teeth

Torcino: Spanish or Mexican bacon

Tostada: flat toasted or deep-fried tortilla

Tortilla Espanola: Spanish potato omelet

Tortillas: flat, thin corn cakes

Total body mass: combination of lean body mass and fat weight

Toxin-mediated infection: infection in human body caused by toxins that exist or passed in foods

Toxoplasma: parasitic disease in undercooked meat and unwashed vegetables; pregnant women are particularly vulnerable

Trachea: windpipe; connects pharynx or larynx to lungs

Traditional Chinese medicine (TCM): range of traditional Chinese medical practices and treatments; includes *zangfu, yin/yang/qi gong, tui na, tai chi* and *shiatsi*

Training heart rate: rate at which heart beats during exercise; should be within target heart rate

Training table: buffet of foods and beverages for athletes in training

Trans bond: chemical bond formed in process of hydrogenation of vegetable oils; form trans fatty acids; implicated with increased blood cholesterol and cardiovascular disease

Trans fatty acids: produced when vegetable oils are hydrogenated, or hardened; used in commercial baked and fried foods and margarines for economy and increased shelf life; implicated with increased blood cholesterol and cardiovascular disease

Trichinosis: parasitic disease; caused by eating raw or undercooked pork or wild game infected with larvae of trichina worm

Triglycerides: major form of dietary lipids; composed of three fatty acids with glycerol backbone

Triticale: hybrid of wheat and rye; first bred in Scotland and Sweden during late nineteenth century; combines high-yield attribute of wheat with disease and environmental strength of rye; found in flour and breakfast cereals

Tropical oils: palm, palm kernel and coconut oils with saturated fatty acids, much like animal foods

Truffles: type of fungi; grows near roots of trees; harvested by dogs and pigs

Tryptophan: essential amino acid; increases brain levels of serotonin and melatonin; converts to niacin

Ts'ai: balance of vegetables and meat in Chinese cooking

Type I or juvenile diabetes: autoimmune disease caused by inadequate insulin production by beta cells of pancreas; usually occurs during childhood; requires insulin injections to control blood sugar levels; no known cure

Type II or adult onset diabetes: condition due to insulin resistance; pancreas produces insulin, but cells resist or do not respond; may not require insulin; therapies may include diet and weight loss

Tzatziki: Greek yogurt and cucumber dip or salad

Ulcers: lesions on eyes, skin or mucous membranes; usually result from inflammation or decreased blood flow

Ultra-heat pasteurized milk: high-temperature processing; gives milk extended shelf life (ESL)

Ultrasound: method for measuring distance between skin, fat and muscle layers; allows measurement of fat, muscle at various body sites

Umami: fifth taste; earthy and savory; often called "deliciousness"

Umbilical cord: cord connecting developing embryo or fetus to placenta

Undernutrition: condition of not meeting nutritional guidelines; examples are eating disorders and malnutrition

Underwater weighing: process for measuring body fat by submerging person underwater; body fat weighs less than lean muscle mass, so the overfat weigh less under water

Unique ratiolytic products: substances that might form during irradiation process

Unpasteurized milk: another name for raw milk; not pasteurized to kill bacteria, protozoa, molds, or yeasts

Unsaturated fatty acids: one or more points of unsaturation in structures; found in both plants and animals; two main types monounsaturated and polyunsaturated

Upper-body obesity: characterized by excessive fat around heart, lungs and abdomen

USDA Choice: grade of meat; less fat than Prime, but still tender and juicy

USDA Prime: grade of meat; well-marbled; covered by a thick layer of firm fat

USDA Select or Standard: grade of meat; even less fat than Choice or Prime; lacks flavor, tenderness of these meat grades

Uterus: female reproductive organ; where fetus develops during gestation

Vegetable broth or stock: stock that does not contain animal protein of any kind

Vegetable gum: fibers include acacia gum and guar gum; can be used in gluten-free foods and diets; supplements available in powdered forms; dissolve easily with little aftertaste

Vegetable juice: liquid extracted from vegetable tissues

Vegetable spreads: generally 20 to 60 percent fat; correspondingly higher amounts of air, water and fewer calories than margarine

Very low-calorie diet: under 800 calories daily; generally medically supervised

Villi: small, finger-like projections; protrude from lining of intestinal wall; increase surface area; allow for increased absorption of nutrients

Vinegar: liquid produced during alcohol (ethanol) fermentation; main ingredient acetic acid; used as condiment and in flavoring and pickling

Visceral fat: fat in abdominal cavity; also called organ fat

Viscous: thickness or resistance to flow

Vitamin B1 (Thiamine): water-soluble B vitamin; involved in energy production and nervous system function; found in fortified grains, pork, legumes and nuts

Vitamin B2 (riboflavin): water-soluble B vitamin; involved in energy production and normal vision; found in fortified dairy products, enriched whole grains and leafy green vegetables

Vitamin B3 (niacin): water-soluble B vitamin; involved in energy release, healthy nervous system and digestive system and vibrant skin; found in fortified grains, legumes, nuts and meats

Vitamin B6: water-soluble B vitamin; involved in protein and fat metabolism; found in leafy green vegetables, protein foods, soy products and whole grains

Vitamin B12: water-soluble B vitamin; involved in DNA synthesis, healthy nervous system and red blood cell formation; found only in animal foods and by-products

Vitamins: organic compounds; required by human body in small amounts; essential for normal growth and development

Vitamins A, D, E, K: fat-soluble vitamins

Vitamin water: water with vitamin fortification

Voluntary muscles (skeletal muscles): create movement by applying force to bones and joints through contraction

Waist-to-hip circumference ratio (WHR): ratio of waist circumference to hips; calculated by measuring waist circumference divided by hip circumference at widest part

Water: one of six essential nutrients for most all body functions; liquid, solid (ice), and gaseous states (water vapor)

Water activity or Aw: amount of water available for microbial growth

Water intoxication (hyper-hydration or water poisoning): potentially fatal disturbance in brain function from water overconsumption; upsets normal electrolyte balance

Water soluble: ability of substance or solute to dissolve in water (solvent)

Water-soluble vitamins: B-complex vitamins: thiamine, riboflavin, niacin, folic acid, B6, B12, pantothenic acid and biotin, plus vitamin C

Weaning: process of withdrawing mother's milk and introducing infants to adult diets

Weight control: eating enough calories and getting enough regular physical activity to achieve and maintain body weight

Weight cycling: repeated loss and regain of body weight

Weight gain: increased body weight over ideal body weight

Weight loss: decreased body weight under ideal body weight

Weight management: management of body weight with diet and exercise over time

Well water: water from rock formation via underground well

Wheat bran: outer nondigestible kernel of wheat; rich in dietary fiber

Wheat flour: 70 percent starch; remaining gluten protein; not pure starch, so does not thicken well; wheaty flavor and cloudy color due to the gluten in protein

Wheat germ: germ or seed of wheat kernel; source of fats, vitamins and minerals

Whey (milk plasma): remaining liquid after milk has curdled and is strained; by-product of cheese or casein manufacture

Whole grains: intact cereal grains that include **husk**, or outer inedible covering; **bran**, or fibrous protective covering; **endosperm**, or starchy interior; and **germ**, or fatty core; considered good sources of fiber, vitamins and minerals and phytochemicals (protective plant substances)

Wilson's disease: genetic disorder; copper accumulation in body tissues

Wine: alcoholic beverage from fermented grape juice and yeast; varieties of grapes and strains of yeasts used depend on wine types

Wok: deep pan with sloping sides; often used for Asian recipes

Womb: uterus; female reproductive organ where fetus develops during gestation

Xanthan gum: gum used in gluten-free baking

Xerophthalmia: medical condition; associated with vitamin A deficiency; eyes fail tear production?

X-ray absorptiometry (DXA): procedure that measures total body composition and fat composition

Yeast: live microorganism responsible for sugar fermentation; includes Baker's yeast for bread production and brewer's yeast for beer fermentation

Yogurt: sour dairy product produced by bacterial fermentation of milk sugar (lactose); yields lactic acid; provides tanginess, texture

Yo-yo dieting: gaining and losing weight; may increase fat cell number over time

Yucca: starchy root similar to cassava; used to make tapioca

Zinc: trace mineral; involved in many human body functions, including enzymes, genetic material, immunity and sexual maturation; found in protein-containing foods, grains and vegetables

Zizaria latifolia: water bamboo cultivated in all parts of Asia; closely related to wild rice

Note: Page numbers followed by "*f*", "*t*," and, "*b*" refer to figures, tables, and boxes, respectively.

634

637

641

647

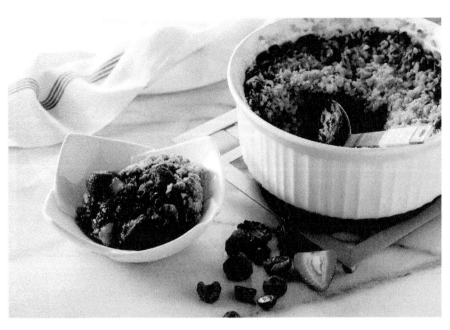

PLATE 4.1
Berry Crumble
© 2014 Grace Natoli Sheldon. Reprinted with permission.

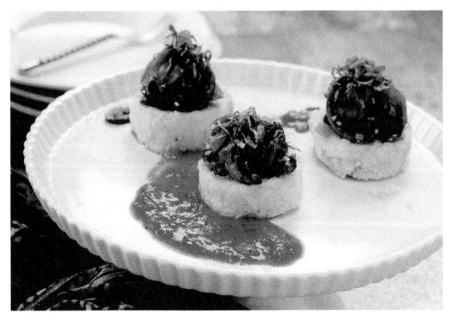

PLATE 4.2
Polenta Bites
© 2014 Grace Natoli Sheldon. Reprinted with permission.

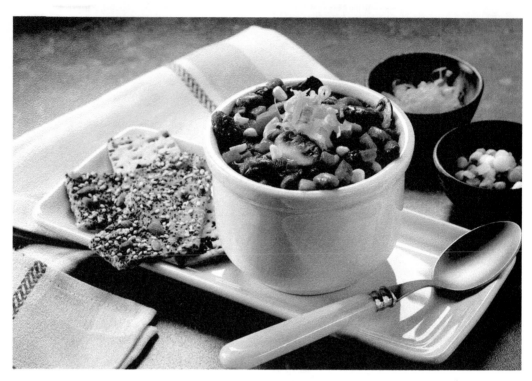

PLATE 4.3
Vegetarian Chili
© 2014 Grace Natoli Sheldon. Reprinted with permission.

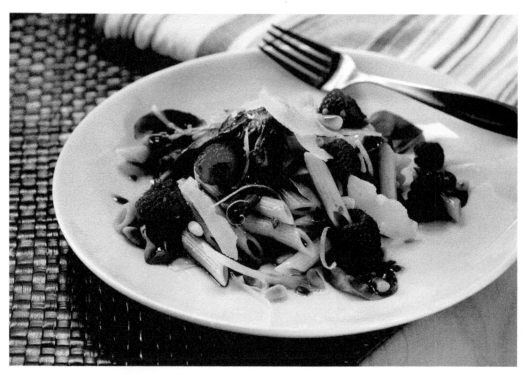

PLATE 4.4
Warm Whole-Grain Pasta Salad with Spinach, Berries and Balsamic Vinaigrette
© 2014 Grace Natoli Sheldon. Reprinted with permission.

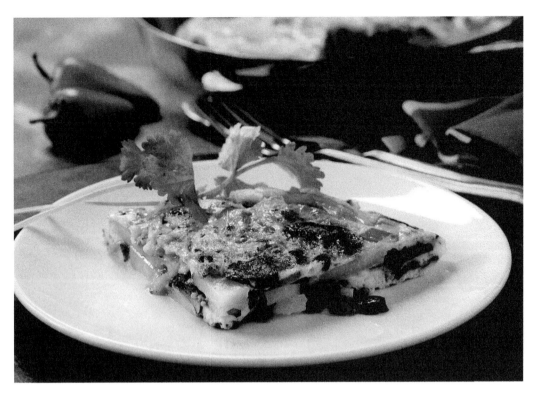

PLATE 5.1
Mushroom and Potato Frittata
© 2014 Grace Natoli Sheldon. Reprinted with permission.

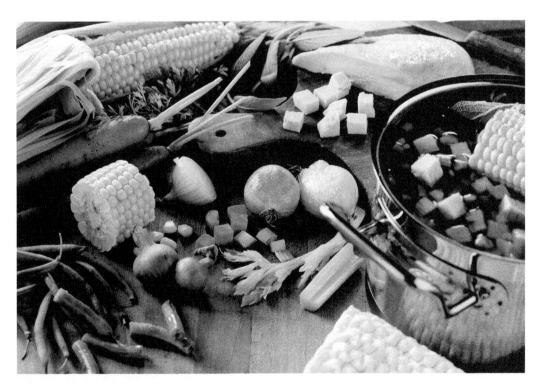

PLATE 5.2
Chicken or Turkey Soup with Corn on the Cob
© 2014 Grace Natoli Sheldon. Reprinted with permission.

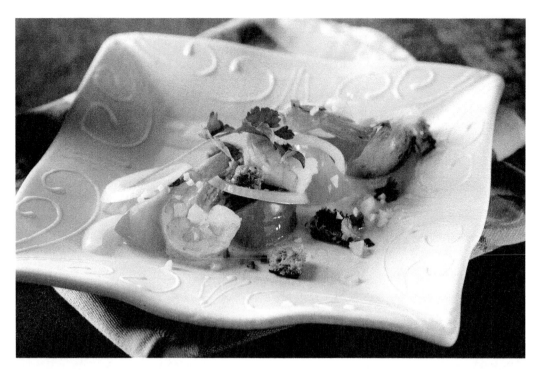

PLATE 5.3
Mixed Tomato and Onion Salad with Grilled Shrimp
© 2014 Grace Natoli Sheldon. Reprinted with permission.

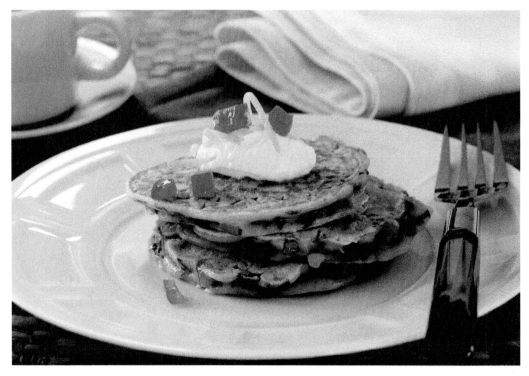

PLATE 5.4
Spinach Pancakes
© 2014 Grace Natoli Sheldon. Reprinted with permission.

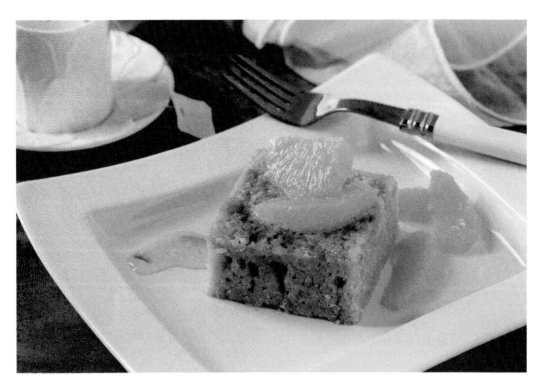

PLATE 6.1
Olive Oil Cake
© 2014 Grace Natoli Sheldon. Reprinted with permission.

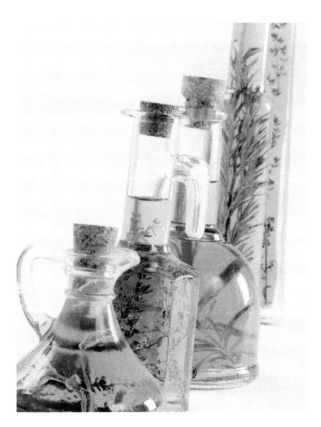

PLATE 6.2
Infused Oils
© 2014 Grace Natoli Sheldon. Reprinted with permission.

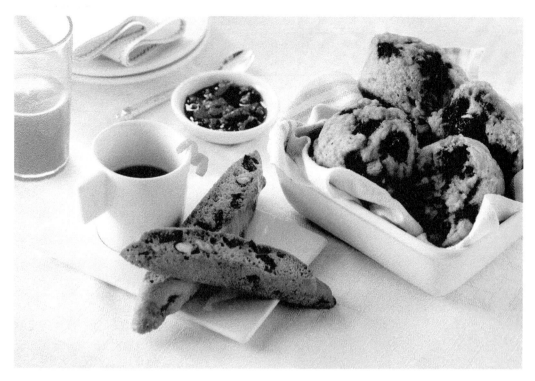

PLATE 6.3
Cherry Pistachio Biscotti (left) and Blueberry-Lemon Muffins (right)
© 2014 Grace Natoli Sheldon. Reprinted with permission.

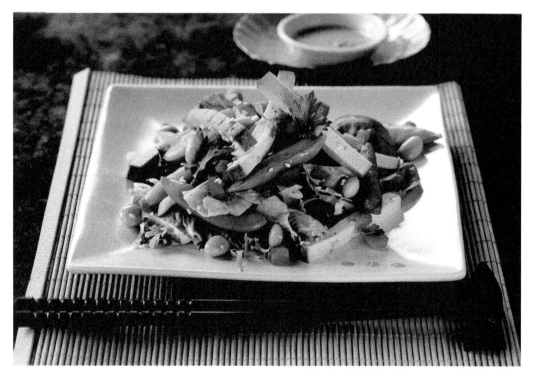

PLATE 6.4
Sugar Snap Peas and Tofu Salad with Tahini Dressing
© 2014 Grace Natoli Sheldon. Reprinted with permission.

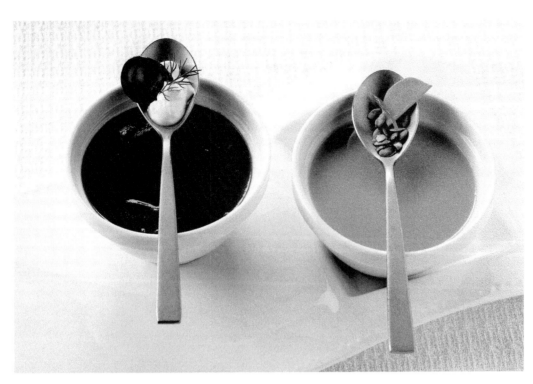

PLATE 7.1
Roasted Beet Soup (left) and Butternut Squash Soup (right)
© 2014 Grace Natoli Sheldon. Reprinted with permission.

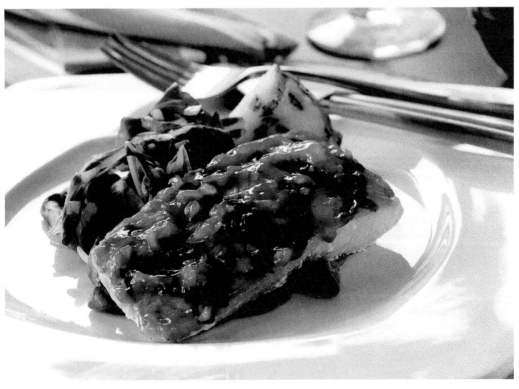

PLATE 7.2
Barbecue Salmon with Sweet and Spicy Sauce and Wilted Arugula
© 2014 Grace Natoli Sheldon. Reprinted with permission.

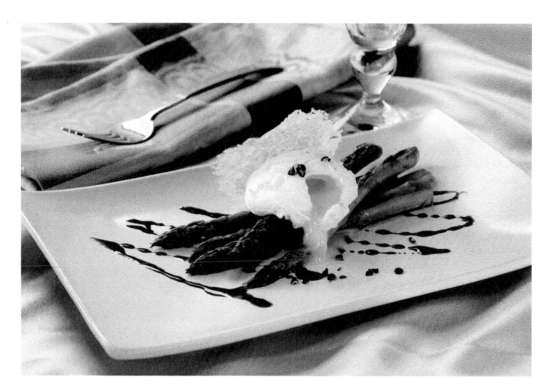

PLATE 7.3
Roasted Asparagus with Parmesan "Crackers" and Eggs
© 2014 Grace Natoli Sheldon. Reprinted with permission.

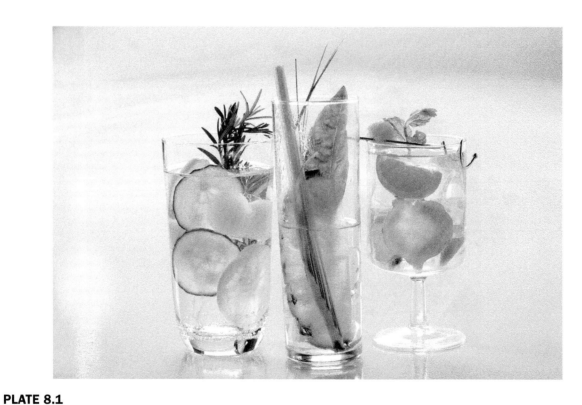

PLATE 8.1
Fruit-flavored Waters: Cucumber, honeydew melon, lemon and rosemary (left); pineapple, basil and lemongrass (center); blood orange, fresh ginger and mint (right)
© 2014 Grace Natoli Sheldon. Reprinted with permission.

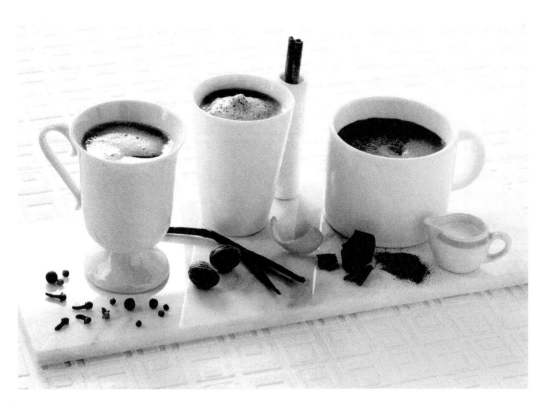

PLATE 8.2
Peppermint Chai Tea (left), Coffee Caribbean (center) and Mexican Cocoa (right)
© 2014 Grace Natoli Sheldon. Reprinted with permission.

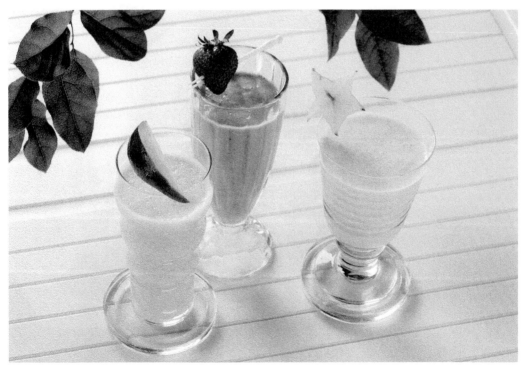

PLATE 8.3
Papaya Yogurt Smoothie (left), Strawberry Soy Milk Shake (center) and Green Tea Shake (right)
© 2014 Grace Natoli Sheldon. Reprinted with permission.

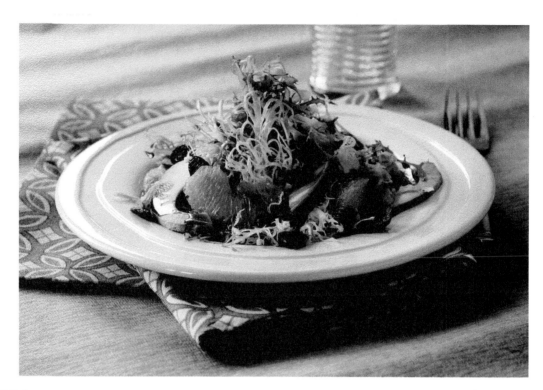

PLATE 9.1
Frisee, Grapefruit, Avocado and Cranberry Salad with Cranberry Vinaigrette
© 2014 Grace Natoli Sheldon. Reprinted with permission.

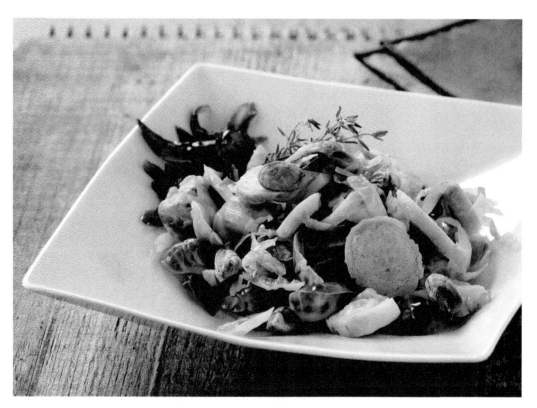

PLATE 9.2
Brussels Sprouts with Caramelized Onions
© 2014 Grace Natoli Sheldon. Reprinted with permission.

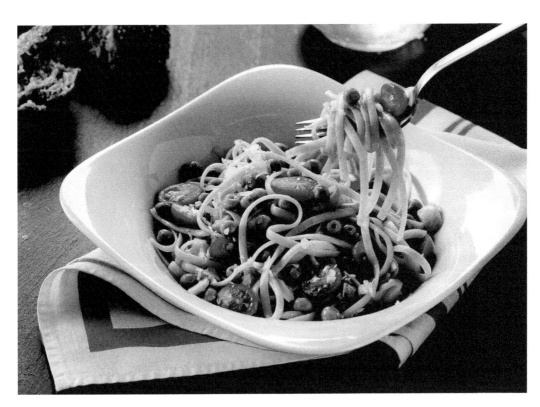

PLATE 9.3
Linguini and Peas with Roasted Garlic Wine Sauce
© 2014 Grace Natoli Sheldon. Reprinted with permission.

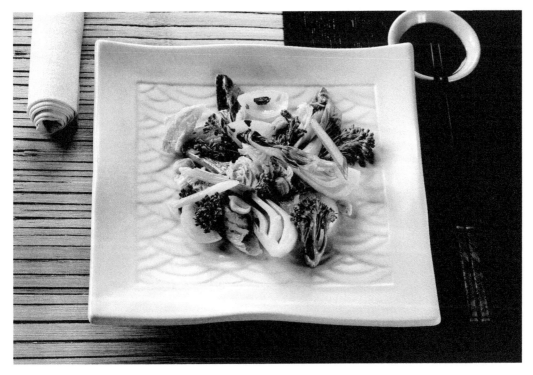

PLATE 9.4
Stir-fried Asian Vegetables
© 2014 Grace Natoli Sheldon. Reprinted with permission.

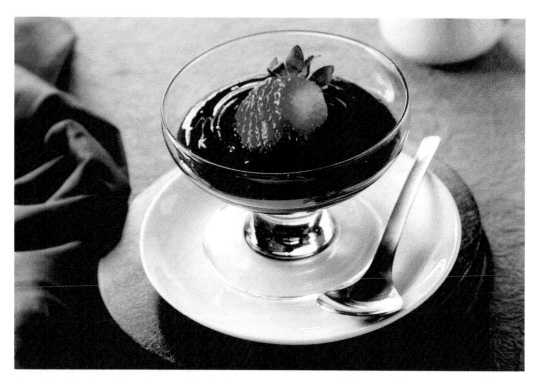

PLATE 10.1
Chocolate Pudding
© 2014 Grace Natoli Sheldon. Reprinted with permission.

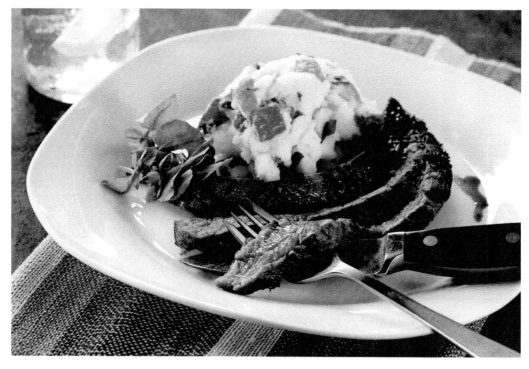

PLATE 10.2
Grilled Flank Steak with Garlic-enhanced Mashed Potatoes
© 2014 Grace Natoli Sheldon. Reprinted with permission.

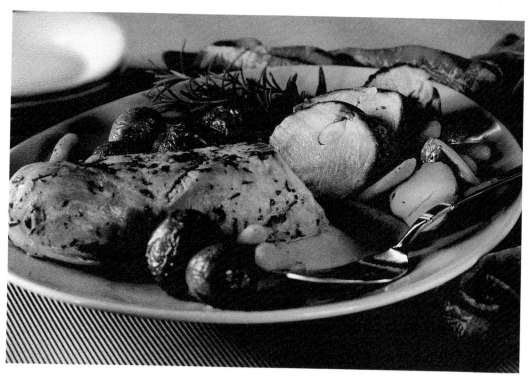

PLATE 10.3

Pork Tenderloin with Root Vegetables

© 2014 Grace Natoli Sheldon. Reprinted with permission.

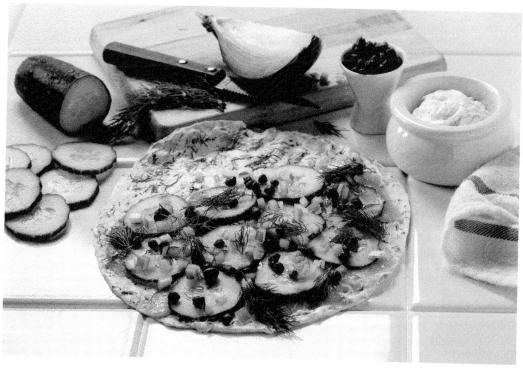

PLATE 10.4

Smoked Salmon Rolls

© 2014 Grace Natoli Sheldon. Reprinted with permission.

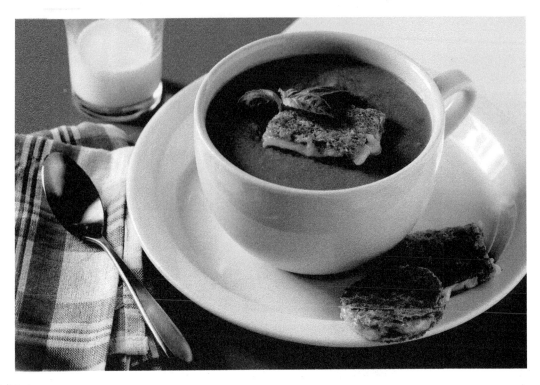

PLATE 11.1
Cream of Tomato-Basil Soup with Grilled Cheese Croutons
© 2014 Grace Natoli Sheldon. Reprinted with permission.

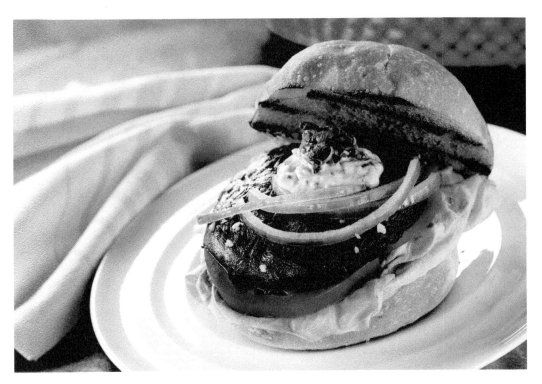

PLATE 11.2
Portobello Mushroom Burgers with Basil-Mustard Sauce
© 2014 Grace Natoli Sheldon. Reprinted with permission.

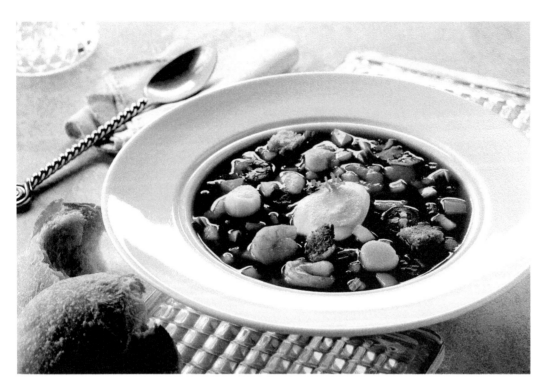

PLATE 12.1
Gazpacho with Baby Shrimp and Bay Scallops
© 2014 Grace Natoli Sheldon. Reprinted with permission.

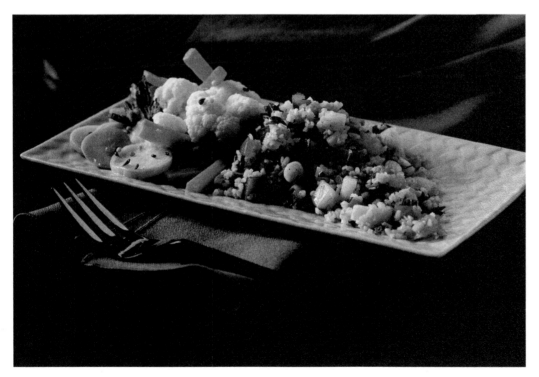

PLATE 12.2
Tabbouleh with Pickled Vegetables
© 2014 Grace Natoli Sheldon. Reprinted with permission.

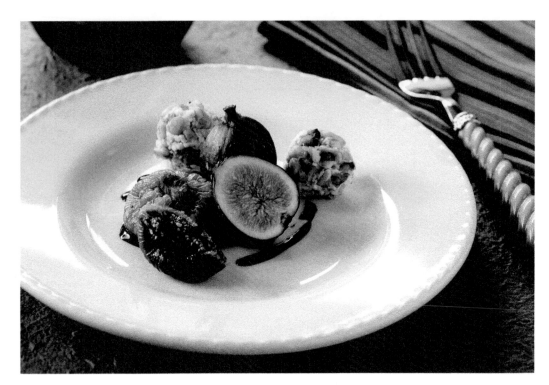

PLATE 12.3
Stuffed Figs in Port Wine Sauce
© 2014 Grace Natoli Sheldon. Reprinted with permission.

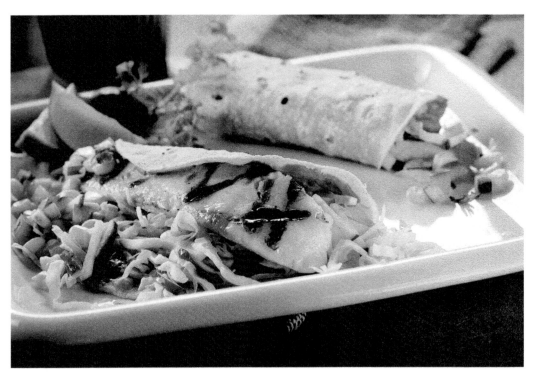

PLATE 12.4
Grilled Tilapia Fish Tacos with Corn Salsa
© 2014 Grace Natoli Sheldon. Reprinted with permission.

Printed and bound by CPI Group (UK) Ltd, Croydon, CR0 4YY

03/10/2024

01040313-0018